The Complete Bedside Companion

No-Nonsense Advice on Caring for the Seriously Ill

RODGER McFARLANE

PHILIP BASHE

SIMON & SCHUSTER

SIMON & SCHUSTER
Rockefeller Center
1230 Avenue of the Americas
New York, NY 10020

SIMON & SCHUSTER and colophon are registered trademarks
of Simon & Schuster Inc.

Designed by Leslie Phillips

Manufactured in the United States of America

2 4 6 8 10 9 7 5 3 1

Library of Congress Cataloging-in-Publication Data
McFarlane, Rodger.
The complete bedside companion : no-nonsense advice on caring for
the seriously ill / Rodger McFarlane, Philip Bashe.
p.   cm.
Includes bibliographical references and index.
1. Home nursing.   2. Caregivers.   3. Critically ill—Home care.
4. Terminal care.   I. Bashe, Philip.   II. Title.
RT61.M38   1998
649.8—dc21   97-43746   CIP
ISBN 0-684-80143-4

The ideas, procedures and suggestions in this book are intended to supplement, not replace, the advice of trained professionals. All matters regarding one's health require medical supervision. A physician or other appropriate trained professional should be consulted before adopting the suggestions in this book as well as about any condition that may require diagnosis or medical attention. All matters regarding one's legal or financial affairs require the advice of a professional. Laws vary from state to state, and if the reader requires expert assistance or legal advice, a competent professional should be consulted.

The authors and publisher disclaim any liability arising directly or indirectly from the use of this book.

Acknowledgments

Rodger McFarlane would like to thank his aunt Kitty, who throughout her life has tirelessly cared for those she loved. There is a special place in heaven for folks like her who give so unstintingly of themselves.

Eternal thanks, too, to Susan Richardson for always believing Rodger could do anything; to Dixie Beckham, Nan Golub, and Brad Miskell for enduring decades of whining and complaining; to Mary Hayes, Bill Vayo, and Jim Rooney for mental and physical health maintenance; to Dr. Kathy Flanagan for helping him make sense out of human suffering; to his brothers, Bob, Dave, and John, for standing together when it mattered most; and especially to Larry Kramer for teaching him to accept personal responsibility for what happens to others around him.

All the insights in this book were gained on the backs of hundreds of remarkable people now dead and the families, friends, and professionals who cared for them. This entire effort is a tribute to their courage, in the hope that it may spare someone somewhere a little of the suffering they endured with such grace.

Philip Bashe would like to thank Robert and Rochelle Bashe and is grateful to the late Evelyn Bashe, Justin Bashe, and, as always, Patty Bashe for everything. And to I'm in a Hurry Pizzeria, for sustenance.

Many thanks to the many physicians, nurses, and other health care professionals who took the time to speak with us: Dr. Bruce Bacon, Christine Beebe, Dr. Kyle Brown, Dr. Christine Cassel, Dr. Lucien Coté, Dr. Steven DeKosky, Perry Ecksel, Dr. Norman H. Edelman, Sarah Eilenberg, Dr. Garabed Eknoyan, Dr. Andrew E. Epstein, Janelle Fail, Lori Fedje, Dan Fish, Esq., Janice Fleischman-Eaton, Dr.

Gerald Fletcher, Dr. Richard A. Gan, Dr. Jam Ghajar, Lou Glasse, Dr. Glen E. Gresham, Dr. Howard Grossman, Dr. Allan R. Hull, Dr. Katherine F. Jeter, Marianne Kelly, Dr. Donald Leslie, Tom Locher, Dr. Jack Lord, Matthew Loscalzo, Audrey MacMillan, Dr. Mary Jane Massie, Dr. Fletcher McDowell, Marge McDowell, Dr. LaMar McGinnis, Suzanne Mintz, Dr. Alfred Munzer, Jane Pilecki, Dr. Thomas G. Rainey, Mary Ann Reeks, Dr. James N. Rogers, Dr. Howard M. Spiro, Daphne Stannard, Allen St. Pierre, Chaplain Christine Swift, Charlie Thomas, Paula Erwin-Toth, Carla Putnam-Veal, Mary Ann Wanucha, Sandra Waring, Dr. William J. Weiner, Ellen Wilson, Dr. Kathleen Wishner, and Dr. Nathan Zasler. Thanks are also due to Dr. Roger W. Enlow for generously reviewing the manuscript for medical accuracy.

Special thanks to our incomparable editor, Rebecca Saletan, whose unflagging enthusiasm for this project from proposal to publication inspired and sustained us daily; also to associate editor Denise Roy, copy editor Rose Ann Ferrick, publicity chief Victoria Meyer, marketing whiz Michael Selleck, art director Michael Accordino, designer Leslie Phillips, their talented teams, and all the hardworking folks in production and sales at Simon & Schuster who lavished on us the kind of attention authors only dream of. Like us, everyone who benefits from reading this book is forever in their debt.

At the risk of permanently damaging his professional reputation, readers should know that our agent, Jed Mattes, is actually a very nice man. The care with which he cultivated this collaboration demonstrates his wisdom and a commitment far beyond his cut of royalties, a true rarity in publishing circles. Not only did he have the foresight to introduce the two of us, but he also had the good sense to take the project to Becky Saletan first. His associates, Fred Morris, Jason Brown, and Adrienne Chew, reflect the good humor, industry, and integrity for which Jed's agency is deservedly famous.

We are especially grateful to the care partners from around the country who generously shared their highly personal and moving stories with such honesty: Sarah Lanier Barber, Naomi Black, Debbie Bryant, Debra Bulkeley, Gerri and Paul Clarke, the Reverend Harry Cole, Gloria Donadello, Louise Fradkin, Suzanne Hardy, Betty Lindstrom, Allene McCool, Lorna McFarlane, Nola J. Miller, Eileen Mitzman, Dr. Alvin Novick, Johnetta Romanowski, Audree Siden, Pat Still, Roslyn Travers, Mary Vitro, and Diane Young; also Karen McFarlane and Darlene Twilley. Through their courage and tenacity in the face of great adversity and their willingness to help all of us learn from their suffering, they are the personification of what we call everyday angels.

Together the authors would like to thank the following organizations and agencies for their help: Abledata, Administration on Aging, Agency for Health Care Policy and Research, AIDS Clinical Trials Information Service, AIDS Treatment Data Network, Alzheimer's Disease and Related Disorders Association, Alzheimer's Disease Education and Referral Center, American Academy of Dermatology, American Academy of Medical Acupuncture, American Association of Blood Banks, American Association of Homes and Services for the Aging, American Association of Kidney Patients, American Association of Retired Persons, American Brain Tumor Association, American Cancer Society, American Cemetery Association, American

College of Physicians, American Diabetes Association, American Foundation for AIDS Research, American Health Care Association, American Heart Association, American Hospital Association, American Liver Foundation, American Lung Association, American Kidney Fund, American Nurses Association, American Pain Society, The American Parkinson's Disease Association, American Psychological Association, American Red Cross, American Society of Anesthesiologists, American Society of Clinical Hypnosis, American Urological Association, The Amyotrophic Lateral Sclerosis Association, Association for Applied Psychophysiology and Biofeedback, Brain Trauma Foundation, Cancer Information Service, CareLinc, Catholic Charities USA, Cemetery Consumer Service Council, Center for Medical Consumers, Centers for Disease Control and Prevention, Children of Aging Parents, Choice in Dying, The Cleveland Clinic Foundation, Community Health Accreditation Program, Cremation Association of North America, Department of Health and Human Services, Eldercare Locator Service, End Stage Renal Disease Network, Family Caregiver Alliance, Federal Trade Commission, Funeral and Memorial Societies of America, Gay Men's Health Crisis, Hemlock Society, Hospice Education Institute/HospiceLink, Huntington's Disease Society of America, Institute for Research in Hypnosis, International Association for the Study of Pain, International Myeloma Foundation, Joint Commission on Accreditation of Healthcare Organizations, Les Turner Amyotrophic Lateral Sclerosis Foundation, Leukemia Society of America, Make Today Count, The Mayday Fund, Multiple Sclerosis Association of America, Multiple Sclerosis Foundation, Myasthenia Gravis Foundation of America, The National Academy of Elder Law Attorneys, National AIDS Hotline, National Association for Continence, National Association for Home Care, National Association of Area Agencies on Aging, National Association of Professional Geriatric Care Managers, National Association of Social Workers, National Ataxia Foundation, National Brain Tumor Foundation, National Cancer Institute, National Center for Health Statistics, National Citizens Coalition for Nursing Home Reform, National Commission for the Certification of Acupuncturists, National Consumers League, The National Council on the Aging, National Diabetes Information Clearinghouse, National Digestive Diseases Information Clearinghouse, National Family Caregivers Association, National Foundation of Funeral Service, National Funeral Directors Association, National Head Injury Foundation, National Hospice Organization, National Health Information Center, National Heart, Lung and Blood Institute Information Center, National Institute of Diabetes and Digestive and Kidney Diseases, National Institute of Mental Health, National Institute of Neurological Disorders and Stroke, National Institute on Aging, National Institute on Alcohol Abuse and Alcoholism, National Kidney and Urological Disease Information Clearinghouse, National Institute on Adult Day Care, National Institute on Drug Abuse, The National Kidney Foundation, National Marrow Donor Program, National Multiple Sclerosis Society, National Organization for Rare Disorders, National Organization for the Reform of Marijuana Laws, National Parkinson Foundation, National Rehabilitation Information Center, National Self-Help Clearinghouse, National Spinal Cord Injury Association, National Stroke Association, Nursing Home Information Service, Older Women's League, Parkinson's Disease Foundation, People with AIDS Coalition of New York, Pharmaceutical Research and Manufacturers of America,

8 ACKNOWLEDGMENTS

Plus One Fitness Clinics, Project Inform, The Simon Foundation for Continence, Skin Cancer Foundation, Social Security Administration, The Society for Clinical and Experimental Hypnosis, Society of Critical Care Medicine, Stroke Connection of the American Heart Association, The THEOS Foundation, Transplant Recipients International Organization, United Network for Organ Sharing, United Ostomy Association, United Parkinson Foundation, United Way of America, U.S. Department of Labor Employment Standards Administration, U.S. Department of Veterans Affairs, U.S. Public Health Service, Visiting Nurse Associations of America, Well Spouse Foundation, and Whitman Walker Clinic Legal Services Project.

Readers are encouraged to share their own caregiving tips and personal experiences. Send E-mail to mcfarlaner@aol.com or letters to THE COMPLETE BEDSIDE COMPANION 779 Riverside Drive #A30 New York, NY 10032-7356.

For my brother David,
who sets the standard for the rest of us.
—R.M.

To my uncle Albert Freeman,
who in caring for his wife, Dollie, truly exemplified
what it means to be an everyday angel.
—P.B.

And to Audree Siden, who so inspired this book
and who died too soon.

Contents

Introduction, 23

How to Use This Book, 31

Part One: Caring for the Sick

1. *The Hospital and the Medical Team: Who's Who and What's What, 41*

When It Is Most Important to Be at an Ailing Loved One's Side, **42**
The Family and Medical Leave Act, **43**
    Set the Stage at Work, **44**
Preparing for a Loved One's Hospital Stay, **45**
    Arranging Blood Donations, **45**
What to Bring to the Hospital (and What to Leave at Home), **48**
    First Stop: The Admitting Office, **48**   Next Stop: The Floor, **51**
The Health Care Team: Who They Are and What They Do, **52**
    Doctors of Medicine (M.D.s), **52**   Nurses, **55**   Nurse's
    Assistants, **56**   Other Hospital Staff, **56**   Hospital Life: "But the
    Doctor Who Was Just Here Already Asked Us That!," **57**
Personalizing the Hospital Room, **58**
Ways to Be Helpful When Visiting Patients in the Hospital, **59**
    Don't Just Sit There, Do Something!, **59**
When the Quality of Hospital Care Is Lacking, **68**
    What Is a Legitimate Complaint?, **68**   To Whom Do You Complain?,
    69

Sidestepping Hospital Visiting Policies, **70**
Making Pitstops Before or After Hours, **71**
Outpatient Appointments and Tests, **71**
Strategic Scheduling, **71**   Preparing for Procedures, **72**
Avoiding Long Waits, **73**   When Accompanying Loved Ones to
Appointments, **73**
Preparing for Discharge from the Hospital, **74**
Postponing or Expediting Discharge Day, **75**
Safety Measures for Around the Home, **76**
Other Steps for Getting Ready, **76**   Modifying the Home, **78**   But Is
It Covered?, **80**
Recommended Reading, **81**

2. Dealing with the Doctors, 82

Choosing a Doctor, **83**
The ABC's of Getting Referrals, **85**   Points to Consider When
Choosing a Doctor, **85**
Seeking a Second Opinion, **86**
How Is a Second Opinon Arranged?, **86**   When Professional
Opinions Collide, **87**   Obtaining Medical Records, **87**
Care Partners, Patients, and Physicians: Ten Keys to Clear
Communication, **88**
Deciphering the Language of Medicine, **90**
Tracking Down the Doctor, **96**
Be Judicious with Questions for the Doctor, **96**
Dissatisfied with the Doctor?, **96**
When It Is Appropriate to Change Doctors?, **98**   The Smart Way to
Make the Switch, **99**   A Final Thought: Dissatisfaction or
Denial?, **100**

3. The Everyday Angel's Cram Course in Essential Nursing Skills, 101

A Caregiver's Basic Daily Skills, **102**
Keeping Patients Hydrated, **102**
Safeguarding Patients Against Infection, **105**
Types of Infections and How to Prevent Transmission, **106**   Special
Care: Increased Susceptibility to Infection, **109**   How Infections Are
Treated, **110**
Daily Hygiene, **110**
Bathing, **112**
How to Give a Four-Star Bed Bath, **114**   Giving a Basin Bath, **115**
Special Care: Bathing a Loved One Who Suffers from Memory Loss,
Confusion, or Intellectual Impairment, **115**
Skin Care, **116**
Moisturize!, **116**   Keep Skin Dry, **116**   Itching, **116**   Symptoms of
Pressure Ulcers, **118**   How to Prevent Pressure Ulcers, **118**   How
Pressure Ulcers Are Treated, **120**

Wound Care, **120**

Three Steps to Sterile Technique, **121**   How to Change a
Dressing, **121**

Oral Hygiene, **123**

Toileting, **124**

When Patients Are Confined to Bed, **124**   When Patients Are
Able to Get Out of Bed, **125**   Special Care: Toileting a Loved One
Who Suffers from Memory Loss, Confusion, or Intellectual
Impairment, **125**   Cleaning Patients After a Bowel Movement or
Urination, **125**   Caring for an Ostomy, **126**

Grooming and Dressing, **127**

Hair Care, **128**   Nail and Cuticle Care, **129**   Shaving, **129**
Dressing Patients, **129**

Turning, Maneuvering, and Lifting, **132**

How to Make an Occupied Bed, **132**   Lifting Patients by
Yourself, **133**   Transferring from a Bed to a Chair or
Wheelchair, **133**   Mechanical Lifting Devices, **134**

Tips for Preventing Falls, **134**

Basic Home Safety, **134**   Basic Walking Safety, **134**   To Prevent
Falls from Bed, **135**   What to Do if a Patient Falls, **135**

Preventing Muscle Contracture and Foot Drop, **135**

How to Perform Passive Range-of-Motion Exercises, **136**   What Is
Foot Drop?, **136**

Measuring Vital Signs, **136**

How to Take a Temperature, **137**   Managing Fever, **138**   How to
Take a Pulse, **139**   How to Measure Blood Pressure, **140**   How to
Monitor Respirations, **141**

Administering Medications Safely, **142**

Before Filling a New Prescription, **142**   At the Pharmacy, **143**
Keeping Track of Medications and Dosing Schedules, **143**   Routes
of Drug Administration, **144**

Allergic Reactions and Anaphylactic Shock, **151**

Managing an Allergic Reaction, **151**

Managing Pain, **152**

Attitudes Toward Pain Relief, **153**   Fundamentals of Pain
Management, **154**   Types of Pain Medications, **155**   Other Methods
of Administering Pain Medications, **155**   Nonpharmaceutical Pain
Management, **156**   What to Do When Pain Is Poorly Controlled, **157**

Essential Skills for Preventing and Managing Specific Complications, **158**

Digestive Complications, **158**

Appetite Loss and Anorexia, **158**   Complications That Inferfere
with Eating, **160**   Indigestion and Nausea, **162**   Difficulty
Swallowing (Dysphagia), **165**   Constipation and Gas, **167**
Diarrhea, **169**

Urinary Tract Complications, **170**

Incontinence, **170**   Urinary-Tract Infections, **172**

Insomnia and Other Sleep Disorders, **172**
Respiratory Complications, **174**
  Difficulty Breathing (Dyspnea), **174**   Difficulty Expelling
  Secretions, **176**   Chronic Coughing, **178**
Circulatory Complications, **178**
  Edema, Blood Clots, Phlebitis, Orthostatic Hypotension, **178**
  Bleeding and Bruising, **179**
Basic First Aid, **180**
  Managing Seizures and Convulsions, **180**   Cardiopulmonary
  Resuscitation (CPR), **181**   The Heimlich Maneuver, **182**
When Should You Call an Ambulance?, **182**

4. *Matters of the Heart, 185*

The So-Called Five Stages of Coping, **185**
  Denial, **186**   Anger, **187**   Bargaining, **190**   Depression, **191**
  Acceptance, **194**
The Fundamentals of Caregiving, **194**
  How to Be Supportive (Without Becoming a Pain in the
  Neck), **195**   Learning to Listen, **197**
Other Sources of Patient Support, **199**
  Patient Support Groups, **199**   Finding Hope and Comfort in
  Faith, **200**
Long-Standing Conflicts, **201**
Caring for People with Special Needs, **201**
  When a Loved One Is Not Conscious, **201**
  When a Loved One Suffers from Brain Function Impairment, **202**
    Memory Loss, **203**   Delusional or Hallucinatory
    Behavior, **204**   Agitated or Paranoid Behavior, **205**
    Combative Behavior, **206**   Restraints, **207**   Wandering, **207**
  When a Loved One Has Impaired Communications Skills, **208**

5. *Mustering the Troops, 211*

Spreading the Work Around, **212**
  The Family Conference, **214**   "If There's Anything I Can
  Do . . . ," **216**   Getting Men Involved, **217**   The Ready Reserves:
  Teenagers and Children, **219**
Long-Distance Angels, **220**
When Friends and Family Disappoint, **220**
  How to Handle Weepers and Wailers, **221**   Cheap Shots and Target
  Practice, **222**   A Memo to Family and Friends Who Want to
  Help . . . , **223**
Community Support Services, **224**
  How to Find Support Services in Your Area, **225** Professional Case
  Management, **227**

6. *The Caregiver as Consumer Activist, 229*

What Are Clinical Trials?, **229**

Who Pays for Clinical Trials, **230**   From Laboratory to Marketplace, **230**

How Do You Find Out About Clinical Trials?, **231**

The Pros and Cons of Participating in a Clinical Trial, **232**   Questions to Ask the Physician When Considering Participation in a Clinical Trial, **234**

A Rational Approach to Unconventional Treatments, **235**

How Do You Find Out About Alternative Therapies?, **237**

When Is Enough Enough? Changing Course from Cure to Comfort, **237**

Making Other Arrangements: Home Care, Hospice Care, and Nursing Home Care, **238**

Why Home Care?, **238**   Home Health Care Personnel, **239**   Home Hospice Care, **240**   When Cultures Collide: Building Rapport Across Class, Race, and Gender, **242**   Nursing Homes and Residential Care, **244**

7. *Care for the Caregivers, 247*

Maintaining Your Physical Stamina, **247**

Tricks for Keeping Your Body Running, **248**

Resolve to Rest; Steal Some Sleep, **248**   Eat and Drink Sensibly and Conscientiously, **248**   Take Steps to Prevent Infection, **250**   Exercise, **251**   Don't Postpone Your Own Doctor and Dental Appointments, **252**   Don't Try Doing It All, **253**   Consider Respite Care or Adult Day Care Services, **253**   Slow Down, Pace Yourself, **254**

Finding the Emotional Strength, **254**

Emotions Common to Caregivers, **254**

"I Feel as if I'm in a State of Shock," **254**   "I Feel So Angry and Resentful," **254**   "I Feel So Guilty," **255**   "I Feel So Isolated and Alone," **256**   "I Worry All the Time," **256**   "I Feel So Helpless," **257**   "I Feel as if He's Already Gone," **257**

Techniques for Managing Stress and Anxiety, **258**   When Depression Strikes, **261**

Caring for the Other Loved Ones in Your Life, **261**

Your Romantic Partner, **261**   Children, **262**

8. *Paying the Bills, 265*

Bookkeeping 101, **266**

Tricks for Maintaining Cash Flow, **267**

Financial-Assistance Programs, **270**

Government-Funded Programs, **270**

Social Security Retirement Benefits, **270**   Supplemental Security Disability Income (SSDI), **271**   Supplemental Security

Income (SSI), **272**   Aid to Families with Dependent Children
(AFDC), **272**   Food Stamps, **272**
Privately Funded Programs, **272**
A Warning About Pensions, **273**
Saving Money on Prescription Drugs, **273**
Buyers' Clubs, **275**   Prescription Drug Patient-Assistance
Programs, **275**   AIDS Drug Assistance Programs, **276**
Paying for Medical Care, **276**
Private Health Insurance, **276**   Government-Funded Health
Insurance, **278**
How to Get the Most out of Health Insurance, **280**

9. *Preparing for the Worst, 282*

Getting Started, **283**
The Paper Trail, **284**
How to Find a Good Lawyer, **286**
Last Will and Testament, **286**
Prearranging the Funeral, **289**
Legal and Financial Power of Attorney, **291**
Other Legal Instruments, **291**
Declaring Someone Incompetent, **292**
Discrimination Against the Sick and Disabled, **292**
Job Discrimination and the Caregiver, **294**
Artificial Life Support and Extraordinary Measures, **294**
Coma, Persistent Vegetative State, and Dementia, **297**
Advance Medical Directives, **298**
Living Wills and Medical Proxies, **299**   Enforcing Advance
Directives, **301**   Resisting the Impulse to "Do Something," **303**
Helping a Loved One Die, **304**
Tough Decisions: Withholding or Withdrawing Treatment, **305**

10. *Journey's End, 306*

Making the Most of Your Time Together, **307**
Making Your Peace, **307**
Ways That Loved Ones Face Death, **308**
Where People Die, **309**
Creating a Comfortable Space for the Dying, **310**   Other Ways to
Create a Comforting Environment for the Dying, **310**
Waiting Room Marathons and Death Watches, **311**

11. *Aftermath, 313*

The Moment of Death, **314**
Phone Calls and Final Arrangements, **316**
The Funeral, **316**   Final Details, **317**
Grieving and Getting On with Life, **318**
"No Regrets," **319**

Part Two: The Everyday's Angel's Cram Course in Adult Medicine

12. *Caring for Someone with Cancer, 323*

What Is Cancer?, **324**

Symptoms of Cancer, **324** How Cancer Is Diagnosed, **325** What Is Staging?, **325**

How Cancer Is Treated, **326**

Surgery, **326** Radiation Therapy and Its Side Effects, **326** What Is Internal Radiation Therapy?, **329** Chemotherapy and Its Side Effects, **329** Other Forms of Cancer Treatment, **334**

Potential Complications of Advanced Cancer, **336**

Recommended Reading, **336**

13. *Caring for Someone with Cardiovascular Disease, 338*

Causes of Cardiovascular Disease, **339**

Types of Cardiovascular Disease, **340**

Heart Attack (Infarction), **340**

Symptoms of a Heart Attack, **340** What Is Angina?, **341** How a Heart Attack Is Diagnosed, **342** How a Heart Attack Is Treated, **342**

Arrhythmias, **344**

Causes and Symptoms of Arrhythmias, **345** How Arrhythmias Are Diagnosed, **345** How Arrhythmias Are Treated, **346**

Congestive Heart Failure, **347**

Pulmonary Edema and Pleural Effusion, **348** Difficulty Breathing (Dyspnea), **349** How Heart Failure Is Diagnosed, **349** How Heart Failure Is Treated, **350** Potential Complications of Advanced Cardiovascular Disease, **350**

Recommended Reading, **351**

14. *Caring for Someone with Cerebrovascular Stroke or Traumatic Brain Injury, 352*

What Happens in a Stroke?, **353**

Ischemic Stroke, **353** Hemorrhagic Stroke, **355**

Traumatic Brain Injury, **356**

What Happens in a Closed Head Injury, **356**

Diagnosis and Treatment of Stroke and Traumatic Brain Injury, **357**

Craniotomy, **358** Carotid Endarterectomy, **358** Aneurysm Surgery, **358** Drug Therapy, **359**

Potential Acute Complications and How They Are Managed, **359**

Impaired Respiration, **361** Heart Attack, **361** Difficulty Swallowing (Dysphagia), **361** Pulmonary Embolism, **361** Incontinence, **362**

Potential Long-Term Effects of Stroke and Severe Traumatic Brain Injury, **363**

Paralysis/Weakness, **363** Contracture, **364** Hemispheric

Neglect, **365**   Persistent Headaches, **365**   Speech/Language Loss
(Aphasia), **365**   Changes in Behavior and Personality, **366**
Depression, **366**
Rehabilitation, **367**
Deciding on the Proper Rehab Setting, **368**   Choosing a
Rehabilitation Program, **369**   How You Can Help During
Rehabilitation, **372**   Potential Life-Threatening Complications, **373**
Recommended Reading, **375**

15. *Caring for Someone with Chronic Obstructive Pulmonary Disease
    (Emphysema and Chronic Bronchitis), 376*

Chronic Obstructive Pulmonary Disease and the Lungs, **377**
What Causes Chronic Obstructive Pulmonary Disease?, **378**
Early Symptoms and Diagnosis, **379**
Symptoms and Complications of Advanced COPD, **379**
Shortness of Breath (Dyspnea), **379**   Chronic Coughing, **384**
Difficulty Expelling Secretions, **384**   Appetite Loss, **385**
Insomnia, **385**   Depression, **385**   Other Potential
Complications, **386**
How COPD Is Treated, **386**
Potential Life-Threatening Complications, **386**
Pulmonary Infection, **387**   Respiratory Acidosis, **387**   Secondary
Polycythemia, **388**   Respiratory Failure/Ventilatory Failure, **389**
Cor Pulmonale, **389**
Recommended Reading, **390**

16. *Caring for Someone with Diabetes, 391*

What Is Diabetes?, **392**
Symptoms of Diabetes, **393**   How Diabetes Is Diagnosed, **393**
How Diabetes Is Treated, **394**
Acute Complications of Diabetes, **404**
Diabetic Ketoacidosis/Hyperglycemic Hyperosmolar Nonketotic
Coma, **405**   Hypoglycemia, **406**
Long-Term Complications of Diabetes, **407**
Peripheral Neuropathy, **408**   Foot Ulcers, **408**   Gastroparesis, **409**
Constipation, **410**   Diabetic Diarrhea, **410**   Incontinence, **410**
Diabetic Retinopathy, **410**
Potential Life-Threatening Complications, **411**
Recommended Reading, **412**

17. *Caring for Someone with AIDS/HIV, 413*

What Is AIDS? What Is HIV?, **415**
The Illnesses of AIDS, **416**
Pneumocystis Carinii Pneumonia, **416**   Tuberculosis, **418**
Mycobacterium Avium Intracellulare Complex, **418**
Cryptosporidiosis, **418**   Toxoplasmosis, **419**   HIV Encephalopathy

(HIV Dementia), **419**   Kaposi's Sarcoma, **419**   HIV Wasting
Syndrome, **420**
How HIV Is Diagnosed, **420**
How HIV/AIDS Is Treated, **421**
Antiviral Therapy, **421**
AIDS Treatment and Prevention, **422**
Clinical Trials and HIV/AIDS, **423**   Managing Symptoms and Side
Effects, **424**
Recommended Reading, **428**

18. *Caring for Someone with Liver Disease, 429*

The Liver, **430**
Causes of Cirrhosis, **430**
Chronic Alcoholism, **430**   Chronic Active Viral Hepatitis, **430**
Early Symptoms and Diagnosis of Liver Disease, **431**
Managing Symptoms of Liver Failure, **432**
Jaundice, **432**   Gallstones, **432**   Edema/Ascites, **433**
Life-Threatening Complications of Liver Failure, **433**
Hepatic Encephalopathy, **434**   Variceal Bleeding, **434**
How Liver Disease Is Treated, **435**
Diet, **437**   Liver Transplantation, **438**
Recommended Reading, **439**

19. *Caring for Someone with Kidney Disease, 440*

The Kidneys, **441**
Causes of End-Stage Renal Disease, **441**
Diabetes, **442**   Hypertension, **442**   Kidney Diseases, **442**
Analgesic Drugs, **442**
Symptoms of Chronic Renal Failure, **443**
How Kidney Disease Is Diagnosed, **443**
Complications of End-Stage Renal Disease and Their Symptoms, **444**
Uremia, **444**   Hyperkalemia, **444**   Hypervolemia/Edema, **444**
Renal Tubular Metabolic Acidosis, **445**   Anemia, **445**   Renal
Osteodystrophy, **445**   Immunosuppression, **446**   Neuropathy, **446**
Dry, Itchy Skin, **447**   Dry Mouth, Altered Taste, and Chronic
Thirst, **447**   Depression, **447**
How End-Stage Renal Disease Is Treated, **448**
But Is It Covered?, **449**
What Caregivers Should Know About Hemodialysis, **450**
Caring for a Fistula or Shunt, **451**   A Typical Hemodialysis
Treatment, **451**   What's in a Number?, **451**   Side Effects of
Hemodialysis, **451**   Our Role as the Patient's Advocate, **452**
What Caregivers Should Know About Peritoneal Dialysis, **454**
Side Effects of Peritoneal Dialysis, **454**

The Renal Diet, **455**
> Protein, **455**   Potassium, **456**   Sodium, **456**   Phosphorus, **456**
> Calories, **456**
The Renal Diet and Diabetics, **457**
Kidney Transplantation, **457**
> But Is It Covered?, **458**   Life Following Kidney Transplantation
> Surgery, **458**
Recommended Reading, **459**

20. *Caring for Someone with a Progressive Neurological Disease,* **460**
> The Central Nervous System, **462**
> Alzheimer's Disease, **462**
> > Early Signs of Alzheimer's Disease, **464**
> Parkinson's Disease, **465**
> > Early Signs of Parkinson's Disease, **465**
> Amyotrophic Lateral Sclerosis, **466**
> > Early Signs of ALS, **467**
> How Neurological Diseases Are Diagnosed, **467**
> How Neurological Diseases Are Treated, **467**
> > Alzheimer's Disease, **469**   Parkinson's Disease, **469**   Amyotrophic
> > Lateral Sclerosis, **472**
> Effects of Advanced Progressive Neurological Disease, **473**
> Effects of End-Stage Alzheimer's Disease, **473**
> > Hyperactivity, **473**   Hiding Objects, **474**   Combative Behavior, **474**
> Effects of End-Stage Parkinson's Disease, **475**
> > Impaired Mobility, **475**   Chronic Constipation, **477**   Dependent
> > Edema, **478**   Eye Irritation, **478**   Seborrhea/Seborrheic
> > Dermatitis, **478**   Dementia, **479**   Depression, **479**
> Effects of End-Stage Amyotrophic Lateral Sclerosis, **479**
> > Impaired Mobility, **480**
> Symptoms Common to Advanced AD, PD, and ALS, **480**
> > Incontinence, **480**   Contracture, **481**   Muscle Cramping, **481**
> > Insomnia, **482**   Speech/Language Loss (Aphasia), **482**
> > Difficulty Swallowing (Dysphagia), **484**   Appetite Loss/
> > Wasting, **485**   Difficulty Expelling Secretions, **485**   Difficulty
> > Breathing (Dyspnea)/Respiratory Failure, **486**
> Recommended Reading, **487**

Appendix A: Recommended Resources, **489**

Appendix B: Miscellaneous Resources, **502**

Appendix C: For Referrals to Home Health Care, Hospice Care, Long-Term
Care, Adult Day Care, Respite Care, and Rehabilitation Facilities, **515**

Bibliography, **519**

Index, **523**

The Complete Bedside Companion

Introduction

As they filed out of Belmany's Funeral Home, one by one the mourners remarked to my younger brother David and me, "Your daddy sure was lucky to have you boys take care of him."

During the last weeks of his battle with lymphoma, a cancer of the immune system, I'd taken leave from my job in New York to help care for my seventy-two-year-old father at his home in Alabama. David, a Manhattan interior designer, had already been with Dad for a month. Bob McFarlane was dying—any time for denial had long since passed—and we were determined to ease his pain and anxiety as much as possible.

Eight months earlier, shortly before doctors discovered his cancer, my father had undergone emergency heart surgery. During the month I spent with him when he came home from the hospital, I'd assured him: "Papa, we know what to do. You don't have to worry. David and I will take care of the house,

the bills will get paid, and you know there is no amount of pain we cannot control. I promise you, you are not going to be alone."

"Yes, sir, he sure was lucky," we heard over and over after the service. "You boys always knew exactly what to do." And I suppose that was true. But then I've probably had more experience with disease and death than most forty-somethings. In the past few years, my stepmother Lynn had died of lung cancer; colorectal cancer had claimed my father's oldest sister, Margaret; and no sooner had we buried Dad than my uncle Billy, caught for years in the cruel grip of Alzheimer's disease, began to deteriorate rapidly. Complications ended his struggle two months later. David and I helped care for them all. In our family that's just what you do.

Perhaps because I grew up surrounded by a large extended family in the small rural town of Theodore, Alabama (just south of Mobile), death had been demystified for me at an early age.

23

My father was a building contractor and a skilled craftsman, so when my maternal grandmother, Vada, and great-grandmother, Josephine, both took ill around the same time, he built them a small two-bedroom home on our heavily wooded property. My visits to the white frame house became a daily routine. Though I was just four years old when they came to live next door, it was my job to assist Josephine out of bed and into her wheelchair, then help her roll up the nylon stockings that she insisted on wearing, no matter how frail she felt.

Because she was also nearly blind, other times I sat on the lid of her bedside commode and read the newspaper to her as well as a beginning reader could. She'd correct my grammar and help me with my alphabet. It was an invaluable education on several levels.

Josephine died at the age of ninety-two. The family physician drove out to the house, put a stethoscope to her chest, and pronounced her dead. My father brought me, David, and our older brother, Bobby, into her bedroom. She appeared to be sleeping, and I remember wondering why my mother was crying.

"Kiss Josephine good-bye," Papa said softly, "because she's gone to heaven now." My mother and grandmother had cleaned her, changed her into a fresh cotton nightgown, and brushed her hair. It all seemed so sweet, so normal, so natural. Only years later did I come to appreciate how unusual this scene really was for 1962.

That early experience left an indelible impression and seems to have set something of a tone for my life. As director of two of America's premier AIDS service groups, Gay Men's Health Crisis and Broadway Cares/Equity Fights AIDS, I assisted countless people with AIDS at the end of their lives, and I continue to do so. In addition, both before and after a four-year hitch aboard a Navy nuclear submarine, I worked as a respiratory therapy technician in the intensive care units at the

University of South Alabama Medical Center. So by the time of my father's terminal cancer, tending to the dying had become all too familiar.

But I was an exception. A loved one's serious illness thrusts most people into the position of caregiver completely unprepared. They feel overwhelmed by expectations and the deluge of information, and underqualified to meet the patient's needs as he or she gets pulled into the vortex of disease and requires more and more assistance. Good and noble intentions, often stoked by the misleading, overly romanticized images of death seen on TV and in the movies, are quickly tested by the harsh reality of what it means to die and what it means to be intimately involved in the daily life of someone who might be dying.

Debbie Bryant, forty-four, of Gulf Shores, Alabama: A year before Mom died, she began having terrible nausea and diarrhea. Her gynecologist suspected cervical cancer and performed a hysterectomy, but no evidence of cancer was found. Three months later an exploratory abdominal surgery revealed the malignancy in her intestine. The tumor was too large to be removed surgically. She underwent radiation therapy, then chemotherapy.

I was twenty-four years old and still lived at home with my parents in Mobile. At first Mom was pretty much able to look after herself, but later on she grew so weak that she couldn't get out of bed. If my mother needed to go to the bathroom, we had to lift her up and place her on the portable potty we kept next to it. I worked the three-to-eleven shift at the hospital, so I'd take care of her in the daytime; my dad looked after her when he came home from work in the evening. Toward the end we hired a home nurse to help us.

Mostly, we took care of Mom's basic needs, like keeping her clean and trying to get her to eat, although she was nauseated all the time. My mother also had a lot of abdominal pain from the

cancer and the chemotherapy. We tried to make her as comfortable as possible, juggling pain medications and adjusting the pillows she kept around her. It was pretty miserable. She died in September, three months before she and my dad would have celebrated their thirtieth wedding anniversary.

I tried to stay strong for Mom, but it was tough. I drank a lot of Scotch.

If you're lucky, you die like my mother, Betty Grace: sitting in her favorite chair at home. A sudden interruption in her heart's rhythm took her without a struggle. My father walked into the house to find her still sitting upright, with the morning mail in her lap. She looked so peaceful that at first he thought she was merely napping.

My stepmother's final months, a blur of trips to and from the hospital, provided a stark contrast. Although the malignant tumor blocking her airway was incurable, doctors ordered radiation treatments to stem its growth. The rays blistered her throat and badly aggravated her chronic cough from emphysema. She grew weak and severely nauseated, tossed and turned, utterly unable to sleep for nights on end, and suffered excruciating nerve pain in her face and neck. At the very end we kept her unconscious on morphine, and she finally died quietly in her own bedroom. It was an ordeal for her and for us, and like so many deaths, an inherently undignified physical process.

In blunt terms, being a caregiver is about wiping your adult brother; carrying your mother to the bathroom and cradling her head as she retches violently into the toilet; bearing painful witness to the loss of control that disease often inflicts on once capable adults. And while there are brave souls who face death resolutely, others lash out at those around them, so consumed are they by fear and rage. How do you reconcile the contradictory, guilt-inducing emotions that a terminal illness stirs up: one day fighting for life, unable to imagine life without your loved one; then, after witnessing another night of unmitigated suffering, praying—for both your sakes—that it will all be over soon.

Tending to the sick is a full-time job. The average caregiver spends thirty hours a week looking after the ill person. In addition, three in ten of us work outside the home, and as many as four in ten have children to raise. Understandably, this staggering load of demands can leave care partners feeling exhausted, depressed, confused, and helpless.

Pat Still, fifty-one, of New York City: My husband had a stroke on July 13, 1984. He was a television cameraman for Good Morning America *and was in San Francisco shooting the Democratic convention. The stroke left him paralyzed on the left side of his body and brain damaged, although one wouldn't necessarily realize it. It was subtle. Our son was seven years old at the time.*

My husband spent four and a half months in a rehab hospital and learned how to walk with a cane, but he was never very steady. A year after the stroke he started having grand mal seizures. The doctors discovered that the arteries carrying blood to the brain were almost completely blocked. They told me he was a walking time bomb, that he was going to drop dead any minute. So I tried to prepare my son for the imminent death of his father. And then it didn't happen! Somehow or other the secondary circulation provided enough blood to his brain.

At that time, we were stuck in the middle-class bind: We didn't qualify for Medicaid because we had too much money, but we didn't have enough money to pay for help ourselves. So I had the twenty-four-hour-a-day responsibility of caring for my husband.

He spent the last three years of his life in a nursing home, after the Medicaid laws changed. It was absolutely essential. By then my son was thirteen years old. We had an electric bed in the middle of our living room. When you walked into the apartment, you never knew what you were going to find. I don't know how many hours my husband spent on the floor, having fallen and been unable to get up, waiting for me to get home. Our apartment wasn't big enough for him to use the wheelchair.

In 1993, when he was sixty-eight, he had a huge cerebral hemorrhage on the other side of his brain. Had he lived, he would have been completely paralyzed and unable to talk. It would have been torment, so l didn't let them put him on life support.

Perhaps you're thinking, *I don't know if I can do this.* To be sure, some people are not able to, for a variety of reasons. Their own health, for one. My twice-widowed father's third wife, Mary, was herself ailing and physically incapable of caring for Dad. What's more, she was then living a concurrent nightmare: an adult daughter dying of breast cancer at Mary's house. Other factors—commitments at home, living far away, time constraints at work—may prevent you from contributing to a patient's daily care.

In my experience, however, circumstances tend to dictate who will be the caregivers. Like Army conscripts, we're not given a choice. One-third of all primary caregivers shoulder the responsibility because they live closer to the patient than other family members.

But human beings are remarkably resilient and resourceful. I can't tell you how many times I have seen spouses, siblings, adult children, parents, lovers, and friends respond to a loved one's critical illness with admirable courage and grace. Some transcend all expectations; I'm talking about folks who used to fall apart at the mere hint of a crisis. I truly believe that most of us possess the compassion and character to pass this test. But caregiving additionally demands that we acquire the necessary practical skills, the strategies for bearing up physically and emotionally,

learning how to get the help we need from others and, above all, the self-confidence to transcend our fears and inhibitions. That is where *The Complete Bedside Companion* can be indispensable.

In clear, practical terms, our book walks you down the road from the onset of symptoms through the very end and afterward. I'm not a registered nurse, but I can prevent bedsores, juggle pain and nausea medications, and flush IV lines with the best of them, and so can you. Likewise, almost anyone can learn to navigate the medical, legal, and insurance mazes. Consider this your map.

A number of the essential caregiving tools and tricks we have gathered come from doctors, nurses, social workers, psychologists, experts in insurance and legal matters, and other professionals, as well as from dozens of caregivers— "everyday angels"—reliving their experiences and sharing their hard-earned insights.

Together they comprise a group that greatly reflects the collective profile of today's American caregivers: 70 percent are women, 55 percent are sixty-five or older, nearly half are the dying person's spouse, and more than 33 percent are adult daughters and sons reciprocating the care their now elderly parents once gave them. There's the Utah wife who tended her husband, an emphysema patient, the last eight years of his life; the Louisiana mother of two whose father was diagnosed with Alzheimer's disease shortly after her father-in-law had died of the same disorder; the medical scholar from Connecticut who nursed his longtime companion throughout a three-year battle with AIDS. In their vivid accounts you will find gold mines of arcane information and practical advice, and the realization that you are not alone. These women and men have been where you are now. This is how they got through.

Above all we hope to convey what it's really like to care for the desperately ill and prepare you for what may arise. We can't always safeguard patients from the ravages of disease, but we can spare them unnecessary pain, suffering, degradation, and other people's psychodramas, and we can free time and energy for *connecting* in a warm, loving environment. Perhaps that means reminiscing, resolving past conflicts, or simply being a comforting presence at the bedside. How we play these scenes will greatly determine how we survive the years after the person's death. Will we look back on this time with a sense of satisfaction or pangs of regret?

Caring for the Seriously Ill: A Lost Art

As recently as the 1930s it was not uncommon for seriously ill family members to be cared for at home. Men, women, and even children were familiar with death and dying; its sights, sounds, and smells did not shock. Chances are, most elderly Americans living today knew of or saw a dying person tended to in the home, where the parlor was reserved not only for social occasions but for funeral services.

With the advent of antibiotics and increasingly effective lifesaving drugs and technology, the hospital soon became the repository for the seriously ill. Certainly the remarkable leaps in medical science and technology over the past half-century have benefited millions, but our dependence on hospitals has led us essentially to quarantine the dying in institutions, physically removing them from our day-to-day lives, and us from theirs. In the hospital, family members find themselves nudged aside —in a maze of impersonal, identical rooms, harsh lights, lack of privacy, tubes, wires, pumps, and high-tech monitors—with the patient's most fundamental needs and concerns overseen by strangers. As a result, many of us have come to assume that nursing a loved one is beyond us and better left to experts in a medical environment.

These changes in terminal care have also shaped physicians' attitudes toward illness and dying. Equipped with such a sophisticated armamentarium, they may tend to view death not as a natural part of life's cycle but as *medicine's failure*. Dr. Howard Spiro, a gastroenterologist for over half a century and director of the Program for Humanities in Medicine at Yale University School of Medicine, observes, "You never hear a doctor say, 'What a great death that was. What a wonderful end to a person's life. It came at just the right moment.'" Instead, Dr. Spiro says, "Death is our adversary." This attitude may manifest in excessive testing or investigational procedures that stand little or no chance of reversing the outcome and ultimately prolong dying.

The cumulative impact of the burgeoning Right to Die movement, the current AIDS epidemic, and the disappointing progress in the long war on cancer seems to be changing doctors' perspectives somewhat, forcing the profession to reexamine its obligations to the dying. For if success is measured solely by conquering illness, how do you define your role when faced with a disease that eludes a cure? Rather than viewing those who are dying as beyond their help, says Dr. Spiro, physicians can assist them in other ways, such as providing practical and emotional support, and adequate pain relief. Dr. Howard Grossman, an AIDS specialist, remarks, "My major goals are twofold: to do whatever I can to make patients' lives as good and productive as possible, and to make their deaths as easy for them as possible.

"AIDS has had a profound impact on bringing the issues of death and dying to the fore in the United States," he reflects. "I think it has also brought out many doctors' compassion." Nonetheless, cautions Dr. Spiro, on both counts "we have got a long way to go."

As does society as a whole. Our modern culture banishes death from life. We broach the subject in the abstract or shrouded in religious and mythological terms, if at all, so that we have lost the art of caring for the dying. But that art is already undergoing a revival as we move headlong into what has been dubbed the Graying of America.

The year 1995 saw a record 2,312,132 deaths registered in the United States. Since the 1970s, the segment of the population age sixty-five or older has doubled, and its growth will continue to outpace all other age groups. According to the U.S. Census Bureau, by the year 2030 the number of Americans over sixty-five will have multiplied to more than 70 million, or one in five. Will we have enough beds in hospitals, hospices, and nursing homes? In light of our already overburdened health care system, most likely not.

This crushing demand for services and spiraling health care costs has left insurers and employers scrambling for alternatives to hospitalization. Home care is infinitely less expensive. And nowadays procedures that were once performed exclusively in medical facilities, such as kidney dialysis, artificial respiration, and IV and oxygen therapy, can be carried out at home. Many other medical measures normally conducted in the hospital, such as chemotherapy, surgery, biopsies, transfusions, and sophisticated diagnostic testing, are all routinely provided on an outpatient basis.

Most significant of all, nine in ten Americans surveyed in a recent Gallup Poll said they wanted to die at home, surrounded by loved ones. In reality, four in five of us die in hospitals or nursing facilities. "I think the greatest blessing one can give a patient," says Dr. Spiro, "is to let him or her die at home.

"Of course," he adds, "it depends on the home."

Clearly, home care is not viable for everyone, such as the nearly 10 million infirm Americans living alone or in situations where the prospective caregiver lacks a support system (for example, a childless aged couple living in a remote town with few community services). And with the average life expectancy inching upward, to seventy-six years as of 1997, increasingly we're seeing families in which elderly adult children of ailing ninety-year-old parents have their own health problems.

Yes, most people can do this, but it's extremely difficult to go it alone. Had my brother and I not been able to take extended leave from our jobs, Dad's final weeks might have been spent in the Mobile Infirmary instead of his beloved house on Rabbit Creek. *The Complete Bedside Companion* will help you formulate a plan for meeting the patient's needs, whatever the setting.

When Denial Masquerades as Hope

A word about the subtitle: *No-Nonsense Advice on Caring for the Seriously Ill.* This book charts the progression of critical illness to its most tragic outcome. (*Critically ill* is defined as acute enough to warrant immediate and continuous medical attention. *Terminally ill* refers to patients considered beyond therapeutic treatment.)

No matter how bleak the prognosis, I don't think we ever stop praying for miracles. And miracles do happen. I've seen more than one comatose patient on life support recover and walk out of the hospital literally days later. At some point, though, you will have to repeat this drill. The cancer patient, after months or years in remission, relapses. An ischemic stroke fells the heart attack survivor. Someone else close to you becomes sick. Being a caregiver can be likened to living on a fault line, with periods of relative calm shattered by seismic episodes requiring mad dashes to the hospital, emergency procedures, and so on.

Few qualities are as essential to caregivers as the ability to recognize when we're genuinely clinging to hope and when our denial is no longer useful, blinding us to reality. Having to acknowledge that someone's condition is irreversible is undeniably heartbreaking. At the same time it brings certain issues into focus and redirects priorities, so that instead of exhorting the sick person (and yourself) to chase after different treatments—to keep up the fight—attention turns to helping him best live out the end of his life.

Bear in mind that regardless of how meticulously you connect the dots, regardless of how competent and composed you are, things will go wrong every day. *Every* day. The cousin who promised to spell you for a few hours just called to say she can't make it. It's Sunday; you've used up all the morphine the nurse left for the weekend, your father is writhing in pain, and the pharmacy with the doctor's orders is closed. When your game plan crumbles, you improvise. This is how most caregivers get through the day, cobbling together support as best they can and moving forward one step at a time.

Mary Vitro, a forty-year-old widow from Clearwater, Florida, spent nearly two years caring for her terminally ill husband while also raising an infant. Just three months after the birth of their son, Douglas, in 1989, Rick, then thirty-eight, was diagnosed with AIDS. He survived an initial bout of pneumonia and lived reasonably symptom free for the next year and a half. But in the summer of 1991 he began to decline, suffering one complication after another. Toward the end, Mary's typical day consisted of tending Rick at his hospital bedside from morning until dinnertime, then going home to take care of Doug. After putting him to bed, cleaning the house, doing laundry, and trying to dig herself out from under an avalanche of medical bills, she would finally collapse into bed around midnight.

"Every morning," she remembers, "I'd wake up with a pounding headache. I look back now and wonder, *My God, how did I do that? How did I keep going?* I don't know. You just do, somehow." She adds, "I would do it again for somebody important to me."

Sarah Lanier Barber, *sixty, of Santa Fe, New Mexico: My parents, both in their eighties, were ill at the same time. My mother was diagnosed with Alzheimer's disease around 1988, although I'm sure she'd had it longer than that. My father insisted on taking care of her by himself, even though he was in failing health and malnourished. I was in New York then, teaching; they lived in Tallahassee, Florida. I would fly down there two or three times a year.*

Then there started to be more than the usual number of crises. My father would mysteriously collapse and have to be rushed to the hospital, and I would be called down to take care of my mother while he was recovering. Each time after he came home, we would talk about the two of them going into a total-care community right there in Tallahassee, where they could have their own apartment and their inde-

pendence. But my mother would get hysterical, and we wouldn't be able to talk about it anymore. There was never any thought of having a person come in and take care of my mother. It had to be me because she wouldn't allow anyone else in the house.

Finally, in 1992, my father went into the hospital for surgery and never came out. He was eighty-six. I was living in New Mexico by then. Because my mother was so demented by this time, I had to put her in the hospital's psychiatric unit, with my father next door in intensive care. The day he died she was transferred to the nursing home. I'd always dreaded that day and had imagined that she would have to be put in a straitjacket and taken off yelling and screaming. But she didn't know what was happening. She's ninety and still lives there, on what is called a total nursing care floor.

I feel as if I've done the best I can. My mother is in a very safe, humane, compassionate place. Each month I obsessively pay her bills and make sure everything is taken care of. I find I have to focus on those day-to-day details, because if I begin to really think about the larger dimension of taking care of my mother, then I start thinking, I need to make this better for her. And there really is no better."

Never do we want to imply that this is easy. To the contrary, caring for a dying person is perhaps the hardest thing you will ever do. It can also be one of the most rewarding, for how many opportunities do we get to be so profoundly meaningful to someone we love? Unimaginable as it may seem, beauty, healing, and growth can flourish amid all the pain and sadness.

"I feel as if I learned a lot about living from observing dying," reflects Audree Siden. When her eighty-eight-year-old mother developed congestive heart failure in 1992, Audree moved her into her Manhattan apartment. That Mae Weisenberg died peacefully there eight months later brought Audree tremendous joy.

"All my life I'd had an extraordinary relationship with my mother," she says. "We were best friends. So taking care of her was as natural as breathing. It was like the completion of a cycle, a giving back. Nothing I have experienced has been as intimate as caring for a dying person."

For me and my brothers there was no greater satisfaction and comfort than to hear my dying father, a man not easily given to expressing his emotions, say to us with tears in his eyes, "I don't know what I would have done without you boys."

How to Use This Book

All it takes is a distraught phone call informing you that a parent has suffered a stroke or a doctor gravely pronouncing that your sister has breast cancer to plunge you into caregiving, where training comes strictly on the job and under duress. Before you've begun to gain your bearings, you're contending with a medical system that has its own conventions and language, and can be hostile to outsiders. It's enough to make even the most competent of us feel out of our depth, helpless, paralyzed.

You see it in the hospital every day: the fear and lack of comprehension on people's faces as the physician sketches the patient's condition in a blizzard of medical jargon. Some words register; others skip off the consciousness, unheard and unrecalled.

As caregivers we are our loved ones' advocates, charged with getting them what they need when they need it. That may be anything from more effective symptom relief or enrollment in an ex-perimental therapy, to information on which to base these and other crucial medical decisions, including whether to utilize or discontinue life-support systems. At some point you may find yourself in the position of having to make those decisions—alone—on the patient's behalf.

The Complete Bedside Companion traces the sequence of events common to a life-threatening illness and examines the innumerable concerns and crises that arise along the way. But we expect you'll skip from chapter to chapter, drawing on whatever information you need to help you get through today.

Accordingly, we've copiously cross-referenced the book to get you speedily from here ("Impaired Mobility," page 475 from chapter 20 on Parkinson's disease) to there ("Tips for Preventing Falls," page 134). Part two, "The Everyday Angel's Cram Course in Adult Medicine," presents crash courses in cancer, cardiovascular disease, stroke, and the other adult diseases or conditions that

31

most commonly result in serious illness or death.* For if we're truly going to aid our ailing loved one, we need to acquire a basic knowledge of the illness—and quickly. The more we know, the more inclined we are to be an active participant in the person's care rather than a spectator. Each chapter outlines

- initial symptoms;
- diagnostic tests and procedures;
- treatment methods and their side effects;
- tips on preventing and managing common complications unique to each disease (chapter 3, "The Everyday Angel's Cram Course in Essential Nursing Skills," centers on the more general medical problems that accompany a number of serious disorders);
- how the illness typically progresses;
- medical terms you are likely to hear, including the names of medications used to control the disease, its symptoms and complications, and the side effects of therapy.

You needn't read all of part two, only the chapters pertaining to your loved one. Bear in mind, however, that many of these illnesses are intertwined. Complications of diabetes, for instance, include kidney disease, heart disease, and stroke. As with my father, patients can also suffer from multiple unrelated ailments in any of a number of ominous combinations.

Disease may erupt as suddenly as a summer storm—heart attack, stroke, acute kidney failure—or gradually erode health like waves lapping at the shore. Alzheimer's disease, one example of a chronic progressive degenerative disorder, persists for eight years, on average. We suspect my uncle Billy had the mind-ravaging disease at least that long. It wasn't until the last year or so, though, that it debilitated him to where he required constant care. And his con-

dition grew critical only weeks before he died from a series of strokes.

Parkinson's disease, another chronic neurological disorder, is not considered fatal in and of itself. Many Parkinson's sufferers live productively for a number of years. But as the disease runs its course, these patients fall prey to a variety of life-threatening complications, among them pneumonia and blood poisoning, two leading causes of death. Our point is that any person whose bodily defenses are impaired by disease or injury—whether he is acutely ill or chronically ill—can take an abrupt turn for the worse, hence our inclusion of Parkinson's and other common chronic conditions.

Other Essential Sources of Information

Information empowers, helping to illuminate our way as we proceed down one unfamiliar path and then another.

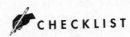 **CHECKLIST**

Things to Do Following a Loved One's Diagnosis

☐ Call organizations such as the American Cancer Society, National Kidney Foundation, Amyotrophic Lateral Sclerosis Association, and so forth, for free written material on a disease.

☐ Ask to receive the organization's newsletter.

☐ Join a support group.

☐ Begin mining information from other caregivers and patients you meet at support groups, in waiting rooms, through on-line computer chat groups and bulletin boards— wherever.

☐ Visit libraries and bookstores.

---

* *The Complete Bedside Companion* does not address the complex age-related issues unique to caring for a child.

For additional reading, consult Appendix A's list of more than two dozen organizations dedicated to assisting patients and families coping with a particular disorder. Most of them run hot lines staffed by trained volunteers who can answer general questions you may have about a disease and its treatment, as well as refer you to services available in your community. When calling, ask to receive the organization's newsletter. Besides providing patients and caregivers with a forum for exchanging perspectives and practical advice, these publications alert readers to medical developments and useful products and services.

That same telephone call can very likely lead you to a support group (see Table A). Support groups, also known as self-help or peer-support groups, bring together people facing a common crisis. Some may be led by a facilitator —usually a social worker or a nurse. Most disease-related organizations conduct groups through their local chapters, and all of them can direct you to smaller independent groups that may meet in your area.

As much as you may surround yourself with friends and family, caring for the dying is an isolating experience. For that reason alone, a support group can be an anchor, bringing sorely needed perspective and some semblance of normalcy to a caregiver's life. Granted, sharing intimate thoughts with a roomful of strangers is not for everyone—men in particular, it seems. I'll confess that I've resisted taking advantage of support groups myself, despite my having helped launch one of the largest networks in the country, Gay Men's Health Crisis. Even if you have no intention of speaking up yourself, by all means *go* just to soak up information. You'll learn how other caregivers structure their care plans, hear best- and worst-case scenarios and every gradation in between, and find out what community services are available and how to plug yourself into the system. Several sponsor pen pal or phone pal programs, which put caregivers and patients in touch with one another—an excellent alternative for those in communities without formal support groups.

Where Else Can You Locate a Support Group?

◆ Hospitals, hospices, nursing homes, kidney dialysis centers; check with a social worker at any of these.

◆ Ask your primary care physician or her office staff.

☎ Your Area Agency on Aging. All AAAs around the country arrange for caregiver groups. To find the number of the agency serving your community, call the free Eldercare Locator referral service (800-677-1116) or check the white pages under Community Service Numbers.

☎ Contact the National Self-Help Clearinghouse (25 West 43rd Street, Room 620, New York, New York 10036; 212-354-8525). It will give you the number of your regional clearinghouse, which maintains directories of all area support groups.

If you're like my aunt Kitty and live in an area without much in the way of support, the group may have to take a less structured form. Although Mobile's population approaches 200,000, she could not find an Alzheimer's-related group during the entire time that she cared for my uncle Billy. But once news of her husband's condition circulated around town, other women going through the same thing began coming up to her or calling to recount their experiences. "I hear Billy's not doing well," someone at church would say. "You know, Alicia's husband had Alzheimer's . . ."

She made a few phone calls, and, in all, about ten people had stories to share. Without ever attending a support

TABLE A
National Support Groups

Organization	Runs Support Groups	For Referrals Only
For Patients with a Specific Condition and Their Caregivers		
AIDS/HIV		
Catholic Charities USA	✔	
☎ 703-549-1390		
Alzheimer's Disease		
Alzheimer's Disease and Related Disorders Association	✔	
☎ 800-272-3900/312-335-8700		
Amyotrophic Lateral Sclerosis		
The Amyotrophic Lateral Sclerosis Association	✔	
☎ 800-782-4747/818-340-7500		
Les Turner Amyotrophic Lateral Sclerosis Foundation		✔
☎ 847-679-3311		
Cancer		
American Brain Tumor Association	P	
☎ 800-886-2282/847-827-9910		
American Cancer Society	✔	
☎ 800-227-2345/404-320-3333		
American Lung Association	✔	
☎ 800-586-4872/212-315-8700		
The Brain Tumor Society		✔
☎ 800-770-8287/617-783-9712		
Leukemia Society of America	✔	
☎ 800-955-4572/212-573-8484		
National Brain Tumor Foundation	✔	
☎ 800-934-2873/415-284-0208		
National Cancer Institute's Cancer Information Service		✔
☎ 800-422-6237		
Cardiovascular Disease		
American Heart Association	✔	
☎ 800-242-8721/214-373-6300		
Cerebrovascular Stroke		
National Stroke Association	✔	
☎ 800-787-6537/303-649-9299		
Stroke Connection of the American Heart Association	✔	
☎ 800-553-6321/214-706-1777		
Chronic Obstructive Pulmonary Disease		
American Lung Association	✔	
☎ 800-586-4872/212-315-8700		
Diabetes		
American Diabetes Association	✔	
☎ 800-342-2383		
Head Injury		
Brain Injury Association	✔	
☎ 800-444-6443/202-296-6443		

Organization	Runs Support Groups	For Referrals Only
For Patients with a Specific Condition and Their Caregivers		
Kidney Disease		
American Association of Kidney Patients ☎ 800-749-2257	✔	
American Kidney Fund ☎ 800-638-8299/301-881-3052		✔
The National Kidney Foundation ☎ 800-622-9010/212-889-2210	✔	
Liver Disease		
American Liver Foundation ☎ 800-223-0179/201-256-2550	✔	
Parkinson's Disease		
The American Parkinson's Disease Association ☎ 800-223-2732/718-981-8001	✔	
National Parkinson Foundation ☎ 800-327-4545/305-547-6666		✔
Parkinson's Disease Foundation ☎ 800-457-6676/212-923-4700	✔	
United Parkinson Foundation ☎ 312-733-1893		✔
Rare Disorders		
National Organization for Rare Disorders ☎ 800-999-6673/203-746-6518	P	
Incontinence		
The Simon Foundation for Continence ☎ 800-237-4666/847-864-3913	✔	
Ostomy		
American Cancer Society ☎ 800-227-2345/404-320-3333	✔	
United Ostomy Association ☎ 800-826-0826/714-660-8624	✔	
Transplant Recipients		
Transplant Recipients International Organization ☎ 800-874-6386/202-293-0980	✔	
For All Patients and Caregivers		
Make Today Count ☎ 417-885-2000	✔	
For All Caregivers		
Children of Aging Parents ☎ 800-227-7294/215-945-6900		✔
National Family Caregivers Association ☎ 301-942-6430		✔
Well Spouse Foundation ☎ 800-838-0879	✔ P	

(P = Pen Pal or Phone Pal Program)

group meeting per se, Kitty discovered that she wasn't the only woman trapped at home with a husband who couldn't feed or dress himself. She also learned that people with Alzheimer's don't improve and what she could anticipate as Billy's condition deteriorated. Now my aunt is the one doling out advice to folks in the situation she was once in.

Information and insight from other caregivers and patients are going to be hugely helpful throughout a loved one's illness, so get into the habit of networking. Ask your patient's doctor for the names of people with the disease who might be willing to talk to you. In the waiting room at the hospital or the doctor's office, don't shy away from striking up conversations with patients and family members. Smile and ask, "What are you doing here?"

A Patient Advocate's Job Description

The term *advocate* sounds more daunting than it really is. Simply, an advocate is the person who looks out for the patient's best interests and sees to it that his needs are met. In a sentence, that's your new job description. The requirements? Proficiency in problem solving, negotiation, diplomacy, and, inevitably, hell raising.

There are countless ways to advocate, including scheduling medical appointments and outpatient procedures and arranging for transportation; accompanying patients to doctors' consultations, taking notes, asking questions, and, afterward, reviewing with them what was discussed; enlisting family and friends or hiring professional nursing care to look after an ill person at home.

Perhaps most important of all is learning what constitutes quality care so that whenever standards fall short— and they will—we know to intervene promptly. I'm talking of taking action to improve not only a loved one's comfort or quality of life but, conceivably, their prospects for survival, as illustrated by the following scenario.

A woman lies in the intensive care unit recovering from open heart surgery and a subsequent bout of pneumonia. Bed-bound patients are magnets for pressure ulcers, better known as bedsores. Even with attentive nursing care, their skin can break down shockingly quickly and turn into a gaping, festering wound that in some cases burrows clear down to the bone. Besides numbing the area, bedsores serve as gateways for germs.

If she's lucky, at least one of her visitors will know to check for evidence of red, cracked, or decomposing skin on her tailbone, hipbone, heels, shoulder blades, elbows—any bony part of the body that presses against the mattress —and to alert the nurse who can then cover the ulcer with an antibacterial cream and dressing, and strategically place pillows around the patient for better cushioning. Granted, this isn't as dramatically heroic as performing mouth-to-mouth resuscitation, but it's a potential lifesaving intervention nonetheless, for in the woman's weakened condition, any infection might well prove fatal.

Having said all that, a caveat: We've written *The Complete Bedside Companion* on the assumption that you or someone you know is in the position of overseeing a loved one's care, perhaps because the person is too incapacitated by illness or side effects of treatment to advocate effectively for himself. But you also see highly capable people, their minds not dulled by illness, who gratefully relinquish decision-making to others. Case in point: my father. Though well educated, he preferred for me and my brother David to orchestrate every aspect of his care. Why? Underlying fear and denial, partly. But then, throughout his life, Dad had always relied implicitly on our mother or Lynn or Mary whenever he injured himself on the job or got sick. His behavior was totally in character.

One of the first lessons you learn as a caregiver is that people usually respond to a life-threatening illness pretty much the same way that they handle other crises. The take-charge types would perform their own surgery if they could, while the passive types will compliantly shake their heads anytime the doctor asks, "Do you have any questions?" The passive aggressives? They'll avoid asking questions, then later grumble that no one ever explains anything to them.

Whatever their nature, people must be encouraged to make as many decisions as they can about their care and quality of life. This is essential because the heartlessness with which a life-threatening illness strips away one's sense of control can wound as gravely as any physical manifestation. Nola Miller, an everyday angel who nursed her husband through eight years of terminal chronic obstructive pulmonary disease, notes, "You have to respect that person the entire time, no matter how drugged or dependent he may become."

In his twenty years as director of the critical care unit at Fairfax Hospital in Falls Church, Virginia, Dr. Thomas G. Rainey has observed the reverse situation, where caregivers get caught up in their advocate role to the point that their positive intentions produce the opposite effect: "They turn into the extreme extension of the busybody who takes over someone else's affairs inappropriately. Ultimately, it's the patient's life. And that person is responsible for his own decision-making up until the point he hands over the responsibility to someone else."

One of the cardinal rules of caregiving is never to infantilize sick people, something we as a society are guilty of in general but particularly when it comes to the elderly and to women. Examples of such behavior include:

- answering questions addressed to the patient;
- phrasing questions that discourage honest replies, such as "You don't want anything else to eat, do you?";
- withholding information the person "can't handle";
- interfering in the person's other personal and professional relationships;
- advising the sick person how she "should" feel about a given situation.

When someone is dependent on you, it's easy to overstep your bounds at times. But try to catch yourself. In practical terms this means that instead of always getting your patient what she needs, *empower* her to get it herself. For instance, if she's up to it, rather than call the Social Security office yourself to uncover the whereabouts of a missing check, hand her the phone number. In this context, then, perhaps you can share with the patient what you are reading here to help her advocate for herself and make informed decisions.

With some folks, however, like my father and Mary, it's best to spoon-feed medically related information. Dad couldn't tell you his oncologist's name; he referred to him only as "that young cancer doctor." In fact, he never did get the hang of the word *lymphoma;* he'd pronounce it "lympha—lympha*noma.*" It was as if he believed that by speaking the cancer's name he might endow it with greater power over his life than it already had.

PART ONE

Caring for the Sick

–1–

The Hospital
and the Medical Team
Who's Who and What's What

Even at seventy-one years of age, Robert Angelo McFarlane was a strapping, vigorous man. Although a retired contractor, my father continued to help renovate antebellum homes in and around Mobile. At six feet two and a bearlike 220 pounds, he still had the build of someone who'd grown up working on the family farm in rural Dawes, Alabama, and later in Granddaddy Mac's lumber yard. Bob was the quintessential southern charmer: dangerously handsome, flirtatious, with a Will Rogers wit and a propensity for reeling off one fishing story after another.

During the winter of 1992–93, my father came down with what appeared to be a stubborn flu that prevented him from working, though in phone conversations he tried not to let on that anything was the matter. We gleaned some insight into Dad's health from his wife, Mary, whom he wed not long after our stepmother Lynn died in 1988, the same year Mary lost her husband, Shorty Foster.

"Oh, son," Mary would fret on the phone. "Your father's not the same. I worry so." I would try to draw information out of her, asking, "What did Dr. Phillips say about Bob's nausea and all the weight he's lost?" But my stepmother was a gentle, elderly country woman and not at all the type to press my father's longtime physician (and fishing buddy) about why the symptoms continued to linger. "I don't know. He just doesn't seem to ever have any energy."

One morning in April, Dad was too weak and winded to get out of bed. Mary called my aunt Kitty, Bob's baby sister; she in turn called an ambulance to take him to the emergency room at the Mobile Infirmary. A battery of diagnostic tests detected congestive heart failure—his heart was pumping weakly and inefficiently, causing fluid to back up into the lungs—brought on by a blockage of the coronary arteries. Bob was immediately admitted to the hospital and scheduled for quadruple coro-

41

nary artery bypass surgery, in which healthy veins from his leg were grafted to the obstructed arteries in order to reroute the flow of blood to the heart muscle. Without the operation, my father was a heart attack waiting to happen.

When It Is Most Important to Be at an Ailing Loved One's Side

Aunt Kitty immediately got on the phone to my younger brother David, who was relaxing on the beach in California after having completed his peak business season. David runs his own firm, designing seasonal showrooms and corporate displays for large companies. He works like a madman from September to mid-January, then divides the rest of the year between traveling and freelance design assignments. Since my brother was on downtime, he was able to fly to Mobile the next morning. "I got there the day before Daddy's surgery," David remembers, "and stayed for the two weeks that he was in the hospital."

Meanwhile, I set about delegating my work duties among my staff at Broadway Cares/Equity Fights AIDS, so I could spend all of May caring for my father. A smooth recovery from bypass surgery can range from a couple of weeks to several months. Between David and me, we had Dad's hospitalization and surgical recuperation covered. Even if subsequent medical problems developed, we could at least get him home and on his feet, and arrange for his future care before I left town. It also gave us a chance—as a family—to tend to the bills, the bank, the house, and the lawyer, something we would later come to appreciate. For Bob, Mary, and Kitty, our timing was perfect. It was also the best use of the limited time Dave and I had. We both kept our trips short, because the two of us quietly suspected

that Dad might be needing us more in the months ahead.

Admittedly, my brother and I enjoyed an extraordinary degree of flexibility personally and professionally. What if your life more resembles that of my other brothers? Bobby, the eldest, lived eight hours away in Shreveport, Louisiana, with his wife, Karen, and their children, Aaron and Lorna. He visited Dad in the hospital but wasn't in a position to take extended time off from work right then. John, the youngest, came right away as well. But he was on active duty in the Army, and he and his wife also have a young son and a daughter.

Upon learning that someone you love is gravely ill, your first impulse is to drop everything and rush to his side. If you live a distance away and have to ration your trips, dashing there at the onset may not be the wisest investment of time unless the person is not expected to survive the immediate storm. With medicine ever more able to pull patients through critical episodes, what begins as an acute crisis frequently stretches out over weeks, months, or longer. Even terminal patients may experience intervals of reasonably good health, during which they require perhaps a single care partner or remain self-sufficient—for the time being.

Generally, the sick person most needs family and friends around during times of transition: when the doctor delivers the diagnosis; during major hospitalizations; at the start of intensive outpatient treatment (kidney dialysis, cancer chemotherapy, radiation therapy) expected to produce unwanted or debilitating side effects; upon being discharged from the hospital in a condition that will require her to rely on assistance with the activities of daily living; upon entering a nursing home; when death appears imminent.

And if circumstances don't permit us to be away from home for every one of these critical junctures, then we prioritize. Yes, it would be wonderful to hold our loved one's hand as the doctor is outlining the diagnosis and prognosis, but I can provide comfort and emotional support over the phone if need be. I can call the primary physician for a long-distance briefing on the sick person's condition, and I can begin alerting family and close friends and neighbors. When pondering the best time to visit, ask yourself, *When can I be most useful?*

Although this is never an easy call, several other factors may influence the answer:

Is there somebody nearby who can be counted on to participate actively in the person's care? If so, then perhaps you assume a *secondary* caregiver's role. Mary, Aunt Kitty, and Dad's next-door neighbor Darlene Twilley were able to take on the logistics of his day-to-day care as long as he was not incapacitated completely. Whenever they sent out an SOS, David and I would fly in. Obviously, for those of us forced to coordinate care from many miles away, it is critical to plan visits as strategically as possible. To help do that, we need to know:

What is the approximate timetable of treatment and recovery? Or, if the odds of survival appear remote, at what point is our loved one likely to become totally dependent? We can't stress enough the importance of learning about the person's illness to gain a fundamental understanding of how the disease characteristically plays itself out and to recognize the landmarks. The other thing to do is develop an open enough relationship with the health care team that you can pump them continually for straightforward information. Personally establishing an ongoing dialogue enables you to assess better what will be required and when. In my experience, nurses and physician's assistants—and especially critical-care staff and hospice workers—tend to be more direct than physicians, more inclined to confide: "If it were my mother, I'd want to be here *now*." But

you'll get that kind of candor only if you've conscientiously built a rapport.

How much time can you take off? And how much advance notice are you expected to give?

The Family and Medical Leave Act

In 1993, Congress enacted the *Family and Medical Leave Act*, which entitles employees to a total of twelve weeks of unpaid leave per year for one or more of the following reasons: to care for an ailing parent, spouse, or child; the birth of a child or placement of a child for

---

You Are Eligible for FMLA Benefits if You

1. work for a public agency or a private business that employs fifty or more workers for twenty weeks per calendar year;

2. have worked there at least one year;

3. have worked a minimum of 1,250 hours over the previous year; *and*

4. work at a location where at least fifty workers are employed by the employer within seventy-five miles.

☎ The booklet "Compliance Guide to the Family and Medical Leave Act" spells out the law's regulations. For a free copy or for answers to questions regarding eligibility, call your local Department of Labor, Employment Standards Administration, Wage Hour Division. Its number appears under "U.S. Offices" in the Government Listings section of the telephone book's white pages. Or call the Department of Labor's public affairs office in Washington at 202-219-8743.

adoption or foster care; a serious health condition that renders the employee unable to work.

It's one of the few pieces of government legislation that genuinely promotes compassion, caring, and self-sacrifice. But realistically the FMLA is going to benefit comparatively few readers. To begin with, only about 5 percent of all U.S. businesses fall under its jurisdiction. What's more, a loophole of sorts permits employers to dismiss so-called key employees (translation: high-salaried) if they can show that reinstating the person following a leave would damage the company financially. More to the point, how many people can afford to forfeit a paycheck for weeks or months on end?

Given the current climate of anxiety over corporate downsizing and tough economic times, it's not surprising that few workers actually take advantage of the law. One year before the federal Family and Medical Leave Act was passed, the state of California instituted a similar mandate. According to a 1994 study, two-thirds of the covered employers reported that less than 1 percent of their employees had taken a leave due to a family medical emergency. Despite the fact that the state measure specifically ensures job security, as does the FMLA, nearly one in ten of the employers surveyed said they could not guarantee leave-takers that their original positions would be waiting for them when they returned.

Set the Stage at Work

Whether the law pertains to your place of employment or not, it's naive to presume that you can abruptly take a prolonged leave of absence. Inevitably, some work will wind up neglected, opportunities will be lost, and business relations strained. The savvy approach is to always have comp time in the bank and a few vacation days set aside for emergencies. More important, have lots of good karma on account with your colleagues.

Your sister calls to say that Dad's inoperable lung cancer has spread to the bones? You would then

- inform your boss and coworkers right away that you anticipate having to take time off at some point in the coming weeks;
- get a jump on projects, putting in nights and weekends if necessary, but do your best to pace yourself;
- make sure everyone understands the extent of your accessibility by phone, fax, and/or E-mail during your absence;
- prearrange for colleagues to take on some of your workload, with the understanding that you'll do the same for them one day.

At Broadway Cares, no one thought twice about covering for me because during the previous year or so, virtually every one of the seventeen people in our office had taken personal leave for weeks at a time for similar crises. Out of sheer necessity, compassion, and mutual respect, picking up the slack for one another became an unofficial company policy. Long before I became a boss, I always took extra shifts or worked weekends for coworkers anytime they asked. That way, when I needed time off, I could call in my chits.

Mapping out a game plan around a life-threatening illness is like trying to construct a tower of toothpicks while white-water rafting: You can expect it to collapse suddenly and often. Our goal is to line up support in advance as best we can. What if the person declines precipitously? We need a backup plan to cover that possibility as well. This is as true for the caregiver who lives a block away as it is for someone who resides on the opposite coast. If a phone call came in the middle of the night saying "We need you here right away," who would look after the kids or feed the cat? Once you can get a grasp on the patient's condition and what the upcoming days and weeks may hold, contact those folks you can depend on.

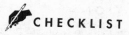

CHECKLIST

**Business to Take Care of *Before*
You May Have to Leave Town
on Short Notice**

❑ Count up your frequent-flyer miles and call a travel agent to get an idea of flight availability and prices over the coming weeks so you can avoid expensive surprises and unnecessary delays.

❑ Have some cash on hand. If you're called away suddenly, it might be a week before you get to a bank.

❑ Get the laundry done, pick up the dry cleaning, stock the pantry, and organize next month's bills.

❑ Leave an extra set of keys with your best friend or good neighbor.

❑ Arrange for someone to pick up the mail.

❑ Set up an automatic payroll deposit at the bank.

❑ Renew your driver's license and pay any traffic tickets. What if you have to rent a car?

❑ Tell your physician what's going on and request prescriptions for yourself for a mild tranquilizer and a sleeping aid—whether you fill them or not—just in case.

At Work

❑ Tell everyone how to reach you quickly and reliably if you're called away.

❑ Brief at least two colleagues on the status of your projects. Show them where everything is and mark everything on your desk clearly, including a list of key documents on your computer.

❑ Brief clients or important customers. Tell them what's up and whom to contact while you're gone.

Preparing for a Loved One's Hospital Stay

While the ultimate outcome of a serious illness may be unpredictable at first, the opening scene frequently takes place in the hospital, whether for an operation, nonsurgical treatment, or diagnostic testing. For patients and visitors alike, the hospital is analogous to a foreign country: full of unfamiliar sights and customs, and a language you may not always understand. Having some idea of what to expect can help ease the anxiety for everyone involved.

Arranging Blood Donations

Preoperative Autologous Blood Donation

My father underwent an emergency bypass graft, so there wasn't sufficient time for him to have one or two pints (*units*) of his own blood stored as a precaution should he require a transfusion during the operation. A coronary artery bypass is one of several surgical procedures for which the National Heart, Lung and Blood Institute recommends that patients provide blood beforehand if their medical condition and time allow. Dad's fragile health would have additionally excluded him from making an *autologous* donation.

Rest assured that the nation's blood supply is extremely safe. Each unit of donated (*allogeneic*) blood is routinely screened for several infectious diseases, including hepatitis B, hepatitis C, and the human immunodeficiency virus (HIV), the precursor to AIDS. There is, however, a window of several weeks or longer between the moment of infection and the point where testing is able to pick up the presence of these viruses, and so it is possible for contaminated

---

INSIDE INFORMATION

More and more hospitals routinely offer preadmission tours to acquaint patients with the facility. If time permits and you think your loved one might benefit from a short visit, call the patient relations department or the department of social work to see if this can be arranged, perhaps on the same day as any preadmission tests the doctor may have ordered.

---

blood to slip by undetected during this incubation period.

We stress that for a seriously ill patient who needs blood and cannot donate his own, the benefits of transfusion overwhelmingly outweigh the negligible danger of contracting a new blood-borne disease. According to a report published in the *New England Journal of Medicine* in 1996, the odds of incurring HIV from a screened unit of transfused blood range is one per million. The figures pertaining to hepatitis C and B are only slightly less comforting: ten per million and sixteen per million, respectively.

Bear in mind that many surgeries carry a low risk of significant blood loss—hysterectomy, mastectomy, and transurethral resection of the prostate are just three examples—and therefore do not warrant preoperative autologous donations. Whether or not your loved one should consider stockpiling blood is a matter to take up with the surgeon. If it is deemed appropriate, expect to be

referred to the hospital blood bank. The donation of blood *(phlebotomy)* can be performed there or at a community blood center such as the Red Cross.

The time factor is bound to rule out a number of patients. Ideally, autologous donations should begin four to six weeks before surgery. However far in advance the process starts, the last unit should be drawn no later than seventy-two hours prior to surgery.

✳ *Ask the doctor about possibly prescribing an oral iron supplement for your loved one during this time.*

New techniques enable the surgical team to salvage blood lost during and immediately after surgery and then re-infuse it into the patient. Although the recovered amount may be equivalent to only one or two units, this is often enough to make donor blood unnecessary.

Directed Blood Donation

Major blood loss during surgery is just one emergency that may call for a transfusion of whole blood or, more commonly, any number of its components, such as red cells, platelets, and the clear liquid portion of the blood, *plasma.* When autologous donation is out of the question, you might want to consider what's called *directed* donation whereby anyone with a matching blood type can designate his blood for a specific patient. Ask your loved one how he feels about this. Some patients find it comforting to know their donor's identity, though studies show no advantage in terms of safety.

Selected Surgeries That May Call for Autologous Blood Donation

- Coronary artery bypass graft
- Major vascular operations
- Primary hip replacement and hip replacement revisions
- Total knee replacement
- Major spine operations with instrumentation
- Selected neurological procedures
- Liver resections
- Prostate removal

TABLE 1
Prevalence and Compatibility of Blood Types

Blood Type	Prevalence (Percent)	Can Receive
O+	38	O+, O−
O−	7	O−
A+	34	A+, A−, O+, O−
A−	6	A−, O−
B+	9	B+, B−, O+, O−
B−	2	B−, O−
AB+	3	All types, + and −
AB−	1	AB−, O−, A−, B−

The hospital blood bank can help make the necessary arrangements for directed donations. Meanwhile, think of the most compulsively organized, detail-oriented person you know and assign her the task of calling prospective volunteers. Obviously, the first question to ask is their blood type—O, A, B, or AB—and whether they are Rh-positive or Rh-negative. This second classification denotes the presence or absence of a particular substance in the blood. More than eight in ten people are Rh-positive. Those with AB-positive blood are known as "universal recipients," able to receive any type and factor of blood. O-negative men and women are "universal donors"; their blood is compatible with all four types, positive or negative.

Blood Platelet Donation

Red cells (*erythrocytes*), which deliver oxygen to all tissues, have a shelf life of five to six weeks, whereas white cells (*leukocytes*), the body's primary defenders against infection, "expire" after only six hours. When someone's white count is precariously low, the physician's initial strategy may be to administer what are called *colony-stimulating factors*—biologic agents that accelerate white cell production. Leukocytes

are transfused only when all other avenues of elevating the white count have been exhausted and the person's life is in jeopardy.

Platelets (*thrombocytes*), manufactured in the red marrow of the flat bones, plug up broken blood vessels. Each cubic milliliter of blood contains about 250,000 to 500,000 of these tiny platelike particles. People with abnormally low levels of platelets are dangerously prone to excessive bleeding and could conceivably hemorrhage to death from even a minor injury or internal rupture. The general rule of thumb among physicians is to order a platelet transfusion when a person's count drops to approximately 10,000 per cubic milliliter; 100,000 if he is scheduled for a surgical procedure.

People whose bone marrow is badly damaged—from leukemia or from aggressive cancer chemotherapy or radiation therapy—may require frequent transfusion support over a period of weeks until their marrow recovers and steps up platelet production. The same is true of bone-marrow-transplant recipients. Typically, it takes weeks before their new marrow begins manufacturing enough thrombocytes that the blood clots normally again. Because donor platelets keep for just five days, hospitals may be harder pressed to maintain a constant supply. This is a time to recruit as many donors as possible. Three donations a day would be ideal to keep a steady stream of deposits flowing into our loved one's "account." Anyone can give platelets, incidentally, regardless of blood type, and you can repeat this good deed twice a week up to twenty-four times per year.

Sometimes when patients receive multiple platelet transfusions, the incremental rise in their platelet count starts to level off. In such cases, family members tend to make better donors, immunologically speaking, because their platelets are more likely to match the recipient's. Think of it as the difference between regular gasoline and high octane.

The process for harvesting platelets is somewhat more involved than a conventional phlebotomy. A nurse inserts a sizable needle in a vein in each arm. While the donor relaxes, plastic tubing routes his blood to a machine called a *continuous blood-cell processor*, then returns it to his bloodstream. Aside from the needle sticks, which hurt momentarily, the ninety-minute procedure is painless.

What to Bring to the Hospital (and What to Leave at Home)

Certainly all parallels between a hospitalization and a vacation end here, but when packing for either one, it's best to travel light. Hospitals do not assume responsibility or liability for lost, stolen, or damaged personal property, so all valuables should be left at home. That includes cash exceeding $20 or so, credit cards, checkbooks, and jewelry, even wedding rings and watches. If your loved one insists on taking items of monetary or sentimental value, have the hospital security office store them for safekeeping.

The ensuing weeks or months may bring additional trips to the hospital, possibly on a moment's notice. Post on the refrigerator a checklist of essentials for your loved one to grab in the event of an emergency. Better still, see to it that she keeps a bag packed and ready to go at all times. The bag should accompany the patient to all medical appointments in the event the doctor decides to send her directly to the hospital. Include the following:

- Water or juice, in cans or plastic bottles—never glass containers
- Nonperishable snacks
- A change of clothing and underwear
- Toothbrush and toothpaste
- Magazines, books, or other reading material
- Important phone numbers, lists outlining the person's health history, medications, and so on

Next, pack a bag for yourself. Being stranded for hours in the ER waiting room is far more bearable when you have something to eat and drink at hand and can freshen up. Add to the above list towelettes, hand towel, sweater, sneakers, chewing gum, and aspirin.

✽ *If you drive, stash the bag permanently in the trunk of your car.*

First Stop: The Admitting Office

Registering at the hospital can be nerve-racking enough for patients without their getting marooned in the admitting office because of missing or incomplete paperwork. Two phone calls, made as far in advance as possible, should enable you to sail right through.

The first call should be to the admitting office. Ask what documentation you should bring with you. Typically, they'll want to see the patient's Social Security card, health insurance card, and copies of any legal documents stating his wishes concerning medical deci-

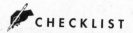 **CHECKLIST**

Packing for a Hospital Stay

Clothing

- ❑ Two pairs of pajamas, nightgowns, or loungewear
- ❑ Fresh underwear
- ❑ A long bathrobe
- ❑ Tennis sneakers or sturdy slippers with nonskid soles
- ❑ A clean set of comfortable clothes to wear home
- ❑ Socks
- ❑ Sweatpants, sweatshirt

Toiletries and Cosmetics

- ❑ Toothbrush and toothpaste, dental floss, mouthwash
- ❑ Deodorant
- ❑ Shampoo and conditioner
- ❑ Brush and comb
- ❑ Shaving kit
- ❑ Any other toiletries that the patient uses daily or would be uncomfortable without: moisturizer, powder, makeup, contact lens supplies, women's sanitary supplies, hand mirror, nail scissors, emery board
- ❑ Eye mask

* Use an indelible laundry marker to write your loved one's name on all clothing and personal items.

Documentation and Other Important Papers

- ❑ The patient's health insurance card
- ❑ A list detailing the dates of past illnesses and surgeries, and any allergies or other health conditions
- ❑ A list containing names and telephone numbers (home and business) of family members to contact in the event of an emergency

- ❑ The doctor's name and telephone number
- ❑ A list of all prescription and nonprescription medications that the patient takes, and the dosages. If he is unconscious or isn't able to remember, bring all the vials from the medicine cabinet with you.

* Record the above information on a note card and place it in the patient's wallet or purse.

Incidentals

- ❑ Containers for eyeglasses, contact lenses, dentures, hearing aids
- ❑ Thermos
- ❑ A small table clock or, better still, a cheap plastic waterproof digital wristwatch with numbers large enough to see without eyeglasses
- ❑ Magazines, books, playing cards, a battery-operated tape recorder or radio with earphones or headphones, and other items for passing the time

* Some medical centers prohibit patients from bringing in anything that runs on electricity; others require the admitting doctor's consent. Even then, all equipment must first be certified by a hospital engineer because shavers, hair dryers, VCRs, and other electrical items may not be properly grounded and could be hazardous. Feel free, though, to pack whatever battery-operated products you wish. Many hospitals provide safety-approved hair dryers, TV, and other appliances. Ask the nurse if any are available.

INSIDE INFORMATION

A typical caregiver makes more phone calls than a campaign worker on election eve, usually from the waiting room or cafeteria. Pack your address book, a telephone calling card, *and several rolls of quarters.* Believe me, at the hospital you'll use them up in no time. As for cellular phones, hospitals usually forbid their use beyond the lobby because they can interfere with medical equipment.

sion-making and treatment. These advance directives include a *health care proxy*, also known as a *durable power of attorney for health care*, and a *living will.* ► See *"Advance Medical Directives,"* page 298.

The next call should be to the patient's employer or health insurer. Increasingly, insurance policies require holders to receive *preadmission certification*—a written statement from the insurer agreeing to cover hospitalization and treatment—and/or a second opinion from another physician prior to admission. Some carriers impose financial penalties on patients who enter the hospital without first obtaining formal approval. Find out beforehand if any such restrictions apply to your loved one.

For a prescheduled admission, call the admitting department early that morning to confirm that a bed is available. True, your loved one has a reservation, but what if the ER had been besieged with emergency cases overnight or someone due to be discharged took a turn for the worse? The last thing you want is an ailing person having to encamp in a crowded waiting room for hours, waiting for a bed to open up.

Ask admitting when they'll have a clearer picture as to when a bed will become free and if you can call then. Jot down the name of the person you speak with (one of the cardinal rules of being an effective advocate for your patient: *always* ask for names), be sure to thank her, and phone back as promised. When she can tell you with reasonable certainty that a bed should be ready in an hour or so, only then do you head to the hospital.

✱ *If a patient entered the hospital via the emergency room, admitting is also the department to call to find out where he has been moved within the facility. Patient information? The main switchboard? They're usually* the last *to know.*

What happens during registration:

An admitting representative interviews the patient or a family member about his insurance coverage.

The patient signs consent forms permitting the hospital to provide treatment and also to release medical information to his health insurer.

The patient can order in-room telephone service. Never leave someone who is conscious without a phone. The department in charge of switching it on is usually open only during the day, so either place the order early in the morning at the admitting office or dial the extension for television and telephone rental before 3:00 in the afternoon and put in the request yourself.

In what is largely a pro forma gesture, your loved one will be handed a copy of the American Hospital Association's "A Patient's Bill of Rights." The one-page sheet outlines his legal rights with regard to consenting to or refusing a particular form of treatment or plan of care, as well as more general concerns such as the right to expect considerate care from the staff.

If the patient hasn't already undergone routine preadmission medical tests, they take place at this time.

EMERGENCY ROOM VISITS

Insurance policies generally give members 48 hours in which to report a visit to a hospital ER. Be sure to call the telephone number on the back of the insurance ID card within that period or else the patient risks having to pay out of pocket.

---

* *Patients must undress from the waist up and don a gown for these procedures; therefore, women may find it convenient to wear a two-piece outfit to the hospital.*

Next Stop: The Floor

Once your loved one is settled in her room, the parade of health care personnel begins. The first person you will probably meet is a unit nurse who will take the handful of paperwork the admitting rep gave the patient and proceed to start a chart, asking about symptoms, current medications, allergies, and so on. But a sick person might not recall the name and dosage of every pill he's taking. Or your elderly aunt may be so embarrassed by talk about bodily functions that she fails to inform the nurse about the abnormal vaginal discharge she's been having. It's up to us, then, to remember for them or to prod them: "Grandma, didn't you say you were short of breath yesterday?"

Whatever we're able to add to someone's health history is bound to prove pertinent in some way: Your father might have forgotten to mention he frequently has bloody bowel movements due to hemorrhoids. This is a significant detail, since blood in the stool is also a warning sign of colorectal cancer. The next thing you know, Dad's undergoing a colonoscopy, unnecessarily. Or it may be that your mom had an angiogram taken and was one of the rare patients who suffers a severe reaction to the contrast medium injected into a vein.

If you can't be at the hospital the day of admission, call the unit nursing desk and give them the necessary information over the phone. While you're at it, is there anything else the person's doctors should be aware of, such as dependency on alcohol or drugs (both legal and illicit)? Where any form of such abuse is concerned, families must dispense with lies or denial and make the medical team aware of the problem up-front. In the midst of a life-threatening illness, the physical complications from abruptly ceasing an addictive substance could compromise treatment dangerously.

* *Ask the nurse to write* on the front of the chart or its inside cover *the following or any other special needs your loved one may have:* "Patient is deaf." "Patient is blind." "Patient is partially paralyzed on the right side." "Patient is allergic to penicillin." *While this information appears on the patient information form tucked inside the chart, not every member of the staff marching into the room for the first time will have had time to carefully read all the papers.*

By the same token, if you intend to be in touch regularly with the staff, request that the nurse write *your* name and number on the front of the chart or tape your business card to it. "Hi, I'm Rodger, Bob McFarlane's son. Please call me night or day if you ever need me to bring something or if Dad needs something or if the doctor's looking for me. Any reason." As soon as the staff comes to recognize you, believe me, they'll call. "Your brother had severe diarrhea last night. Could you drop off some clean underwear in the morning?" The anonymous "emergency contact" listed on the patient information sheet generally gets called only when the sick person has declined sharply, is transferred to intensive care, or dies.

The Hospital:
Land of 1,000 Initials

ER: *Emergency Room*—where trained staff offer immediate care to those with life-threatening illnesses and injuries.

CCU: *Coronary Care Unit*—an intensive care unit for patients with life-threatening heart disease. Both the CCU and the ICU usually maintain stricter visiting hours than the hospital at large and permit visits from family members only.

ICU: *Intensive Care Unit*—a specially staffed floor or section that houses critically ill patients requiring continuous attention. The unit is divided into *SICU* (surgical ICU, for people awaiting or recuperating from an operation or who are seriously injured) and *MICU* (medical ICU, for patients being treated nonsurgically).

OR: *Operating Room*—where the surgery takes place. Afterward, patients spend time in the *recovery room* before being returned to their room.

On your way home that first day, stop at the nurse's desk and ask to speak to the unit clerk, who is in charge of filing and updating all patient records. "Hi, I'm Rodger McFarlane. Do you have my father's chart handy? I just want to make sure my name's on there." Know for certain this has been done. Then hand the clerk a card as well.

Introduce yourself to the charge nurse, the intern, and the medication nurse—anyone who comes in the room. Point out your name on the chart and encourage them to call you with any questions that might arise. (Left unspoken: more likely you'll be calling them.) Establishing a rapport while we have the opportunity to be *a face* will serve us well on those days when we can't be at our loved one's side and must solve

problems or procure information over the phone—which is most of the time.

Our initial contact with the health care team sets the tone for the relationship and greatly shapes their perceptions of just how actively we will participate in the patient's care. Don't underestimate the lasting impact of first impressions, especially poor first impressions. We want to earn people's cooperation and trust from the get-go and not have to strive to win them over. Having once been a member of the team myself, I can tell you that the folks entrusted with your loved one's health will be silently assessing the kinds of questions you ask and your helpfulness, your intelligence, your attentiveness, your composure under stress—in short, whether you are going to be an ally or a pain in the neck.

The Health Care Team: Who They Are and What They Do

Throughout the day, other medical and hospital personnel stop by the patient's room: this one to take temperature, pulse, and blood pressure; that one to start intravenous fluids. Who are these strangers? Not all will introduce themselves or explain the purpose of their visit. They should. "A Patient's Bill of Rights" states: "Patients have the right to know the identity of physicians, nurses, and others involved in their care, as well as when those involved are students, residents, or other trainees."

✱ *If any health care provider fails to identify himself, patients and caregivers should not hesitate to ask (preferably with a smile), "Now, which one are you?"*

Doctors of Medicine (M.D.s)

Attending Physicians. Although patients are usually seen by many doctors

EMERGENCY ROOM VISITS

Paramedics, the personnel who staff ambulances and work alongside physicians and nurses in the ER, are trained to manage the sick or injured during transport to the hospital. Under a doctor's orders they can administer injections and IV fluids, read electrocardiograms, and perform heart defibrillation and other life-support measures. They are also called *emergency medical technicians,* or *EMTs.*

while in the hospital, the attending physician is responsible for supervising that person's care. He could be the patient's longtime internist or family practitioner if he has *privileges* (permission to practice) at the hospital. Or he could be someone you've never met—a staff member at the hospital to which the patient was referred.

Generally, patients can expect their "attending" to check in on them once a day. (They can also anticipate being charged for the visit even if it consists of nothing more than a "How are we feeling today?" and a signature on the chart.) In a group practice, two or more attendings typically "cover" for each other: One sees the patient today, the other sees the patient tomorrow. But ultimately one member is in charge of overseeing that person's progress.

In a teaching hospital, the attending physician and the senior house physicians supervise a staff of certified M.D.s at various levels of additional training —*fellows, residents,* and *interns*—who join him on his daily rounds. On a day-to-day basis your loved one will undoubtedly see these physicians more than she does her attending.

Interns. At the bottom of the pecking order are medical school graduates serving a one-year hospital apprenticeship. They can do everything a veteran doctor is allowed to do but must have any order they write reviewed and co-signed within twenty-four hours by the attending or *chief resident.*

Residents. These doctors have completed their internship and are training in a specialized area of medicine for anywhere from three to five years. While the attending physician heads the team hierarchy, the residents actually order many, if not most, tests and medications. They are accountable to a chief resident or the *chief of service.*

Fellows. To attain this title resident doctors go on to study a subspecialty. For example, to become a vascular surgeon requires a five-year residency in general surgery followed by a three-year fellowship in vascular surgery.

Medical Specialists. Did the attending physician say he was referring your uncle to a "nephrologist" or a "neurologist"? Medical specialists' designations *can* sound confusingly alike.

Medical Generalists. A *family practitioner* provides comprehensive, continuous health care for all family members, regardless of sex or age.

An *internist* diagnoses and treats diseases in adults.

A *general surgeon* is qualified to perform a number of common operations.

Physician's Assistants. Nowadays the person ordering medications or postsurgical testing may not be an M.D. at all but a senior nurse or a *P.A.* With two to four years of college and two years in a physician's assistant program, P.A.s are eminently capable of carrying out these and routine procedures that were once the exclusive domain of doctors, though a physician must review and co-sign their orders.

Medical Specialists Directory

Type of Physician	Specializes in Preventing, Diagnosing, and Treating
Cardiologist	Diseases of the heart
Dermatologist	Diseases of the skin
Endocrinologist	Diabetes and other disorders of the hormonal (endocrine) system
Gastroenterologist	Diseases of the digestive tract
Geriatrician	Disorders in older people
Gynecologist	Diseases of the female reproductive organs
Hematologist	Leukemia and other diseases of the blood and blood-forming tissues
Hepatologist	Diseases of the liver
Immunologist	Human immunodeficiency virus (HIV)/acquired immunodeficiency syndrome (AIDS), allergies, and other diseases and disorders of the immune system
Infectious Diseases Specialist	HIV/AIDS, infections of postoperative wounds, pneumonia, tuberculosis, Lyme disease, malaria, other tropical diseases, et al.
Nephrologist	Diseases of the kidneys
Neurologist	Diseases of the nervous system
Oncologist	Cancer (This category is further broken down by subspeciality: gynecologic oncologist, urologic oncologist, etc.)
Ophthalmologist	Defects, injuries, and diseases of the eyes
Orthopedist	Deformities of and injuries to the musculoskeletal system
Otolaryngologist	Diseases of the ear, nose, and throat
Proctologist	Disorders of the anus, rectum, and colon
Psychiatrist	Mental, emotional, and behavioral disorders
Pulmonologist	Disorders and diseases of the lungs and chest
Rheumatologist	Arthritis and other disorders of the joints, muscles, tendons, and ligaments
Urologist	Disorders and diseases of the male reproductive organs (penis, testicles, prostate, et al.) Diseases of the male and female urinary tracts
Vascular Surgeon	Peripheral vascular disease, phlebitis, thrombophlebitis, and other diseases of the blood vessels (though a surgeon, may also use nonsurgical techniques)

Type of Physician	Specializes in
Anesthesiologist	Administering anesthesia during surgery and using anesthetic drugs or agents to alleviate pain
Pathologist	Identifies diseases through microscopic study
Physiatrist	Physical medicine and rehabilitation
Radiologist	Performing and interpreting X rays, sonograms, CT scans, MRI scans, and other imaging studies for viewing internal organs and systems
Radiotherapist	Using X rays and other forms of radiant energy to treat cancer and other diseases

Medical Students. The galley slaves of the hospital may tag along during rounds to take medical histories, conduct physical examinations, and draw arterial blood for blood-gas analysis—always while under the watchful eye of an intern or resident.

✻ *Patients should know they have the right to request someone more experienced to perform a particular procedure.*

Nurses

Registered Nurses. Among their other duties, *R.N.*s administer medications and treatments, and teach patients (and us) how to take care of themselves once they go home. Some have acquired specialized skills. Chemotherapy nurses, for instance, are experienced in the nuances of safely administering the toxic cancer-fighting drugs, while veteran IV nurses are expert at inserting a needle into a suitable vein.

Nurse Practitioners. The *N.P.*'s education goes beyond the R.N.'s two to four years of nursing school. Within their area of specialization (critical care, gerontology, midwifery), nurse practitioners might as well have an "M.D." after their names. They are authorized to order tests and even plan treatment. The truth is that the N.P. is often as proficient, if not more so, than the attending physician, who usually sees a broad range of patients and may not have as much practical experience handling certain health problems.

Licensed Practical Nurses. In today's hospitals you'll find fewer and fewer *L.P.N.*s, nurses with twelve to eighteen months of training. While practical nurses are allowed to give routine oral or intramuscular medications, the task of starting an IV always falls to an R.N. or N.P. When a patient is critically ill, a senior nurse will usually take over administering even the most commonplace drugs, though some highly experienced L.P.N.s do work in the ICU, ER, and OR.

Depending on hospital policy, the nursing staff works eight-hour or twelve-hour shifts, with one nurse serving as your loved one's *primary nurse.* He is responsible for coordinating his patients' care around the clock and gives instructions to the nurse who comes on duty to relieve him, called the *designated primary nurse.* Hospitals try to assign patients the same core of rotating nurses throughout their stay as much as possible, for the sake of continuity.

Since these nurses see your loved one regularly, get to know them, for they are invaluable sources of information. You want to find out when your patient last received pain medication? An explanation of that test the resident has scheduled for tomorrow? The primary nurse will be able to tell you.

If she's busy, ask the *charge nurse*, also known as the *head nurse*. This person, usually a senior R.N., juggles the nurses' room assignments in the event of emergencies, keeps an eye on newer nurses, and in general keeps things running smoothly. Should the need arise, the charge nurse cares for patients, but most of the time you'll find her stationed at the nurse's desk or "floating" on the unit.

Continuing up the ladder of seniority, each unit has a *nursing director*, while a hospital *nursing supervisor* oversees the entire nursing staff during a given shift. You probably won't have much communication with either one unless you need to register a complaint, a matter we address later in this chapter.

Nurse's Assistants

Nurse's Aides. At the other end of the hierarchy are the folks who bring our loved ones their meal trays, remove bedpans, change the sheets, and tend to many of their most personal needs. I have seen family members treat aides dismissively. Don't you dare! Nurse's aides deserve your utmost respect. They're constantly observing and handling your patient—more than perhaps anyone else on the health care team—and are frequently the first to spot problems and changes in his condition. You'll come to depend on them for feedback and to relay requests to the nursing staff. The aides, along with the nurses, are also experts at knowing how to navigate the hospital bureaucracy and get what you need.

Nursing Students. In a teaching hospital, student nurses perform an array of procedures—under the guidance of a nurse instructor or a member of the hospital nursing staff—from changing dressings to inserting urinary catheters, to suctioning congested airways.

Other Hospital Staff

Unit Clerk. The clerk, usually a layperson, serves as unit secretary, pushing the paperwork, maintaining the patient charts, and requisitioning lab work, tests, and drugs. Don't overlook this prolific source of information. She'll know the whereabouts of the doctor or the medication nurse; that your sick friend won't return from X ray for three hours because radiology is backed up; and when you can realistically expect the results of that important thyroid scan.

Technicians and Technologists. These health care professionals are trained and certified in a specific area of diagnostic testing or therapy, be it nuclear medicine, respiration therapy, electroencephalography, radiation therapy, or lab work. Depending on the complexity and sophistication of the procedure, they either perform it themselves—drawing blood at the bedside, taking conventional X rays, carrying out electrocardiograms—or assist the doctors.

Social Workers. People often equate "social worker" with "counselor" or "therapist." While a hospital social worker certainly can provide short-term crisis counseling, her main responsibility is to sit down with patients and family and help make preparations for the sick person's discharge. As care partner you'll rely on her for assistance with coordinating whatever services need to be in place the day your loved one leaves the medical center. That might entail arranging for nursing care at home or a nursing home; applying for

Social Security disability insurance or other government entitlements; and routing you to community services such as meals on wheels. ▶ See "Preparing for Discharge from the Hospital," page 74.

Patient Representatives. The patient rep, also known as a patient advocate, will introduce himself the first day. Ostensibly, patient representatives attempt to resolve complaints concerning the quality of care or hospital policies and procedures. They *can* be helpful for dealing with minor problems on the order of bending visiting hours or allowing overnight vigils in the patient's room. But remember this about patient advocates: First, few medical centers have more than one or two on staff, so they're inundated with complaints. Second, they work for the hospital. ▶ See "To Whom Do You Complain?" page 69.

Registered Dietitians (R.D.s). Early on in a hospital stay, a staff dietitian will visit your loved one to discuss his nutritional needs not only for the time he is hospitalized but afterward. Like most cardiovascular patients, Dad was counseled to cut down dramatically on fat, salt, and cholesterol once he recuperated from surgery. If you're the person who'll be preparing most of the meals, the dietitian will want to go over the dietary plan with you, too. In my experience, this is usually cursory at best—perhaps a ten-minute consultation at the end of which you're handed a pamphlet.

Orderlies. These male hospital attendants tend to the personal needs of male patients: bathing, cleaning up accidents, assisting with urinary catheterization, and so on. They also do general work that demands a degree of physical strength, such as turning and lifting obese patients.

Transport Attendants. Trained in CPR, these escorts wheel patients to and from tests and other procedures. Remember that person's face. What sometimes happens is, you accompany your loved one to X ray for a heart catheterization, and while you're thumbing through a magazine out in the waiting area, she has already been taken back to her room, still under sedation—only no one thinks to tell *you* this. They don't realize you're sitting there. The nurse's desk and the reception desk may not know your "missing" loved one's whereabouts, but the attendant will.

Hospital Life: "But the Doctor Who Was Just Here Already Asked Us That!"

Sometime during the first twenty-four hours in the hospital, a staff physician comes by to examine our loved one and take a detailed history for the purpose of forming a medical profile. This usually happens after the nurse and the charge nurse have already asked several of the same questions, and the charge nurse has conducted a cursory physical exam. Why the multiple histories? And didn't the doctor who admitted the patient forward his medical records to the hospital days ago?

Yes, but the attending physician isn't here now. Suppose she makes her daily rounds at, say, 8:00 A.M., and our patient was admitted at noon: He therefore won't see the attending physician until the following morning—later still should one of her other patients have an emergency. As far as the hospital is concerned, it is responsible for the care and safety of someone it has never seen before, and so one of its doctors must evaluate the person's present condition. If a procedure requiring anesthesia is slated for the next day, he can anticipate a late-night visit from the anesthesiologist and going through the same routine yet again. Tiring and exasperating as it may seem at times, this information overlap ensures that everyone tending to the patient has a complete, accurate overview of his condition. Resist the temptation to give shorthand answers.

It's all too easy for hospitalized patients to lose track of time, and the days may blend into one another. Each unit of the hospital follows a basic daily routine: regular meal deliveries, visiting hours, doctors' rounds, and times for nurses to dispense medications and take vital signs (pulse, respiration, temperature).

✻ *Anytime you visit your loved one, jot down the next day's "calendar of events," including the date and day of the week, and tape it to the bedside table.*

Having chronological landmarks can help patients stay focused and retain a sense of control. Encourage them to ask the nurse to outline the day for them each morning. When can they expect to see the attending physician? Are any tests scheduled? What other doctors or health care professionals may visit today?

Personalizing the Hospital Room

In light of the many serious issues to contend with, decorating the hospital room may seem a minor concern. It's not, as anyone who has had to stare at an empty wall of indeterminate color will attest. Bring in blankets, throws, a favorite chair, photos.

"We've seen some very creative solutions to making the hospital room homey," says Daphne Stannard, an intensive care nurse at the University of California at San Francisco Medical Center. One family, she recalls, placed photos of the patient's beloved dog around the room; another family made a tape recording of their dog barking. "One woman brought her husband a favorite pillowcase that she'd sprayed lightly with his favorite perfume." Stan-

nard believes that comforting reminders of home, of *normalcy*, are "crucial to healing." When her own father, a botanist, was hospitalized, she and her two sisters filled his room with flowers.

✻ *If you're thinking of saying it with flowers, clear this with the nurse first. Fresh flowers, plants, and fruit carry bacteria and are generally not allowed in areas of the hospital that house patients prone to infection due to compromised immunity, such as bone marrow recipients, people with AIDS, and those receiving cancer chemotherapy. Some chemo agents also make patients hypersensitive to smell, so much so that the scent of flowers can bring on nausea. Silk flowers trap dust, so send small potted plants instead. They don't topple over when bumped, as might happen with a top-heavy floral arrangement, and they last.*

Decorating the room is also a way of personalizing an ailing loved one to the hospital staff. Don't be shocked to overhear doctors and nurses refer to the people under their care as "the patient" or according to their disease. It's not a sign of callousness, just a mechanism for coping with the emotional demands of their jobs. "I've heard nurses say, 'Take this down to the appendectomy in room 302C,' " says the Reverend Harry Cole. As a pastor, Cole has spent countless hours in hospitals visiting the sick. When his wife, Jackie, suffered a cerebral hemorrhage and lay in a coma for six weeks, Cole "made sure that wasn't going to happen. Jackie is a very beautiful woman. I wanted people to know what she looked like before the stroke. So I placed her picture on the windowsill. I would look at her lying there in the bed, then at the picture, and hope that the person in the picture would return. The staff, too, would look at the picture. And even though things seemed pretty dire, we could look at her and see that person in the picture"—not the tortured woman curled up in a fetal position, tethered to a breathing machine and fed through a stomach tube. Also, anytime the Reverend Cole spotted an instruction that referred to his wife as "patient," he instinctively crossed it out and wrote "Jacqueline."

Ways to Be Helpful When Visiting Patients in the Hospital

Numerous studies have suggested that hospitalized patients who are surrounded by visitors are more likely to show improvement than those who lie in their rooms alone and unattended. However, this correlation between frequency of callers and prospects for recovery is probably attributable more to the law of averages than to the healing power of love. The more time that family and friends spend with the sick person, the greater the chance that one of them will notice a medical warning sign early on ("Excuse me, nurse. Does she feel feverish to you?") or point out an oversight on the part of the staff ("Excuse me, but shouldn't my friend have received his antianxiety medication by now?"). *Being there* also gives us added leverage should signs of trouble arise.

Although most health care professionals would probably deny it, the patient fortunate enough to have plenty of company during a hospital stay tends to receive better care. The room is usually a little cleaner, the nurses and aides a little more attentive. It's not a matter of favoritism. For one thing, heavier traffic simply brings more calls to the nurse's desk for assistance; in the course of a typical day, that could mean several additional pairs of eyes looking in on your loved one.

Another reason? Nurses like to make a good impression. They're proud of their profession, by and large, and are keenly aware of how comforting it is for family members to know that at least their seriously ill loved one is in skilled, caring hands. What's more, I firmly believe that when a patient languishes in the hospital alone, it's easier for the staff to slip into that mind-set of viewing the sick according to their disease and losing sight of the person. What is more humanizing than for a nurse to witness a terminally ill man silently holding his wife's hand or a woman on oxygen playfully asking her granddaughter what she did at school today? The person in the bed suddenly acquires an entire history—a life—beyond that found on the medical chart.

✳ *Sitting with the patient when no one else can get to the hospital is an ideal assignment for that family member or friend who wants to be of help but perhaps isn't comfortable handling more demanding tasks.*

Don't Just Sit There, Do Something!

Organize the Room Efficiently

Place the trash basket near the head of the bed, not at the foot of the bed so that the nurse, the doctor, and the orderly all bump into it. If your loved one can't reach the basket, tie a small plastic garbage bag to the bedside rail.

If other visitors are expected, arrange the chairs so that one side of the bed is clear enough for staff to reach the patient.

Remove food trays that haven't been bused.

Organize the top of the bedside vanity and the windowsills, and clear off the rolling table that extends across the bed.

Slide bedpans, drainage bottles, and the like under the bed where no one will kick them.

Fold extra bed linens and towels neatly over the foot of the bed or the back of a chair. Hang the person's robe on the bathroom door. Store everything else in the closet or the lower drawers of the vanity.

Love Thy Loved One's Neighbor

Since insurance doesn't routinely pay for private accommodations, most patients are going to be sharing the room with someone else. Get to know the roommate and any regular visitors; you may be able to depend on them to spot for you when you're not there. Let's say you walk into the room to find your father half-dozing and groggy from morphine.

"Dad, was the doctor here yet today?"

"Uh-huh," he murmurs drowsily. Roomie catches your eye and emphatically shakes his head. That knowledge could spare you the aggravation of leaving too soon and missing the physician when you need to speak with him.

Assist Patients with Ordering Meals

Ask your loved one if she has filled out the next day's menu; if not, help her do so. When the tray arrives, always check to see that the dietary department sent up the correct order, especially if your loved one is on a restricted diet (see sidebar). The slip of paper on the tray will clearly indicate what type of meal it is. Countless times I've seen a patient receive dinner when he is scheduled for surgery or a test first thing in the morning and is supposed to be fasting. The doctor wrote out an NPO order (the Latin words *nil per os*, meaning "nothing by mouth") but the NPO sticker was not posted on the chart, the door, and over the bed, or the physician's instructions weren't relayed to dietary in time. For a patient to eat prior to a test or operation would almost certainly scuttle the procedure, especially if it entails general anesthesia. The doctor wants the stomach empty in order to minimize the risk of an unconscious patient regurgitating and inhaling vomit into the lungs, which could trigger the potentially deadly inflammation called aspiration pneumonia.

* *"Nothing by mouth" means no food and no liquid. Sucking a piece of hard candy, a tiny ice cube, or a glycerin swab is allowed, however.*

Assist and Befriend the Staff

A hospital is not a hotel, and nurses are not maids. Ask someone to show you where to find refills of water and where basic supplies, blankets, and pillows are stored, and fetch them yourself. I always try to take as much of the workload off the staff as I can. The TV's malfunctioning? Let's not pester the nurse with that. We can check the hospital directory for the number of the department responsible and call ourselves. Not only will the staff love you for it, but it feels good to actively participate in a loved one's care instead of sitting idly by. And seeing family and friends work in tandem with the health care team can strengthen the patient's trust and confidence in them.

Perhaps because folks tend to defer to the busy, important doctor, they sometimes vent their frustration and sense of powerlessness on the nurses and aides. Understandable but not acceptable, for you need these men and women on your side.

Engage them! Say "Hi, how are you doing? Boy, you guys are busy today." Everyone is overworked and underpaid (especially in this era of nursing staff cutbacks), so show some empathy and acknowledge their effort. You don't have to bring flowers and presents, as I sometimes do, but after a nurse has spent time holding your loved one's hand or made sure the pain medication arrives on time, a simple "thank you" is appreciated.

Let the Staff Know How the Patient Really Feels

"Family members serve as the conduits between the patient and health care providers," says ICU nurse Daphne

Restricted Diets Commonly Prescribed in the Hospital

Clear Liquid Diet—every 1 to 2 hours on average.

Consists of water; tea; black coffee; fat-free broth; seltzer; ginger ale; apple, cranberry, or white grape juice; plain gelatin; sugar and sugar substitutes; honey; and sucking candy.

May be prescribed

- following surgery, particularly of the gastrointestinal tract. By the time the person is ready to be discharged, he has usually progressed to solid food or at least to a full-liquid diet or soft diet;
- to help clear the bowel in preparation for endoscopic or X-ray examinations of the colon (sigmoidoscopy, colonoscopy, barium enema);
- during bouts of extreme acute illness or infection;
- for patients temporarily unable to digest solid food.

Full Liquid Diet—every 2 to 4 hours on average.

Consists of all the liquids found in the clear-liquid diet plus milk, strained soups, fruit and vegetable juices, gelatin, custard, eggnog, ice cream, sherbet, oatmeal, and other cereal gruels.

May be prescribed

- as a transition between the clear-liquid diet and the soft diet;
- postsurgery;
- during spells of fever, infections, or stomach inflammation;
- for patients temporarily unable to digest solid food.

Soft Diet—3 easily digestible meals per day with or without between-meal snacks; no roughage.

Consists of all liquids, strained cereals, tender or pureed cooked vegetables, seedless and skinless cooked fruits, ripe bananas, ground or minced meat, poultry or fish, eggs, mild cheeses, plain cake, puddings, and moderately seasoned foods.

May be prescribed

- as a transition between the full-liquid diet and the normal hospital meal plan;
- for patients who have difficulty chewing or swallowing;
- following an acute illness;
- for patients suffering from GI disorders or acute infections.

Other Specialized Diets Served to Patients.

Low-Fat, Low-Salt, or Low-Cholesterol Diet—typically prescribed for patients with atherosclerosis and hypertension, as a means of helping to lower their risk of heart attack, stroke, and chronic kidney disease.

Diabetic Diet—high-cholesterol, low-fat, moderate protein. ► See "Caring for Someone with Diabetes: The Diabetic Diet," page 397.

Renal Diet—calorie rich but prohibitively low in protein, potassium, salt, and phosphorus. ► See "Caring for Someone with Kidney Disease: The Renal Diet," page 455.

Vegetarian, Kosher, and Other Special Diets—when approved by the physician.

Stannard. "The more everyday practical knowledge that we have about this person, the better we'll be able to care for him. It could be simple things that don't seem terribly important but may end up being important later. So if you know, for example, that your loved one has a low threshold for pain but tends to be stoic, share that information early on. 'My husband's probably not going to complain about pain, but you should be aware that his tolerance is really quite low.'"

Get Out of the Way!

One thing that drives the hospital staff to distraction are visitors who get in the way. They cluster around the bed, chattering away. In walks the physician. The guests glance at him, then resume their conversation, making no effort to move. The doctor might be there to speak to the patient in private. Or maybe he needs to perform a bedside examination that the person finds embarrassing even with the curtain drawn.

Anytime a doctor or nurse enters the room, ask "Would you like us to step outside?" And if you're with some of the oblivious types described above, say to them "How about our taking a walk while the doctor's here?" or "Let's grab a cup of coffee in the cafeteria"—unless, that is, you're a true hands-on caregiver, in which case offer to stay and help. When I'm sitting with a friend and an intern shows up to insert a nasogastric feeding tube, I don't go flying out the door. I hold my buddy's hand and pat his brow. The point is, never assume that your presence is needed or wanted. Ask.

✻ *Be sensitive to the roommate's right to privacy as well. Offer to leave the room whenever a doctor or nurse comes to see the other occupant, or if the person needs to use the bathroom, and so forth.*

Tend to Your Patient's Personal Care

Johnetta Romanowski: I was the only person Dennis allowed to do anything for him in the hospital. He wouldn't let the nurses give him a sponge bath; he wouldn't even let them get him out of bed. It had to be me. Not that I could do these things better than the nurses, but Dennis trusted me. He'd call me at seven in the morning and say "I want to get out of bed. Please come get me."

Patients can appear to have split personalities at times: cheerful and cooperative toward the nurses, seldom asking for a thing; demanding and needy whenever we're around. Don't be surprised if your loved one prefers that you tend to some of his personal needs during visits. He may draw the line at toileting and other intimate matters, but if anything, people often feel less self-conscious with those close to them than with strangers.

My aunt Margaret was a painfully modest churchgoing woman. When she was dying of colon cancer in a hospice outside Mobile, it horrified her to be naked in front of nurses and aides, much less have them touch her. Even after she'd faded into a semicomatose state, the sensation of air on her body would cause her to grimace as if in pain, and she'd tug frantically at the bed sheets in an attempt to cover herself.

That's when Aunt Kitty, David, or I used to close the door and say "It's okay, Margaret. I'm just going to rub some lotion on your legs." Her face would relax, and she'd drift off to sleep.

Although officially nurses are discouraged from letting visitors assist patients, Daphne Stannard says, "We push that boundary all the time, especially when we see that someone genuinely wants to get involved." Learn the basic nursing skills described in chapter 3, and you shouldn't meet any resistance.

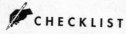

CHECKLIST
A Typical Hospital Visit: Patient Care

❑ See to it that the person drinks plenty of fluids. Hydration is our number one concern in the dehumidified environment of the hospital. The combination of being ill and dehydrated creates a breeding ground for germs. Each year more than 2 million patients, or 1 in 20, contract what are called *nosocomial* infections while hospitalized.

* *Ever taste the juice hospitals serve? It's usually either watery pineapple-orange or syrupy apricot nectar. Bring your loved one the good stuff: designer water, a six-pack of Coke, 100 percent orange juice in plastic bottles—whatever she likes to drink. But be sure to observe any dietary restrictions imposed by the doctor.*

❑ To relieve dry mouth, give the patient ice chips; a cold, wet washcloth; or a glycerin swab to suck on.

❑ Gently moisturize the skin, including the feet, back, and butt. This doubles as a relaxing massage. Apply lip balm, too.

❑ Check for evidence of bedsores, particularly on the tailbone, heels, shoulders, elbows—anywhere bony protrusions come into prolonged contact with the mattress or bear weight. Should patches of skin look as if they're breaking down, alert the nurse immediately.

❑ Remind your loved one to change position, or turn her yourself every 30 to 60 minutes.

* *Anytime she shifts in bed or gets out of bed, fluff the pillow and tighten those sheets. Wrinkles in the bed contribute to skin deterioration.*

❑ If the person is too ill or weak to use utensils, spoon-feed her yourself.

❑ Escort her to the bathroom if she's able to walk or help position her to use a bedpan or urinal.

❑ Give the person a bed bath or assist her with taking a shower.

❑ To aid circulation, help an ambulatory patient out of bed and into the room's most comfortable chair. Or accompany her on a walk around the unit.

* *When helping someone in and out of bed, always use the automatic controls to lower it first and help her avoid tripping over any tubes or wires winding around the bed.*

Be the Patient's Advocate

Patients should always feel entitled to assert themselves while in the hospital, yet few do. Perhaps it isn't their nature; perhaps they're too ill. Whenever visiting loved ones, think of yourself as a troubleshooter, there to make things better for them in terms of both comfort and safety. Even if the person is eminently capable of speaking up for herself, sometimes it's preferable for us to do the negotiating. The roommate keeps blaring the TV? Let *me* ask him to turn it down or, if that fails, complain to the nurse. After all, I don't share a room with this person.

Pat Still, an everyday angel from New

York, fell into this pattern during the three years her late husband had to live in a residential care facility due to severe disabilities from a stroke. "I was the bad guy so he could be the good guy," she says. "He would be nice to everyone in the nursing home, give me his complaints, and I would run around solving them."

If we're observant, virtually every visit to the hospital presents situations that call for us to intervene.

The Situation: Too Many Visitors or Folks Who Overstay Their Welcome.

In the hospital or at home, patients need someone to make sure the procession of well-wishers doesn't get out of hand. At the same time we don't want to give the appearance of keeping friends and family at arm's length, which will only inspire resentment all around.

This was no small challenge when my stepmother was dying at home of lung cancer. Lynn was seventy-eight, though you'd never have guessed it. Spirited and vivacious, she was a "hot thang" who loved to dance, laugh, and talk-talk-talk in a staccato delivery that left no doubt she was a country girl from the hills of Tennessee. When Bob married Lynn in 1980, three months after Mom died, my brothers and I were surprised but thrilled. I offer as proof the fact that I let her charm me into singing at the wedding.

A life of chain-smoking had afflicted Lynn with emphysema some years before. But around 1987 her hacking cough worsened, and she began losing weight and experiencing chest pain. X rays revealed a massive inoperable tumor in one lung. Over the next year she received radiation once a week, primarily to slow the inoperable cancer's progression and permit her to breathe.

My stepmom was one of those people who feels obliged to perpetually entertain the world, and dying only accentuated this trait. The radiation treatments had seared her throat, making it painful to swallow or speak. Nonetheless, whenever company came, Lynn held

court in the living room or on the front porch for hours—in full makeup, hair styled, fingernails polished—chatting animatedly and telling jokes until she'd collapse. Dad, a raconteur himself, used to get upset with her for exhausting herself, though someone like my stepmother might argue, quite convincingly, that there would be plenty of time to "rest" soon enough.

A good way to avoid standing-room-only audiences at the bedside and interminable encores from visitors who refuse to leave is to set the parameters for the visit ahead of time on the phone. "Could you come by around six? Great. Just so you know, Bob's had five people by already today, and he's getting worn out, though of course he'd never admit it. He'd love to see you, but I'd appreciate it if you could keep the visit to half an hour or so." Then when you walk into the room after thirty minutes, wink, and gesture at the clock, the visitors don't feel insulted or that they're being tossed out. Most folks take the hint.

Those who don't, we evict, albeit ever so sweetly: "Mrs. Hunter, I'm going to have to interrupt here. It's really nice to see you, but right now Mom has to have her dinner" or her medication or her sleep. *Make up an excuse if necessary.* When Dad was ill, I regularly ran interference for him with a certain elderly gentleman who used to settle himself in a chair and meander up and down memory lane until my father's eyelids were drooping. Citing one of the reasons above, I'd politely escort him out the door while Dad flashed me a look of heartfelt gratitude.

The Situation: Venipunctures.

When you're seriously ill, getting stuck with needles can be a daily routine. Perhaps a *phlebotomist* comes by the room to draw blood from a vein in the arm for any number of tests. The respiratory therapy department might request a sample of arterial blood for a blood-gas analysis to measure the balance of oxygen and carbon dioxide in the circulation. If the doctor has ordered intravenous fluids or medication, expect yet another needle stick.

Inserting a needle into a vein or artery demands considerable skill. Even the most accomplished IV nurse or phlebotomist can't score a direct hit every time, particularly if disease, old age, or repeated stickings have ravaged vessels near the skin's surface, causing them to collapse, or "blow." Obesity, too, makes it more difficult to target an accessible healthy vein.

All the more reason for us to insist that venipunctures be performed *only* by experienced medical providers. Unless they're all busy elsewhere, most hospitals will accommodate your request. It's rare for nursing students to be assigned this task, but medical students and interns practice on patients all the time. My personal ground rule is simple: Three strikes and you're out. I'll say "Please stop. Let's not do this now." Then I'll bring my loved one an ice pack. And if he cannot tolerate even one clumsy attempt, we ask that somebody else try again later.

Suzanne Hardy's twenty-eight-year-old daughter, Kristin, has been in and out of hospitals most of her life due to an assortment of serious diabetes-related complications. Her mother says firmly, "I've let it be known that I won't even allow third-year medical students messing around with Kristin. My kid has been through enough. Let them practice on someone else."

Besides lobbying for experience and calling time-out in the middle of an inept venipuncture, there are other strategies to help spare loved ones as much discomfort as possible. Before an IV injection or a phlebotomy, try these tricks for enlarging blood vessels and improving circulation:

1. Just prior to the procedure, warm up the site with your hands or wrap it in a warm, wet washcloth.
2. See to it that the person eats healthily and drinks plenty of fluids if possible.
3. Encourage her to walk around and to exercise her arms and hands daily by squeezing a rubber ball or lifting one-pound weights.

  ✱ *Cans from the pantry work just fine for "pumping iron."*

4. Regularly moisturize the lower arms, hands, and fingertips. Stickings are less painful when the needle doesn't have to penetrate dry, hard skin.

Many patients find venipunctures far more bearable if they don't look at the needle. In addition, the deep-breathing exercises and relaxation techniques described in chapter 3's discussion on pain management can ease anxiety and the perception of pain as well.

Try to coordinate blood drawings and IV's. When checking in on the floor, ask the nurse if blood can be taken the same time the IV is started. The person placing the intravenous line simply inserts a catheter into the vein, withdraws however many units are needed, and then detaches the cylinder containing the blood and connects the needle to the plastic tubing. Congratulations. Your thinking ahead just saved your loved one from an unnecessary needle stick.

You might also ask the doctor or nurse about alternatives to venipunctures:

Finger sticks: Blood platelet counts, blood sugar counts, and several other blood tests call for only a drop or two of blood, which can be obtained by pricking a fingertip or an earlobe with a pinlike needle.

A central venous catheter or permanent port: Men and women expected to undergo frequent blood tests and IV procedures over a length of time—such as those on cancer chemotherapy, or kidney dialysis, and those with AIDS—should consider intravenous catheters or permanent blood-access ports. These devices allow the hospital staff or home care nurse to deliver drugs, fluids, and nutrients without having to puncture a vein every time.

The central catheter—a small, flexible plastic tube—is surgically implanted into a large vein in the arm or the chest, where it can remain for months. When the nurse wants to administer medication, for example, she injects it directly into the portion of the tube that protrudes from the skin. In similar fashion, surgeons can create a permanent venous-access site during a minor operation. Here a small round metal disc is placed under the skin, typically in the chest, and connected by way of a small tube to a large vein. Needles must pierce only the skin to draw from or discharge their contents into the port.

In addition to eliminating the need for repeated venipunctures, both types of indwelling catheters provide another advantage in that they feed into large central veins, which can better withstand the caustic chemicals used to fight cancer than the smaller peripheral vessels utilized for conventional IVs. ▶ See *"Central Venous Catheters," page 150; "Caring for Someone with Kidney Disease: Caring for a Fistula or Shunt," page 451.*

The Situation: A Loved One Needs Prompt Relief for Pain, Nausea, Anxiety, and Other Symptoms or Side Effects. Remember the scene in the Oscar-winning tearjerker *Terms of Endearment* where Shirley MacLaine begs for someone at the nurse's desk to relieve the dying Debra Winger's cancer pain?

"It's past ten o'clock," she says calmly. "Give my daughter the pain shot, please." But when the staff fails to respond immediately, her tone escalates into a full-scale shriek: "Give her the shot, you understand? Do something! All she has to do is hold on till ten! Give her the shot, do you understand? GIVE HER THE SHOT!!!" Finally a petrified nurse scurries to deliver the injection.

"Thank you very much," Shirley says, quickly composing herself. "Thank you."

The outburst worked for the moment: Debra Winger received her medication; Shirley MacLaine, an Academy Award. In the long run, hysteria, condescending attitudes, or abusive language prove more disruptive than effective. The staff will permit you one or two tantrums—chalking them up to the care partner's daily cocktail of too much stress and too little sleep. But create too many scenes, and the patient is going to suffer. While hospital personnel are too professional to overtly "punish" someone for a caregiver's behavior, the offending party can expect to get shut out of the information loop.

I'll admit to having pulled a Shirley MacLaine at times, but only in situations where someone's inefficiency or negligence threatened to endanger my patient, and only after I'd exhausted the preventive measures below.

Anticipate symptoms and delays. At the first sign of discomfort, mosey on down to the nurse's desk and politely nudge them for relief *now*, not when the patient is miserable. Likewise, if your loved one is on a medication schedule (typically every four hours), "contact the nurse when it's coming up on the four-hour mark," advises nurse Daphne Stannard, "not when we already have an out-of-control situation."

Suzanne Hardy: *The patient's family doesn't always understand why it's often so hard to get pain medication on time in the hospital. It could be that the nurse has six other patients and one of them just came back to the floor from surgery. Or if the drug is a narcotic, they may not have it on the unit; the nurse might have to go to the pharmacy to get it.*

Anytime a patient enters the hospital, ask the primary physician to order all pain, antinausea, antianxiety, and insomnia relief PRN. Patients and families also don't always appreciate that the nurses are not authorized to modify drug dosages or schedules. So if 50 milligrams of Demerol every four hours doesn't seem to be taking the edge off your father's postoperative pain, you're going to have to appeal to the nurse to convey your request for a new order to the doctor. But what if she can't get him on the phone right away? A PRN order leaves it up to the nurse's discretion to dispense medication as needed. (PRN stands for *pro re nata*, Latin for "according to circumstances.") Even if a patient never has to ask for more relief, what a comfort it is to know that should his symptoms become unbearable, he doesn't have to wait out the clock. ▶ *See "Administering Medications Safely," page 142.*

Catch flies with honey, or how to get the patient what she needs. I don't think I've ever strolled up to the nurse's desk feeling happy with the staff's speed or efficiency. That's usually why I'm there in the first place: something is late, someone forgot something, and so forth. But I remember the caregiver's mantra, *This is about the patient, not about me*, and set aside my anger and frustration before politely making my request (which is essentially a demand phrased as a question): "Who do I talk to about getting Mr. McFarlane his four o'clock pain shot?"

Or when you walk over and the nurse is counting pills, don't launch into "I need a blanket." She's going to reply "Just a minute." You stand there, she glances up, and you say "When you get a minute, may I please ask you a question?" According to basic human psychology, the response more often than not is "Sure, what is it?"

While you don't allow anyone to trample the patient's rights, always keep your sights on what's truly important: getting her what she needs while preserving your relationship with the staff. Another term for patient advocate is case manager. As with any manager, the bottom line is getting the job done.

The Situation: Foul-ups. Trust in the medical team is essential. If you're so

uncertain of the staff's competence that you feel compelled to question their every decision—or maybe you're wary to a degree that's not in anyone's best interest—then you and your loved one ought to be discussing a change in venue.

As in any field, however, no one is infallible, not even the most conscientious, experienced health care provider. According to a major study published jointly by the Harvard School of Public Health and the Harvard Law School in 1990, roughly 1 percent of all medical care is tainted by negligence. An estimated 100,000 people die annually due to medical mistakes, with hundreds of thousands more seriously injured.

"I could write a book about hospital errors," Suzanne Hardy says with a sigh. "There have been at least thirty times when Kristin has been hospitalized for hyperglycemia—her blood sugar was really high—and a nurse hung an IV bag containing glucose instead of saline." Infusing glucose, a simple sugar, into her bloodstream could conceivably have sent the young woman's blood-glucose level skyrocketing and landed her in a coma. Since Kristin lost her eyesight to diabetes, Suzanne worries more about slipups going undetected.

"If you want to help the person in your family get well," she emphasizes, "you have to be there with the person and know what's going on." During visits, pay attention to what's being said and done so that if a nurse came in waving an order to draw arterial blood for a blood-gas analysis—when you know darn well that a respiratory therapy technician just carried out that unpleasant procedure thirty minutes before (as happened another time while Suzanne sat with Kristin)—you can point out the mistake in the event that your loved one cannot do so for herself.

"I don't mean to sound as if I'm putting down the medical profession," Suzanne Hardy says, "but doctors and nurses are human beings with a lot on their minds and too many patients. Very rarely is Kristin in the hospital now that

I'm not there with her. If my being there can help prevent an accident, that's what I'm going to do."

* *Tutor your loved one on the details of his medical care so he'll be able to advocate for himself when family and friends aren't around. For instance, before an operation, say "Dad, remember not to eat or drink tonight. Even if they bring you a tray, you're not supposed to swallow anything until after the procedure tomorrow."*

Before You Go Home for the Night

• Refill the person's water pitcher and replenish the supply of foam cups and straws.
• Ask what else you can get him before you leave. If he wears dentures, clean them for him.
• Place items the person uses most often within easy reach, such as the call bell, the phone, the controls for the bed and the TV, juice, water, something to eat, tissues, and so on. Put hairbrushes, reading glasses, breath fresheners, magazines, headphones, and the phone book in the top drawer. Fold an extra sheet and blanket over the foot of the bed or the rail.
• Reorganize the room for efficiency, just as you did when you arrived. Water any plants.
• Remind the person to call you if the doctor comes in.
• Ask what you can bring the next time you visit. Patients underestimate how stultifyingly boring the hospital can be day after day. But what would be a perfectly thoughtful gift for someone convalescing at home may not be practical in the cramped confines of a hospital room. Giving an artist a coloring book and crayons seems like a clever idea except that the minute somebody moves the bed tray, the crayons roll off onto the floor. Save games, jigsaw puzzles, and anything

with lots of pieces for after the person is discharged.
• Remind the person to call you if she thinks of anything else before you return, then call her around bedtime and review the list.

When the Quality of Hospital Care Is Lacking

An acquaintance of mine, now deceased, once checked himself out of the hospital at two o'clock in the morning, incensed that he hadn't received dinner because the kitchen was long since closed. Looking back, the man's behavior can probably be attributed partially to the beginnings of AIDS-related dementia, but in any event, he was not choosing his battles judiciously. A delayed meal is not something we go to the mat about. If your loved one is that hungry, go down to the cafeteria and buy a bagel or apple to tide him over.

What Is a Legitimate Complaint?

• Rude, disrespectful, or abusive behavior from anyone on staff and
• Failure to respond *at once* to any of the following life-threatening emergencies: respiratory distress; chest pain; cardiac arrest or sudden changes in the heart rate or rhythm; critically elevated blood pressure; a sudden drop in blood pressure, as from internal hemorrhaging *(circulatory shock)* or a bacterial infection *(septic shock);* an apparent high fever; a seizure; choking on secretions; critically elevated intracranial pressure, as may be seen following a stroke or traumatic brain injury; a fall; malfunction of a mechanical respirator or other piece of life-support equipment. These machines, as well as many monitoring devices, are equipped with alarms that sound

should they break down or detect a significant change in a crucial bodily function (heart rate, breathing, blood pressure).

- Having to wait more than *five minutes* for a nurse or aide to arrive after someone has alerted the desk that the patient is in severe pain or severely agitated or nauseated or throwing up, or that a nasogastric tube, drainage tube, or IV tube has become disconnected; an intravenous drip stops, the bag is empty, or you notice swelling at the injection site; a kidney hemodialyzer appears to be malfunctioning; a dressing peels off or is soaked with blood or fluid; the patient is lying in vomit, urine, or feces.

* *That said, we don't just sit there fuming. While waiting for assistance, we either change the patient and the sheets ourselves or at the very least place a towel under them.*

If your loved one requires intensive, round-the-clock care that the nursing staff cannot realistically provide, you might consider hiring *private duty* nurses, aides, or sitters for one-on-one attention.

Hospital nursing departments often maintain files of freelancers. Bear in mind that they are not hospital employees. You must negotiate fees individually and pay each person directly, typically at the end of the shift. Since insurance virtually never covers private duty care, this is beyond most people's means and rarely a feasible option except perhaps to give the primary care partner a temporary break.

Other contacts for locating private in-hospital nursing care:

☎ The Visiting Nurse Associations of America (888-866-8773) or look under "Nurses" in the Yellow Pages.

The staff's response time to a non-life-threatening situation like those given above depends on whatever else is happening in the unit at that moment. Under normal circumstances your loved one should not have to wait an hour for someone to reinsert an IV line that wriggled out of the vein when he rolled over in bed. But if a kidney patient down the hall just went into uremic convulsions, obviously his needs take precedence. Switch off the flow-control clamp on the tubing until the nurse can get to him.

"One time in our CCU," recalls Daphne Stannard, "there were three codes [a *code* denotes someone in cardiac arrest or respiratory failure] going on simultaneously, and every single nurse was at one of them. I'm sure there were some patients lying in urine, but we just couldn't deal with that right away."

To Whom Do You Complain?

First, confront the person you're unhappy with. From the nurse's perspective, it is far preferable to have the patient or care partner complain directly to her than to be called on the carpet by the doctor about a problem that could have been easily rectified face-to-face. When you must say "My patient Mr. Jones says he had to wait two hours to get his pain shot," well, maybe there was a gap in communication. Maybe no one ever relayed your request to the nurse. Ask a second time to give the nurse a fair chance to fix the mistake.

If you don't receive satisfaction at that level, begin working your way up the hospital chain of command: Report to the *primary physician* and the *charge nurse* rude, disrespectful, or abusive behavior by any member of the hospital staff; staff negligence in responding to a medical emergency or a call for help; dissatisfaction with the caliber of patient hygiene, skin care, and so on, and all other issues relating to patient comfort and safety.

Throughout a hospital stay, advises Dr. Jack Lord of the American Hospital Association, "the attending physician is the patient's primary advocate and should be involved in any complaint or concern [including grievances against residents, interns, specialists, or subspecialists]. He or she usually has the most leverage within the health care facility."

When our unhappiness is with nursing, the charge nurse, too, can be an effective mediator. She's also the person to approach if an inconsiderate roommate has been asked to keep the noise level down but to no avail. She can speak to the uncooperative party or, possibly, transfer your loved one to another room.

Report to the *patient representative* all complaints not corrected at the previous level.

This is purely a formality. The patient advocate can certainly be a useful ally, but in matters pertaining to medical care, his primary function is to defuse the situation (that is, minimize the threat of litigation), which is rarely the same thing as seeing to it that whatever prompted you to complain doesn't happen again.

Climb this rung anyway because if you have to appeal to the next level, the first question you'll undoubtedly be asked is "Have you filed a complaint with the patient representative?"

Report to the *unit nursing director* or the *nursing supervisor* on duty any continuing complaints with a particular nurse.

Report to the *hospital administrator* on call (immediately) and the *chief administrator's* office (during business hours) if the facility refuses to honor a valid advance directive or power-of-attorney for health care.

At no point in this entire process should you threaten to sue for malpractice. Maybe you will take the hospital to court—but later, after this is all over. Only one in eight people injured by medical negligence files a claim. In order to win a malpractice suit, one must prove gross negligence or malicious intent, and this is no simple feat. As I once heard a veteran attorney put it, "There's a big difference between malpractice and damn bad medicine." A doctor who misdiagnoses your loved one's illness may be guilty of poor judgment, but poor judgment does not necessarily connote malpractice.

More important, hurling threats does nothing to improve services *now*. And don't even waste your breath on "I'm taking my mother out of this miserable hospital!" No you're not. The only valid reasons for transferring elsewhere in the midst of a hospitalization for a life-threatening condition are: when another institution offers potentially lifesaving therapy not available at the present hospital or if your hospital refuses to comply with the patient's advance directive or the wishes of the health care proxy or next of kin regarding life support. Otherwise, stay put for the time being and work within the system to remedy the problem.

Should you feel you're not getting anywhere, though, be aware that you can request your state regulatory agency to intercede. This office usually operates under the *department of health*. By law it must send an investigator to the medical facility within twenty-four hours of your complaint.

☎ Look for the state department of health's telephone number under "State Offices" in the Government Listings section of the white pages.

Sidestepping Hospital Visiting Policies

Hospitals tend to be flexible about visiting hours, particularly when a patient is seriously ill. Just don't wait until eight o'clock to announce that you'd like to stay a few extra hours. Clear early arrivals, late departures, and underage visitors ahead of time with the charge nurse. For overnight visits the facility may ask for authorization from the attending physician. Inquire about its policy when checking in at admitting.

Some hospitals set aside a limited number of rooms furnished to accommodate a family member. These are usually available on a first-come, first-served basis. In New York University Medical Center's Cooperative Care unit, "you're in a hotel-like setting," says Eileen Mitzman, whose daughter Marni was hospitalized there several times due to complications from AIDS. "I lived with her for a couple of weeks at a time. You eat your meals together, and the caregiver can even get the patient her medications. It was the kindest, most humane thing I've ever seen in hospital care."

✱ *The admitting doctor must make these arrangements for you.*

Making Pitstops Before or After Hours

What if it's more convenient for you to drop off clean pajamas on your way to work than wait until the start of visiting hours in the afternoon? This is rarely a problem as long as you've gotten the charge nurse's permission ahead of time. Should you run into resistance, don't retreat out the door. Instead, pick up a house phone, dial the operator, and ask for the extension of the appropriate nurse's desk. No house phone? Call the operator from a pay phone.

I always make it a point to greet the security guard and the clerk at the visitor's desk. Once they recognize my face, I can go flying in past the automatic doors—"I just need to run this upstairs. Can I bring you some coffee on the way down?"—and they wave me on toward the elevators. The other trick to gliding in and out of the hospital easily is to walk purposefully and carry yourself as if you belong there.

Outpatient Appointments and Tests
Strategic Scheduling

For someone who is ill and frail, trips to and from the doctor's office, hospital, or outpatient clinic can be profoundly exhausting and as anxiety provoking as any medical procedure. "What if I trip and fall?" "What if we get stuck in traffic on the way to the medical center and I have to go to the bathroom?" The worrying types expend themselves mentally before they even leave the house.

Finesse in scheduling and coordinating outpatient visits will make the difference between patient and caregiver getting through the day relatively easily and straggling home feeling worn out and stressed out. The key is to consider all the what-if's and to plan accordingly while looking to minimize walking distance, travel time, and waiting time. The following tricks should help:

Ask the doctor if any upcoming tests could be done while the person is hospitalized. This will save a return trip soon after discharge.

Try to avoid late-afternoon appointments. The reason is that the waiting room tends to clog with traffic as the day wears on. Postponements don't happen often, but if we're the 4:30 appointment for a CT scan on the day the machine breaks down and takes two hours to repair, and the ER fills up with two stroke victims and a case of severe head trauma, the possibility exists of getting bumped to the next day.

Schedule appointments around the person's sleep pattern. I always prefer getting in and out early, but serious illness and medications frequently disrupt patients' sleep cycles. If a loved one lies awake night after night only to finally doze from dawn to mid-morning, let's not court disaster by rousing him for a 10:00 A.M. lower GI series when he's liable to be cranky and weary from sleep deprivation.

Don't squeeze too much into one day. You're rearranging your week so you can drive a friend to the hospital this Thursday at noon for a pulmonary exercise test. She's also due for a mammogram. It's tempting to try to work it in later in the day. After all, you're going to be at the hospital anyway.

If the two of you are confident she has the physical and emotional stamina to handle both, go for it. Otherwise you may wind up regretting it. You thought you'd have a two-hour break between procedures. No. The exercise test takes two hours instead of one and proves far more tiring than your friend anticipated. Several times she pedals the stationary bicycle for a few minutes, then complains of shortness of breath and leg pain and must rest before continuing. Plus, breathing into a mouthpiece so unnerves her, the technician has to calm her down repeatedly. She returns to the waiting room winded and on edge.

Now the two of you trek to the mammography suite in a pavilion the equivalent of two city blocks away. Her appointment time comes and goes. Mammograms are always stressful; the longer you wait, the more she frets. This procedure, too, lasts longer than expected. The technologist isn't satisfied with two of the exposures and has to reposition one breast between the platform and the compression paddle. In her fatigued, agitated state, your friend feels sorer than usual on the car ride home. By the time you drop her off (after sitting in rush-hour traffic you hadn't counted on), she's drained and miserable. The price paid is that she spends the next two days flat on her back.

Be sure to know your loved one's limitations and what the procedure entails, and anticipate delays before deciding whether or not to add that extra stop.

✳ *Always allow for rest time between appointments.*

When scheduling appointments, know which days and times are convenient. The office person in charge of the date book is going to offer the next most convenient appointment for *them*. That's not the way to make an appointment. First, state your business:

"I'm calling to schedule a follow-up exam for Mr. McFarlane. He's Dr. Smith's patient."

"I have an opening next Wednesday at three o'clock."

"No, it needs to be in the morning." Save the explanations as to why. Be specific. Be linear. "If you don't have anything Wednesday morning, then Thursday or Friday morning is good. We can be there at whatever time you want us."

Remember, the person on the other end of the phone is not trying to inconvenience you, she's simply telling you the time slots available. If you've been pleasant and straightforward, she might say, "We're pretty well booked up those two days, but let me see if I can squeeze you in Thursday morning." Maybe she can; maybe she can't. But that response is far different from a curt "Can't do it Thursday. We're all booked up."

Preparing for Procedures

Ask the doctor or his assistant to describe the procedure in detail. The old expression "What you don't know won't hurt you" does not apply to patients facing medical procedures. It's always better to have some idea of what to expect. Most folks set to undergo a lumbar puncture, for example, would probably tremble upon glimpsing the four-inch hollow needle used to withdraw cerebrospinal fluid from the central canal of the spinal cord. In reality, the insertion of that needle between two vertebrae in the lower back produces pressure but little pain as such; if anything, it's the stinging sensation from the injection of a local anesthetic to numb the area that hurts, and then only for about ten seconds. A patient should know this ahead of time.

Anxiety over an upcoming medical procedure usually has several layers. Besides the fear of pain, patients worry about receiving upsetting news or having to endure any number of indignities. Then there's the nervousness that can set in before any unfamiliar situation. If you think your patient is open to it, suggest he "rehearse" the procedure in his mind from start to finish. Granted, visualization doesn't work for everyone, but those who practice the technique often find it helps them relax and feel less disoriented.

Request medication for anxiety and/or nausea in advance—ideally at the same time the test or procedure is ordered. On the related issues of managing anxiety, nausea, or pain (each explored at length in chapter 3), heed your instinct. Though the doctor may assure you that no sedation is necessary for a lumbar puncture, you know from past experience that your husband's stomach churns and his nerves jangle prior to any procedure involving needles. You also know he's not likely to ask for a short-acting sedative himself.

Do it for him. Given the background information, it's a rare doctor who will deny the request—unless medication somehow interferes with the procedure. (Example: Patients are not sedated before needle biopsies of the lung or kidney except in cases where someone is *extraordinarily* anxious, because the medical team needs the person alert and able to cooperate by holding deep breaths at various intervals as the physician positions the needle.) When you call to schedule the appointment, ask if the premedication has been ordered. Then—erring on the side of caution—double-check again while you're signing in.

* *Patients should never drive themselves to any outpatient procedure that calls for a sedative or a narcotic painkiller.*

Avoiding Long Waits

The appointment at the doctor's office is at 1:00 and the trip takes you about an hour door-to-door? Call the receptionist at 11:30 and ask, "Does it look as if the doctor is *really* going to see us at one sharp? Mom isn't feeling well, and I'd like to bring her in at the last minute if possible." The receptionist should have a reasonable idea of how close to schedule the physician is running.

When Accompanying Loved Ones to Appointments

If you've never been to the office or medical facility before, call to inquire about parking and whether or not wheelchairs are available in the lobby or the garage. Also find out if there are take-out coffee shops, delicatessens, and so forth, nearby.

Be efficient. Plan your itinerary for the ill person's optimum comfort. In the event that your loved one suddenly had to use a bathroom, are there gas stations and fast-food places along the way? Purposefully load up the car, turn on the heat or the air-conditioning, and make sure you have everything you need before helping the sick person to the car.

Know exactly where you're headed. If you're driving Grandma to a city hospital where parking is scarce, pull up in front and escort her inside the building, then go park and meet her in the lobby. For the return trip, the same routine: Bring the car around and assist her outside. (If you're traveling by taxi, have her wait inside while you hail the cab.) Preserve the ailing person's stamina as much as you can.

As with any medical visit, stash the patient's suitcase of essentials and your own emergency bag in the trunk. There's always the chance that the physician will decide to admit your loved one into the hospital immediately.

If you're bringing children, take along games, coloring books, and other quiet distractions, plus drinks and snacks. See to it that everyone has eaten beforehand (except a patient who's been instructed to fast). What if you're detained past mealtime? The last thing you want in the waiting room is a crew that's cranky, hungry, and bored.

Keep a vomit bag or bucket in the car as well as paper towels and mouthwash, just in case. After an angiogram, my father would always feel profoundly nauseous from the opaque solution injected to highlight the blood vessels on the X ray. By contrast, patients receiving cancer chemotherapy may throw up on their way *to* treatments, a curious phenomenon dubbed "parking lot syndrome."

During X rays, sonograms, CT scans, and other imaging procedures, don't press the person running the test to tell you what they see. Technologists are not supposed to reveal anything to patients or care partners, with good reason: Only a radiologist or physician-specialist is qualified to accurately interpret the films.

See to it that the patient and any other passengers use the bathroom before leaving. Your loved one will probably be anxious to head straight home, so try to avoid side trips. For the same reason, keep snacks and cartons of juice on hand. Another suggestion: Everyone's bound to be tired, you included. Prepare dinner the night before or get takeout.

Preparing for Discharge from the Hospital

By law, before a hospital releases a patient, it must have an appropriate *discharge plan* in place to ease the transition home or to another facility, and to maintain the continuity of care. Although one of the medical center's social workers usually coordinates this process, "it is a collaborative effort," stresses Mary Ann Wanucha, manager of the patient and family services department at Bayfront Medical Center in St. Petersburg, Florida.

The attending physician determines the care setting and writes orders for medications and home medical equipment, if necessary. The primary nurse reviews the doctor's instructions with both patient and care partner(s), and teaches them the nursing skills needed to ensure the person's safety and comfort at home. Rehabilitation specialists, a dietitian, and a mental health professional may round out the team that tailors aftercare around the patient's support system—or lack of one.

Thus the discharge plans for two seventy-year-old men recovering from triple bypass heart surgery may be markedly different. The widower who lives alone would probably be transferred to a short-term nursing facility until he was healthy enough to look after himself. His hospital roommate, blessed with a healthy wife and adult children and grandchildren to lend help, could recuperate at home. The social worker would have already arranged for a nurse and a nurse's aide to visit several times a week for as long as was medically necessary.

"We begin to gather information about the patient almost at the point of admission," Wanucha says. Some hospitals ask new arrivals to fill out a form detailing the circumstances at home when they check in. During the hospital stay, the social worker comes by the room to interview the ill person. "At our hospital we try to see patients within seventy-two hours. We also contact the family. Let's say the person is married. We need to talk to the spouse and get a sense of what life is going to be like when the patient goes home. If the patient lives alone but has relatives in another state, we call them to make sure they're aware of what's going on. Oftentimes they're left out of the loop until just before the patient is to leave the hospital, and it comes as quite a shock to them to discover that perhaps medical insurance doesn't cover all his needs."

In Florida, with its sizable population of transplanted retirees, Wanucha routinely discusses the discharge plan with family members via long-distance phone calls. She describes a common scenario: "The family travels here at the onset of the illness, but then they have to go back to their own families, jobs, and other obligations. In that case we'll work out the arrangements and keep them informed of what is going on." Those arrangements may include

- lining up home nursing care or home hospice care;
- transferring the patient from the hospital to a nursing home or hospice facility;
- seeing to it that medical supplies and equipment ordered by the physician are delivered to the home in time for discharge day;
- filing the necessary forms with Medicare, Medicaid, or the patient's private medical insurer and/or disability insurer;
- applying for any government benefits the person may be entitled to, such as supplemental security income, Social Security disability insurance, unemployment insurance, public assistance, or worker's compensation insurance;
- referring patients and caregivers to meal delivery services, adult day care centers, and other support services and limited financial aid that may be available through private and government-funded community service agencies such as Catholic Charities USA and the patient's local Area Agency on Aging, and through patient support organizations like the National Kidney Foundation and the American Lateral Sclerosis Association.

Social work departments have different styles. Some handle every preparation themselves, down to the smallest detail, whereas others set the process in motion but delegate a certain amount of responsibility to the patient and family.

✳ *Should several days go by in the hospital without a visit from the social worker, contact the department yourself. Everyone needs ample time for making important arrangements and pivotal decisions that could affect several lives.*

Postponing or Expediting Discharge Day

This is the story: Your younger brother is set for discharge from the hospital on Thursday, five days from now. You're leaving on a business trip on Wednesday, though, and your sister in Ohio can't travel here until Friday evening. The patient, an alcoholic on the mend from major surgery, will be visited by a home nurse, but only for a few hours a day several days a week. Never one to take good care of himself, your brother is still weak; the thought of his having to take a taxi home and spend even just one night alone in his apartment has the entire family worried.

Ask the primary physician to please keep him in the hospital one more night, and explain why. Expect to be turned down, for with the increase in managed-care health plans, the current trend among insurers is to trim hospitalizations, not extend them. Although a longshot, make the request anyway. You just might pull it off, particularly if you've established that all-important rapport with the doctor.

In the opposite situation, you're planning on driving your loved one home from the hospital first thing in the morning, but the nurse informs you that she'll have to stay all day until the attending comes by on rounds and checks the results of her blood-gas analysis. Only then will he write the discharge orders. Rounds? That could be as late as dinnertime. With three school-age children, you need to be home far earlier than that.

Get in touch with the primary physician and ask if he can't write a provisional discharge in advance, stating that the patient may go home in the morning after the test results are in and are determined to be in the desired range. The house physician can then write the final orders to send your loved one on her way.

That morning, while you're waiting, call the admitting department and the business office. "Mrs. Johnson is checking out in an hour. Do I need to stop by for any reason?" Don't wait until the patient is fidgeting in her wheelchair, restless to leave, for the nurse to tell you, "Oh, you have to pick up a signed release from the cashier before you can go."

Safety Measures for Around the Home

In the days leading up to Dad's discharge from the Mobile Infirmary, my brothers David and John, and John's wife, Sheri, went on a house-cleaning spree because it was hard to predict how feeble Bob would be and, consequently, how much time we would have for housework once he went home. They washed, folded, and put away all the laundry; scrupulously scoured the refrigerator and all surfaces where food would be prepared; cleaned the windows, window screens, and the air-conditioner filter—all traps for bacteria and molds; and stocked up on groceries as well as salt substitutes, antacids, and other essential supplies (see checklist).

When shopping at the pharmacy, envision the worst-case scenario: At 3:00 A.M. your loved one awakens with violent diarrhea, and the hospice nurse on call instructs you to give him Imodium to control the diarrhea and Gatorade to restore electrolytes. What will you do if you don't have either, you're there by yourself, and the drugstore in town is closed?

Other Steps for Getting Ready

Post by the phone or on the refrigerator a list of important information and telephone numbers:

- each doctor's name, medical specialty ("Dr. Jones—neurologist"), the condition she is treating, and telephone number;
- the schedule and dosage for every medication;
- the number of the pharmacy and the pharmacist's name;
- the number of the nearest twenty-four-hour pharmacy;
- the number of the home health agency and the principal contact there if you're using home nursing care or home hospice care;
- the local emergency number;

* *If you're from out of town, don't assume that it's 911. Check to be sure.*

- the number of the local fire department;
- the number of the local Poison Control Center;
- the twenty-four-hour number of the company supplying oxygen or other medical equipment, such as a mechanical respirator or a kidney dialysis machine.
- *your* home and work telephone numbers and those of other family and friends involved in the person's care.

Move the bed away from the wall for easier access.

Clear off a bedside table and keep near the bed a heavy chair, a plastic urinal or commode, the person's cane or walker, a flashlight, and a nightlight.

Since seriously ill people frequently fall into irregular sleep patterns, install room-darkening shades to facilitate daytime naps.

✒ CHECKLIST

Have These Essential Supplies on Hand

- ❏ Hydrogen peroxide
- ❏ Sterile gauze pads
- ❏ Paper adhesive tape
- ❏ Triple antibiotic cream or ointment (Neosporin)
- ❏ Cortisone cream for itches, rashes, skin irritations
- ❏ Antacid
- ❏ All prescription medications for sleep, nausea, anxiety, and pain, which you should request *before* your loved one goes home
- ❏ Plastic urinal or portable toilet (commode)
- ❏ Disinfectant spray
- ❏ Isopropyl (rubbing) alcohol
- ❏ Cornstarch or baby powder
- ❏ Band-Aids
- ❏ Alcohol swabs
- ❏ Over-the-counter pain medications: acetaminophen (Tylenol, Excedrin), aspirin (Ecotrin, Bayer Aspirin), *and* a nonsteroidal anti-inflammatory agent (Motrin, Advil)
- ❏ Thermometer
- ❏ Inexpensive stethoscope
- ❏ Inexpensive blood pressure gauge
- ❏ Syrup of ipecac, used to induce vomiting
- ❏ Over-the-counter antinausea medication
- ❏ Over-the-counter diarrhea medication
- ❏ Glycerin suppositories
- ❏ Stool softener
- ❏ Benadryl elixir, used to counteract severe allergic reactions
- ❏ Unscented premoistened wipes
- ❏ Cotton balls
- ❏ Q-Tips
- ❏ Latex gloves, available in pop-up dispenser boxes
- ❏ Water-based lubricant gel
- ❏ Canned nutritional supplements such as Ensure
- ❏ Gatorade or a similar sports drink for replacing crucial electrolytes
- ❏ Extra sheets and pillowcases if necessary
- ❏ Electric hospital bed

Place small plastic trash cans with liners at strategic locations—by the bed, a favorite chair, the dinner table. This way the patient can spit up phlegm or vomit without having to get up.

Obtain a cordless telephone with a two-way intercom feature. These can be purchased, rented, or borrowed and will help make it unnecessary to holler back and forth. A sick person's having to yell or repeat himself saps his energy, and the noise is stressful for everyone.

The intercom saves us countless steps as well. Dedicated intercom systems and baby monitors also do the trick, although the latter affords only one-way communication, and the former doesn't free you nearly as much as a portable phone.

✳ *Giving the patient a hand bell seems like a lovely idea until about the second day—when the incessant ringing begins to grate on your nerves.*

Move or rearrange items to prevent tripping. Take up scatter rugs and move decorative objects, glass tables, coffee tables, furniture with sharp corners, and anything else that could conceivably cause an accident. Most of us will be caring for someone who has some difficulty getting around. Bob, for example, was physically weak. What's more, the surgeon had constructed the coronary graft using a vein taken from my father's left leg, leaving a painful incision that ran from groin to knee.

My brother and I cleared a circuit around the house for Dad: from his bedroom to the bathroom; from each of those two rooms to his favorite chair in the living room; from the living room to the kitchen table; and an unobstructed path to the front door. We paid attention to door frames and sturdy furniture so that he never had to take more than two or three steps without finding something to grab onto that could support his weight: the back of a sofa, the footboard of the bed, and so forth.

✱ *For people with Parkinson's disease or those who have trouble lifting their feet, consider removing all door thresholds, a common cause of stumbling.*

Modifying the Home

My father stood six feet two. I'm six feet six and a world-class triathlete. The first time I tried helping him into the bathtub, we teetered precariously over the edge. I was convinced that either I

Equipment and Supplies

Hospital beds, bedside commodes, walkers, wheelchairs, oxygen tanks, suction machines, air mattresses, and any other necessary equipment can be rented or bought outright from home-care agencies or their contractors.

---

was going to drop him, he was going to pull me in with him, or I was going to accidentally knock the hair dryer into the water and electrocute us both. (Most household accidents, incidentally, occur in the bathroom.)

The next day I installed a foot-long metal "grab bar" next to the tub. Building codes generally require that they be capable of supporting 250 pounds of force—more if the person weighs in excess of 200 pounds. The American Association of Retired Persons recommends anchoring grab bars into wall studs or into blocks of wood screwed directly into the studs. Fastening the bars to tiles or Sheetrock, or using nails, clamps, or Molly bolts, says the AARP, are not adequate.

Mounting a grab bar, available at many pharmacies and through mail-order companies that specialize in assistive/adaptive devices, is one of literally thousands of ways to improve home safety and comfort. What a difference it made for my father, who from then on could bathe himself safely. More labor-intensive and costly customizations include building a wheelchair ramp and installing an adjustable-height sink. Below is a room-by-room tour of sample home modifications, ranging from simple to extensive. It is not intended to be comprehensive, only to show you some of the helpful assistive products available.

Products and Modifications for the Bedroom

By "bedroom" we mean wherever the patient stays. Sometimes moving the ill person's bed to a centrally located room

---

Assistive Technology: Where to Find It and How to Comparison Shop

The National Rehabilitation Information Center's Abledata database of approximately 21,000 patient products enables you to comparison shop at home. A free service, Abledata will research specific categories of products for you—grab bars, stair lifts, space-saving doors—and send you up to 20 product descriptions at no cost. For up to 100 product reports, NARIC charges $5, and $5 for each additional 100 reports thereafter.

☎ Call Abledata at 800-227-0216/ 301-608-8998.

► See Appendix B: "Adaptive Technology," page 504.

---

on the ground floor—off the living room or the kitchen, for instance—proves more convenient for everyone. The patient feels less isolated, a part of things, and the care partner doesn't have to schlep all over the house quite as much.

- Hospital beds
- Metal trapeze bars hung from the ceiling or vertical ceiling-to-floor poles to help patients maneuver in and out of bed
- The Clapper (whose TV commercial has been the butt of jokes for years) and other noise-operated bedroom lights
- Motorized ceiling lifts for hoisting and transferring patients from bed to wheelchair and back again
- Long wooden tong devices that allow patients to pick up small items a foot or two away without having to get out of bed

Products and Modifications for the Bathroom

- Water-pressure-powered bath lifts
- Grab bars in the shower, opposite the shower, and by the toilet
- Shower benches or tub chairs for use in stall showers or tub showers
- Tub-transfer benches that permit the person to slide into the tub from a sitting position
- Handheld shower heads
- Power-operated bath lift
- Shower curtains to replace glass shower doors
- Elevate seats for toilets so patients don't have to squat down as far (but since sitting too erect can impede bowel movements, one solution is to combine the raised seat with a footrest)

Products and Tricks for Hallways and Stairways

- Wood or metal handles on walls adjacent to heavy or difficult-to-open doors so patients can grip them with one hand while turning the doorknob with the other
- Sturdy railings or vertical grab bars on both side of steps
- Stairway elevator

Methods for Modifying Furniture

- Tilt chairs forward by placing two-by-four wooden blocks under the rear legs, thus making it easier for the disabled to sit down and rise from a sitting position
- Remove caster wheels from chairs

Miscellaneous

- Adequately lit rooms, hallways, and stairways
- Magnetic door latches instead of cylinders to eliminate the need to turn doorknobs or press levers
- Soft-plastic sleeves over doorknobs, making them easier to turn by those

with Parkinson's disease, Lou Gehrig's disease, and other conditions that weaken hand muscles
- Remove area rugs altogether or spray the underside with a nonskid spray, apply two-sided tape, or place nonslip mats beneath them
- Portable or permanent wheelchair ramps

But Is It Covered?

Usually not. Medicare, Medicaid, and private insurers typically pay for what is termed *durable medical equipment* —wheelchairs, oxygen equipment, commodes, seat-lift chairs, lifts, tilt chairs, prosthetic devices—if prescribed by the doctor. However, they rarely cover home modifications without a fight. (See "How to Get the Most out of Health Insurance" in chapter 8, "Paying the Bills.") Of the three, the Medicaid program for indigent men and women is the most generous. While guidelines vary from state to state, most approve payment for items such as bath and shower chairs and grab bars.

Funding for assistive technology and home remodeling can take many forms: grants and loans from state and local agencies such as the state division of rehabilitative services, the state protection and advocacy agency, and community action agencies; the Veterans Administration; Lions Clubs, Rotary Clubs, and the Knights of Columbus; and church, synagogue, and other religious organizations, to name but a few.

Unfortunately, says Carla Putnam-Veal of the Assistive Technology Funding and Systems Change Project, few patients or caregivers pursue available aid. For one thing, most folks aren't even aware that financial assistance exists for people who are disabled by illness. "But also," she observes, "a lot of times patients and their families don't consider themselves as disabled per se."

The Assistive Technology Funding and Systems Change Project, a free re-

> **Writing an Effective Proposal for Funding**
>
> The American Association of Retired Persons suggests keeping your letter to two or three pages and addressing the following points: why you need to modify the home, your proposed solution, an estimate of the project's total cost as well as a breakdown of individual materials, and the amount, if any, that the patient is able to contribute.

ferral service sponsored by the United Cerebral Palsy Association, can save you time and effort in trying to locate an agency that will fund or arrange home modifications for patients. "The first thing we would do," says Putnam-Veal, "is refer the person to their state Tech Act Agency, which can then direct them to whatever resources are available." The difference between ATFSCP and many other information and referral programs is that it works with callers long term until they obtain the assistance they need. If one agency denies your succinct proposal requesting funding—be it for a grab bar, a wheelchair ramp, or a computerized communications aid—the project returns to the drawing board with you to target another prospective source of funding. In Putnam-Veal's experience, people who commit to seeing this often tedious and frustrating process through—making the necessary phone calls and writing the necessary follow-up letters— "generally are successful at getting what they need."

☎ Call the Assistive Technology Funding and Systems Change Project at 800-827-0093, Monday through Friday, 9:00 A.M. to 5:00 P.M. ET.

Dad hobbled out of the hospital escorted by his wife, Mary, Dave, and John. Dave drove Bob home in a sepa-

---

MONEY SAVER

The Internal Revenue Services allows patients to deduct equipment, furnishings, and permanent home modifications for access as medical expenses on their federal tax return.

---

rate car, unencumbered by suitcases, flowers, or other passengers. "I just want to get in my own bed," he said wistfully as he looked out the car window. When they rounded the clover leaf exit to Tillman's Corner, he relaxed visibly.

My father's house roosted high above the canal on wooden pilings. In his weakened condition, climbing those thirty steep steps must have felt like ascending a Mayan ruin, but Bob made it —one at a time, clutching the rail, and John steadying him from behind. (Your loved one should always go first. *Then* you collect the luggage.)

When my father finally collapsed into bed, he smiled and sighed, "Damn, that feels good."

Recommended Reading

Available free to members and nonmembers from the American Association of Retired Persons (800-424-3410) is "The Doable Renewable Home: Making Your Home Fit Your Needs." Whether you plan to hire a professional or do the job yourself, we recommend this excellent thirty-six-page book that describes and illustrates dozens of ways to modify the home for safety and convenience.

—2—

Dealing with the Doctors

Louise Fradkin, *seventy, of Levit-town, Pennsylvania: My mother was an executive secretary at a private school; she was a rather authoritarian figure who could instill terror in the teachers just by raising an eyebrow. But when it came to her doctor, she was completely passive. Like many older people, she put physicians on a pedestal and wouldn't dream of questioning them. I went with her to all her doctor appointments. She'd say, "If you have any questions, ask my daughter."*

Aside from the bond we share with our ill loved one, no relationship is more important during this time than the one between us and the primary doctor. Having a strong personal affinity is not necessary. However, mutual respect and trust are essential to building a rapport that feels comfortable—and comforting—to both us and the patient.

"Ideally, a patient has a physician who has known him for a long time and shares his values, or at least under-stands them," observes Dr. Howard Spiro of Yale University School of Medicine. But between our national propensity for relocating and the increased reliance on health care specialists, "medicine," he believes, "has largely become strangers taking care of strangers."

Whether your doctor is an old family friend or a hospital resident meeting the patient for the first time, it's been my experience that people's attitudes toward the medical profession fall into three categories—two of which can interfere with those all-important lines of communication.

1. *The Doctor as Deity.* By its very nature, the balance of power in the doctor-patient-caregiver triangle decidedly favors the physician. Seriously ill people can shrink from asking questions for fear of "bothering" or "offending" the doctor, subconsciously worrying that if they "misbehave," he may punish them by withholding treatment. When family

82

and friends also act beholden to the doctor, the patient is left without an effective advocate.

Senior citizens especially tend to regard physicians as omnipotent, a holdover from a time when choices regarding medical care were few, and doctors truly did know best. But today we can expect to encounter M.D.s who have given over the traditional sole lead for a part in a larger ensemble. Even the most prominent physician now sees his orders critiqued by a hospital review board (not to mention second-guessed more than occasionally by insurance companies) and interacts daily with other health care professionals from a cross section of disciplines.

Our expectations of doctors have changed, too, stemming from the public's prudent insistence on exercising its rights as consumers. "I find that caregivers today are much more aware of what's going on, ask more questions, and are far more assertive than my parents' generation," says Louise Fradkin, who cofounded the caregivers' support organization Children of Aging Parents. Regrettably, some folks miss the crucial distinction between healthy assertiveness and counterproductive antagonism, which leads to the other extreme:

2. The Adversarial Stance. The contentious care partner continually puts the doctor on the defensive, creating an us-against-them atmosphere and greeting each new development with a barrage of extraneous questions and uninformed opinions. Talk that could undermine the patient's confidence in the doctors or the treatment plan must be halted at once, no matter who the source is. That includes well-meaning friends with medical backgrounds.

If anyone sincerely believes better care can be found elsewhere, he should do his homework before broaching the matter with the patient. If you saw a segment on a TV newsmagazine program about a new therapy for heart disease, send away for a videotape or a transcript of the show. Comb newspapers and medical journals for information about this breakthrough. Have published articles to show your loved one or a concrete plan of action to propose, rather than firing off such vague charges as "I don't think your doctor knows what he's doing." ► *See "When Is It Appropriate to Change Doctors?" page 98.*

3. The Team Approach. In the ideal relationship, caregivers and physicians work in partnership.

Choosing a Doctor

The reality is that few people with a life-threatening illness shop around for medical care as they might for another professional service. Entry into the medical system typically follows either of two scenarios: an acute illness that abruptly lands you in the hospital for an emergency procedure or your regular physician suspecting a health problem and referring you to a specialist.

Once the process has been set in motion, folks usually stay on the conveyor belt as it carries them from one medical professional to another, whether they're pleased with the quality of care or not. The reluctance to get off in mid-ride is justified. Most patients (and caregivers) feel ill prepared to undertake the search for a new doctor.

I've generally found that if you share a history and a rapport with your primary physician, you can follow his recommendation and feel confident you're going to be in capable hands. In determining which course to pursue, everyone involved in the decision must honestly evaluate the goals of treatment. Based on our understanding of the diagnosis and the disease—limited though it may be at this point—is it realistic to hope that the ailment could possibly be brought under control, either permanently or temporarily, and with a quality of life acceptable to the patient? If the evidence suggests yes, then the foremost qualification we look

---

INSIDE INFORMATION

Not every community has a major medical center. One approach to obtaining state-of-the-art care locally is to arrange for a consultation at an institution known to be on the cutting edge of research and treatment for a particular condition. Doctors there design the blueprint for therapy, which many times can be carried out at a facility nearer to the patient's home. ► *See "Seeking a Second Opinion," page 86.*

---

for in a physician is experience with our loved one's particular problem.

By "experience" we mean that if your mother suffers from, say, a gynecologic cancer, the doctor sees dozens, if not hundreds, of women like her every year so that he is thinking constantly about this group of cancers and is skilled in the newest, most effective treatment techniques. We're not implying that you reflexively rule out general practitioners, but as numerous studies indicate, having an experienced physician behind you can improve the outcome. According to a 1995 study of 220,000 Medicare patients, heart attack victims who were treated by a cardiologist were 15 percent less likely to die within the following year than those cared for by a general practitioner, while in a ten-year study of people with the human immunodeficiency virus, going to a physician experienced in HIV treatment nearly doubled those patients' survival time, from fourteen to twenty-six months.

When it is acknowledged that the aim of treatment isn't therapeutic but *palliative*—that is, intended to keep a terminally ill person comfortable—the physician's bedside manner and accessibility eclipse clinical expertise on our list of priorities. For a feeble eighty-five-year-old woman with irreversible emphysema, osteoporosis, and the stirrings of Alzheimer's disease, the "best" doctor may well be the local internist she has trusted for thirty years, who knows her medical history and her family, and returns phone calls on the weekend.

You could apply the same yardstick to choosing a hospital, which is the other route some folks take to accessing medical care. Instead of researching individual physicians, they seek an institution that specializes in cancer care, AIDS care, poststroke rehabilitation, and so forth. These tend to be larger teaching hospitals affiliated with a medical school. What they offer are high-tech facilities, cutting-edge therapies, and round-the-clock critical care in all subspecialties.

However, if we're beyond the point of heroic interventions, a smaller nonteaching facility—often a community hospital—may be a more practical choice. What it lacks in sophisticated technology and specialists of every stripe it often makes up for with more warmth and personalized attention. When we're seriously ill with hopes of getting better, we appreciate the fact that the attending physician and the resident and the intern are all keeping their eyes on us. But when we're terminally ill, an audience of doctors in training at the bedside to observe even the most minor procedure can seem an unnecessary intrusion and an indignity.

❋ *If your loved one wishes to be treated at a particular medical center, you can ask the primary physician to make the referral for you, or you can do so yourself by contacting the facility's physician referral department. Perhaps you or the primary physician have a doctor there in mind; if not, the department will route the patient to someone appropriate. Should you make these ar-*

rangements yourself, you'll need to send the primary physician a written request for him to transfer all medical records and notes to the new hospital.

The ABC's of Getting Referrals

Ask your regular physician and/or nurses at the hospital or doctor's office or other caregivers and patients you meet.

* *An effective technique for getting a straight answer from medical professionals is to personalize the question this way: "If you were sick with [cancer, cardiovascular disease, and so forth], where would you go for treatment or which doctor would you choose?"*

* *Ask other patients and caregivers what they liked and didn't like about the doctor or hospital.*

Browse the *Directory of Physicians in the United States* or the *Official American Board of Medical Specialties Directory of Board Certified Medical Specialists.* These multivolume reference books, available in most libraries, list physicians alphabetically by state, along with their specialties, subspecialties, type of practice, the hospital(s) where they have privileges, recognition awards, and other information that can help you select the right doctor for your loved one.

Call patient support organizations (American Liver Foundation, National Stroke Association, American Lung Association, and so forth) and government-funded health hot lines such as the CDC National HIV/AIDS Hotline and the Cancer Information Service, which routinely refer callers to specialists and specialty hospitals for that particular illness. ▶ *See Appendix A, "Recommended Resources," page 489.*

Points to Consider When Choosing a Doctor

Much of a patient's time is spent answering questions. When considering a doctor, however, it's *her* turn to do the asking. Certainly you can set up an office appointment to meet a new physician and get a feel for his style and how his practice operates. But in the interest of saving time (and money—expect to be charged for the visit, which insurance may or may not cover), feel free to call the office with the following questions. And when you call, you can determine whether the staff seems courteous and cooperative. This is important because you'll be dealing with them a lot.

- Is the doctor currently accepting new patients?
- Does the patient's insurance plan allow him to see this doctor?
- Is the doctor board-eligible or board-certified in his specialty?
- Is this a solo practice or a group practice? If the latter, how does the patient feel about not always seeing the same doctor?
- Approximately how many cases like our loved one's does the physician see per year?
- Is the doctor's office conveniently located? Don't underestimate the importance of proximity.
- At which area hospital(s) does the doctor have privileges? Is that an issue for our patient?
- Does the physician accept Medicare or Medicaid?
- Will the doctor honor the patient's advance directive?
- Is he receptive to caregivers participating in discussions about the patient's care?
- Will the doctor continue to oversee our loved one's care if she moves to a nursing home or hospice?

None of these questions addresses the quality we want most in a doctor:

**Questions to Ask About
a Doctor's Office Policies**

- What days/hours is the office open?
- How far in advance must we schedule appointments?
- How are medical emergencies typically handled, and how quickly can we see the doctor?
- Who can answer our questions if the doctor is unavailable?
- Who cares for patients after hours or when the doctor is away?
- How are bills and insurance copayments handled?

---

the ability to communicate. I can "rent" clinical expertise by the hour. When I'm sick, I need someone who takes the time to explain matters clearly and patiently, who puts me at ease, and who listens to my concerns and treats them seriously. The only way to gauge a doctor's communication skills in advance is to interview him, as we said; otherwise, the best we can do is rely on the recommendations of others.

Seeking a Second Opinion

Your loved one's health insurer may insist on a second opinion before okaying surgery or other major procedures, unless, of course, the medical problem demands immediate attention. The purpose could be to have a consensus on the proposed plan of treatment or to verify the diagnosis.

Whether or not insurance requires a second opinion, "it is always appropriate to get one," says Dr. Tom Rainey, especially when the condition is life-threatening. Obviously, no number of concurring opinions guarantees a treatment's success. But it's a good idea to solicit another physician's opinion if only to alleviate any nagging doubts and to discourage second-guessing.

How Is a Second Opinion Arranged?

Insurance may designate a doctor to review medical records, examine the patient, perhaps order additional tests, and then render a written opinion to the company. (The patient won't receive a copy unless she requests it.)

Or you may ask the primary physician for a referral to another doctor. Many times patients and caregivers are reluctant to request a second opinion. What if the doctor feels his competence is being questioned and takes offense? In Dr. Rainey's view, any physician who acts insulted or discourages you from seeking another opinion "is an immediate question mark." Consider this grounds for changing doctors.

* *If you're uncomfortable broaching the subject with the doctor, fib! Say the insurance company requires a second opinion.*

INSIDE INFORMATION

From a logistical standpoint, it's best to obtain a second opinion while the person is still hospitalized and all pertinent medical records and test results are available to a broad range of doctors. That may not be possible. Some physicians won't confer with someone else's postoperative patient until he's fully recovered from surgery, which could take months. Similarly, a person in the middle of a drug regimen—cancer chemotherapy, for example—may have to wait until the completion of treatment to schedule a second opinion consultation with another doctor.

Using the ABC's of gathering referrals, you can also find another physician yourself. One school of thought advocates pursuing an *independent* second opinion on the premise that it's human nature for doctors to lean toward recommending colleagues who share similar beliefs and professional biases.

When Professional Opinions Collide

For all the advances in medical knowledge and diagnostic accuracy, medicine remains as much an art as a science, which is why two doctors can analyze the same evidence and arrive at vastly different conclusions. Conflicting opinions regarding the problem or the solution shouldn't send us into a frenzy or necessarily undermine our confidence in the medical team. Much of the time an apparent "fork in the road" merely divides alternate routes that run side by side to the same destination. In other words, both positions might have merit.

The ideal situation is to have a trusted primary physician to help us sort through and interpret seemingly contradictory recommendations. These are daunting decisions, to be sure, but let's not get trapped into seeing things as either/or. In medicine the choices are rarely that clear-cut.

Obtaining Medical Records

A new physician will want to review the patient's medical records as well as any relevant films (X rays, scans, angiograms, and so on) and slides of diseased tissue removed during surgery or a biopsy. Get on this right away because it can take days—sometimes weeks—to assemble everything you need.

Call the consulting doctor's office. Ask them to send you a list of the medical records the doctor needs and ask the following:

- Does he need any films and/or pathology slides? If so, please specify which ones. Do we need to order duplicates?
- Which of these must arrive at your office prior to our appointment? May we bring any materials with us?

Call the primary physician's office or the hospital's department of medical records. Ask the following:

- What is your policy for requesting medical records and films? Must letters be notarized? What other information should I include? Typically, this would be the patient's name, date of birth, Social Security number, date of hospitalization, a list of the reports you want, plus the name, address, and phone number of the party receiving the records.
- Is there a charge for having copies made? What forms of payment do you accept?
- If you plan to pick up the records in person, ask: When will the records be available? Where do I pick them up, and from whom?
- If you plan to have the records sent to the physician or the patient, ask: When can we expect to receive them? How will they be sent? Then call back the consulting doctor's office and say, for example: "The hospital said it will Federal Express the records to you by Monday."

Written reports of X rays, scans, and biopsies are typically on file, but usually not the films or slides themselves. To get these duplicated you may have to write additional letters: for most films, to the department of radiology; and for pathology slides, to the department of pathology.

A word of advice to patients and caregivers: Resist the temptation to read the reports yourself. The language is so technical, you're likely to misinterpret the doctor's notes or invent your own meanings and alarm yourself and everyone around you unnecessarily. A

MONEY SAVER

Copies run anywhere from a few dollars to well over $100 per exposure.
Ask the consulting physician's office to specify, if possible, which films or slides it needs.

✳ *Should the medical facility allow you to pick up the originals, never send them through the mail. Hand-deliver them in a clearly marked envelope.*

---

good example would be a patient spotting "R/O carcinoma of the uterus" at the top of the page and taking this to mean she has cancer, when in fact "R/O" stands for "rule out." Translation: The physician has *discounted* cancer as a possible cause.

Care Partners, Patients, and Physicians: Ten Keys to Clear Communication

Talking to doctors doesn't come naturally to most of us. It takes practice. The following suggestions can help ensure that we and the medical team get in tune from the beginning and stay that way.

1. When several people are actively involved in someone's care, it's wise to designate one of them, two at most, as the point person for conferring with the primary physician. Ideally, these instructions come from the patient. Dad always told his doctors, "I want you to talk to Rodger or David." The rest of the family was free to speak to the internist or the surgeon or the oncologist whenever they wished, but all important news was to go directly to me or my brother, to alleviate confusion and lessen the chances of some crucial message getting translated inaccurately.

2. At the outset, tell the doctor you'd like to be informed *in detail* about your loved one's condition. "I got frustrated sometimes," says Naomi Black, whose daughter Nancy died of complications from liver disease, "because I didn't feel the doctors were telling us everything

that we wanted to know." Physicians are frequently accused of withholding information from families. In all fairness, many times the blank or distraught face before them tells doctors that the person simply cannot accept hearing the reality of the patient's condition or needs the prognosis softened with euphemisms. Relay your preferences clearly, and your doctor is likely to respond in kind.

✳ *Taking the initiative to educate ourselves about a loved one's illness sends a message that we welcome information and can be entrusted with it. Ask the physician to recommend any books, pamphlets, and videos she thinks would be enlightening. Informed questions elicit more precise answers.*

3. Specify *how* you would like updates on the person's condition to be relayed. Over the phone? In person only? Whenever possible, it's preferable for the ailing loved one and the caregiver to *hear the physician's words together*. During consultations, patients' minds can wander or snag on one statement the doctor made so that they miss his next point entirely. Or they're too frail, frightened, medicated, or mentally impaired to grasp what's being said. If your loved one responds better to written instructions, let the physician know.

Another consideration: How does the person react to distressing news? We don't want someone who is utterly terrified of being sick or prone to hysteria or emotionally unstable to be asked to sign a Do Not Resuscitate order without a family member or friend present. Believe me, it happens. Ask the doctor to hold off delivering word of any major developments until you can be at your loved one's side. The information should come from the physician's mouth, however, for several reasons:

A doctor's words carry an authority ours do not, especially when the message is one that nobody welcomes hearing. My telling a patient secondhand that "The doctors say there's nothing more they can do" is more likely to leave the door of denial ajar than if his physician looks him in the eye and says his condition is terminal.

Few of us are trained to relay this kind of information. While there are doctors who lack sensitivity, the physician has played this scene many times. She's also there to field the difficult questions that may follow.

Being the bearer of grim news sets us up as a lightning rod for anger or bitterness at a time when we want to be a source of comfort and support.

Our loved one must always feel confident that no one is keeping the facts from him and that ultimately he—unless unwilling or unable—is at the helm.

4. Take notes at doctors' appointments. It's up to us to help the person hear what was said and integrate it into the overall medical picture. Bring a journal for taking notes, but do so inconspicuously. With doctors' apprehension about malpractice claims at an all-time high, discretion is advisable. When you reach for your notebook, just say "I'll never remember this unless I write it down."

Likewise, I know folks who taperecord meetings with the physician. This is too intrusive. Although he probably won't object to being recorded, you're more likely to receive a guarded, formal interview than a candid impression of the case. You don't have to get every word down on paper, just the major points. It's better to concentrate on listening and ask for clarification than get extensive written notes.

5. Come prepared. List your concerns and questions beforehand. As questions pop into your head—you read a relevant article in the newspaper or a problem recurs that you'd forgotten to mention—jot them down in your journal, which you should carry with you to every appointment and patient visit. "I used to walk around the hospital with my notebook full of questions," recalls Johnetta Romanowski, who cared for her fiancé throughout his fight against lung cancer. "If Dennis's doctor didn't have time to answer them, he would take the notebook and give it back to me the next day with the answers written in it."

6. In your journal, keep a daily log of the person's symptoms. When describing symptoms to the doctor, "you need to be specific," says Dr. Tom Rainey, who suggests recording the following details:

- How frequently does the symptom occur?
- When did it start? How long did it last?
- Describe the symptom as accurately as possible—its appearance and what it felt like.
- If the symptom has occurred before, how did it compare to this most recent episode?
- Is the symptom confined to its original area? Has it spread?

Many people find it difficult to verbalize symptoms and side effects. Help them pinpoint the right word. Whereas a "burning" sensation in the chest may be indicative of nothing more serious than heartburn, "pressure" could signal the heart condition angina pectoris. Whatever the symptom—pain, diarrhea, forgetfulness, labored breathing—Dr. Rainey recommends expressing its severity on a scale of one to ten, with one denoting least severe and ten most severe.

Alert the doctor to anything else you think might help provide clues or a pattern to the problem. For example, if nausea is a recurrent symptom, what did your loved one eat today and when? From this information the physician may conclude that the person's diet is too high in fried or fatty foods (which can upset the digestive tract) or that he's taking his antibiotic on an empty stomach.

7. When speaking to the doctor, be concise and stick to the issues. "For many physicians," says Dr. Rainey, "the most frustrating patients or caregivers are those who go so far off track during a consultation that it's not helpful. The doctor has to spend his energy trying to redirect the interview into something more constructive instead of focusing on the patient's issues."

8. See to it that the patient is included in discussions about his care. Should you observe a physician excluding your loved one or treating him as if he were invisible, take it upon yourself to redirect the conversation to the patient. "Excuse me, Doctor," you say, making eye contact with your father. "Dad, did you understand that?" Or, "Mom, what do you think about what the doctor just said?"

9. If you don't understand something the doctor said or you have a question, speak up immediately. "The only stupid question is the one you don't ask" stresses Dr. Jack Lord of the American Hospital Association. I know I've interrupted doctors countless times to ask "Wait, can you go back a minute? What do you mean by that?" And if you're still unclear after hearing his answer, ask him to explain it again, until you're confident you understand. Doctors are accustomed to repeating information for patients and loved ones, so don't worry that he'll think you're a nuisance.

❋ *To test your understanding of what was said, repeat it back to the doctor in your own words. "So what you're saying is, my husband is going to need surgery to clip the aneurysm in his brain to prevent another stroke."*

10. After discussions with the doctor, "debrief" each other. Review your notes with the patient and reflect on the meeting later that day and the following day. Chances are you'll find that each of you came away with different interpretations of what the doctor said, raising new questions to note in your journal and to ask the physician the next time you see her.

Deciphering the Language of Medicine

In any situation, be it accompanying a loved one to a doctor's appointment or bringing in a car for repairs, understanding the terminology is perhaps our first step to gaining a sense of control. Don't worry: You needn't memorize an entire medical dictionary; mastering the rudimentary word elements in Table 2.2 will enable you to follow most conversations. For example, the suffix *-oscopy* appended to a noun denotes an endoscopic examination; *-otomy*, surgery. Knowing this, should Mom's gynecologist tell us she's scheduling a laparos-*copy*, we won't confuse it with a lap-aro*tomy*, as laypeople frequently do. The difference between the two surgical procedures? A hospital stay of about one week. In a laparoscopy, a flexible viewing instrument called a laparoscope is passed through a tiny incision in the abdomen, and the patient typically goes home within four hours. By contrast, a laparotomy is major exploratory surgery, with a recuperation period of approximately six weeks.

Inquiries to Make at the Time of Diagnosis

- Please explain the disease to us.
- How is it generally managed or treated?
- How will this impact on the patient's daily life?
- Can you suggest reading material for learning more about the disease?
  ◀ See "Seeking a Second Opinion," page 86.

TABLE 2.1
Questions to Ask About Upcoming Tests and Treatments

Question	Tests	Surgery	Other Treatment
What will this procedure tell us and why do you feel it is necessary?	✔	✔	
What is this treatment's success rate?		✔	✔
Are there other treatment options available?		✔	✔
Is this an outpatient procedure? An inpatient procedure? If the former, will the person be able to drive himself there and back? If the latter, how long will the patient be hospitalized?	✔	✔	✔
When will treatment begin? How long will the patient be undergoing treatment?			✔
How far in advance must the procedure be scheduled?	✔	✔	✔
Is any preparation necessary (fasting, enema, discontinuing medications, etc.) beforehand?	✔	✔	✔
Please explain the procedure from start to finish.	✔	✔	✔
Who performs the procedure?	✔	✔	✔
Is a family member or friend allowed in the room with the patient during the procedure?	✔		✔
Does the procedure require sedation and/or anesthesia? Can we request either one if we wish?	✔	✔	✔
How long does the procedure usually take?	✔	✔	✔
Does the procedure cause pain, discomfort, claustrophobia? If so, what can be done to make my loved one more comfortable?	✔	✔	✔
Are there any common side effects and complications? If so, how are they managed?	✔	✔	✔
Are there any serious health risks involved? What can go wrong?	✔	✔	✔
When will we know the test results?	✔		
How accurate is the test? Will further testing be required?	✔		
How much does the procedure cost? Does my loved one's health insurance cover it?	✔	✔	✔
How long is the average recuperation from this surgery?		✔	
Will the patient need someone to care for him at home?		✔	✔
Is follow-up care needed?		✔	✔
How will we know if we're making progress?		✔	✔

TABLE 2.2
Key Medical Prefixes, Suffixes, and Root Words Worth Knowing

Word Element; Refers to	Examples
Pertaining to Medical Procedures	
-centesis procedures in which a syringelike instrument is used to pierce and drain one of the body's hollow spaces	• *Thoracentesis:* aspirating fluid from the thoracic cavity housing the heart and the lungs • *Abdominal Paracentesis:* aspirating fluid from the abdominal cavity
-ectomy surgically excising part or all of an organ	• *Mastectomy:* surgically removing part or all of a breast • *Lobectomy:* surgically removing a section of the lung, brain, or liver
-gram/-graphy recording images, sound, electrical activity	• *Pyelography:* an X-ray study (pyelogram) of the kidneys and ureters • *Electrocardiography:* a recording of the heart's electrical activity
-ology the study of	• *Radiology:* the branch of medicine that uses X rays, radioactive substances, and other forms of radiant energy to diagnose and treat disease • *Oncology:* the branch of medicine that deals with diagnosing and treating tumors
-ostomy the surgical creation of an artificial opening, or stoma	• *Colostomy:* an opening in the large intestine for the purpose of evacuating the bowel • *Tracheostomy:* an opening in the trachea (windpipe) to facilitate breathing and removing secretions
-otomy any surgical incision	• *Craniotomy:* incision through the skull • *Laparotomy:* incision through the abdominal wall
-plasty plastic surgery to restore, reconstruct, or improve the appearance of body parts that are diseased, damaged, malformed, or missing	• *Angioplasty:* surgically repairing a vessel that carries blood or lymph fluid • *Esophagoplasty:* surgically repairing the esophagus
radio- procedures utilizing high-energy rays	• *Radiography:* making X-ray films of internal body structures • *Radiotherapy:* using X rays or other forms of radiant energy to treat diseases such as cancer

Word Element; Refers to	Examples
-scopy a visual examination conducted with a viewing instrument	• *Bronchoscopy:* inspecting the large airways of the lung through a bronchoscope • *Laryngoscopy:* inspecting the larynx (voice box) through a laryngoscope

Pertaining to Medical Conditions

-algia	pain	• *Neuralgia:* nerve pain • *Hepatalgia:* liver pain
dys-	something abnormal or functioning improperly	• *Dysrhythmia:* an abnormal heartbeat or other rhythmic disturbance • *Dysphagia:* difficulty eating or swallowing
-emia	a condition of the blood	• *Septicemia:* blood poisoning • *Uremia:* a buildup in the blood of urea, the principal component of urine
hyper-	a high or excessive condition	• *Hyperglycemia:* an abnormally high concentration of sugar in the blood • *Hypertension:* chronically elevated blood pressure
hypo-	something low or deficient	• *Hypoglycemia:* an abnormally low concentration of sugar in the blood • *Hypokalemia:* an abnormally low concentration of potassium in the blood
-itis	inflammation	• *Phlebitis:* inflammation of the blood vessels • *Colitis:* inflammation of the inner lining of the colon
-megaly	enlargement	• *Cardiomegaly:* enlargement of the heart • *Heptamegaly:* enlargement of the liver
-oma	a benign or malignant tumor	• *Leiomyoma:* a benign tumor of the uterus • *Carcinoma:* cancer
-osis	disease or an abnormal increase	• *Toxoplasmosis:* a protozoal infection • *Acidosis:* a dangerous accumulation of acid in the blood and body tissues
-pathy	a noninflammatory condition or disease	• *Cardiopathy:* any disease of the heart • *Neuropathy:* any disease of the nerves

(continued on next page)

TABLE 2.2 *(cont.)*
Key Medical Prefixes, Suffixes, and Root Words Worth Knowing

Word Element; Refers to		Examples
Pertaining to Medical Conditions *(cont.)*		
-penia	a deficiency	• *Thrombocytopenia:* a deficiency of blood platelets • *Leukopenia:* a deficiency of white blood cells
-plegia	paralysis	• *Paraplegia:* paralysis of the legs • *Hemiplegia:* paralysis on one side of the body
-pnea	breathing	• *Dyspnea:* difficulty breathing • *Apnea:* temporary suspenson of breathing
-sclerosis	hardening	• *Atherosclerosis:* hardening of the arteries • *Myosclerosis:* hardening of muscle tissue
Pertaining to Body Organs and Body Systems		
aden-	glands	Adenectomy
angi-	blood vessels	Angiogram
arteri-	arteries	Arteriogram
arthr-	joints	Arthroscopy
cardi-	heart	Cardiogram
cephal-	head	Cephalitis (also known as encephalitis)
cerebr-	brain	Cerebrovascular accident (CVA, or stroke)
cervic-	neck, cervix	Cervicectomy
col-	colon (bowel)	Colectomy
colp-	vagina	Colpectomy
cyst-	bladder, cyst	Cystectomy
derm-	skin	Dermatitis
encephal-	brain	Encephalopathy
gastr-	stomach	Nasogastric tube
hemat-/hemo-	blood	Hematoma (contusion), hemodialysis
hepat-	liver	Hepatitis
immuno-	immune system	Immunotherapy (therapy aimed at bolstering the body's immune response against infection)
laryng-	larynx	Laryngectomy

Word Element; Refers to		Examples
lymph-	lymphatic system; also lymphocytes, a type of white blood cell	Lymphoma
mast-	breast	Mastectomy
my-	muscle	Poliomyelitis
nephr-	kidneys	Nephrectomy
neur-	brain and central nervous system	Neurosurgery
ophthalm-	eye	Ophthalmologist
orchi-	testicles	Orchiectomy
oste-	bone	Osteoporosis
pharyn-	pharynx (throat)	Pharyngectomy
phleb-	vein	Phlebotomy (drawing blood)
pneumo-/ pulmo-	lungs	Pneumonectomy, pulmonitis (also pneumonitis)
proct-	rectum	Proctoscopy
splen-	spleen	Splenomegaly
thorac-	chest	Thoracoscopy
thyr-	thyroid	Thyroidectomy
tracheo-	trachea	Tracheopathy
ureter	ureter	Ureterectomy
urethr-	urethra	Transurethral resection
uro-	urinary tract	Urologist
uter-	uterus	Uterine cancer
vesic-	the bladder or a small bladderlike cavity filled with fluid	Seminal vesicle

Tracking Down the Doctor

Unless we're able to accompany our loved one to appointments, arranging a face-to-face audience with the physician may require sleuthlike skills. You can station yourself in the patient's room until the doctor stops by during rounds, except that an emergency or a procedure that runs longer than anticipated could delay the doctor's visit. You might wind up waiting there all day, only to give up and go home just minutes before he strolls into the room. Try tracking the physician through the hospital operator or make an appointment for a private consultation at the doctor's office.

If you have a burning question that can be answered over the phone, call the office secretary in the morning and ask her how the doctor's schedule shapes up for the day. During what hours does she think you'll have your best shot at getting through to him? Or you can ask the patient to call you from her hospital room when the doctor walks in and hand him the phone.

Be Judicious with Questions for the Doctor

While we have a right to expect the primary physician to be reasonably accessible in person and by phone, let's not waste our time and his time with calls about day-to-day management that other health care personnel can answer just as readily—and certainly more quickly. It might take days for the doctor to get back to you with the name of the antidepressant he just prescribed for your husband, while the room nurse, the charge nurse, and the physician's assistant all have that information in the chart. Save calls to the attending for discussions related to big issues such as an explanation of the diagnosis, a change in the prognosis, a new symptom that arises (and you want to know if the doctor wishes to see the patient immediately), or a medication that doesn't seem to be working.

If you want information about a hospitalized loved one's condition after hours, when patients' phones have been turned off and the attending has gone for the night, call the nurse's desk and ask for the primary nurse. She is more than familiar with the case and highly capable of answering your questions herself or finding out the answers for you.

Dissatisfied with the Doctor?

With a loved one's life at stake and people's emotions wound tighter than a

---

Tips for Avoiding Phone Tag

Missing the doctor's call can have serious ramifications. Whoever is in charge of speaking to the doctor should consider purchasing or borrowing

- an answering service or machine, which is useful when the phone rings while you're helping the patient shower and you can't leave him alone;
- call waiting, so that the doctor's office doesn't have to try your number repeatedly because you're on another call;
- a portable phone, for when you need to take calls in private, perhaps away from the patient or others;
- a cell phone, so the doctor can reach you when you're in transit;
- call forwarding, so you don't have to wait beside the phone for a call.

And when you tell the doctor's secretary you'll be at a certain number at a certain time, be there! It shouldn't be the physician's responsibility to track you down.

TABLE 2.3
Questions and Answers

Questions About . . .	Concerning a Patient in the Hospital	Concerning a Patient Receiving Home Care
	In Lieu of the Primary Physician, Try Asking	
Upcoming tests and procedures	• Physician's assistant • Room nurse • Charge nurse • Resident doctor • Nurse or technician/technologist in the department that performs the test or procedure	• Home-care nurse or hospice nurse • Physician's office nurse or assistant • Nurse or technician/technologist in the facility that performs the test or procedure
Medications and dosages	• Physician's assistant • Room nurse • Charge nurse • Medications nurse • Resident doctor	• Home-care nurse or hospice nurse • Physician's office nurse or assistant
The long-term care plan *(When is the patient expected to be discharged? Will home care be necessary? A nursing home?)*	• Any nurse • Hospital social worker • Resident doctor • Physician's assistant	• Hospice nurse • Nursing home staff • Hospice or nursing home social worker

tourniquet, misunderstandings and disagreements are inevitable. Physicians are human beings making discretionary judgments in a complex, unpredictable setting, and we are one of many individuals demanding their time and attention. We don't run off to someone else the first time we're unhappy with the doctor—or the second or third time. Like a marriage, the physician-patient partnership requires commitment. Changing doctors is always an option, but we want to preserve the continuity of medical care whenever possible.

If there's one piece of advice for averting a "divorce," it's to address conflicts as they arise. The biggest mistake patients and care partners make is swallowing complaints rather than risking a confrontation. Smoldering anger and resentment eventually ignite. Meanwhile, the physician may not even be aware that a problem exists. Should you feel that a doctor has handled a situation poorly, speak your mind, following the guidelines below:

1. Compose yourself—at least overnight. Never act in the heat of the moment, but don't wait so long that details become blurry, the urgency fades, and you ultimately neglect to pursue the matter.

2. Compose your thoughts. If you're the type that's easily flustered, put them in writing. State your case concisely and logically, addressing such points as:

• your exact grievance: for example, "You didn't call back when I rang to remind you that you hadn't ordered the pain medication for my father, as we'd discussed."

- how this made you or the patient feel: for example, "Pop was furious and hurting pretty badly, and I was up with him all night."
- how you would like to see the situation rectified. State your goal and offer solutions, such as, "What's the best way to reach you in the future? If I can't get in touch with you, who else can I speak to?"

3. Include the patient in the discussion—for two reasons: so the physician understands you're expressing the patient's feelings, not your own, and so the ailing person doesn't have to worry that perhaps you said something to offend or alienate the doctor.

4. Substantiate your claims. Don't hurl vague charges like "The nursing care at this hospital is terrible!" Offer concrete examples: "Yesterday my brother pressed the call button for an hour before the nurse's aide brought his bedpan."

5. Phrase your comments as objective statements or questions, not indictments. Instead of griping "The sedative you prescribed didn't work," which is likely to prompt a defensive response, say "My sister was tossing and turning all night. Could we discuss the possibility of either increasing the dosage or trying something else?"

6. Be persistent. Should the physician seem to be dodging the issue, don't let him off the hook. Repeat how you feel.

When It Is Appropriate to Change Doctors

Changing the primary physician in the middle of treatment for a life-threatening illness should be viewed as a measure of last resort, one that is warranted in but ten situations and then only after you've made your displeasure known

and repeatedly attempted to rectify matters.

1. The doctor habitually fails to return calls within a reasonable period of time. Naturally our notion of "reasonable" is likely to differ from the physician's. When you've left a message with the answering service at midnight saying that your elderly mother is so agitated she can't sleep, any amount of waiting for a callback seems interminable. From the doctor's perspective, though, a patient's anxiety does not constitute an emergency; he is not being negligent by getting back to you in the morning.

What constitutes an unacceptable delay? When you call from home or the ER stating explicitly that it is an emergency, and you don't receive a timely callback. ▶ *See "When Should You Call an Ambulance?," page 182.*

2. The medical team refers your loved one to another physician or facility. No matter how much you depend on him or how comfortable he makes the patient feel, your primary doctor may recommend a sophisticated or experimental treatment available exclusively at a different hospital and under another physician's care. Or the patient may be at the stage of illness where care would be best carried out by a home-care agency, a hospice, a nursing home, a rehabilitation clinic, or a family practitioner.

3. Gross negligence or indisputable medical incompetence. Examples of gross negligence or clear incompetence include amputating the wrong leg, enucleating the one good eye, or administering a substance that triggers a severe reaction when the physician was explicitly informed about the allergy in question. Anyone can make a mistake, and many common medical errors can be overcome or reversed quickly. But it's time to change doctors when a blunder that could have been avoided causes permanent harm or when an irreconcilable breach of trust develops.

4. The doctor refuses to honor the patient's advance directive stipulating that no extraordinary measures be taken to prolong her life, or the wishes of the next of kin or medical proxy.

5. Repeated clashes with the doctor over the issue of adequate symptom control. It's one thing for a physician to disagree with us about when to move from therapeutic treatment to palliative care, but quite another when escalating requests for symptom management are ignored. Only the patient or his designated advocate can decide how much pain, nausea, anxiety, sleep deprivation, immobility, dependence, and indignity he is willing to endure. While we should value the experience and advice of health care providers, when a doctor says "It isn't *that* bad" or "My other patients don't complain so much," move on.

A lack of personal chemistry doesn't necessarily preclude patients and physicians from treating each other cordially and communicating openly. *Toxic chemistry*, on the other hand, is sufficient cause to leave a doctor even if doing so disrupts treatment temporarily. "Toxic" connotes a physician-patient relationship that is irredeemably detrimental as in the following situations.

6. The doctor appears uncomfortable discussing issues related to a life-threatening illness, which in turn presents a barrier to communication for the patient and family.

7. The doctor seems overly fatalistic about the value of therapy. If faced with this dilemma, having explored the patient's treatment choices will help you differentiate between a physician who is being unduly pessimistic when he says "there's nothing we can do" and one who is being bluntly realistic.

8. The doctor dismisses your questions, including those regarding a second opinion or a different course of treatment. A physician can disagree with you. He can ultimately decline your request for, say, medication. But it is his professional obligation to hear

you out and respond thoughtfully and respectfully.

9. The doctor tries to make you feel guilty or irresponsible when you insist on doing what you feel is best. Any physician who implies that a decision you make will cause the patient's death has neither you nor your loved one's best interests at heart.

10. The patient feels, *for whatever reason*, that communication with the doctor has crumbled permanently. There are doctors who never call back, speak to patients and their care partners condescendingly, refuse to answer questions, become defensive at the slightest prodding, and repeatedly ignore requests, both major and minor. You can find among the ranks of physicians flagrant sexists, racists, homophobes, religious fanatics, and self-important jerks. *Find a better doctor right away.* This is not someone you'll be able to deal with effectively when the patient's condition deteriorates or the decisions grow tougher or the pressure mounts or you're worn out, confused, and brokenhearted—and your loved one needs you the most.

The Smart Way to Make the Switch

Never drop one doctor until another has accepted the case, for once you inform the current attending of your intentions, expect to tumble to the bottom of his administrative priority list. What would happen, then, if the consultation with the new physician was delayed for some reason, and in the interim the patient grew sicker?

Rarely is this a comfortable situation for either party, though by no means should that deter you from proceeding with your plan. Our goal is not only to avoid winding up in limbo but to forgo or at least minimize a period of transition from doctor A to doctor B. Here's how:

Once the prospective doctor has reviewed the case, examined the patient, and offered her medical opinion, explain that you're considering changing attendings. Be specific as to why, such as, "We feel that Dr. A. is overly conservative when it comes to prescribing medications for pain, nausea, and so forth, and that Dad has been suffering unnecessarily as a result. Could you please tell us your position on symptom relief?"

Next ask if she would take the case and whether doing so would place her in an awkward position. For all you know, she might be your erstwhile physician's sister-in-law, golfing buddy, former classmate, or subordinate in the hospital or medical center hierarchy.

After the new physician has accepted the case, write Dr. A. a short letter from the patient. Without going into the reasons why, simply state: "I've decided to continue treatment with Dr. B. She will assume the responsibilities of primary physician and will be supervising my care henceforth. Thank you for your cooperation." Have the patient sign it if he's able. If not, sign it on his behalf and attach a copy of your medical power of attorney. Forward a copy of the letter to the new attending.

✳ *If the person is hospitalized at the time of the change, personally hand additional copies to the charge nurse and* *the admitting office, and send copies to the chief of medical services and the nursing supervisor.*

Before you notify the present primary physician, make sure you have adequate supplies of all essential medications, especially those for controlling heart conditions, hypertension, emphysema, pain, nausea, anxiety, and insomnia.

A Final Thought: Dissatisfaction or Denial?

Understandably, a patient's loved ones may feel betrayed when treatment fails or the outcome is far worse than they were led to believe. Those of us involved in the decision to change doctors need to assess honestly the justification for contemplating such a move, especially in cases where an ill person isn't responding to treatment. Are we genuinely unhappy with the caliber of medical care—after all, it can be difficult to have good feelings about a doctor who always seems to impart depressing news—or are we subconsciously hoping to find someone to paint us a sunnier picture whether the medical reality supports such optimism or not?

—3—

The Everyday Angel's
Cram Course in Essential
Nursing Skills

The day of discharge from the hospital is often one of conflicting emotions, both for the patient and for the person shouldering responsibility for his day-to-day care.

Naturally we're elated to have our loved one home, but beneath the joy bubbles an undercurrent of anxiety. Here there's no nurse or lifesaving technology just down the hall. Even if the person's condition warrants visits from a home health care provider, for all but perhaps those dozen hours a week he is completely dependent on *us*.

What's more, it is now routine for patients to be sent home before they're fully recovered, a trend that began in 1983. That was the year the federal government restructured Medicare to pay fixed fees for specific medical conditions, assigning each to one of some five hundred "diagnosis-related groups," or *DRGs*. Whether a seventy-year-old Medicare patient takes one week or two to recuperate from gallbladder surgery (DRG No. 198), the hospital's reim-

bursement is the same. Inpatient stays have shrunk ever since—from an average of 7.2 days in 1980 to 5.7 days in 1995.

If you've never taken care of a seriously ill person before, the enormous responsibility ahead is bound to seem overwhelming. What kind of nurse will you make? Will you know what to do in an emergency?

You'll do fine. In Dr. Gerald Fletcher's years as a cardiologist at Atlanta's Emory University Hospital, he has found that "the type of people who are willing to care for someone at home usually manage quite well." Ellen Wilson, a home hospice nurse in the Seattle area, makes a similar observation: "I'm always amazed at the power people have to overcome obstacles and to perform tasks that they never would have thought they could do."

The trick, Dr. Fletcher advises, is to "learn everything you can while you're with the patient in the hospital, where there are doctors and nurses to back you up. Get the hands-on experience there so you won't be frightened when the person comes home. Think about situations that might arise and ask whatever questions come to mind, no matter how silly they may sound to you."

Hospital nurses consider patient and family teaching an integral part of their job, whether it's to demonstrate how to inject a diabetic's daily insulin or how to suction mucus from the throat of a person with end-stage emphysema. Paul Clarke, father of two, underwent kidney transplant surgery in 1992 at Hartford Hospital in Connecticut. Throughout his three-week hospitalization, says his wife, Gerri, "the entire staff worked to prepare us for going home." As a transplant recipient, Paul now faced a lifetime of immunosuppressant therapy to reduce the threat of rejection. "Every time the nurses walked into the room carrying a medication," recalls Gerri, "they sat down and talked to us about it until we could identify each pill and why Paul was taking it. [At one time, her husband took thirty pills a day.] And before they walked out the door, they always asked us if we had any questions to ensure that we fully understood what was going on. It was fabulous preparation for caregiving and made us far less fearful."

This is an ongoing education. Throughout an illness's progression, other health care professionals—homecare nurses, technical support personnel from companies that lease medical equipment, and anyone else who enters the picture—will help you handle problems as they arise. In home hospice care for the dying, says Nurse Wilson, "a lot of our focus is on teaching the family and empowering them to do most of the care. When we see a medical problem developing, we'll explain what complications might crop up and how they can manage them."

I've yet to meet a care partner who didn't blanch the first time someone showed him how to change an ileostomy bag or clean a tracheostomy tube. With guidance, though, you'll gain confidence until such tasks become second nature to you. Trust us: You're about to surprise yourself.

A Caregiver's Basic Daily Skills

Most of us will find our days focused on the tasks, precautions, and nursing skills listed below, whether a loved one is on the way to recovery or near death.

1. Encouraging the person to drink plenty of water.
2. Safeguarding against infection.
3. Assisting with daily bathing, toileting, and dressing.
4. Keeping skin clean and moisturized.
5. Turning bedridden loved ones at least every one to two hours.
6. Seeing to it that the patient exercises his limbs four times a day.
7. Checking vital signs in the morning, at night, and anytime a new symptom emerges.
8. Administering medications.
9. Knowing when to call the doctor or the local emergency number.

Keeping Patients Hydrated

"Ask the average person if they drink a lot, and they'll say they do," observes Paula Erwin-Toth, a nurse at the Cleveland Clinic Foundation Medical Center. "But when we take their fluid history, we usually find they don't drink nearly enough water."

Surprisingly few folks, healthy or sick, appreciate the importance of drinking the equivalent of six to eight

16-ounce glasses of liquid a day. The body can function without food for weeks on end but can survive only a few days without H_2O, which tours the circulatory system as part of blood and lymphatic fluid and permeates tissue spaces to bathe literally every cell.

Water comprises more than half our weight. A physically active person excretes about two and a half quarts a day, most of it through urine, feces, perspiration, and respiration. Unless an equal amount of fluid is replenished, he will quickly become dehydrated.

Seriously ill patients are prone to dehydration for a double-barreled reason: Not only can common symptoms such as chronic diarrhea and vomiting deplete the body of water, but to anyone who is sick and weak and nauseous, the thought of drinking anything can seem unpalatable. Consequently, the problem is often one of excessive output compounded by insufficient intake.

Conditions That Can Lead to Dehydration

- Nausea/vomiting
- Diarrhea
- Profuse perspiration due to fever
- Any neurological disorder that leaves someone confused, forgetful, or unable to feed herself

- Unusually frequent urination (*diuresis*), a side effect of some medications
- Dry mouth or an unpleasant taste in the mouth
- Conditions that make swallowing difficult
- Abnormally high respiratory rates
- Mechanical ventilation

Conditions That Dehydration Can Lead to

- Fluid and electrolyte imbalance
- Uremia
- Urinary tract infection
- Bedsores
- Respiratory tract infection
- Constipation
- Acidosis

Signs of Dehydration

- Infrequent urination with little output
- Thirst
- Dry mouth, gums, throat, tear ducts
- Dry or cracked skin that has lost its elasticity
- Dry, sunken eyes
- Elevated temperature (water helps regulate body temperature)
- Brownish or rust-colored urine

✱ *If you pinch a fleshy area on the person's body, does the skin stay raised, resembling a pup tent? This is evidence of severe dehydration.*

Some 60 percent of the fluid we lose daily escapes as urine. To know for sure whether or not you have a case of *fluid-volume deficit* on your hands, measure the volume of each urination over a twenty-four-hour period by having your loved one relieve himself into a plastic urinal or similar collection device. Pour it into a one-quart measuring cup. Someone who is dehydrated would expel significantly less than the approximately forty-eight ounces, or six cups, of urine normally produced.

✚ *Notify the doctor, home-care nurse, or hospice nurse promptly if twelve hours go by without urination.*

Should a noticeable deficit persist over the course of a day or two, point it out to the nurse. Dehydration can snowball into a life-threatening crisis. The water in the body delivers crucial minerals called *electrolytes:* sodium, potassium, calcium, magnesium, chloride, bicarbonate, and phosphate. While too much or too little of any electrolyte can seriously disrupt body functions, we are most concerned with the concentrations of sodium and potassium, which regulate the balance of water within and outside the cells. Electrolyte values are determined by analyzing the blood serum. A blood drawing can be carried out at home by a home health care company, and the lab results faxed directly to the doctor.

A person suffering from dehydration will likely have elevated levels of sodium and chloride but deficits of potassium, calcium, and magnesium. Potassium deficiency can trigger abdominal pain, dimmed reflexes, and irregular heart rhythms, or cardiac *arrhythmias.* It can also lead to *acidosis.* Here the equilibrium between the body fluid's acid base content tilts toward acidity, bringing on still more complications. Inadequate calcium or magnesium can produce equally serious symptoms, including arrhythmias.

Remember, however, that diminished output is not always indicative of dehydration. Our patient may be consuming plenty of liquid but is retaining fluid on account of incipient kidney failure, peripheral edema, or pulmonary edema brought on by congestive heart failure.

Tricks for Getting Patients to Drink

Handing an ill loved one a tumbler of water and expecting him to drink it down is like asking a healthy person to chug the contents of a fish tank. How many of us actually finish a full glass in one sitting?

Patients will find it much easier to drink if they sip gradually throughout the day instead of taking big gulps. Mary Ann Reeks, a home hospice nurse from Atlanta, suggests filling the glass only halfway. "A full glass can be intimidating to patients," she says. "They feel as though they have to drink it all right away. We encourage caregivers to pour just a little bit of liquid over ice and keep it next to the bed."

For basic hydration, you can't beat water. But here are some alternatives: ice chips, ice pops, electrolyte freezer pops, sherbet, sorbet, and Jell-O. Freeze favorite beverages into ice cubes, then break them into ice chips for sucking. For variety, serve Kool-Aid, lactose-reduced milk, soy milk, nonfat soups

---

MONEY SAVER

Mix this homemade brew concocted by sports nutritionist Nancy Clark, author of the *New York City Marathon Cookbook:*

1/4 cup sugar
1/2 cup hot water
1/4 cup orange juice
1/4 teaspoon salt
3 1/4 cups cold water

In a quart jar or pitcher, dissolve the sugar in the hot water. Add the remaining ingredients and stir. Makes 4 cups.

and broths, and juices and nectars diluted in water. Citrus juices should be used sparingly, however, says Nurse Erwin-Toth, "because they can set patients up for a urinary tract infection." Flavors that are easiest on the digestive tract include grape, apple, and cranberry juices, and apricot, mango, and peach nectars.

You can also fill a glass equally with water and a sports drink such as Gatorade or Endura, which helps to restore sodium, potassium, sugar, and calories. You can offer drinks with straws and spoons. But do not serve beverages containing caffeine, such as coffee, black tea, chocolate milk, and most sodas. They are diuretics, which exacerbate fluid loss. Try hot beverages, including caffeine-free pekoe or black teas and broths.

Never, never, *never* torment a patient over how much or how little he's eating or drinking. Encourage him to drink whatever he can tolerate comfortably, then back off. In the worst-case scenario, the doctor will order home intravenous replacement therapy, consisting of water and dextrose (IV glucose, or sugar), plus any electrolytes that need replenishing. Sodium bicarbonate, an alkali, may also be added to the mix to neutralize acidosis.

Safeguarding Patients Against Infection

Infections pose one of the gravest threats to the ailing. Pneumonia, for example, is the fifth deadliest of all illnesses, killing 82,317 men and women in 1995. And those are just the deaths *directly* attributed to the inflammatory lung disease; many mortalities from cancer, AIDS, stroke, and so on, are the result of secondary lung infections that arose following long illnesses, hospitalizations, or surgery.

An infection develops when microorganisms infiltrate the body through a break in the skin, mucous membrane, or other point of entry and manage to evade an armada of defenses. "Good" microbes, or normal *flora*, that inhabit our skin and organ linings prevent small numbers of *bacteria*, *viruses*, *fungi*, and *protozoa* from proliferating, while the body's chemistry creates a similarly hostile environment. Should germs slip past this initial line of protection, the immune system's white blood cells join the attack.

Sickness weakens both these barriers to infection. Just being immobile, in

---

The Warning Signs of Septic Shock

Every year more than 20,000 people die of blood infections, also referred to as *septic shock, septicemia,* and *blood poisoning.*

✚ *Notify the doctor, home-care nurse, or hospice nurse immediately if the following symptoms occur:*

- Diminished urine output
- Sustained fever above 101 degrees
- Chills
- Weakness
- Nausea and vomiting
- Diarrhea
- Tiny skin abscesses
- Red-and-blue streaks along the skin over blood vessels leading to and from the initial site of infection

fact, increases one's susceptibility. A major function of stool, urine, saliva, and mucus is to eliminate infectious agents. If you're debilitated and confined to bed, you're prone to constipation, you don't relieve yourself as often, your mouth can dry out, and you may find it difficult to raise phlegm; in effect, your body acts as an incubator for bacteria and other microbial opportunists to grow, multiply, and eventually injure cells. Dehydration and malnutrition, too, interfere with our immune response.

Once infected, the body tries to protect itself through a series of physiologic changes known as *inflammation*. The classic signs are redness, swelling, and pain. Any infection can progress into a life-threatening condition, especially in patients with limited resistance. A sore throat, if caused by streptococcal bacterium (strep throat), can evolve into rheumatic fever of the heart; likewise, a case of influenza can lead to viral pneumonia. Should the microorganisms make their way to the circulatory system—perhaps via an open sore—infection may take hold anywhere in the body: the heart valve (endocarditis), the brain (encephalitis), the abdomen (peritonitis), and elsewhere.

Types of Infections and How to Prevent Transmission

Of the four main types of infection, the two most prevalent are bacterial and viral. Bacterial infections produce disease-causing toxins; they tend to be more dangerous than viral infections, though not always. But whereas bacteria characteristically respond to a class of drugs called *antibiotics*, few viruses can be tamed medicinally. The common cold springs from a virus. As you surely know from experience, there's no medication to prevent it from running its course, only agents to control fever and other symptoms.

Fungal infections such as thrush *(Candida)* come on slowly by and large. Though tricky to diagnose and harder still to treat, they are rarely deadly except in the severely immunocompromised. Protozoal infections include several diseases, like the *pneumocystis carinii* pneumonia frequently seen in AIDS, as well as the intestinal abscesses and life-threatening diarrhea associated with common amoebas. Pneumonia, incidentally, can assume any of the four identities: bacterial, viral, fungal, and protozoal.

Microorganisms are resourceful, hitching rides on people's bodies, inanimate objects, even the air. There are three main modes of transmission.

1. ***Direct contact*** with someone who is infected. For instance, kissing someone with a cold sore; grazing someone's infected wound with your hand, then touching your eyes or nose; touching an open wound with unsanitary hands, introducing infection; or from a person with a cold who has absentmindedly rubbed his nose and then shaken the patient's hand.

Handwashing Hints

- To cut down on the spread of germs, use a liquid soap in a pump bottle and dry hands with paper towels.
- Lather with soap and running water for a good 30 seconds, all the way up to your elbows. Also be sure to wash any jewelry you may be wearing on your hands. Feel free to make the water as hot or as cold as you like. It's the flushing action that does away with microbes, not the temperature of the water.
- Keep a pump bottle of inexpensive lotion by the faucet and moisturize your hands after each time you wash to cut down on cracks in the skin due to dryness.

How to Prevent Direct Transmission

♦ **Wash your hands** thoroughly with soap and water before and after contact with your patient; going to the bathroom; touching your mouth, nose, or eyes; and cooking and eating.

Hand-washing is the single most important infection-control measure a care partner can practice. Even if you slip up and get blood, fecal matter, or pus on your skin, soap and water reduces your risk of infection to a statistical zero. So go ahead and be obsessive about it.

♦ **Cover any cuts or sores** on your skin with sterile dressing.

♦ **Avoid close contact if you develop a skin infection** such as boils, cold sores, fever blisters, or shingles. Or be sure to wear vinyl or latex gloves. The same holds true should a patient's skin become infected.

♦ **Practice sterile technique** when cleaning around openings in the skin, such as surgical wounds, pressure ulcers, and catheter sites, and when changing dressings. ► See "Three Steps to Sterile Technique," page 121.

2. Indirect contact with a contaminated inanimate substance or object. For instance, a germ-laden doorknob or faucet, infected blood or other body fluids that enter a mucous membrane or a break in the skin, and ingesting contaminated water or food.

How to Prevent Indirect Transmission

♦ **Never share personal items** that could conceivably be infected with germs, blood, or other body fluids: toothbrushes, razors, hairbrushes, combs, makeup, contact lens containers, denture cups, eyebrow tweezers, pierced earrings, soap, and used towels, washcloths, handkerchiefs, or tissues.

♦ **Don't eat off someone else's plate** or drink from his glass.

♦ **Spray disinfectant** on doorknobs and faucets at least once a day, and on bedpans, toilet seats, and the flushing lever after each use.

♦ **Wear latex gloves** when handling blood, urine, feces, mucus, vomit, and other body fluids, or when cleaning an infected wound or drainage site. ► See "Cleaning Patients After a Bowel Movement or Urination," page 125.

♦ **Observe safety measures for preparing and storing food.** All of us contract at least one food-borne disease each year, but for most healthy people it amounts to little more than an acute episode of nausea or diarrhea, and perhaps a low-grade, short-lived fever. But nearly ten thousand Americans die each year from highly common food-borne infections such as salmonella and E. coli.

Many of the people who die from food poisoning are in some way immunocompromised: cancer patients undergoing heavy chemotherapy, people with AIDS, transplant recipients whose immune systems are pharmaceutically suppressed. But many of the worst cases of food poisoning are also seen in the elderly or people otherwise constitutionally depleted by the ravages of disease. Sloppy kitchen habits developed over a lifetime can place an ailing loved one in mortal danger.

• Wash your hands fastidiously before preparing food and immediately after touching raw meat, fish, or eggs. Use plenty of hot running water and soap. Dry your hands thoroughly with paper towels.
• Use a solution of hot water and chlorine bleach (one tablespoon per gallon of water) to disinfect food-preparation surfaces such as cutting

boards and countertops, as well as kitchen spigots, drawers, cabinet handles, and refrigerator doors. Remember that sponges are breeding grounds for germs, too. Leave them to soak in disinfectant each night and exchange them for new ones frequently.

- Peel all fresh fruits and vegetables, then wash them under running water.
- Set the thermostat in the fridge at or below 40 degrees Fahrenheit, and the freezer at zero degrees Fahrenheit.
- Store all refrigerated food in air-tight containers, particularly raw meat and dairy products. Clean up spills immediately and disinfect interior surfaces of the refrigerator often.
- Never use canned or prepackaged foods that are leaking, bulging, or dented. Remember to clean and disinfect the cutting edge of the can opener, too.
- Never set out food to thaw at room temperature. Keep it covered and thaw in the fridge or in the microwave.
- Give leftovers one, two days at most, then toss in the trash.
- Cook meat and eggs thoroughly: Meat should have no pink in the middle; eggs should not run. When eating out, avoid dishes with raw or undercooked eggs or meat.

◆ *Serve only purified water* to avoid contracting giardia and cryptosporidiosis. While the latter disease is rare (fewer than one thousand cases annually), this step is advised for severely immunodeficient men and women with T cell counts below 200. The water should be used for drinking, making ice, brushing teeth, diluting juices, and washing fruits and vegetables. In lieu of having to boil tap water—for five minutes, then let it cool—you can buy bottled spring water or install a water filter, a cheaper alternative.

✱ *Before purchasing a filtration unit, be sure that it filters to 2 microns or less, to trap the microscopic protozoa.*

3. *Airborne transmission,* such as being in the path of an infected person's sneeze, cough, or droplet spread while he is speaking (examples are strep throat, flu, and viral pneumonia) or inhaling infectious microbes that stay suspended in the air and can travel distances greater than three feet (examples are tuberculosis and chicken pox).

How to Prevent Airborne Transmission

◆ *Chronically ill patients and anyone age sixty-five or older should consider an annual flu vaccination* in the early fall, as recommended by the U.S. Public Health Service.

◆ *The National Institute on Aging additionally recommends pneumococcal vaccinations* for the same age group, who are two to three times more likely than the general population to contract pneumococcal pneumonia. It is also strongly advised that anyone with a chronic illness or compromised immunity ask his physician for the vaccine, which protects against other pneumococcal bacterial infections as well. (Medicare pays for the vaccine, and one shot usually lasts a lifetime.)

◆ *Keep sick rooms well ventilated,* with plenty of fresh air.

◆ *On days when you have a cold or the flu* and can't line up someone else to look after your loved one, wear a surgical mask whenever you enter her room.

◆ *If a patient with an infectious disease such as a bad cold, the flu, pneumonia, or tuberculosis is coughing or sneezing,* wear a surgical mask anytime you're in the same room.

It's important to understand that we represent a far greater health risk to patients than they do to us. We are walking cultures transporting germs from the outside world, and if we transmit an infection to someone who is severely ill, we may endanger his life, whereas most infections contracted by an otherwise healthy person are easily resisted or, at worst, an inconvenience.

Making a big deal about infection control by calling attention to your efforts or to others' slip-ups only reinforces a patient's feelings of contamination, isolation, and vulnerability. So if you need to wear a mask because your husband has tuberculosis, slip it on nonchalantly. Suggest that visitors tell him as they enter, "I can't kiss you because I've got the sniffles" or "I have a cold, so I'm going to sit over here"— lest your husband interpret their reticence as fear or revulsion.

Special Care: Increased Susceptibility to Infection

When disease, treatment, and/or malnutrition has impaired the immune system of the person in our care, we need to be extra conscientious to minimize opportunities for infections.

Anyone taking an immunosuppressive drug, such as cancer patients and bone marrow or organ transplant recipients, faces a heightened risk of infection. (Radiation therapy, too, can inhibit production of white blood cells.) Diabetes, if not managed adequately through diet and medication, attenuates the immune response. AIDS patients whose T cell counts have dwindled are especially vulnerable.

When white counts fall below normal, encourage loved ones to heed the following safety measures.

Avoid nicks, cuts, scrapes, and skin irritations. Do this by

- using an electric shaver instead of a razor;
- using a soft-bristle toothbrush;
- using baby wipes after bowel movements; they clean thoroughly without having to wipe too harshly. Bidets or

a quick rinse with a handheld shower attachment are also ideal;
- keeping skin well moisturized;
- cleaning cuts and scratches immediately with water, soap, and antiseptic;
- using cuticle cream or remover instead of cutting or tearing nail cuticles;
- refraining from squeezing or scratching pimples, blackheads, and insect bites.

Avoid potential carriers of infection:

Consider wearing a surgical mask to the doctor's office or hospital. ◀ See "Strategic Scheduling," page 71, for tips on how to avoid lengthy waits during medical visits.

Stay away from anyone with a contagious disease, such as a cold, measles, or the flu. Never allow anyone with chickenpox in the same room as your patient until all the small red spots have completely scabbed over. This ironclad rule also applies to shingles, or *herpes zoster.* Contact with shingles or chickenpox can touch off a potentially fatal outbreak of chickenpox in a person who has never had it before.

Zoster is one of the relatively few opportunistic infections that can readily outfox a healthy immune system. In the event that you come down with shingles, which usually erupts across the chest, be sure to cover all blisters thoroughly and wear gloves around your loved one.

(Here's a question to ask would-be visitors over the phone: "Were you exposed to chickenpox or measles anytime in the last nine to twenty-one days?" During this incubation period, a person could be infected yet not exhibit any symptoms.)

✚ *Notify the doctor, home-care nurse, or hospice nurse immediately should an immune-impaired patient be exposed to chickenpox, shingles, or measles.*

Normally, the antiviral drug *acyclovir* must be given within twenty-four hours of contagion to chickenpox in order to prevent serious complications. (The window for shingles is seventy-two hours.) Since immunocompromised people's bodies take longer to mount a defense against viruses, they can still benefit from drug therapy (with *famciclovir, ganciclovir,* or *valacyclovir*) beyond those time parameters. With measles the opposite is true. Whereas healthy people have up to six days after infection for *immune globulin* to prevent or at least temper the disease, immunocompromised patients need a shot immediately.

Get inoculated yourself. If you are caring for or living with a severely immunocompromised patient, ask the primary physician if you need to be inoculated against the so-called childhood diseases of polio, chickenpox, measles, and mumps.

Take precautions when it comes to animals. Pets can transmit infections, too. For instance, cats carry the *toxoplasma gondii* protozoan, which is transmitted through contact with their feces. *Psittacosis,* a contagious disease common to parrots and other pet birds, also presents a hazard. More to the point, fur, feathers, and claws harbor a host of germs picked up around the house and outside.

Accordingly, have patients wash hands with soap and water after petting or holding animals. Empty litter boxes every day and wash them in hot water with unscented chlorine bleach. (Do not allow patients to help with this task.) Make sure pet inoculations are up to date and call a veterinarian at the first indication of illness. If you're an animal lover, then you know what comfort and joy pets can bring. Observe the above precautions, and there should be no need to isolate pets from someone who is ill.

✚ *Notify the doctor, home-care nurse, or hospice nurse immediately of any signs of infection: fever, chills, sweating, diarrhea, severe cough or sore throat, unusual vaginal discharge or itching, or redness or swelling, particularly around a wound, sore, pimple, or boil. What might be a passing bug in you or me could be fatal to a loved one with damaged immunity.*

How Infections Are Treated

Antimicrobial agents work in a variety of ways to kill microorganisms outright or prevent them from reproducing or growing. Antibiotics, used to treat bacterial infections, are the largest group. When taking an antibiotic, finish the prescription—even if the symptoms have subsided—unless the doctor instructs otherwise. Discontinuing an antibiotic prematurely allows the germs to multiply again, possibly as a fierce new strain resistant to antibiotics.

Don't badger the doctor for antibiotics if he says they aren't warranted. Overusing antibiotics can accelerate the evolution of drug-resistant strains. Furthermore, even the most innocuous antibiotics, such as tetracycline and penicillin, often produce nasty gastrointestinal symptoms.

Daily Hygiene

Tending to a loved one's most personal physical care requires transcending any inhibitions we may have about touching another person's body and bodily functions, and overcoming our initial squeamishness. There are also new and complex emotions to deal with: perhaps a grown man's awkwardness at seeing his ailing mother naked and vulnerable, and her subsequent feelings of embarrassment; or the reversals of identity that may shake up a marriage defined by traditional sex roles, where the subordinate partner suddenly finds herself in the unfamiliar position of making decisions for her debilitated spouse. What's more, our taking over these intimate tasks for a patient is a sharp reminder to everyone involved of just how ill and dependent he is.

The following suggestions can help you get past the discomfort that many folks feel the first few times they bathe someone in bed, change a urine drainage bag, or wipe a loved one's bottom.

1. Imagine you're caring for a baby. No one freaks out if a baby has an accident in his diaper; if anything, we chuckle about it. Adopt a similar mindset: *I'm changing a diaper. Whose it is doesn't matter.* Keep your focus on the act of love you're performing.

Audree Siden changed her eighty-eight-year-old mother's diaper four to six times a day. "Most of us are terribly inexperienced handling another body except in a sexual context," she reflects. "I chose to view it simply as part of the cycle of life and told myself that I was doing for her exactly what she had done for me when I was an infant. It became as if I were changing my own child."

2. Never infantalize the person. Be sensitive to the fact that your loved one may be mortified by his reliance on you and mourning the loss of his independence. You may be spoon-feeding your sister as you would a child, but the person in that bed is still an adult. Always make the extra effort to preserve her dignity and self-respect.

Ask permission before tending to personal care. "I asked my mother how she felt about having me changing her diapers and whether or not she would prefer using a bedpan," says Audree. "At this point she really had no choice, but I felt it was important to acknowledge to her that I was thinking about any possible embarrassment for her. She said, 'I trust you.' It was a very sweet moment."

Respect the person's privacy. Bodily functions should never be turned into public spectacles. "Whenever I had to change my mother's diaper," Audree recalls, "no one was allowed in the room, including her grandchildren."

If you're in the hospital, ask any visitors to step outside, then close the door and draw the curtain around the bed.

Don't expose loved ones unnecessarily, yanking the bedsheet down from their neck to their ankles. A capable care partner should be able to clean a patient's genital or anal regions while letting her stay covered from the waist up.

Explain what you're about to do, step by step. Example: "Mom? Now I'm going to roll you over on your side while I pull the old bedsheets out from under you. Just hang on to the side rail for a minute, okay?"

3. Practice makes perfect. Efficiency and confidence go a long way toward defusing a patient's self-consciousness and agitation. Someone who has just thrown up all over himself is probably going to be impatient and enraged at the indignity of his situation. Now is not the time to be fumbling with the vomit basin because we forgot to put on gloves or shuffling in and out of the room a half-dozen times before we've assembled all the cleaning supplies.

The key to gaining confidence is experience so that you grow progressively desensitized to the sights, smells, and sounds of disease and dying. Start by assisting the nurses and aides when they bathe or toilet patients, either at the hospital or at home. Rehearse each skill with another person present the first couple of times, then try it by yourself. Don't get discouraged; you'll get the hang of it.

4. Detoxify and normalize the situation for the patient. As an ICU respiratory therapy technician, one time I had to change the diaper of a grandmother with degenerative arthritis. At four hundred pounds she was simply too heavy to be maneuvered by the female nurse who was tending her. She was an old churchgoing woman from Satsuma, Alabama, and the idea of having a male stranger touch her in this way was traumatic for her.

"Oh, son," she sobbed, "this is so embarrassing."

"Miz Holman, you hush now," I said. "I'm just gonna change a diaper here and get your butt cleaned up real quick. I'm not even gonna look, okay? Now, you grab onto the bed railing . . ."

Dispense with euphemisms. Frame what you're about to do in a positive light, as in *I'm here to do something that's going to make you feel better.*

5. Whatever the scene, play it cool. We walk into our loved one's room and find him lying in urine. Overreacting with needless melodrama ("Oh my God! What happened here?") will heighten his self-consciousness and distress. De-escalate the atmosphere. In your calmest, most comforting tone of voice, assure him that everything is under control—even if the thought of yet another load of laundry is enough to bring tears of exhaustion. "Don't worry, dear, we'll get you cleaned up right away. We have to keep your bottom dry."

6. A sense of humor helps. The ability to laugh in the midst of any crisis is a tremendous asset, one that will get you through countless tough moments. For example, I can't help gagging spontaneously whenever someone throws up noisily. My father and I nearly laughed ourselves into a state of altered consciousness every time he heaved and I retched along sympathetically.

7. Try these techniques for overcoming the "ickies":

Roll up your sleeves and put on gloves. You'll feel far more confident wiping feces, vomit, or urine if you're not all apprehensive about getting some on you. Reusable vinyl gloves are adequate, but the disposable latex kind that doctors and nurses use are best. They come in pop-up dispenser boxes, much like tissues. We suggest stashing several boxes around the house. If you do use vinyl gloves, check to see they don't have holes or cracks in them. (You might also want to slip on a smock or apron. Or wear a man's button-down shirt backward.)

Inhale through your mouth instead of your nose. Taking slow, deep breaths helps ease physical aversion reactions. Don't try to hold your breath. You'll rush whatever you're doing and make a mistake, or you'll faint.

Suck on a mint or butterscotch candy. The odors associated with disease and dying can send you reeling sometimes. Because the senses of smell and taste are so intertwined, sucking on candy or chewing gum offsets even the funkiest odors.

Dab wintergreen oil on a surgical mask and wear it. This will help if you absolutely cannot tolerate the smell of feces, vomit, and so forth. The wintergreen oil, by the way, will blister your sinuses, but it works. I've walked through morgues filled with bodies that had been lying out in the Gulf Coast sun following a hurricane, and three days later it still felt as if I had a cheap air freshener inside my head.

8. Keep your sights on what's important: the patient's health, comfort, and dignity. Anytime I get upset, frustrated, or frightened while caring for a seriously ill loved one, I always repeat this little mantra: *It's worse for them than it is for me.* Whatever our fears, discomfort, and embarrassment, imagine what the patient is feeling.

9. Find someone who can handle these intimate tasks if they are too much for you. It can be either a layperson or a home-care professional.

Bathing

For patients who are ambulatory, one of the truly delicious pleasures of the day is to relax under a warm shower. The first time my dad showered following his discharge from the hospital, he lowered himself onto the stool I'd placed in the tub, closed his eyes, and grinned as the spray caressed his head and back. "I think I'll just sit right here a little while, son," he purred. "This is better than sex!"

Bathing sick people, like maneuvering them and changing the bed with the person still in it, is always easier if you have someone to help you. But since the reality is that care partners must frequently carry out these tasks without assistance, our instructions are intended for one person.

- Should you have a choice, a stall shower is preferable to a tub shower. Having to step over the high side of the tub is more likely to lead to a fall.
- Purchase a waterproof shower stool or chair, available at almost any surgical supply store. Or save money by buying a plastic lawn chair, which works just as well.
- Outfit the tub or shower with a grab bar; a nonslip textured-rubber bath mat (adhesive-backed strips or flowers are not as effective); a handheld shower head; a shower caddy; soap on a rope or a bar of soap placed in a nylon stocking, which you tie to a towel bar; a long-handled bath brush or sponge.

☎ Special adjustable-handle brushes, suction-cup-mounted soap holders, and other adaptive devices make showering more manageable. For written descriptions of the many products available and where to order them, call the National Rehabilitation Information Center's free Abledata database at 800-227-0216/301-608-8998. ◄ *See "Modifying the Home," page 78.*

- Clear shelves and countertops of all breakable objects and make room for towels, surgical dressings and supplies, medications, and all your other "stuff," so there's no fumbling around while wrangling a cold, wet sick person.

- Substitute plastic drinking cups for glassware.
- To prevent accidents, mop up any spills at once.
- Remind loved ones not to lock the door when bathing or using the toilet unassisted.
- For patients who have been experiencing difficulty catching their breath, leave the bathroom door or window open and turn on the exhaust fan, if there is one, to prevent steam and humidity from building up.
- Water should be no warmer than approximately 100 degrees. Hot water dries out the skin and can cause the blood pressure to drop, leading to dizziness or fainting. Test the temperature with a bath thermometer, available in the baby's department of most drugstores.
- Slipping on a long terry cloth robe after bathing eliminates the need for vigorous towel drying. Cracks and creases can be tended to while moisturizing.

Helping a Loved One into the Tub

Wrap an arm around the trunk of his weaker side. Normally, that would be the left side for a right-handed person —and the reverse for a lefty—unless a stroke, arthritis, or some other condition has disabled that side of the body. To determine your loved one's stronger side, ask him to squeeze your hands. Or have him extend both legs and try to keep them straight while you push down on them.

Have him step into the tub, strongside leg first, while holding on to the grab bar mounted on the wall.

With your free hand, help him lift his weaker leg over the side.

For a bath, support him with two hands as he eases himself down.

How to Give a Four-Star Bed Bath

Bed baths aren't strictly for the bedbound. Caregivers should consider this option anytime tub or shower bathing becomes too physically demanding or hazardous. Betty Lindstrom gave up on showers for her husband, a six-foot-tall outdoorsman, long before Parkinson's disease rendered him immobile.

"I always had a fear of Clarence's falling," she recalls, "because I knew I wouldn't be able to hold him up. Once a week or so a nurse's aide used to come to the house and help me get him into the shower. But eventually it became so dangerous that they didn't want to do it anymore, and I didn't think it was wise, either. So we started bed baths."

- First of all, don't rush. Set aside thirty minutes, although with practice you should be able to trim a good ten minutes off that time.

- Set out your supplies:

  Two plastic basins or small buckets filled with warm water;

  Two washcloths (preferably bath washcloths because they're thinner and softer than conventional ones);

  Three towels—two for drying and one for placing under the water basins;

  Bar soap that contains no detergent, perfume, or antibacterial agents because they all dry out the skin; "super-fatted" or glycerin soaps are less harsh;

  Two clean sheets—one flat, one fitted;

  Nonscented moisturizer or emollient;

  Latex gloves;

  A bath blanket or large beach towel.

- Our main concern is to prevent the person from catching a chill. Close the windows to keep out drafts and make sure the room temperature is comfortably warm.

- Before you begin, ask your loved one if he needs to use a urinal or bedpan.

- Strip top linens and blankets and cover the person with the bath blanket or large towel.

We always want to encourage patients' autonomy as much as possible. If your loved one is so inclined, let him clean his genitals and anus and any other areas within reach in private. Then take over washing the back, the feet, and anyplace he might have missed. The instructions below assume that your patient needs you to bathe him completely:

- Imagine the person's body is divided into ten sections: face, neck, left arm, right arm, chest, abdomen, left leg, right leg, back, and genital/anal area. Concentrate on washing and drying one area at a time, top to bottom, all the while keeping the rest of the body covered. Start with the eyes. (Note: Here we refrain from using soap.) Then proceed to the face and neck.

Place a dry towel under each area to be cleaned.

- Designate one basin for soapy water and one for clean water. Lather up your washcloth and cleanse the exposed skin, making sure not to scrub hard. Use a clean wet cloth to wash off all the soap residue, then wring it out.

- Thoroughly dry each section before you move on to the next, paying special attention to skin folds and crevices where germs love to hide, such as between the toes and beneath a woman's breasts—wherever skin touches skin.

- When you're finished drying each area, gently rub emollient or moisturizer into the skin.

- Should your clean water turn cool or soapy at any time, change it. Likewise, retire soggy towels in favor of fresh ones.

- Last of all, tend to the genitals, the anus, and the perineal area in between.

♂ *Masculine Care: Clean carefully under the testicles and, in uncircumcised patients, the foreskin. "That's something a lot of family members neglect to do," says home hospice nurse Ellen Wilson. "It's a highly sensitive area, and if it becomes infected, soreness develops. Don't be afraid to gently pull the foreskin back."*

♀ *Feminine Care: Similarly, wash the folds of the labia. When cleaning the anus, remember to wipe from front to back so as not to introduce germs into the vagina or the urinary tract.*

- In order to reach the back of a patient who cannot sit up, use a *drawsheet*—a sheet folded into thirds—to easily roll him over onto his side.

- When you're done, put on crisp, fresh cotton sheets. The drawsheet enables you to do this with the person still in bed. Cotton linens and blankets are preferable to synthetic fibers because

they permit air to circulate and sweat to evaporate more freely.

▶ *See "Turning, Maneuvering, and Lifting," page 132.*

Giving a Basin Bath

Consider this a cross between a shower and a bed bath. Basin baths are ideal for folks who can walk to the bathroom but may not have the strength or steadiness to risk a bath or shower. The patient sits in front of the sink, either in a chair or on the toilet, wrapped in a warm beach towel, while you bathe and dry her, one area at a time as with a bed bath.

Special Care: Bathing a Loved One Who Suffers from Memory Loss, Confusion, or Intellectual Impairment

The fragmentary memory and limited cognitive function characteristic of dementia (what was once referred to as senility) further complicates bathing. Brain-impaired patients may no longer remember how to wash themselves, or they might scrub the same spot repeatedly, forgetting they just cleaned there. It goes without saying that we never leave a loved one suffering from dementia in the bathroom unattended.

The safety tips below come from the Pittsburgh Alzheimer Disease Research Center. Bear in mind that dementia is a complication of conditions other than Alzheimer's, such as stroke, traumatic brain injury, and AIDS.

- Since dressing brain-impaired people can be time consuming, schedule bath time for the morning, before putting on their clothes, or at night, after they undress for bed.

- Clear the bathroom of extraneous items, which may confuse or distract.

- Turn down the thermostat on the hot water tank to eliminate the danger of the person accidentally scalding himself.

- Remove the door lock.
- If your loved one seems agitated and refuses to bathe, let it go until later or skip it altogether and try again tomorrow.

* *Don't always leave bathing for the evening when loved ones (and caregivers) are most likely to be tired or cranky, and inclined to put it off. A person who is well hydrated and up and about can get away with bathing every other day; sicker folks, however, require cleansing and moisturizing at least once a day.*

Skin Care

The skin is the body's largest organ as well as a natural barrier against infection. Maintaining its integrity is as essential to our loved one's well-being as any medication. Dry, cracked, or ulcerated skin becomes a gateway through which microorganisms enter. This is a particular concern with older people, whose skin secretes less oil and has lost some of its thickness.

Moisturize!

After each bath, smooth a hypoallergenic, unscented moisturizer or emollient over every inch of the body to restore and lock in the moisture washed away by soap and water. This doubles as a relaxing, loving massage. But keep your touch light. If the surface layer has sustained damage, Reeks explains, "rubbing too hard further injures the tissue underneath."

When we say to leave no area untouched, take it literally. Get in between those toes and fingers, and the creases between the buttocks, upper thighs, and groin, the insides of the elbows and behind the knees. Exposed mucous membranes—the anus, vulva, and inside the nostrils—also require our attention.

Don't overlook the lips, which can become dry and cracked in dehydrated patients. Lip balms are adequate, although, as Nurse Wilson points outs, "if somebody isn't producing much saliva, they tend to cake, and that isn't very comfortable." Her recommendation? Vitamin E capsules. "They're the best," she says, "because they have an oilier consistency and stay on better. You just pierce the capsule and occasionally apply the gel inside to the lips." A smear of petroleum jelly will also do the trick. If our loved one's mouth dries out, coat his tongue and gums as well.

* *Also moisturize affected areas each time you wash them; for instance, after toileting, hand-washing, and so forth.*

Keep Skin Dry

Urine, stool, perspiration, and wound drainage, all highly acidic, chemically erode the skin. It is imperative that accidents be cleaned up straightaway using a soft cloth or sponge, and the skin coated with a protective barrier cream or salve. Barri-Care, Nu-Gard, Peri-care, and Triple Care are just several of the many brands available. Should urinary or fecal incontinence become a chronic problem, we suggest lining the bed with a quick-drying absorbent cloth pad to draw moisture away from the skin. It's time to also consider adult diapers. ▶ *See "Incontinence," page 170.*

Itching

Among the many causes of red, itchy skin are dehydration, allergies, numerous common medications, fungal infections, jaundice, radiation treatments, and autoimmune disorders. Our main tasks are to eliminate the source of irritation, to soothe the itching or burning, and to prevent infection and further breakdown of the skin.

◆ *Keep your loved as thoroughly hydrated and well nourished* as possible.

◆ *Maintain scrupulous personal hygiene:* bathing, hair, skin, and nail care.

◆ *Systematically eliminate any chemical irritants coming in contact with the skin.* Common culprits include urine and feces; various brands of soaps and skin-care products such as moisturizers or oils; deodorants and other personal hygiene products; scented toilet paper; and laundry detergent or chemical fabric-softener residue in sheets and clothes.

◆ *Opt for cotton sleepwear and underwear* rather than polyester and other synthetic fabrics, which promote fungal infections. Change and wash them frequently. Sheets and blankets should also be changed, washed, and thoroughly rinsed regularly.

◆ *Soothe itchy, irritated skin with a cool bath containing baking soda or oatmeal.* Dust skin, particularly creases and cracks that retain moisture, with cornstarch after baths and showers.

◆ *To relieve acute episodes of itching, give your loved one a mild over-the-counter oral antihistamine* such as Benadryl or Actifed, or smooth on a nonprescription cortisone cream. However, itching, flaking, and redness that persists more than a few days should be reported to the nurse or doctor.

✳ *Skin rashes of sudden onset, particularly when accompanied by itching and swelling around the face and neck, often indicate the beginning of a life-threatening allergic reaction. This demands immediate medical intervention.*

▶ See *"Allergic Reactions and Anaphylactic Shock," page 151; "Caring for Someone with Cancer: Radiation Therapy and Its Side Effects—Skin Inflammation," page 327.*

Common Sites of Pressure Ulcers

From Lying on the Back
- Back of the head
- Shoulder blades
- Backs of the elbows
- Spine
- Lower back (sacrum)
- Hips
- Buttocks
- Ankles
- Heels

From Lying on the Side
- Side of the head
- Shoulder
- Hip bone
- Side of the thigh, leg, knee, ankle
- Insides of knees and ankles from pressing against each other
- Side of foot

From Sitting in a Wheelchair
- Shoulder blades
- Lower back
- Buttocks
- Backs of the knees
- Heels

Pressure ulcers, more commonly known as *bedsores,* imperil anyone confined to bed or a wheelchair. "A bedsore," explains Dr. Donald Leslie, associate medical director of the Shepherd Spinal Center in Atlanta, "is a breakdown of the skin resulting from unrelieved pressure over any bony prominence." The areas of the body most prone to ulcer formation are those that bear weight when we're lying down or sitting (see the sidebar). If a loved one remains in the same position for too long, the tiny blood vessels that nourish the skin become compressed. Deprived of oxygen and nutrients, the tissue begins to die, and a pressure sore starts to develop.

Symptoms of Pressure Ulcers

A caregiver must examine the skin meticulously at least once a day for evidence of emerging bedsores. Be especially vigilant if you are looking after someone who has lost sensation in the lower limbs or some other part of the body, as can happen to stroke survivors and diabetics. They won't feel the pain that signals a pressure ulcer's onset. Similarly, patients who are brain-impaired may not be able to process pain or alert you to what they are feeling.

Physicians and nurses employ four stages to grade the severity of a pressure ulcer. At stage I the skin has not deteriorated, although the patch will appear red or purple and may feel warm to the touch. What you're seeing, says nurse Mary Ann Reeks, "is just the tip of the iceberg. The skin underneath is damaged."

Most pressure ulcers are reversible if caught early on. Should they progress, however, "they're extremely hard to clear up," she stresses. Bedsores in stages III and IV, which are usually infected, may resemble a festering craterlike black hole and emit a fetid odor.

"My dad had horrible three-inch-wide bedsores on his hips from not being turned in the nursing home," says Diane Young, a caregiver from New Orleans. "You could see clear down to the bone." The open sores became infected and funneled germs directly into the bloodstream. "That's what took his life," she adds. "The death certificate read 'septicemia': blood infection."

✚ *Notify the doctor, home-care nurse, or hospice nurse immediately upon detecting a bedsore.*

How to Prevent Pressure Ulcers

Prevention is critical—and not only in terms of our loved one's comfort. The caliber of skin care telegraphs to medical professionals your ability as a care partner. If you bring someone to the emergency room and the nurses discover bedsores the size of a quarter on both heels, your credibility as a patient advocate just evaporated. They will assume that either you don't know what you're doing or you don't care about the patient. Caregivers, too, should view skin care as a barometer for gauging the attentiveness of the staff, whether at home or in a hospital or nursing home. To be sure, bedsores can arise despite the best efforts of the most skilled professional, but finding a bedsore on a patient (which you point out immediately to a nurse) definitely warrants keeping an even closer watch on the overall level of care.

Reposition the person in bed every one to two hours to relieve the pressure. "People underestimate how little time it takes for a bedsore to form," says Dr. Howard Grossman, an internist at New York's St. Luke's–Roosevelt Hospital. "Lie on one side for just fifteen, twenty minutes, and skin already starts to break down."

The key to preventing bedsores is to see to it that your loved one shifts position regularly. "If patients can't move by themselves, you have to do it for them," says nurse Sarah Eilenberg, patient care manager of the Visiting Nurse Association of San Diego County, California. "That includes when they're sleeping. A lot of times family members don't want to disturb the person. But you're not doing them any harm; you're sparing them future pain."

Repositioning every one to two hours is sufficient for patients with no skin damage. When skin shows signs of deteriorating, however, no more than an hour should pass without a change in position. It's wise to get into the routine of repositioning every time you enter the room. By repositioning we don't mean rolling patients like logs or contorting them like figures in a cubist painting. Tilt the head this time, next shift a leg, then lift the right shoulder

INSIDE INFORMATION

Check to see if your loved one is receiving adequate support by gently sliding your hand between the patient and the mattress, palm up, to the site of the pressure point. The support surface there should be at least one inch thick.

blade off the mattress, and so on. Placing pillows or foam wedges strategically will help the patient to maintain postures comfortably. But do make it a priority to get loved ones off their buttocks once an hour.

Other preventive measures include:

◆ *When moving someone in bed or to a chair, lift, don't drag,* for the friction can abrade the surface layer of skin and damage the tiny blood vessels underneath. (To reduce friction when lifting, first dust the skin lightly with cornstarch.)

◆ *Invest in a special pressure-release mattress* like the egg-crate type that hospitals often use. The irregular-shaped, form-fitting foam distributes weight more evenly. According to Nurse Eilenberg, "To be effective, the mattress should be at least four inches deep." Air, gel, or water mattresses can also be beneficial.

◆ *Natural or synthetic sheepskin bedpads* "reduce the rubbing and friction against the skin that can cause bedsores," says Eilenberg. The machine-washable pads, available at most surgical supply outlets, come in various dimensions or in rolls that you cut to the desired size.

☎ To find stores and mail-order companies that sell or rent medical equipment, look in the Yellow Pages under "Hospital Equipment and Supplies," "Physicians' and Surgeons' Equipment and Supplies," and "Surgical Appliances and Supplies."

◆ *When loved ones are lying on their side,* place a foam wedge between the lower shoulder blade and the upper hip, to alleviate pressure on the hip. Also, check to see that the person isn't unknowingly lying on his arm, impeding circulation.

◆ *A number of companies also market elastic-mesh or foam protectors* for wearing on the elbows or heels.

◆ *Elevate the head of the bed no more than 30 degrees* from the horizontal position. Too sharp an angle may cause patients to keep sliding down, further damaging their skin. Exception: Patients who have trouble catching their breath often need the head of the bed raised for improved respiration.

◆ *At every opportunity, swipe the bed* with your hand and tighten the sheets. Even wrinkles and crumbs contribute to bedsores.

◆ *When patients cannot move their legs,* keep their ankles and knees separated with pillows or foam wedges. "The heels should not rest on the bed," emphasizes nurse Mary Ann Reeks. In lieu of slipperlike heel protectors, place pillows under the ankle-to-midcalf region, "and let the heels hang off them." The feet should be suspended high enough so that you can slip a sheet of paper beneath them. Do not, however, put pillows directly under the knee; this impedes circulation.

◆ *When in a chair or wheelchair,* a person able to shift her own weight should modify position every fifteen minutes. A person who cannot should be repositioned hourly, with pillows or wedges inserted between the knees and ankles. Use foam, gel, or air seat cushions two to three inches deep. Avoid doughnut- or ring-shaped models, which actually heighten the risk of developing pressure sores by reducing blood flow and causing tissue to swell.

How Pressure Ulcers Are Treated

In some cases, pressure ulcers are so extensive, it takes electrotherapy— applying electric current to the skin— or minor surgery to mend the damage. This is not something to attempt on your own. "It's best to let a nurse evaluate the severity of the wound and what needs to be done," says nurse Sarah Eilenberg.

Generally, you'll be instructed on how to clean the lesion, remove dead tissue, and place a protective dressing over the area (see "Wound Care," below). Relieving pressure at the affected site and encouraging loved ones to eat a balanced diet, which promotes healing and helps in preventing new sores from forming, are also important during this time.

Irrigating a Pressure Sore

Pressure sores are usually irrigated with water rather than cleaned by hand, although you may use a solution-moistened pad to gently wipe away loose debris and old drainage.

1. Wash your hands and glove up.
2. Fill the bulb syringe or other implement with saline.
3. Hold the irrigation device one to six inches away and spray the wound with enough force to rinse off dead tissue and pus but without damaging healthy new tissue. You'll probably refill the syringe several times before you're through. *Cleaning bedsores can be painful. Offer loved ones a mild over-the-counter analgesic such as aspirin, Tylenol, or Motrin thirty to sixty minutes before you start. If your patient is already on a regular medication schedule to relieve pain or anxiety, hold off until these have kicked in.*
4. Remove the basin.
5. Pat the surrounding skin dry with a clean towel.

Wound Care

Pressure sores; leg ulcers due to poor circulation; incisions; insertion sites for intravenous catheters, feeding tubes, and postoperative drainage tubes; and surgically created openings, or *stomas* —any opening in the skin must be viewed as a potential conduit of infection. Thus caregivers need to learn *sterile technique* to safeguard against unwittingly transferring germs from the environment to their loved one or to themselves when tending to a wound or the immediate area around it.

"Sterile technique" may conjure images of a lab technician in a bubble helmet and bulky white suit, but it really

---

Make Your Own Saline Solution

Saline solution is used for many purposes, such as flushing intravenous lines, so this recipe should come in handy and save you money:

1. Boil 1 gallon of tap water for 5 minutes or use 1 gallon of distilled water.
2. Add 8 teaspoons of table salt.
3. Sterilize a spoon by boiling it. Use it to mix the solution until the salt dissolves completely.
4. Let the solution cool to room temperature before using.
5. Store in a tightly sealed, sterilized glass or plastic container.

The solution keeps for up to 1 week.

amounts to little more than sensible hygiene. Familiarize yourself with the routine because you're also going to be employing it prior to injecting medications, wiping a patient's bottom, and any other task that could conceivably result in contamination. ▶ *See "Caring for an Ostomy," page 126.*

Three Steps to Sterile Technique

1. *Wash hands thoroughly* with soap and warm running water, rinse, then towel dry.

2. *Set up all supplies* on a clean, flat surface such as a bedside dresser on which a clean towel has been placed. Open all containers and packages now, taking care not to touch their contents with your bare hands.

3. *Don a pair of disposable gloves.* Anytime you come into contact with a germ-laden substance (urine, feces, blood, pus from a wound), discard the soiled gloves in a plastic bag, wash and dry your hands again, and put on a new pair to continue the job.

That's all there is to it.

✱ *Find it difficult to pull on a pair of surgical gloves? Don't tug too hard— you may tear the latex. Sprinkle your hands with baby powder or cornstarch first, and they'll slip on like a, well, glove.*

How to Change a Dressing

Dressing is a broad term that refers to any material used to cover and protect a wound. *Wet dressings* encompass saline (salt water), gels, or ointments for creating a moist environment for healing; *dry dressings* are the sterile pads, gauzes, sponges, tapes, and bandages placed over the site. *Wet-to-dry dressings,* such as saline-saturated gauze layered with dry gauze and taped in place, are typically ordered for gaping pressure ulcers and other more serious skin wounds; when peeled off, they remove

dead tissue and debris, which is essential to healing. One popular brand of dressing, Duoderm, consists of a padded bandage bordered by self-sticking adhesive; wet-to-dry Duoderm pads contain an inner layer of healing gel that rests against the wound.

"Every kind of wound, whether it's a bedsore or a surgical incision, requires a different kind of dressing," says Nurse Eilenberg. "A very wet wound may be treated with a dry dressing, whereas a dry, sticky wound may be treated with either a wet dressing or an ointment. Use the wrong treatment, and you can make them a lot worse." The doctor or nurse will tell you which type and size to buy.

The extent of the wound also determines how frequently we'll need to change dressings. For a noninfected bedsore, "sometimes just cleaning it and leaving a Duoderm control-gel pad

---

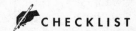

CHECKLIST

Supplies for Changing Dressings and Cleaning Wounds

- ❑ Dressings the physician has prescribed
- ❑ Paper adhesive-backed tape
- ❑ Clean towel or plastic bag for protecting bed linens
- ❑ Sealable plastic disposal bag
- ❑ Cleansing or rinsing solution
- ❑ Disposable plastic cups
- ❑ Latex or vinyl gloves
- ❑ Scissors that have been washed with soap and water, then wiped with rubbing alcohol
- ❑ Bulb syringe or other irrigation device for gently spraying away dead tissue and old drainage if necessary; a turkey baster works fine for folks with feeble hands or a weak grip
- ❑ Basin (for irrigating only)

in place for three to seven days is often sufficient." More severe wounds, she continues, "may need to be packed and dressed two or three times a day."

Preparations

1. Wash your hands.
2. Make sure your loved one is comfortable.
3. Tear open the paper jackets containing all dressings to be used, but don't take them out yet or touch them with your bare hands. If any of the dressings becomes dirty or wet, toss out the entire package.
4. If necessary, lay a towel or plastic garbage bag under the part of the body on which you'll be "operating."
5. Cut however many pieces of paper tape you'll need. Each should be at least four inches longer than the width of the dressing.
6. Open the plastic disposal bag and place it within easy reach.
7. Lay out all the other supplies.
8. Put on your gloves.

Remove the Old Dressing

1. Carefully peel the ends of the tape toward the center of the dressing. If the tape sticks, soften the adhesive with a few drops of baby oil.
2. Remove the old dressings, one layer at a time, and drop them into the plastic bag. If the dressing sticks, moisten it with sterile lukewarm water.
3. Dispose of the gloves and wash your hands again.

Inspect the Wound

✚ *Notify the doctor, home-care nurse, or hospice nurse immediately* should you notice

- bleeding;
- pus, thick green or yellow drainage, warmth, redness, hardness, tenderness, or swelling around the site—all indications of infection;
- the patient complains of worsening pain;
- the wound does not appear to be healing. Pressure sores, for example, usually begin to heal within two to four weeks, shrinking in size and depth and exuding less drainage.

Clean the Wound

1. Put on a new pair of gloves.
2. Fold the gauze pad into quarters and dip it into the cleansing solution recommended by the doctor. *Don't clean wounds with iodine or alcohol. Not only do they sting like the devil, they both dry out sensitive tissue.*
3. Clean the wound softly, being careful not to touch another part of the skin. For nonsurgical wounds, stroke outward from the center. For surgical wounds, stroke in a circular motion from one end of the incision to the other. Never rub back and forth across the sutures.
4. Use fresh gauze pads liberally—for each new step and as soon as a pad becomes soiled—so you don't ferry germs from one area to another. Keep cleaning until the wound is immaculate.
5. With a clean towel, pat the wound and neighboring area dry.

Cold water is great for slowing minor external bleeding, while warm water works better when you need to soak through a scab or crusty discharge.

Apply the New Dressing

1. Strip off the old gloves, wash your hands, and put on the new gloves.
2. It never hurts to rub a little nonprescription antibacterial cream around wounds. Popular brands include Polysporin, Neosporin, and Garamycin.
3. Moisturize the surrounding skin, paying particular attention to areas that have been covered by tape or dry dressings. Change the angle of the tape each

---

Oops . . .

Anytime you think you may have fouled a freshly sterilized site, start all over: Wash everything off, change gloves, dress the wound again. No exceptions.

---

time you apply a new dressing to give the skin an opportunity to breathe.

4. When using a nonadhering dressing, gently place one or two layers of gauze over the wound. *When using an adhesive dressing,* apply with a rolling motion, making sure not to stretch the material. Then smooth around the edges with your fingers.

5. While holding the dressing(s) in position with two fingers, place one piece of paper tape along one edge and onto the skin. Then do the same on the opposite side. Use just enough tape to secure the dressing. Paper tape is preferable to cloth tape; it doesn't hurt as much when you peel it off.

6. Place all used materials, including gloves, into the plastic bag. Seal it and place it in an outdoor trash can with a secure lid.

✱ *When caring for someone with a contagious disease, ask the doctor or nurse to outline the local regulations for disposing of potentially infectious waste and materials, or check with the local health department or department of sanitation.*

7. Wash your hands.
Note: *Never reuse dressings.*

Changing a Dressing Covering a Tube or Drain. To accommodate the tail of plastic tubing protruding from the skin, cut a small slit in one side of a gauze pad and fit it around the tube, then make a slit in the bottom side of a second gauze pad and conform it around the tube to wedge it snugly in place. Add one or more layers of gauze and tape the dressing down.

Oral Hygiene

Mouth dryness, or *xerostomia,* is a chronic nuisance for many ill people. Diseases (such as diabetes), radiation therapy to the head and neck, and many medications can slow down production of saliva. Since this secretion rinses away teeth-decaying germs, xerostomia also predisposes patients to cavities and periodontal disease. Regular oral hygiene, therefore, is a must.

Brush the person's teeth after every meal and before retiring, using a soft-bristle brush and a mild fluoride toothpaste or a paste of baking soda and water. Rinse the brush thoroughly and store it in a dry place.

Many commercial mouthwashes contain excessive sodium and alcohol, which only dry out the mouth further. Stir half a teaspoon of salt and half a teaspoon of baking soda in one cup of warm water and have the person swish it around in his mouth four to six times a day.

✱ *Patients who feel nauseous and can't brush without gagging should rinse with baking soda and water or salt water until they're able to tolerate a brush in their mouth with stronger tastes and smells.*

Men and women who have difficulty gripping a regular toothbrush may find it easier to hold a wide-handled brush or electric toothbrush.

For cancer patients slated to undergo chemotherapy or radiation therapy: If possible, make an appointment with the dentist prior to treatment. Now is the time for a cleaning and taking care of any cavities, gum disease, abscesses, or ill-fitting dentures. ▶ *See "Dry Mouth," page 161.*

INSIDE INFORMATION

Upon discharge from the hospital, remember to bring home the urinal, bedpan, vomit basin, and plastic beaker for measuring urine issued to the patient upon admission. Why not? He has already paid for them.

Toileting

When Patients Are Confined to Bed

Using a Urinal

Plastic urinals make it relatively easy for bedridden men to urinate while sitting up or lying supine or on their side. They simply place the narrow container between their legs and insert their penis in the opening. Women aren't as fortunate in this regard for obvious anatomical reasons. When a woman is able to sit up, a female urinal is ideal. Unlike a conventional bedpan, which has a deep rim, forcing the person to hoist up her hips three to four inches, the female urinal tapers almost flat so that she need only raise her hips slightly in order to slide the device under her.

Using a Bedpan

As almost any nurse will tell you, plastic bedpans are preferable to metal because the latter type can feel as jarringly cold against one's bare bottom as an outhouse seat on a winter morning. If a metal bedpan is all you have, remember to run warm water over it and then dry it before using. To prevent either kind from sticking to the person's skin, liberally sprinkle it with talcum powder or cornstarch.

Ideally, loved ones should be sitting up when using a bedpan, not only for comfort's sake but to enlist the force of gravity in moving their bowels. Prop them up with pillows or raise the head of the hospital bed.

If the person is able to arch her hips

a few inches, have her lie on her back, upper torso elevated, knees bent, and heels flat against the mattress. Then slide the bedpan underneath her, with the rounded part to the rear.

If this is too physically demanding or the person is unconscious, roll him on his side. If you're by yourself, use a drawsheet. Place the bedpan up against his backside and then return him to his back.

✳ *Center the pan under the person so that it doesn't tip. The tapered front should extend about four to five inches. Most important of all, make sure the orifices in question are well over the catch basin.*

Anticipate messes. Sick people dribble urine, they have diarrhea, they squirt and splatter fecal matter. Let watery stool seep into a mattress just once, and you'll have a heck of a time trying to get out the stain and dispel the odor. Protect the mattress with multiple layers by making the bed from the top down with a drawsheet placed under the person's midsection; a large disposable plastic-lined pad, popularly known as "chucks," or a large washable absorbent pad; a fitted bedsheet; a heavy-duty plastic pad covering the middle of the mattress (a folded shower curtain or large lawn or leaf bag tucked in works equally well); and an absorbent mattress pad for cushioning.

Never leave a bedpan under a patient for long stretches. It seems obvious, but according to nurse Sarah Eilenberg, "I've seen caregivers stick them under Mom and come back eight hours later. By then, of course, she has a bedsore."

MONEY SAVER

Instead of buying a commode at a surgical supply store, set a bedpan on a solid chair and place a chuck under it.

When Patients Are Able to Get Out of Bed

Using a Commode

A portable commode stationed at the bedside spares patients the indignity of toileting in bed and the risk incurred from trekking back and forth to the bathroom. Shaped like a chair, a commode consists of an aluminum or plastic frame that supports a toilet seat and seat cover. The removable plastic basin underneath is emptied after each use.

* *For a more aesthetically pleasing look, adorn the commode with a colorful cloth or throw.*

Perhaps your loved one finds the idea of a commode unappealing and is determined to use the bathroom. The urge to urinate awakens many older patients, particularly men, in the middle of the night. To minimize the chances of a fall, leave a light on in the bathroom and the hallway, or illuminate the way by plugging in several night-lights. You might also consider shifting the person's bed as close to the bathroom as possible.

Special Care: Toileting a Loved One Who Suffers from Memory Loss, Confusion, or Intellectual Impairment

One night, a few weeks before Dad died, he got out of bed to use the toilet. Half asleep and disoriented, he urinated behind his bedroom door, thinking he was in the bathroom. My brother and I were concerned that he could have fallen. We often took turns sleeping in a makeshift bed just outside his room so that he would awaken us if he tried to walk to the john.

A person suffering from dementia, whether drug-induced or organic, can sometimes have trouble locating the bathroom during the day. Help him recognize the door by taping a drawing or photograph of a toilet to it, or post a sign reading TOILET in block letters. Keep the bathroom free of magazines and other unnecessary objects to reduce potential distractions.

Cleaning Patients After a Bowel Movement or Urination

As with any task involving personal hygiene, encourage loved ones to clean themselves as long as they feel up to it. But when that's not possible and this responsibility falls to you, the goal is to quickly reestablish the person's dignity and comfort.

First get a cross-draft going, to dissipate the odor. Unless it's too cold outside, open two windows and turn on a fan, without calling undue attention to the act. Next say something like "Hold on, I'll be right back and get you all cleaned up." A minute later you return with a tray containing your supplies: unscented baby wipes rather than toilet paper, which can irritate, a basin of lukewarm water, soap, washcloth, towel, moisturizer, clean sheets and chucks, a plastic garbage bag, a bucket for all the soiled items, and gloves.

♀ *Feminine Care: Remember, always wipe the vulva, vaginal area, or rectum from front to back.*

When you're through wiping the genitals and rectum, wash between

---

INSIDE INFORMATION

To throw out soiled chucks without dirtying yourself, turn a plastic garbage bag inside out, reach inside, pick up the mess, then simply invert the bag around it.

---

the person's legs as you would when giving a bed bath. There are a number of soapless, nonirritating cleansers on the market specifically for dissolving urine and fecal matter. Brand names include Confident, Hygiene 1, and Orchid Fresh.

Empty the contents of the bedpan down the toilet. Baby wipes are thicker than adult towelettes and can clog plumbing. Deposit each used towelette in your plastic bag, along with other nonflushable items such as paper towels, tampons, and sanitary napkins. Seal the bag and place it in a covered outdoor trash can.

Toss soiled clothes and bed linens in the wash right away, along with your usual detergent and half a cup of full-strength chlorine bleach, which will sterilize almost anything. (Use one cup for badly soiled linens.) So-called color-safe bleach does not disinfect, however.

Don't leave a bucket of excrement-stained laundry lying around the house. Not only will stains set in, but that sickroom smell won't dissipate. If you normally do your wash at a laundromat and can't get there for a day or two, rinse the clothes in cold water and pour detergent directly on the stains.

Caring for an Ostomy

Ostomy refers to any surgically constructed opening in the body. A *colostomy* or *ileostomy* allows a patient to evacuate stool through an opening, or stoma, in the lower abdomen, perhaps as a result of the removal of a sizable portion of the intestines due to an obstruction, perforation, bowel cancer, or other diseases of the digestive tract. People who require *urostomy* surgery may have had their bladder removed or were born with deformities of the urinary tract.

"An ostomy isn't artificial," emphasizes nurse Paula Erwin-Toth. "It's the person's own organ." Erwin-Toth, head of enterostomal therapy at the Cleveland Clinic Foundation, has had a urostomy since she was ten years old. To create an ostomy, the intestine or urinary-tract diversion is brought through the abdominal wall, then sutured into place. The stoma, which measures up to one inch across, protrudes slightly above the skin level. Erwin-Toth describes it as resembling "a red cherry tomato. It's the same type of tissue as inside your mouth."

Emptying and Changing Ostomy Bags

Some people with ostomies may have a sense of fullness or pressure near the stoma when urination or bowel movements are coming on, but they have no voluntary control over the flow of these functions. Therefore they must wear a pouchlike collecting device over the ostomy at all times.

"With a colostomy," says Erwin-Toth, "you may need to empty it only once or twice a day. An ileostomy, though, may need to be emptied anywhere from five to ten times a day, depending on how liquid the output is. The colon reabsorbs fluid back into the body," she explains. "So the higher up the intestine you go, the more watery the stool becomes." As for a urostomy, "it usually must be emptied every couple of hours, on average."

Caregivers and ostomy patients are often concerned about odors and leakages. Perfect fit of the drainage bag can eliminate most problems. Many models feature vents that allow gas to escape from the bag while deodorizing it in the

---

How to Get Rid of Stains (Blood, Feces, Urine, and Vomit)

Consumer Reports recommends using various combinations of everyday household cleaning products to remove stains left by blood and bodily waste.
   Use in the order specified:

Blood	Ammonia, mild detergent, enzyme detergent
Fecal Matter	Mild detergent, ammonia, vinegar
Urine (new)	Mild detergent, ammonia, vinegar, enzyme detergent
Urine (old)	Mild detergent, vinegar, ammonia, enzyme detergent
Vomit:	Vinegar, ammonia, mild detergent, enzyme detergent

---

process. A tight seal between the skin around the stoma and the bag is also essential because urine and stool can irritate the skin, leading to pain and infections.

There is a wide array of ostomy-care products and appliances available through pharmacies, medical supply houses, and catalogs. Finding the best system of adhesives, drainage bags, and skin-care products for your loved one requires experimentation and expert advice. Ask your physician or home-care agency for a consultation with a nurse specializing in ostomy care, or contact the United Ostomy Association, which publishes an informative quarterly magazine and sponsors support groups nationwide. The American Cancer Society also runs support groups for people with colostomies or ileostomies. ► *See Appendix B: "Ostomies," page 510.*

☎ United Ostomy Association, 800-826-0826 or 714-660-8624.

☎ American Cancer Society, 800-227-2345 or 404-320-3333.

Whatever type of ostomy and drainage system your loved one has, a few basic rules apply:

◆ Wash your hands with soap and water before and after assisting your loved one with ostomy care, being careful not to spread germs. As with toileting, strict sterile technique is not required, but latex gloves will certainly allow you to work more confidently, without worrying about soiling your hands. Also, a well-ventilated room quickly dispels any unpleasant odors. ◄ *See "Daily Hygiene," page 110.*

◆ Wash the stoma gently but thoroughly with soap and water when changing drainage bags. Some stomas tend to bleed easily, so a gentle touch is required. Erwin-Toth says not to worry, though. "You're not going to hurt the stoma; they're hardy little guys."

✚ *Notify the doctor, home-care nurse, or hospice nurse immediately if you notice any signs of infection around the stoma, including swelling and redness or an unusual discharge. Let the medical team know right away whenever someone with an ostomy spikes a fever.*

Grooming and Dressing

Being seriously ill chips away at a person's sense of self- and body image. For my stepmother, the most upsetting aspect of having terminal lung cancer was that it prevented her from fulfilling the cherished roles that, in Lynn's mind, defined her: doting wife, mom, stepmom, grandmother, and great-grandmother, as well as desirable woman, lover, and natural-born hostess. Although the disease certainly exacted a toll on her famous good looks, keeping up her physical appearance was a way for Lynn to temporarily elude this new, unwelcome identity—*cancer patient*—which followed her like a shadow.

Whenever Lynn expected visitors, out came her makeup, nail polish, rollers, and hair spray. Dressed in slacks and a casual top, she insisted on greeting company in the living room. My father would have preferred that she conserve her energy, but he understood how important this was to her.

Anything that enhances self-worth and allows loved ones to feel more like their old selves and remain life-focused should be encouraged. The simple act of exchanging that sick person's uniform of pajamas or gown for street clothes and getting spruced up does wonders for a patient's spirits. Plus, you just plain feel better when your hair isn't all matted and oily, and you don't have two-day-old stubble sandpapering your shoulder every time you lie on your side.

Another argument for taking the time to groom and dress patients whenever possible is that if more of us had experience caring for the ill and dying, a loved one's sickly appearance wouldn't get in the way of emotional intimacy. For some folks it can. "The nursing home sometimes would have Dad dressed in a hospital gown or in someone else's clothes," recalls Diane Young. The sight of her father looking so disheveled used to bring her to tears. "Then we started putting jogging suits on him, which looked real sharp! Seeing him dressed neatly, as he used to look, was very helpful for me."

Every day, assist your loved one with grooming. "How about letting me give you a shave?" "Feel like putting on a little makeup this morning?" Propose that you help him get dressed. In my experience, relatively few patients take to their sickbeds to passively await death. Most want desperately to stay alive and find comfort in the routines of normal daily life. If the reply is no, however, let it go.

Hair Care

- Use mild shampoos and conditioners, such as baby shampoo. And remember, excessive shampooing will dry out the scalp. Untangle snarls by wetting the hair with a cream rinse or conditioner, or use a children's spray-on detangler.
- To shampoo hair in bed, purchase a plastic shampoo tray, which resembles the "splash" that one sets under an outdoor drainpipe to carry away rainwater from the house. Place an empty basin on a chair, several inches lower than the bed. The person lies back, with her head in the tray. As you pour warm water over her hair—sparingly, to minimize the mess, but enough to thoroughly rinse out the suds—the tray channels the overflow down into the basin. Or you can position your loved one's head slightly over the edge of the bed, with a towel and plastic garbage bag underneath, and a dishpan on the floor to catch the runoff.

✽ *As with giving a bed bath, wash hair before you plan to change the bed.*

- To give a shampoo at the sink, sit the patient in a chair facing the sink and have her lean forward, gripping the edge for stability.
- Let's say the person has a cold but his hair needs cleaning. Try one of the dry shampoos on the market. Caregiver Nola Miller used it on her husband, bedridden with chronic obstructive pulmonary disease. "You just rub the shampoo in, wipe it off, and comb the hair," she explains.

Some other suggestions for your loved one's hair care:

- Encourage loved ones to brush their hair themselves. Besides fostering independence, even minimal physical exertion stimulates the circulation and helps avert contracture of muscles and joints.
- On days when loved ones don't feel

like fussing with their hair, popping on a baseball cap, bandana, turban, or scarf lets them feel more "presentable" while at the same time expressing their individuality.

- Avoid elaborate hairdos that require extensive blow-drying and styling for chronically fatigued patients or those with a respiratory ailment. Think *practical*.
- When someone has severe emphysema, never use hair spray—or, for that matter, any aerosol, including deodorants—which can further impair breathing.
- Ask the patient's barber or beautician, or your own stylist, if he or she makes house calls. You'll be surprised how many will, especially for a regular client. (A generous tip helps.) The staff at the hospital, nursing home, or home health care agency can usually recommend local hair cutters who routinely visit sick people at home; ask around at patient/caregiver support group meetings as well. ► *See "Caring for Someone with Cancer: Hair Loss (Alopecia)," page 333.*

Nail and Cuticle Care

Keep fingernails short, to reduce the chances of patients inadvertently scratching themselves. And anyone who is immunocompromised shouldn't cut or tear her cuticles but should use cuticle cream or remover instead.

Don't neglect the feet. Long, ragged toenails peeking out from under the covers are not only unsightly but they turn thick and brittle, split and break, and snag on bedclothes and socks. In cases of extreme neglect, the nails may curl under and break the skin, inviting infection.

The best time to cut toenails is after bathing and drying the feet, when the nails are softer. Trim them straight across—using toenail scissors rather than clippers—and then file down the corners with an emery board. Suggestion: Spring for a pedicure kit. Extremely thick or brittle toenails are best left to a physician, nurse, or podiatrist.

Shaving

In general, an electric shaver is easier and safer than a razor for shaving bedbound patients. For those prone to excessive bleeding due to blood platelet deficiency, or *thrombocytopenia*, an electric model is a necessity. Loved ones suffering from tremors, as seen in Parkinson's disease, should also go electric.

Dressing Patients

On a purely practical level, it's actually best if men and women confined to bed don't wear any clothes, but most folks probably aren't going to be comfortable lying naked under the sheets—not only for reasons of modesty but because it may compound their feelings of vulnerability.

Forget about long pants or full-length nightgowns that go on over the head. Ever try tugging a person's pants on and off while he is lying down? It's exhausting. As for long nightgowns, patients get entangled in them all the time. And what if the person urinates or defecates herself? We'd have to cut the soiled gown with a scissors, since we're not about to pull it up over her face.

The most practical garment for everyone concerned is a hospital gown, which falls to about mid-thigh on an average-size person and ties in the back. They're designed specifically to leave your butt exposed.

When selecting clothes for someone able to get out of bed, comfort and convenience take precedence:

Dressing Do's

Attire should be easy to remove in the event of a bathroom emergency. Examples: wide skirts and pants with elastic waistbands or drawstrings.

Attire should also be easy to put on—wraparound skirts as opposed to styles you have to step into or pull down over the head.

Lean toward lightweight fabrics, weather permitting.

Dressing Don'ts

Clothing made of rough, abrasive material can irritate the skin.

Tight, restrictive clothing can constrict the chest and abdomen. For similar reasons, don't bother with belts, brassieres, and girdles. If your loved one complains of feeling naked without a belt or a bra, suggest suspenders or a camisole.

Socks or stockings with elastic bands and panty hose can impede circulation in the legs.

How to Assist a Patient with Getting Dressed

1. Have the person sit on the side of the bed.
2. Help him on with his undershirt and shirt so he doesn't catch a chill. If it's a pullover top, don't make a sick or disoriented person hold his arms over his head with his face covered while you struggle to get his arms in the sleeves. Use the same technique as a parent dressing a squirming child: Run your hands up the sleeves, take his hands, and pull his arms through each sleeve. Gather up the excess material, then pull the garment over his head in one smooth motion.
3. Slip on socks or stockings.
4. Place underwear or panties inside pants and pull them on together over the ankles.
5. Put on the person's shoes or slippers.
6. Ask the patient to stand—wrapping his arms around your neck for support if necessary—while you pull up his pants and fasten them.

Dressing Patients with Special Needs

When a patient has difficulty using his hands, you might consider the following:

- Replace buttons with button hooks, Velcro strips, or elastic cuffs or waistbands.
- Tie cloth or leather pull tabs onto zippers for easier gripping.
- Suggest oversized pullover shirts, blouses, sweaters, and sweatshirts instead of button-down tops.
- Consider tennis shoes with elastic laces or Velcro straps.

When a patient suffers from memory loss, confusion, or intellectual impairment, he can easily become flustered trying to decide which clothes to wear or may no longer remember

IN THE HOSPITAL

Street clothes aren't practical in the hospital, where the staff needs convenient access to patients' bodies. A lightweight robe, button-down house dress, kimono, or caftan from home covers up a person better than the hospital-issue gown. Patients should feel free to wear their own tennis shoes or slippers and headgear as well, all of which help to reinforce their individuality with the health care team.

how to get dressed. "Once," recalls Diane Young, "after giving my father a bath, I handed him a pair of socks and told him to put them on while I straightened up the bathroom. When I came back, he was just staring at them. 'Daddy,' I said, 'why didn't you put your socks on?' And he said, 'I don't know what to do with them.' "

The tricks below are intended to make dressing a mentally impaired loved one easier. Still, there's no getting around the fact that this can be an immensely frustrating task. The best advice we can offer is to set aside extra time and do your best to keep your impatience in check because dementia patients become easily upset, which only serves to confuse them more.

- If cognitive impairment is relatively mild and the person can dress herself with supervision, organize apparel by type: underwear in this drawer, socks in that drawer, and so on. Then label each drawer clearly.
- Too many choices can be overwhelming. Weed out clothing that is seldom worn, no longer fits well, or is out of season. You'll save yourself aggravation if you also store away garments that have complicated fasteners.
- Offer no more than two choices of clothing at a time. Hold up two blouses and ask, "Which would you like to wear? This one or that one?" If this proves too perplexing for the person, select an outfit for her.
- Set out clothing on the bed in the order it's to be put on. Hand the person one article at a time.
- Loose-fitting clothing is best, especially for patients who wear adult diapers for incontinence, as did Diane Young's father. "The jogging suit was ideal," she says. "It had an elastic waistband so he didn't have to fool with a zipper. It was easy to launder, and the fullness in the pants helped accommodate the bulkiness of the diaper."
- Tops should have zippers, buttons, or snaps down the front. Having a sweatshirt pulled over his head can be frightening for the patient.
- If your loved one wants to wear the same clothes a second day in a row, don't argue. However, be sure dirty clothing goes directly into the hamper or at least out of sight so you don't find yourself trying to dissuade a stubborn patient from putting on a soiled pair of pants.
- Keep jewelry and other accessories to a minimum or omit them altogether.
- Because Alzheimer's patients sometimes wander off, sew or iron name labels in all clothing.

Adaptive Grooming and Dressing Aids

Innovative devices such as combs with easy-to-grasp extension handles and gadgets for pulling up socks and stockings help ailing loved ones maintain their independence. For written descriptions of the myriad products available and manufacturers' phone numbers, call the National Rehabilitation Information Center's free Abledata database at 800-227-0216/301-608-8998.

Turning, Maneuvering, and Lifting

The purpose of learning the proper ways to maneuver patients is to ensure not just their safety but yours, too, as well as to save wear and tear on your back. If you haven't received instruction in these techniques, ask your loved one's doctor to approve a visit by a home health care nurse, through the hospital, the health department, or the local Visiting Nurse Association.

Ever wonder how petite ninety-pound nurses shift patients three times their size about the bed without so much as breaking a sweat? The answer is *drawsheets*, a must for those of us tending loved ones who are bedridden or incontinent. Actually, we recommend them in all circumstances. Your back will be eternally grateful.

To make a drawsheet, simply fold a sheet in thirds, place it lengthwise across the bed and under the patient's hips—from approximately the shoulders to mid-thigh, the body's center of gravity—and then tuck in the ends so they're not bunched up on the floor. Now you have the leverage to reposition without having to lift the person.

Let's say your patient asks to be repositioned from her back onto her left side:

1. Untuck the drawsheet on the right side of the bed.
2. Standing on the opposite side of the bed—in this case, the patient's left—pull her right leg and right arm across her axis.
3. Then reach across her, grasp the end of the untucked drawsheet and pull it toward you, rolling her gently onto her side. If the bed has side rails and the person is able to lend a hand by holding on to them, this becomes easier still.

Drawsheets also allow us to slide patients toward the head or foot of the bed without the sheet rubbing against their skin:

1. Ask the patient to lie prone, with her knees bent and both feet flat on the mattress.
2. Untuck both ends of the drawsheet.
3. Stand on the person's weakest side or at the head of the bed.
4. Untuck and gather both ends of the drawsheet over her midsection.
5. On the count of three, have her push off the mattress with her feet while you assist by pulling the drawsheet up.

If your loved one is unable to help:

1. Untuck the drawsheet.
2. Stand at the head of the bed.
3. Slide your arms along each side of the person's body, palms to the ceiling. The insides of your forearms should be supporting the backs of her shoulders.
4. Grasp the drawsheet on each side of the patient.
5. Knees bent, push with your legs as you pull her toward you on the drawsheet.

The drawsheet serves a dual function in that it keeps urine, fecal matter, and so forth relatively contained. This spares you from having to remake the entire bed every time there's a spill or an accident—which, when someone is seriously ill, can be a recurring event. Sometimes my stepmother used to cough so hard that she'd soil herself. All I had to do was roll her to one side, clean her, pull out the dirty drawsheet and absorbent pad beneath it, put down new chucks and a clean drawsheet, and return her to a comfortable position.

How to Make an Occupied Bed

The first time you do this correctly, you'll feel like the magician who has yanked the tablecloth out from beneath a fully set dinner table without disturbing a single spoon. Once you have the sequence down, it shouldn't take more than five minutes.

1. Stand on the patient's right. Using the drawsheet, roll him toward you, as close to the edge of the bed as safety allows.
2. Walk around to the opposite side of the bed so that you're now facing the patient's back. Pull out all tucked-in linens: fitted bottom sheet, plastic liner, mattress pad, drawsheet.
3. Hold the edge of the used bedding and begin rolling it up tightly away from you until the roll touches the patient, who is still lying on his side.
4. Make the stripped half of the bed, including a clean mattress pad and plastic liner (if necessary), bottom sheet, chucks, and drawsheet.
5. Roll up the excess fabric in the middle of the bed but fold the material over itself (toward you) this time. You're left with two parallel tubes of rolled-up bedding running down the center of the bed from head to toe.
6. Turn the patient toward you, over the two humps of material and onto the clean side of the bed.
7. Now go around to the unmade side of the bed and strip it.
8. Unroll the clean bed linens and finish making the bed.
9. Reposition your loved one in the middle of the bed and cover him loosely with a top sheet and one or two blankets.

Lifting Patients by Yourself

Whether we're transferring someone from the bed to a wheelchair or helping her to her feet after a fall, the basic body mechanics are the same. So that you don't wind up taking a spill yourself, remember to observe the three most important rules for lifting another person—or any heavy object—safely:

1. Always keep your knees slightly bent for a low center of gravity. This incorporates the large muscles in the thighs and hips into the maneuver and lets you get your whole body weight into the act, radically reducing the mechanical stress across your back.

2. Always plant your feet squarely on the floor, about shoulder-width apart, for support and balance.
3. Don't hold your breath. Plant and pause. Before you move the person, take a deep breath, then squeeze your abdominal muscles tightly and exhale forcefully as you pull the weight toward the axis of your body in one smooth motion—every time.

Transferring from a Bed to a Chair or Wheelchair

1. First help your loved one sit upright on the side on the bed. Have her lie on her side, facing you, with her knees bent.
2. Swing her legs over the side of the bed.
3. With one hand gently supporting her upper back, gently pull her upright. "Never pull a patient by the arms," stresses nurse Mary Ann Reeks.
4. Place the chair on the person's strong side.
5. When lifting, we rely mainly on our leg muscles, which are far stronger than those in the lower back. Stand directly in front of the person, then move in close. "Put your knees against theirs," says Reeks, "and grip the patient under the arm, by the armpit, or around the waist." Have the patient hold onto your shoulders.
6. On a count of three, pull the person to an upright position, straightening your legs as you rise with her. Now the two of you rest for a minute. Some older folks experience attacks of *orthostatic hypotension* upon standing—their blood pressure drops abruptly, and they become temporarily weak and dizzy. Continue to brace her knees with yours.

✳ *One trick for avoiding orthostatic hypotension is to have the person stimulate circulation down below by flexing her ankles and wiggling her toes before getting up.*

7. The fear of falling can virtually paralyze patients. According to Nurse Reeks, "They tend to do better following instructions than attempting this on their own. Tell them what to do next: 'Take a step. . . . Now lock your knees.' And so on." Reassure them that you won't let them fall.

8. Carefully turn the person until the back of her knees are touching the chair. As the two of you pivot, always face her; never twist your body.

9. Have the person grasp the arm of the chair with her strong hand.

10. Gingerly lower her into the seat, remembering to bend your knees instead of bending from the waist. ▶ *See "Edema, Blood Clots, Phlebitis, Orthostatic Hypotension," page 178.*

Mechanical Lifting Devices

Consider mounting a trapeze bar on the ceiling, to give patients something to grab onto when getting out of bed.

When patients are completely immobile, a ceiling-mounted mechanical lift may be necessary. Insurance may cover lifts and other equipment for moving disabled patients if authorized by the doctor. ◀ *See "Modifying the Home," page 78.* ▶ *See Appendix B: "Adaptive Technology," page 504.*

Tips for Preventing Falls

Every year 250,000 older Americans fracture their hips, usually due to falls. Many of us will be caring for elderly women with the degenerative bone disease osteoporosis, or cancer victims whose primary tumor has migrated to the bones, or other patients at risk for broken bones. Prolonged use of the widely prescribed class of hormonal drugs known as *glucocorticoids* (brands include Deltasone, Aristocort, and Medrol) can cause long bones to snap during ordinary physical activity.

A bone fracture may prove fatal to people in frail health. The long convalescence in bed predisposes them to infection, and many ultimately die of pneumonia or septicemia. Preventing mishaps is therefore one of a caregiver's prime concerns.

Basic Home Safety

In addition to modifying the home for safety, as outlined in chapter 1, there are several other measures you can take:

- Don't wax bare floors.
- Throw out all throw rugs.
- If the person is unsteady on his feet, rearrange furniture so that he's not forced to navigate narrow pathways.
- As if child-proofing a house, either temporarily store away furniture with sharp edges or pad the corners heavily with utility tape. Banish glass tabletops as well.
- Make sure electrical cords aren't left coiled on the floor.
- Since the glare of the sun on a floor can disorient and lead to an accident, hang sheer curtains, which let in sunlight but do away with glare.

Basic Walking Safety

Two words: sensible shoes! Many folks make the mistake of wearing tennis sneakers or walking shoes because they're soft and comfortable. As any podiatrist will attest, a solid shoe that fits snugly and supports the ankle and arch is a far safer choice. Avoid crepe and rubber soles and heels, which can stick to the floor, prompting a fall. Conversely, if the underside is too slick, scuff it with sandpaper. Shoes should have low heels.

A great way to break in leather shoes is to lightly coat the person's feet with mineral oil and have him wear the new pair—sans socks—around the house for two or three days. This conforms the shoes to the shape of the foot.

If your loved one requires assistance,

walk alongside her, gripping her forearm with one hand and supporting her back with the other.

Ask the doctor if he recommends that the person use a cane or walker.

✻ *For people with Parkinson's disease, a cane or walker can actually get in the way and cause an accident.*

To Prevent Falls from Bed

Raise the side rails on the hospital bed. You can also rent rails that attach to a regular bed. One word of warning, however: A patient who is confused or delirious may try to scale the rails and sustain a worse injury than if he fell out of bed with the rails down.

"When patients constantly try to get out of bed," says Mary Ann Reeks, "we tell the family to put a baby monitor in the room or tie a bell to the bed rails." Another approach is to disassemble the bed frame and place the box spring and mattress—or just the mattress—on the floor so the person can't get seriously hurt. ▶ *See "Caring for Someone with a Progressive Neurological Disease: Parkinson's Disease—Impaired Mobility," page 475.*

What to Do if a Patient Falls

Don't grab the person and try to stop the fall. You could injure your back or go tumbling to the floor with her. If you can, break the fall by guiding her down along the length of your body and trying to protect her head.

Before helping her to her feet, check for bleeding, bruises, and broken bones. If you suspect injury, call the doctor. If you suspect serious injury, summon an ambulance. Don't attempt to move the person yourself, just make her comfortable with pillows and a blanket while you await assistance. If there is minor bleeding, use a sterile gauze pad to apply gentle but firm pressure to the wound. Once the bleeding stops, clean and dress the cut or laceration.

Watch your loved one for signs of a head injury. Does she seem disoriented or listless? Other symptoms to report to the physician: dizziness, blurred vision, headache, nausea, and numbness in the extremities.

✻ *The doctor will most likely instruct you to observe the person regularly for the next several hours or over the next twenty-four hours if she hit her head. When she is sleeping, wake her up every four hours just to be certain she is conscious and alert.*

✚ *Call 911 under the following circumstances: loss of consciousness even if only momentary, fractured bones, convulsions, and blood or fluid seeping from the ears, nose, or mouth.*

Preventing Muscle Contracture and Foot Drop

Don't let our warnings about falls in the home scare you. We *want* our loved one up and about if possible. Like a self-winding watch, the human body has to move in order to function properly. Getting those arms and legs in motion winds it up again: Circulation improves, which in turn promotes quicker healing and helps prevent blood from pooling in the legs. The bladder and bowel resume their normal schedules, reducing the threats of urinary tract infection and constipation. We breathe better, digest better, and think more clearly when we're moving around.

Mobility also safeguards against *contracture*, the atrophying of muscles and joints that endangers anyone confined to bed for an extended period of time. "Even after a week in bed with the flu," nurse Ellen Wilson points out, "if you don't keep everything moving, you'll experience stiffness." True contracture, once it sets in, can be permanently crippling: Hands curl up like claws, and shrinking muscles often pull patients into a fetal position. "A contracture can get so tight," says nurse practitioner Audrey MacMillan, "that to try to move it feels as if you're breaking a bone." Our goal is never to get to that stage.

When patients are bedridden, a physical therapist or nurse can come to the home and teach them how to keep muscles and joints pliable through simple exercises. Sit in on the lesson so you'll be able to coach the person through his in-bed workout. In cases where a loved one is unable to exercise on his own—perhaps due to weakness, paralysis, or intellectual impairment—we manipulate the major joints of the body for him. The health care professional will show you how.

Even if a patient is unconscious, these passive range-of-motion exercises need to be carried out, ideally four times a day. Severe contraction makes the everyday tasks of caregiving that much harder. Despite a caregiver's most diligent efforts, some loss of muscle tone is inevitable. Nevertheless, you're performing a wonderful service, for the contorting of the toes, knees, shoulders, and other joints can cause painful cramping. And, says Wilson, "just the touch of another person is very beneficial."

How to Perform Passive Range-of-Motion Exercises

The fundamentals of passive range-of-motion (ROM) exercises can be summed up in three words: *rotate, flex,* and *extend.* To rotate is to turn; flex, to bend; extend, to straighten. "Never try to force movement," stresses MacMillan, clinical coordinator at the Pittsburgh Alzheimer Disease Research Center. Maneuver limbs slowly, gently, rhythmically, while keeping attuned to your loved one's comfort.

Pay attention to fingers, wrists, elbows, shoulders, neck, hips, knees, ankles, and toes. Ask a nurse or physical therapist at the hospital or from the home-care agency to demonstrate these

basic movements to you. Repeat each movement six to eight times per joint several times a day, with each session lasting no more than five to ten minutes. "It's better to do these exercises several times in short intervals," says Wilson, "than in one long exercise routine."

✱ *To help ward off contracture of the hands and fingers, you can buy soft grips that strap around the patient's hand. They not only keep the fist from closing but prevent skin breakdown by separating the fingers.*

What Is Foot Drop?

Foot drop is another serious concern. "When you're lying down, your foot naturally flexes down, with the toes pointed downward," explains Nurse Wilson. "If you don't keep the foot bending up and down, using those muscles, it eventually gets stuck in that position." For years, nurses placed an L-shaped board under the mattress at the foot of the bed to keep the feet resting upright. One of the drawbacks of *footboards,* says Wilson, is that they can be uncomfortable, causing patients "to scrunch their knees as they naturally slip down in the bed."

Wilson and many other health care pros suggest simply fitting bed-bound loved ones with high-top sneakers. That's what an ICU head nurse told the Reverend Harry Cole when his wife was in a coma from a massive cerebral hemorrhage. "So I bought Jackie a pair of red high-top Reeboks," he says, laughing gently at the image of his wife, who regained consciousness a few weeks later. "You'd lift the sheets, and there she was in a hospital gown and sneakers."

Measuring Vital Signs

Vital signs include a patient's temperature, blood pressure, pulse, and breathing rate. For someone in stable condition, it's usually sufficient to check these in the morning and again in the evening, as well as anytime a new symptom emerges or an existing one worsens.

How to Take a Temperature

1. Sterilize the bulb end and shaft of the thermometer by wiping it with a gauze pad saturated in alcohol, then rinse it under cool running water. Some digital thermometers come encased in a disposable plastic sheath, which you replace before each measurement.

2. *If you're using a mercury thermometer*, grasp the glass end and with a snapping wrist motion shake down the mercury to below 95 degrees Fahrenheit.

3. Insert the bulb end (see Table 3).

4. Leave the thermometer in place for approximately . . . (see Table 3).

5. Remove the thermometer and read the temperature. Bear in mind that "normal" temperature varies slightly from the 98.6 degrees we memorized in grade school.

To read a mercury thermometer, hold it at eye level and turn it slowly until the dark line comes into view. If you can't get the hang of it, buy a digital-readout model that displays the temperature in numbers.

6. Clean and dry the thermometer, then store it in its protective case.

An elevated temperature, or *hyperthermia*, doesn't necessarily indicate fever per se. Our internal thermostat

TABLE 3

Insert Thermometer		Leave in Place		Normal Temperature
		Mercury	Digital (Listen for tiny beep)	
Orally				
Under the tongue as far back as possible		4–5 minutes	45–60 seconds	96.8°–99.5°
Rectally				
Gently into rectum, about 1 1/2 inches, after first lubricating thermometer with petroleum jelly and positioning patient on side, top leg bent at knee. *Make sure you're using a rectal mercury or digital thermometer; likewise, use only an oral thermometer for taking temperature orally or under the arm.*		3 minutes	45–60 seconds	97.8°–100.5°
Under Armpit				
Under armpit, then fold arm across chest to hold thermometer in place. *This is the least accurate route for taking a temperature and should be used only when oral and rectal methods are out of the question.*		10 minutes	45–60 seconds	97.8°–98.5°

routinely "turns up the heat" when we're exercising, sunning at the beach, and sometimes in response to emotional stress. If you suspect a loved one has a fever (see sidebar listing common symptoms), take her temperature every hour or two until it falls to within normal range, or more frequently if the readings keep getting higher. Elderly folks need to be monitored especially carefully: The body-heat regulator in the brain loses sensitivity as we age so that an older patient's temperature may soar dangerously without her realizing it.

A fever usually harbingers an underlying infection or inflammation, though not always. Medications can induce a reaction called "drug fever." Malignant tumors of the bone, kidney, and other parts of the body often ignite noninfectious fevers, probably by releasing substances that act to raise the setting of the natural thermostat. The body, laboring to maintain what it now perceives as normal temperature, accelerates heart rate, respiration, muscle activity, and metabolism. Nurse Mary Ann Reeks notes, "Some cancer patients tend to spike a temperature once a day," frequently around the same time. "We usually give them Tylenol and watch them closely."

Another example: Quadriplegic men and women, paralyzed from the neck down, experience a curious phenomenon dubbed "quad fever." According to Dr. Donald Leslie, associate medical director of the Shepherd Spinal Center in Atlanta, "Many patients will run a fever without having an infection. Typically it's treated just by cooling the person off."

Nonetheless, given the potential dangers of infection, we should notify the physician, home-care nurse, or hospice nurse if our loved one sustains a *low-grade fever* (between 99.5 and 101 degrees) for twelve hours or if she develops a *high-grade fever* (101.1 degrees and above), regardless of how it was measured—though be sure to mention which method you used. Once the problem has been identified, ask the

---

Symptoms of Fever

- Skin feels warm to the touch
- Flushed cheeks
- Listlessness
- Aching muscles and joints
- Headache
- Patient complains of feeling extremely hot or cold
- Appetite loss or thirst
- Shivering, chills, profuse sweating
- Watery eyes
- Nausea, vomiting, diarrhea, constipation—all of which may be triggered by a rise in temperature.

At excessively elevated temperatures (approximately 103° or higher):
- Rapid heartbeat
- Shortness of breath
- Confusion, delirium, seizures

---

doctor what body temperature and/or underlying symptoms merit a phone call in the future.

Managing Fever

Unless we're reporting a high fever, the physician may hold off prescribing a fever-reducing medication, or *antipyretic*, until he's determined the source of the problem. If it's an infection, the person will probably be put on an antimicrobial drug. Elevated temperatures can usually be brought under control with an over-the-counter antipyretic such as *acetaminophen* (Tylenol), *naproxen* (Aleve), *salicylic acid* (aspirin), or *ibuprofen* (Motrin), all of which also ease fatigue and aching.

Our task is to keep our loved one comfortable, thoroughly hydrated, and nourished.

When a patient complains of feeling hot:

- *Cover him with only a sheet*, while making sure the room is free of drafts.

- *Give him a* cool *sponge bath or apply a* cool, *damp washcloth*—never cold. One reason feverish patients feel hot is that their blood vessels dilate in an attempt to dissipate the heat; therefore, pay special attention to areas where the vessels lie close to the surface of the skin: forehead, neck, armpits, and groin. Nurse Reeks suggests that when sponging a patient, "let the water evaporate on the skin; that tends to cool them down. An old-fashioned alcohol rub also helps to lower a temperature," she adds. "Rub it on the chest and the arms for about five minutes." Witch hazel liniment works well for this purpose, too.
- *Change clammy bed linens and bedclothes promptly.* Sweat-dampened sheets against the skin paves the way for bedsores. Mary Vitro, who nursed her husband with AIDS, recalls that it wasn't unusual for her to change the sheets four or five times a night.

When a patient complains of chills:

- *Cover him with blankets*, though sometimes no amount of warmth seems to relieve the chills. "Rick could be under four comforters, yet still he would say, 'I'm so cold,' " says Mary, crying at the memory. "I would lie on top of him." If using a hot-water bottle, fill it with warm, not hot, water.
- Chills generally precede a rise in temperature. *After the chills and shivering subside, take the person's temperature.*
- Between perspiring profusely and breathing rapidly, a feverish person loses more water than normal. According to the American College of Physicians, caregivers should *encourage patients to drink two to three quarts of* cool *liquids every twelve hours—twice the normal amount.* ◄ *See "Tricks for Getting Patients to Drink," page 104.*
- Fever forces the body to expend extra energy. If its nutritional needs aren't met, the body will begin breaking down its own tissue for fuel. Since our loved one may not have much of an appetite, the trick is to *maximize calories and carbohydrates.* Try enticing the person with bread, pasta, peanut butter, potatoes, and fruit. ► *See "Tricks for Stimulating Appetite," page 159.*
- *Keep a record of a loved one's fevers:* How frequently do they occur? When? For how long? The pattern can often lead doctors to the cause.

At temperatures of 103 degrees or higher, fever enters the danger zone. Brain cells become overstimulated, which can bring about confusion, delirium, and convulsions. The heart pumps eight to ten beats faster per minute for each degree above normal; for someone suffering from cardiac or respiratory disease, the heightened pulse and respiration could conceivably prove fatal.

Your loved one's doctor may instruct you to summon an ambulance or bring the patient to the emergency room. Or she may advise you to place ice packs in the groin and under the armpit at twenty-minute intervals (twenty minutes on, twenty minutes off) until the fever breaks. You can use store-bought ice packs or make your own: Simply fill a plastic food-freezer bag with ice and wrap it in a damp towel. ► *See "Managing Seizures and Convulsions," page 180; "Delusional or Hallucinatory Behavior," page 204.*

✚ *Notify the doctor, home-care nurse, or hospice nurse immediately if your patient suffers severe shaking chills lasting twenty minutes or complains of shortness of breath.*

How to Take a Pulse

A pulse is used to determine a patient's heart rate, which is expressed as the number of beats per minute. (The most accurate method for doing this is to place a stethoscope against the upper chest or back and listen to the heart directly.) Usually a pulse is taken by palpating large arteries near the surface of the skin; in other words, actually feeling the steady *thump-thump-thump* with your fingertips. The four vessels used most reliably to count a pulse are the *carotid* arteries on either side of the windpipe, in the front of the neck, and the *femoral* arteries in the crease of the groin. Even much smaller arteries provide a palpable pulse, for example, the *radial* artery inside the wrist near the base of the thumb. The radial pulse can be hard to find in the sick or frail, however. Swelling in the hands can also hinder the effort.

Two rules to remember when counting heart rate:

Don't use your thumb, which has an artery near the skin's surface. Your own pulse will interfere with an accurate count of the patient's.

Don't press down; the pressure can restrict the normal flow through the artery, distorting the count.

Instead, gently rest the tips of your index and middle fingers against the skin over the artery. If you have trouble finding the pulse because the person is obese or has low blood pressure, choose one of the larger arteries instead. When in doubt, use a stethoscope to listen to the heart directly.

If the heartbeat is strong and regular, counting the pulse for fifteen seconds and multiplying by four will yield a fairly accurate one-minute rate.

If the pulse is irregular, count for a full minute.

In order to assess whether someone's pulse is abnormally high or low, we have to know her usual *resting heart rate*, the baseline against which we compare subsequent counts. Resting heart rates vary according to a patient's age, physical fitness, medical condition, and any medications he's on.

To ascertain the resting heart rate, *count the pulse after your loved one has been sitting quietly or lying down for at least fifteen minutes.* Repeat the procedure at approximately the same time each day under the same conditions, and you'll quickly determine a normal range for your patient's resting rate.

One of the heart's many miraculous features is that it adjusts its rate automatically to compensate for the demands placed on the body. For instance, you'd expect the pulse to beat much faster after struggling to get on a bedpan, stepping out of the shower, drinking coffee, or eating a large meal; conversely, you'd expect it to slow noticeably during a nap or following a dose of strong pain medicine. Likewise, coughing fits, shortness of breath, fever, vomiting, or acute anxiety can increase the pulse rate, whereas various medications, shock, loss of oxygen to the brain, and *bradycardia*, a slowing of the heart's pumping action, can decrease the rate profoundly.

How to Measure Blood Pressure

If the pressure of the blood against the blood vessel walls falls too low, the brain and other vital organs are dangerously deprived of essential oxygen and toxic waste removal services. Let it climb too high, and blood vessels big and small start to break down, which can trigger life-threatening problems such as stroke and kidney failure.

Blood pressure is expressed in two numbers, such as 120 over 80, or 120 mm Hg/80 mm Hg (mm Hg stands for millimeters of mercury, or the height of the column of mercury on the manometer). The first number reflects the peak force generated when the heart muscle contracts, driving blood into the large arteries that carry it throughout the body. This is called *systolic* pressure. The second number represents the lowest pressure within the arteries while the heart chambers are refilling (*diastolic* pressure).

Blood pressure measurements provide the medical team with valuable information about the overall health of the circulatory system as well as how the body compensates for physical stress. For example, cardiovascular disease is often first detected because blood pressure remains abnormally high even when the patient is resting. Similarly, plummeting blood pressure might signal internal hemorrhaging or shock related to a drug reaction or a disturbance in the normal cardiac rhythm *(arrhythmia)*.

As when taking someone's pulse, it's important to determine first the patient's normal range of blood pressure in order to know whether a given measurement falls on the high or low side. To get a baseline blood pressure, we take a reading while our loved one is at rest, then repeat this over several days under similar physical and emotional conditions.

Depending on her condition and the medications she's taking, the medical team will instruct you how often to measure blood pressure and under what circumstances. They'll give you an upper and lower range so you'll know when to report abnormal readings to the doctor or nurse.

These days you can find a wide variety of electronic devices for measuring blood pressure at drugstores, surgical supply houses, and through mail-order catalogs. They're highly accurate when used according to the instructions and with fresh batteries, and less cumbersome than the traditional inflatable cuff and stethoscope. To verify the accuracy of the electronic pressure sensors— which should be done at least once a week—there's no substitute for an old-fashioned manometer and a pair of human ears.

Step-by-Step Instructions for Measuring Blood Pressure

1. Have the patient sit in a chair and rest her forearm on a table. If she is bed-bound, be sure that her arm lies at approximately the same level as the heart, not elevated too high or allowed to hang off the bed.
2. Fasten the inflatable cuff around the upper arm, high enough to clear the bend in the elbow. The cuff should be wrapped snugly enough that it doesn't slip up and down, but loose enough that you can slide two fingers under it while deflated.

✻ *A poor-fitting cuff can throw off the reading. For extremely thin patients, a pediatric cuff provides a more even fit. Likewise, an obese person might need a special oversized cuff.*

3. Place the drum of the stethoscope over the *brachial* artery located just inside and just below the crook of the elbow, and hold it there gently with one hand.
4. Place the earpieces of the stethoscope in your ears.
5. Close the handheld air valve and inflate the cuff by repeatedly squeezing the rubber bulb until the gauge reads about 30 mm higher than your previous top readings.
6. *Slowly* deflate the cuff by slightly opening the valve. Note the precise reading on the gauge when you first hear the pulse. That's the systolic pressure.
7. As you continue slowly to deflate the cuff, note the point at which the sound of the pulse disappears. That's the diastolic measurement.

✻ *Don't hesitate to repeat the procedure to double-check your readings.*

How to Monitor Respirations

The rate of breathing also holds important clues for caregivers and the medical team. Normal respirations increase when our bodies demand more oxygen; they slow considerably when we're resting. Rapid breathing might indicate anything from anger, pain, or physical exertion to a drug reaction, blood loss, or heart problem. An extremely slow respiratory rate might be normal for someone who's sedated; it could also harbinger a drug overdose or neurological damage.

The best way to count respirations is by placing a stethoscope against the chest, back, or ribs, and literally listening to the air rushing in and out of the lungs. It sounds exactly like wind. Another reliable technique is to rest the palm of your hand on the patient's diaphragm—just below the breastbone, where the ribs meet—and count the muscle contractions for one minute. For a patient whose chest clearly rises and falls with each breath, you can simply count visually.

When counting respirations, pay attention to the sounds and patterns of breathing, too.

- A *"wet" chest with audible gurgling* during each breath indicates congestion, perhaps from a lung infection such as pneumonia, or *pulmonary edema*, where a failing heart causes blood to back up into the lungs.
- *Audible wheezing or rattles* indicate restricted or obstructed air passages as seen in lung diseases like asthma and emphysema, or during a severe allergic reaction *(anaphylactic shock)*.
- *Irregular breathing*—for instance, several quick, shallow breaths interrupted by long pauses—can signal profound neurologic or metabolic problems.

Administering Medications Safely

It is not unusual for a seriously ill person to be taking ten, twenty, or more prescribed medications daily. All powerful medicines have potentially life-threatening side effects, while allergic reactions and interactions between incompatible drugs disable and kill hundreds of Americans every year. Many people also take several over-the-counter products for various symptoms, along with food and food supplements, vitamins, and minerals—not to mention alcohol or illicit drugs. The number of unpredictable and potentially dangerous combinations is endless. Further complicating matters is the fact that each patient reacts

slightly differently to various drugs and drug combinations.

Underlying medical conditions can cause some medicines to have a more profound effect than anticipated. Some exert no effect at all when certain organs fail; or a patient may build up tolerance following repeated doses. Women's bodies react to many drugs differently from men's. And as age weakens the body, drugs can have all sorts of unanticipated effects.

Human foul-ups can be equally deadly. When more than one doctor is writing a patient's prescriptions, the likelihood of mistakes and oversights increases. Did you know that as many as one in five prescriptions is written or filled incorrectly? In addition, confused or harried caregivers and patients mix up drugs and dosages or don't follow directions correctly.

Clearly, among the caregiver's most important responsibilities are keeping track of medicines and doses—or helping the patient do this—and closely monitoring reactions to any new medication.

Before Filling a New Prescription:

- Make sure the doctor is aware of all prescription and over-the-counter medications the patient is currently taking. Don't assume he read it in the chart.
- Remind the doctor and the pharmacist of any known allergies or past reactions to a specific drug.
- Ask the physician the following questions and write down the answers:

What is the name of the medicine and what is it supposed to do? Most drugs have both brand names and generic formulations. So the physician might say, "I'll give you a prescription for Xanax," an antianxiety agent, but the druggist may refer to it by its trade name, alprazolam. Also bear in mind that many drug names sound similar, like the antibiotics clarithromycin and erythromycin, to cite one example.

When do I give it? How often and how much?

In what form is it administered? Pill, capsule, liquid, patch, suppository, injection?

What restrictions should I observe? Should specific foods, alcohol, or other drugs be avoided when taking it? Should it be taken on a full stomach or before eating? Is there anything else we should know?

What side effects should I look out for? Dizziness, upset stomach, fever, fatigue, mood swings, constipation, diarrhea, fluctuations in blood pressure? Will it make my loved one groggy, forgetful, or hypersensitive to sunlight, for example?

How long should we continue giving the medicine?

✷ *Warning: Abruptly stopping certain regimens can cause life-threatening symptoms or serious relapses of disease. Except in the case of an acute allergic reaction, first check with the medical team before discontinuing any medication.*

What should I do if we miss a dose? What if we accidentally give too much at once or give the dose too often?

How should we store the medicine?

✷ *If you forget any of the doctor's instructions or become confused, don't hesitate to call back. Or ask the pharmacist to repeat the information.*

At the Pharmacy

Before leaving the pharmacy, check the label to make sure you've been handed the right medicine at the correct dose and that you clearly understand the directions. Read the "Contraindications" and "Precautions" sections on the printed package insert before you administer the first dose at home.

Discard all prescription medications that are not used at least occasionally, as well as all expired over-the-counter drugs. Never give your loved one medicine that was prescribed for someone else even if your patient has the same symptoms. ► *See "Allergic Reactions and Anaphylactic Shock," page 151.*

The neighborhood pharmacist is an often-overlooked but key member of your health care team. If you use the same pharmacist to fill every prescription, she can keep an eye out for errors or potentially dangerous drug combinations as well as clarify the physician's instructions. In a pinch, the pharmacist can get on the phone with your doctor and take orders for new prescriptions or refills, saving you a trip to the office or hospital.

Pharmacists also possess a wealth of practical tips on managing specific symptoms. "Clarence had a bad cough once," Betty Lindstrom recalls, "and the pharmacist suggested a cough medicine that worked very well. He also suggested a soothing powder for clearing up bedsores and other items that helped with his skin."

Many pharmacists will allow regular customers to run up a monthly bill, easing pressure on limited cash flow, and provide computer printouts of medications and cash outlays for insurance claims. Betty's drugstore "used to make deliveries at practically any hour of the day or night without charge," she says gratefully. "And frequently the druggist would say, 'Maybe you'd like to try some free samples.' I always got discounts on chucks and adult diapers, which I appreciated."

Keeping Track of Medications and Dosing Schedules

Toward the end of my stepmother's struggle with emphysema and lung cancer, Lynn was taking more than a dozen medications each day. There were two bronchodilators to ease her breathing —one a pill, the other an inhaler—a beta-blocker to steady her heart's rhythm; a diuretic to reduce congestion and edema; a pill to prevent ulcers; various antacids for indigestion and heartburn; a laxative and fiber supplement to prevent constipation; pills for diarrhea and cramps; a regimen of heavy pain control, including morphine and a mild tranquilizer; antinausea pills, patches, and suppositories; a sleeping pill and more pain meds at night. Keeping track of it all was a full-time job.

My brother Dave drew up a large easy-to-read daily chart that included

- the name of the drug;
- what it was for;
- a description of what it looked like (tape a sample to the chart to eliminate any confusion);
- how much to give and when;
- any special instructions, such as "never on an empty stomach."

A spiral notebook will suffice. Leave extra space to record the time each dose was actually administered or an explanation of why it was skipped; for example: "too nauseous to swallow pills." Or you can do what hospital nurses do and use a large calendar with space following each hour of the day, like an appointment book. Every morning list each medication dose and when it is due. After you've given one dose, check it off and reset your alarm clock for the next one.

Pharmacies and medical supply catalogs offer an array of gadgets to help simplify the task of tracking multiple medicines. There are pillboxes for presorting medications by hour or by day and hour, as well as pocket electronic timers that can be set to go off when it's time for the next round of medications.

As careful as Dave and I were, we made our share of mistakes while caring for Lynn and for Dad. We'd miss a dose, thinking the other had already given it. Or we'd double-dose, not realizing the other caregiver had just administered the drug—or that Bob had taken the medicine himself. Only by keeping scrupulous written records were we able to keep errors to a minimum and to spot a mistake immediately when one did occur. The point is to set up an *uncomplicated* system that works for you and is readily understood by the patient and your fellow caregivers.

Routes of Drug Administration

How rapidly a drug takes effect is determined chiefly by the route of administration. For instance, when you swallow a pill or capsule, thirty minutes or more elapse before the medicine dissolves in the stomach and starts being absorbed into the bloodstream (longer if taken with a large meal). A liquid oral medication gets down to business faster since there's no delay waiting for it to dissolve.

Nausea, difficulty swallowing, or unconsciousness frequently rule out oral administration. Many common oral medications also come in suppository form, which deposits the dose directly against a membrane in the rectum. The bullet-shaped suppositories melt in the rectum and are absorbed twice as fast as oral drugs.

Some medicines break down chemically or cannot be absorbed in the digestive tract, or faster delivery into the bloodstream is needed. One method is to inject the drug *subcutaneously*, or directly into the layer of fat just below the skin. Absorption is gradual through this route, making it ideal for the hormone insulin and other medications where a relatively constant concentration in the bloodstream is desired. Faster still are *intramuscular* injections, which deposit the drug directly into a muscle so that large concentrations are absorbed into the bloodstream within just minutes.

By far the fastest route is injecting

drugs directly into a vein. *Intravenous* administrations have the advantage of almost instantaneous effects, but they carry increased risks. The reason most IV meds are given at the hospital—and then only by doctors or registered nurses—is that adverse side effects, drug interactions, or allergic reactions also occur instantly, requiring extremely close monitoring of the patient. However, routine IV medications that the patient has tolerated safely before can be administered at home by experienced caregivers who have received special instruction.

Some drugs, such as nitroglycerin, which is taken to reverse the heart condition angina pectoris, are held under the tongue *(sublingual)* and rapidly absorbed by the dense tangle of blood vessels in the mouth. The effect is virtually immediate. Medications inhaled into the lungs in the form of a mist (aerosol), as for relieving asthma, also enter the bloodstream within seconds.

Oral Meds

The easiest and most common way of taking medicine is by swallowing it. A secondary advantage of oral medications is that the effects are gradual, affording caregivers or the medical team time to take corrective action should an adverse reaction develop.

When giving any oral medication, be it liquid, tablet, or capsule, have your loved one sit upright or with the head of the bed elevated in order to minimize the risk of choking. The person's head should be level, not tilted back. Dry pills, tablets, or capsules can be difficult to swallow. To make them go down more easily, suggest that the patient try the following:

- Take a sip of water, then place the pill on the tongue and wash it down with another sip.
- Insert the pill in a small slice of banana.
- Crush the pill or empty the capsule and mix it with applesauce, ice cream, pudding, or any other easy-to-swallow food. If you don't have a mortar and pestle, place the pill between two spoons and press down on the top spoon while twisting slightly. *Voilà!* The crushed pill will be contained neatly in the bottom spoon.

* *However, pills with enteric coatings to protect the stomach should not be crushed.*

- If your loved one finds capsules easier to swallow, ask the pharmacist to sell you empty gelatin capsules and insert a pill in each.

If a pill lodges in the throat or esophagus, have your loved one sit upright and encourage him to relax. Offer a few sips of a carbonated beverage (or water if there's no carbonated drink on hand). He should continue to take sips until he feels the medicine dissolve.

If someone is choking or coughing, the pill may have become trapped in the windpipe. With the patient leaning for-

---

MONEY SAVER

One little-known fact about prescription pills is that larger doses often cost no more than smaller ones. For example, the wholesale price of Zocor, a cholesterol-lowering agent, is exactly the same for a 40-milligram (mg) tablet as a 20-milligram tablet. Thus, if your loved one's daily dosage is 20 milligrams, you can buy an inexpensive pill splitter and cut the 40-milligram tablets in half, realizing substantial savings. Ask the doctor about ordering higher concentrations of expensive drugs to be divided at home.

ward, cup your hand and firmly thump her on the back, between the shoulder blades. This should dislodge the pill and allow it to be expelled. If the person is having trouble breathing, perform the Heimlich maneuver to attempt to clear the airway. ▶ *See "The Heimlich Maneuver," page 182.*

When a patient is unconscious or too nauseous to keep down an oral medicine, ask the doctor if you can give it as a suppository. Coat the pill with Vaseline, K-Y Jelly, or another lubricant and insert it in the rectum. This is especially useful with patients who are vomiting but need to take antinausea or pain medications.

Suppositories

Suppositories are designed to melt quickly at body temperature, so keep them refrigerated until it's time to administer them. You'll need to wear a sterile latex glove, not only to avoid introducing germs into the rectum but to grip the medication, which quickly becomes slippery. It also helps to apply a water-based lubricant such as K-Y Jelly to the suppository before inserting.

With the patient lying on his side, draw the top knee up toward the chest about 90 degrees, just enough so that you can see the anus. For folks with big bottoms, you may need to use your free hand to lift the upper cheek in order to gain access to the orifice.

Introduce the tapered end of the suppository into the anal opening and gently push it up into the rectum with the tip of your finger. The average adult's anus is about one inch deep. You'll feel the end of your finger clear the anus and enter the larger space of the rectum. If you have any doubts, ask a nurse to demonstrate this technique for you or try inserting a plain glycerin suppository into your own rectum.

Sometimes the suppository slips out, particularly if the person is unconscious or has poor bowel control, so check to see that she didn't expel it after you've removed your finger. Conscious patients should be reminded to squeeze their anus tightly for several minutes until the medication has had time to liquefy.

Transdermal Patches

Transdermal patches, applied directly against the skin, are ideal for delivering antinausea and pain medications to anyone requiring round-the-clock symptom control. Once the drug seeps into the bloodstream, the level remains constant until all of it has leached out of the patch.

Patches should be applied to clean, smooth areas of the body because dry, flaky skin delays absorption. The adhesive backing can irritate delicate skin, which is why we change locations each time we put on a new patch. Allowing the patch to get wet will dilute the medicine or dissolve it completely. Consequently, the area must be covered with a waterproof dressing whenever patients bathe or shower.

To double a dose, apply two patches; to reduce the dose by 50 percent, cut a patch in half. (You'll have to throw away the unused piece once you've broken the seal.) Patients with faulty memories need to be closely monitored when using patches. They might forget they're wearing one and ingest additional medication, thus risking an overdose, or they may forget to replace the patch after it has run out of medicine.

✳ *Keep written records of exactly when and where each patch is applied.*

Injections

Some caregivers and patients balk at the idea of administering injections. Most people, though, can quickly learn how and, with a little experience, overcome any aversion to needles. Heck, diabetics do this every day. A nurse will instruct the patient and the family until they perfect the technique, usually by practicing on an orange.

Most injectable drugs come in single-dose glass vials. You hold the tiny bottle upright, tap it until all the medicine has drained from the top chamber, break it open, then withdraw the prescribed amount into your syringe by pulling back the plunger. Any medicine left in the vial gets poured down the sink.

For powdered injectable drugs you attach a syringe filled with *diluent*, then inject the clear diluting fluid into the vial. After gently swirling the bottle—with the needle still in it—you withdraw the medicine into the syringe, then push the plunger to the correct volume mark prescribed by the physician. Discard the vial.

For rubber-topped vials, you must inject air into the bottle equal to the volume of medicine you need to withdraw. Remember to sterilize the rubber stopper with an alcohol swab before inserting the needle through it. The prescription calls for a dose of 2 cubic centimeters. First inject 2 cubic centimeters of air. Failing to do so will create a vacuum, making it virtually impossible to withdraw the medicine.

Once you've drawn the medicine into the syringe and removed the needle from the bottle, you'll need to eliminate any air bubbles before injecting the medicine. Hold the syringe with the needle pointing upward and tap the body of the syringe until the bubbles gather at the top. Carefully advance the plunger enough to expel the air. Check the gradients marked on the syringe to make sure the syringe now contains the correct amount of medicine. If not, repeat the procedure.

General tips on giving injections:

- *Wash your hands* and gather your medication, alcohol swabs, syringe, and needle.
- *Check the label to ensure that you have the right drug.* Make sure it's the right concentration, expressed as milligrams (mg) per cubic centimeter (cc). Check the expiration date on the vial.

- *Rotate injection sites.* Never use the same site twice in a row because repeated injections can irritate tissue. This can slow the absorption of the medicine as well as lead to *phlebitis*, a painful inflammation of the blood vessels. Ask the doctor where to give the injections.

* *Make a note of where each injection was given and choose an alternate site for the next one. Don't return to a site until you've used up all your other sites.*

- *Once you've selected the injection site, sterilize the skin* with an alcohol swab. Use a circular motion, beginning in the center of your target and rotating outward. Allow a few seconds for the alcohol to evaporate because alcohol in the puncture site stings like crazy.
- *After you've inserted the needle but before you inject the drug, check your position by aspirating.* Once a needle pierces the skin, there is always the possibility that it has inadvertently landed in a blood vessel. Injecting a drug directly into the bloodstream can be extremely dangerous. To determine whether you've hit an artery or vein, pull back slightly on the plunger. If blood appears in the syringe, withdraw the needle, dispose of the syringe and its contents, and start again.

Intramuscular (IM) Injections

Drugs that need to be injected in large concentrations (such as antibiotics) and drugs that cause local tissue damage (such as many pain and nausea medications) are injected deep into the meat of a large muscle. The rich vascular bed of muscle tissue allows for rapid absorption, and the relative amount of damage done to the surrounding tissue is minimized by the muscle's sheer bulk.

No matter how thin your patient may be, you should be able to easily feel a large muscle on the upper two-thirds of the thigh *(quadriceps)*. The upper, outer quadrants of each butt cheek *(gluteus maximus)* are also highly reliable injection sites. Most adults also have well-developed hip muscles. Shoulder muscles can be used occasionally, but few people's arms are large enough to tolerate repeated shots. The nurse will show you how to locate these big muscles.

To give an IM injection:

1. With your free hand, gently stretch the skin taut around the injection site.
2. Holding the syringe and needle in your other hand like a dart, insert it at a 90-degree angle to the skin with a quick, even thrust, all the way to the hilt.
3. Pull back on the plunger to aspirate for blood. If you see no blood in the syringe, slowly and evenly depress the plunger until the syringe is empty.

Subcutaneous Injections

When slower absorption is desired, as with growth hormones given to beef up wasted or anemic patients, medicine is injected into the layer of fat between the skin and the muscle. The procedure for giving a subcutaneous, or "sub-Q," injection is much the same as for IM injections, except a much shorter needle with a very narrow bore is used, and the injection sites are chosen differently.

The easiest places to give sub-Q injections are around the waist and on the top of the upper thigh—anywhere we can pinch a layer of fat between our fingers and pull it away from the underlying muscle. Love handles and the belly are ideal. With a fold of skin and fat held firmly between the thumb and index finger, the short needle is driven to its hilt into the center of the fold.

After You've Delivered the Medicine

- *Gently press an alcohol swab* against the injection site as you withdraw the needle in one smooth, quick motion.

Then gently massage the injection site briefly. This helps diffuse the medicine and reduce pain.
- *Inspect the injection site.* If you notice bleeding or oozing, press an alcohol swab against the site until it stops.
- *Never resheathe needles!* The most frequent source of accidental needle jabs is when a nurse or caregiver tries to reinsert the needle into its protective sheath following an injection. Even with steady hands and perfect vision, health care workers often prick themselves, which can infect them with whatever germs are in the patient's blood.

The home-care company or pharmacy will provide you with a plastic biohazard disposal unit, often called a "sharps" container. The entire needle and syringe should be dropped into this widemouthed plastic receptacle, needle first. You'll also receive instructions for discarding the disposal unit itself.

✳ *Never throw needles, syringes, or biohazardous waste disposal units into the regular garbage. Not only is it illegal, it places unsuspecting people at serious risk of injury. Seal and return full disposal units to the home-care nurse, doctor's office, or hospital for proper destruction.*

Tricks for Minimizing the Pain and Fear Associated with Injections

- *Suggest your loved one not watch.* Often the anticipation and the sight of the needle are far worse than the actual injection. Experienced nurses always have shots drawn up before they enter the room, and they approach you from behind whenever possible.
- *Tap or gently slap the skin* at the injection site two or three times just before you put in the needle. Stimulating the skin's local nerve endings minimizes sudden reflex movements and blunts the stinging sensation caused when the skin is pierced.

- *Encourage the person to fully relax* the muscle at the injection site. Injecting into a flexed muscle often results in bruising and a painful cramp that can last for days.
- *Remind the patient* not *to close his eyes or hold his breath.* Instead, instruct him to look away and take a deep breath, then exhale deliberately through pursed lips. Stick him as he exhales. Perceived pain is far lower, and the person is less likely to jump, jerk, or faint.
- *The injection site feels sore?* If the shot was given that day, apply a cold compress or an ice pack. Soreness and knots that are a day or more old call for warm, moist towels and a gentle massage.
- *An ounce of prevention:* Needles penetrate smooth, healthy skin far more easily than dry, brittle skin. Make sure your loved one stays well hydrated and the skin is kept clean and thoroughly moisturized at all times.

Intravenous (IV) Injections and Infusions

Glucose, saline, electrolyte solutions, blood, and blood products are infused continuously through flexible catheters threaded directly into a vein, usually in the hand or arm but anywhere else a large vessel can be located near the body's surface, such as the neck and legs. In addition, antibiotics, chemotherapy agents, pain and nausea medications, and many other compounds can be mixed into these solutions, which come in plastic bags that are hung from a metal pole. In emergencies, powerful drugs can be injected directly into a vein in order to achieve a faster and more profound effect than through any other route.

Rarely will lay caregivers be expected to administer drugs or fluids intravenously, and then only after receiving plenty of training and supervision from a nurse. (Never will you be

---

Alert the nurse if an IV line

- stops;
- slows down or speeds up noticeably;
- becomes disconnected or leaks;
- causes swelling or redness at the injection site;
- has blood backing up into the tubing.

---

called on to start an IV, a procedure that requires considerable skill and constant practice.) It falls to us, however, to alert the hospital or home-care nurse if a problem should develop with the intravenous line and to keep an eye peeled for glaring errors, such as a nurse hanging a bag of sugar water *(dextrose)* on a known diabetic or rapidly infusing a large volume of fluid into someone with impaired kidney function or congestive heart failure.

Infusion rates are regulated by adjusting the small plastic clamp along the clear, flexible tubing while counting the actual drops dripping from the bottom of the hanging bottle of IV fluids. Many IVs are controlled by electronic pumps set to deliver a specific number of drops per minute; whenever the infusion is interrupted, an alarm sounds.

Although the persistent beeping can quickly become annoying—especially with a temperamental IV or a patient who constantly changes positions in bed or bends his arms a lot—resist the impulse to turn it off, and insist that the nursing staff leave it activated as well. Investigate each alarm until its cause is identified and corrected.

You may encounter some of the following common problems with IV lines:

All too frequently an IV catheter will wriggle out of a vein or perforate the fragile wall of the blood vessel, particularly in the very sick and the elderly. When this happens, the fluid continues to drain into the surrounding tissue, causing obvious and immediate local swelling. This *infiltration* should be called to the nurse's attention at once and the IV turned off until a new catheter can be inserted into another vein. *To turn off an IV*, simply close the clamp on the plastic tubing. (If there's a pump, switch it to "off" and then close the clamp.) *Don't hesitate to shut down an infiltrated IV:* The swollen tissue is prone to develop phlebitis, it hurts, and it makes starting future IVs or drawing blood at that site impossible for several days, if not permanently. Don't worry about interrupting the infusion; it's not going in the vein anyway.

The presence of blood in the tubing is usually a sign that the IV bag is empty and needs to be replaced. If a new bag isn't attached within a few minutes, a clot can solidify within the catheter, blocking the IV and forcing us to start another one. *Alert the nurse when an IV bag is running low*, well before the problem develops.

Backflow of blood also occurs when the IV tubing is accidentally disconnected. It makes a mess but is quickly corrected: Simply reconnect the tubes where they came apart. A crimp in the tubing can also cause blood to backflow; check for a crimp somewhere along its length.

Tiny air bubbles in an IV line pose no threat to the patient, but large air bubbles in the bloodstream can create problems not unlike blood clots, interrupting circulation to part of the brain, lungs, or heart muscle. There are two methods for removing air:

1. Temporarily clamp off the line at the patient end by crimping the tubing with your fingers. Quickly disconnect the tubing at any junction downstream of the air bubble. Allow the fluid to dribble into a waste can until the bubble passes. Reconnect the tubing and release the crimp.

2. Crimp the tubing near the patient. Insert a sterile syringe needle into one of the tubing's rubber-capped injection ports, near the bubble. Draw out the air manually.

＊ *Remember to first swab the injection port with alcohol to reduce the risk of introducing germs.*

IV injection sites (and, by extension, all IV tubing and connections) grant germs direct access to the bloodstream. Dressings and bandages over the site should be kept clean and dry, and changed daily or anytime they become soiled. When changing dressings, remember to tape several inches of the tubing securely to the patient's skin near the bandage so that an inadvertent snag doesn't rip out the IV. ◄ *See "How to Change a Dressing," page 121.*

Central Venous Catheters. For seriously ill patients on long-term IV antibiotics or repeated doses of harsh chemicals administered intravenously, a long, flexible catheter can be implanted in a large vein, usually in the chest or abdomen. The exposed end protrudes several inches and is capped with an injection port. Not only does this spare them from having to endure hundreds of additional needle sticks, it provides a reliable port for delivering critical medications. These *central lines* go by a variety of brand names, including Hickman, Port-O-Cath, and Broviac. Many people suffering from renal failure have a *shunt* permanently implanted in an arm for routing their blood through a hemodialysis machine, which performs the functions of a kidney, drawing off fluid and filtering out toxins.

Central venous catheters require especially meticulous sterile technique, for a bug that slips inside can not only destroy the port but cause a life-threatening infection. The nurse will instruct you and your patient on how to clean and dress the site where the catheter enters the body, as well as how to keep the line clear by periodically flushing it with a sterile anticlotting solution such as Heparin. Although a tube in the chest or abdomen can damage a sick person's body image, Dr. Howard

Grossman favors the torso over the arm as a catheter site. As the New York internist points out, "If the tube is in your arm, cleaning it becomes much harder because you have only one hand free."

Permanent ports can also be implanted surgically just under the skin so that no tubing protrudes externally. Drugs are injected through the skin directly into the small reservoir, which leads to a large vein. Here, too, avoiding infection becomes a matter of life and death. ◄ *See "Three Steps to Sterile Technique," page 121.* ► *See "Caring for Someone with Kidney Disease: Caring for a Fistula or Shunt," page 451.*

Allergic Reactions and Anaphylactic Shock

Anaphylaxis is the medical term for the immune system's exaggerated reaction to a foreign agent, or *antigen.* Virtually any chemical introduced into the human body has the potential to provoke a severe allergic reaction. In the medical world, common culprits include many antibiotics, codeine, and contrast dyes used to highlight organs on X rays.

Allergic reactions are first noticed as localized swelling, redness, and itching, like the welt caused by an insect sting, the burning rash that follows a brush with poison ivy, or the stuffy, irritated sinuses associated with hay fever. In some people, however, an allergic reaction can rapidly cascade into a life-threatening crisis.

The best way to protect your loved one is to know which, if any, medications or foods have triggered a reaction in the past and to notify the doctor prior to starting a new medicine. Read the "Contraindications" and "Precautions" sections on the printed package inserts of all meds before giving the first dose.

As our bodies change with age, disease, and treatment, however, various drugs, food, and other antigens that were well tolerated in the past can also cause unpredictable reactions. One of a caregiver's most essential lifesaving skills is to recognize an allergic reaction and know how to treat it immediately. Allergic reactions can occur astonishingly rapidly, escalating to anaphylactic shock before you have time to get the patient to the hospital or wait for an ambulance.

Initial symptoms:

- Redness, puffiness, and itching at the site of administration
- A rapidly disseminating rash anywhere else on the body *(hives)*
- Sudden nausea or vomiting
- A sudden pounding headache
- Flushed skin
- Rapid heartbeat and breathing

Advanced symptoms:

- Swelling, most noticeably around the eyes, face, and neck
- Heart palpitations
- Chills and tremors
- Blurred vision
- Difficulty breathing due to swelling of the airway
- Audible wheezing due to bronchospasms
- Clammy skin
- Falling blood pressure
- Loss of consciousness
- Urinary or bowel incontinence
- Dangerously depressed respirations and heart rate, leading inexorably to circulatory collapse and respiratory arrest ► *See "When Should You Call an Ambulance?," page 182.*

Managing an Allergic Reaction

The good news is that most allergic reactions can be defused quickly and treated effectively at home if caught early. *Monitor patients carefully when beginning a new drug.* Keep in mind that an allergic reaction might not flare

---

VOICE OF EXPERIENCE

"My daughter once had an allergic reaction to Compazine, a nausea medication. Luckily, she was in the hospital for some tests when it happened. Her eyes rolled back in her head; it was the scariest thing I ever saw.

"The doctor picked up what was happening and gave her an injection of Benadryl, which took away the effects of the Compazine immediately."—Eileen Mitzman

---

up immediately following the first dose. Promptly discontinue use of any medicine or food you believe may be triggering the reaction.

For mild, early reactions, an over-the-counter *antihistamine* such as Actifed or Benadryl will do. Benadryl liquid is best because unlike with a pill, you don't have to wait for it to dissolve in the stomach before the antihistamine starts to reach the bloodstream. If a pill is all you have, crush it and dissolve it in half a glass of water for faster absorption.

* *If the symptoms do not improve noticeably within fifteen minutes, repeat the dose and head for the hospital or call 911.*

Severe reactions must be treated immediately and more aggressively. Injectable *epinephrine* in a bolus designed for self-administration can be purchased from your pharmacist. For people who have a history of severe allergic reactions, this is an essential item to keep on hand at all times.

If you are in doubt, treat the person for anaphylaxis and call for help. Antihistamines might leave your loved one feeling sleepy, and epinephrine can cause short-lived palpitations and rapid pulse. Still, it's better to err on the side of caution than wait until your patient is gasping for breath. Never underestimate anaphylaxis: Any allergic reaction that does not respond immediately to antihistamine therapy constitutes a life-and-death medical emergency. ▶ *See "Cardiopulmonary Resuscitation (CPR)," page 181.*

Managing Pain

Uncontrolled pain is an abiding terror for every seriously ill person. Sadly, in a majority of cases their fears are justified. Upward of 60 percent of critically ill people report moderate to severe pain that is inadequately managed. Equally tragic is the fact that this suffering is largely unnecessary. It's not intractable pain that prevents most patients from finding relief, it's misconceptions and ignorance about pain medications—on the parts of patients, their loved ones, and health care professionals alike—that most often stand in the way. It frequently falls to the caregiver to make sure the patient gets whatever she needs.

Pain comes in an endless variety of forms, with many different causes:

- *Visceral pain* is common with diseases or medications that interrupt normal digestion and excretion.
- There can be severe *local pain* due to direct damage to soft tissue, following surgery or a fall.
- *Pains in bones, joints, and muscles* can result from fractures in folks with brittle bones, bruises from clotting disorders, disuse, and atrophy while bedridden or during a raging fever.
- Many different kinds of *headaches* are caused by a wide range of diseases and drugs, such as tumors and steroid therapy.
- Patients may experience excruciating nerve pain (*neuralgia*) following radiation therapy or surgery, or as a re-

sult of an infection such as shingles or nerve damage caused by a lifesaving drug.

All of these and more can occur in any number of sinister combinations and vary in intensity over the course of a day. Each person also has a different threshold for various types of pain, while other factors—anxiety, sleep deprivation, nausea and vomiting, constipation, and diarrhea—can allow an already bad situation to spiral totally out of control.

Attitudes Toward Pain Relief

Far too many doctors and nurses arbitrarily withhold pain medications or strictly ration what they do give. This can be attributed partly to their own ill-informed notions about dependence and addiction. Sometimes it's just frank ignorance of current standards of pain management. "Things are getting slightly better," anesthesiologist Dr. James Rogers says cautiously, "but there hasn't been a big change because this is still not taught in medical schools."

Dr. Rogers, director of the pain clinic at the Audie L. Murphy Veterans Administration Hospital in San Antonio, Texas, has a dual perspective on the inadequacies of pain control. In 1978, as an Arizona police officer, he was broadsided by a car that had run a stop sign. The impact crushed his left leg, leading to a two-month hospitalization during which he underwent *ten* amputations. "Slowly my leg kept getting shorter and shorter," he says.

According to Dr. Rogers, at least half of every day was spent in what he describes as "severe pain." Yet the nursing staff refused to step up his pain medication, despite his pleas. The experience inspired him to attend college, then medical school, and to specialize in pain management.

It is crucial that we discuss symptom control with the primary physician at the beginning of a loved one's disease,

well before symptoms escalate. Refusal to medicate pain or other adverse symptoms *to the patient's satisfaction* is one of the rare circumstances that justifies changing doctors.

Patients—and caregivers—can harbor antiquated or misguided attitudes as well. Many believe that taking narcotics is shameful ("They're afraid they'll be thought of as a drug addict," observes Dr. Rogers) or will leave them addicted for life. While temporary physical dependence can happen, patients weaned off opiates or other controlled substances rarely if ever develop a psychological addiction. Decades of clinical experience have shown that fewer than 1 percent of patients given narcotics for medical reasons become addicted.

Others fear that the doses of medication needed to blunt pain will render them zombielike, unable to communicate or think clearly. With the many drugs and techniques available these days, sedation to the point of stupor is rarely required, and then only in the final hours of end-stage disease when being rendered "out of it" would be regarded by many as a blessing. The medical term for this is *terminal sedation*.

Some people believe that tolerating pain is courageous or that suffering is somehow a test of spiritual faith; in fact, unremitting pain only leaves an ill person weaker and sicker, even hastening death in the worst cases. My dad resisted taking pain medicine until the last few days of his life because he believed he was being "strong" by tolerating as much pain as he could. Pop didn't view pain medicine as part of his arsenal for fighting disease and maintaining vitality; to him, starting the morphine symbolized his concession to disease, that he had lost the battle.

My stepmother Lynn was more typical. She was willing to try anything to attain relief from her cancer pain, but she and her doctor were simply unaware of all the tools at their disposal. A mild tranquilizer first thing in the morning, a sleeping pill at night, along with low doses of morphine and an anti-nausea agent throughout the day usually kept her fairly comfortable. But when radiation treatment to her throat brought about unbearable neuralgia in her face, none of the usual meds did the trick, and her oncologist didn't know what else to do. Only because I called in an anesthesiologist friend did she receive the aggressive, expert treatment she needed (including injecting a numbing medication directly into the irritated nerve root in her neck). Without an advocate, she would have suffered needlessly or been forced to take enough morphine to knock her out completely.

Fundamentals of Pain Management

Patients can quickly develop a surprisingly high tolerance to any medication, so that progressively higher doses are needed to achieve the same effect. To derive the maximum benefits from a pain medicine, try the following:

- *To learn a loved one's drug-tolerance level, give the highest dose prescribed by the doctor first.* Then reduce subsequent doses by 25 to 50 percent until you determine the least amount of drug that provides adequate relief. In other words, work your way down to the lowest acceptable dose. As tolerance develops, you'll increase the dose from there.
- *Raise the dose whenever necessary.* You'll need to consult with the doctor or nurse first, but the primary goal remains getting the patient relief, not minimizing drug intake. If the person becomes temporarily physically dependent on the drug, we'll wean him off it later should he no longer require it.
- *Mix pain meds from different families.* You'll need the doctor or nurse to monitor your decisions, but you'll often find that narcotic doses can be lower when other analgesics or anti-

inflammatory drugs are given at the same time. ▶ *See "Types of Pain Medications," page 155.*
- *Don't wait until someone is complaining of pain to medicate.* Pain prevention requires lower doses than does attempting to alleviate pain after it has crossed the patient's pain threshold.
- *Notice patterns of pain.* Sometimes people hurt worse late at night when they're trying to fall asleep or first thing in the morning when many meds have worn off. Many hurt more when they're tired or stressed out. Administer pain meds prophylactically before the pain returns, and you'll get away with less medicine *and* less suffering.
- *Instead of increasing the dose, try administering pain medicine more often.* For example, the doctor has prescribed 20 milligrams of morphine every four hours for your mom. Two hours after the first dose, she's already hurting, and the clock seems to stand still in anticipation of the next dose. Try giving 10 milligrams every two hours instead. Over an eight-hour period she'll receive the same total amount of morphine (40 milligrams), yet you might find that the more frequent doses are all that's needed to avoid pain breakthrough.
- *Try administering pain medication through different routes.* Transdermal patches or pain meds diluted into IV fluids can deliver a continuous dose. Suppositories and shots kick in faster than drugs taken orally. Experiment until you find what works best for your patient's unique constellation of symptoms.
- *Medicate for nausea at least half an hour before giving pain meds.* Most patients find repeated doses of any strong medicine leaves them constantly sick to their stomach, leading some to avoid taking the pain relief they need. If your loved one is complaining of feeling queasy, use a suppository or patch to deliver the meds.

Many antinausea drugs also help patients relax as well as chemically bolster the effects of narcotics.

- *Medicate anxiety, depression, and sleep disorder aggressively.* As director of social work oncology at Baltimore's Johns Hopkins Oncology Center and a former member of the pain team at Memorial Sloan-Kettering Cancer Center in New York, Matthew Loscalzo reminds us, "Worry, sadness, and stress do not cause pain, but they do make it worse. By controlling these, you can often reduce pain and instill a sense of control."
- *Concentrate on restoring the patient's sense of control over the circumstances instead of absolute alleviation of pain.* Often, if we can just take the edge off a sick person's discomfort and prevent it from intensifying, he is better able to tolerate a moderate level of pain with fewer drugs. Effective medication and cognitive-behavioral interventions for concurrent symptoms such as insomnia, anxiety, and nausea go a long way toward combating feelings of impotence or desperation. ▶ *See "Nonpharmaceutical Pain Management," page 156.*
- *Anticipate constipation.* Any drug strong enough to take the edge off pain also slows down the smooth muscles of the digestive tract. Patients regularly taking pain meds should also ingest a fiber supplement (Metamucil, for example) every day. Add a mild laxative if they miss their regular bowel movement, and encourage them to drink plenty of water and get up and move about as much as possible. Should two days pass with no bowel movement, alert the medical team. ▶ *See "Constipation and Gas," page 167.*

Types of Pain Medications

We start with *nonprescription pain relievers:* aspirin, acetaminophen (Tylenol, Excedrin), and nonsteroidal antiinflammatory drugs (NSAIDS), which include Advil, Motrin, and Nuprin.

If nonprescription drugs are inadequate, a *mild narcotic* (codeine, Percocet/Percodan, Darvon) would be additionally prescribed, depending on the cause of the pain.

If the pain increases or remains severe, a *stronger opioid* (morphine, fentanyl, dilaudid) is added.

"Narcotics are certainly the mainstay in most pain treatment," says Dr. Rogers. However, the effect of narcotics, or opioids, is improved considerably by adding complementary drugs from other rungs on the "analgesia ladder." These include antidepressants, anxiolytics, sedatives—even antiemetics, which not only alleviate nausea and tension but enhance narcotics' effect. The doctor can choose from literally hundreds of medications in order to find the optimum combination for any given patient. "There are more ways to treat pain than you could ever imagine," says Dr. Rogers.

As with all strong medicine, side effects and toxicity are not uncommon, particularly in the elderly and sick. These include kidney damage, liver dysfunction, clotting disorders and bleeding, and ulcers in the stomach and esophagus. Pay careful attention to the doctor's instructions for monitoring patients taking repeated doses of pain meds. Read the "Contraindications" and "Precautions" sections on the printed package inserts. Many patients will also be prescribed a drug to prevent ulcers, such as Tagamet or Zantac.

Other Methods of Administering Pain Medications

One of the great innovations in pain control of the last few years is *patient-controlled analgesia systems,* or *PCA,* which consists of a computerized infusion device that piggybacks into the IV tubing or central venous line. The patient presses a button to administer a predetermined dose of narcotic anytime he needs it. Anticipating the fears of families and patients, Dr. Rogers points out, "The patient-controlled pumps really are very safe. The worst thing that can happen if the patient gives himself too much is that he'll fall asleep and stop pushing the button."

PCA systems are programmed with a short delay between cycles to prevent inadvertent overdoses. They also provide a printout of how often and how much medicine is administered, so that the optimum dosage can be calculated for future administrations.

For chronic, unremitting pain, a catheter can be inserted into the space around the spinal cord (epidural) or into the spinal canal (intrathecal) to deliver medication directly to the affected nerves. This prevents the pain signals from ever reaching the brain and has the added advantage of not passing through the bloodstream. Patients can remain more highly functional and clearer headed, even when taking large doses.

Nonpharmaceutical Pain Management

In addition to the vast armamentarium of drugs and drug delivery systems, there are a number of techniques patients can learn to enhance the effectiveness of their medications: acupuncture, guided visualization, biofeedback, hypnotherapy, and so on. What's more, they can help alleviate other symptoms, such as nausea and anxiety. According to Dr. Rogers, these methods are finding greater acceptance within the medical community as useful adjuncts to traditional interventions.

"When it comes to pain control, no single thing helps everybody," he emphasizes, "and so the doctor has to tailor an individual treatment to the patient. The bottom line is to enable the person to have a good quality of life, and whatever it takes to get there is what needs to be done."

At the present time these pain management techniques are limited primarily to your more sophisticated medical centers, and so it will require some digging on your part to locate experienced practitioners who can help impart these skills to your loved one. To obtain referrals, contact the psychiatry department at a major teaching hospital or call the professional organizations listed here and in the appendix.

Deep Breathing, Progressive Relaxation, and Guided Visualization/Imagery

The adrenaline rush and muscle tension that grips us when we're upset or in pain can be mitigated by taking a series of slow, deep breaths. For example, coach your loved one to inhale for a count of four . . . then exhale evenly and deliberately for a count of eight. Guided visualizations or imagery can also be extremely helpful. Here the patient is taught to concentrate on a relaxing, comforting thought or scene during the breathing exercises.

Biofeedback, Hypnosis, and Meditation

Working with a trained nurse, psychologist, social worker, or psychiatrist, the patient is taught to relax deeply using predetermined cues. In biofeedback an electronic device indicates to the patient when his pulse slows down or his skin temperature lowers. Hypnosis uses a customized audiotape to talk a patient through a rehearsed progressive-relaxation or deep-breathing exercise, or through a series of verbal cues that reminds him how to relax.

For referrals to experienced practitioners in your local area, contact:

☎ Association for Applied Psychophysiology and Biofeedback, 10200 West 44th Avenue, #304, Wheat Ridge, CO 80033-2840.

☎ American Society of Clinical Hypnosis, 2200 East Devon Avenue, Suite 291, Des Plaines, IL 60018; 847-297-3317.

Acupuncture

This ancient Chinese healing art is thought to work by interrupting specific paths of electrical currents coursing through the body by inserting hair-thin needles into the skin in precise locations. If your doctor or local hospital can't recommend a trained medical acupuncturist, contact:

☎ American Academy of Medical Acupuncture, 5820 Wilshire Boulevard, Suite 500, Los Angeles, CA 90036; 800-521-2262.

☎ National Certification Commission for Acupuncture and Oriental Medicine, 1424 16th Street, Suite 501, Washington, DC 20036; 202-232-1404.

Cold Compresses or Ice Packs

Overstimulated nerves, swelling, and inflammation can be calmed profoundly by applying cold in the form of a compress or ice pack. Always remember, though, that cold slows circulation to the affected area. Place a towel between the skin and the ice pack to prevent frostbite, and limit all treatments to no more than twenty minutes. They can be repeated as soon as normal circulation returns. To test circulation in the extremities, press on the nail bed, then quickly release. If it turns pink instantly, you have got the green light to apply cold to the area again.

Moist Heat and Gentle Massage

For injuries that are one or more days old, increasing circulation to the area promotes healing and reduces local pain. Placing warm, moist towels over the site and gently massaging the muscles almost always makes folks feel better. If heat or touch makes the pain worse, revert to cold packs. A hot-water bottle wrapped in a towel is a great way to ease abdominal cramps.

A word about giving a massage: A gentle touch is essential. Patients can suffer serious internal bruises if they have a blood-clotting disorder or are taking anticoagulant drugs, while in the very old or calcium-depleted, brittle bones can break surprisingly easily. Leave deep-tissue massage strictly to trained professionals working closely with the medical team.

Splinting

When muscles have been cut, as during surgery, or when ribs have been broken or bruised, just the movement associated with normal breathing can be excruciating. Coughing or vomiting? Sheer hell. Encourage your loved one to practice holding a pillow, firm cushion, or thick rolled-up towel firmly against the sore area when taking a deep breath, coughing, sneezing, throwing up, or changing positions. Mechanically shore up the weak spot.

Transcutaneous Electrical Nerve Stimulation (TENS)

Pain signals radiating along the path of a nerve can often be interrupted by applying a weak electrical current to the skin above. TENS is a favorite of physical therapists treating chronic pain associated with orthopedic injuries or a pinched nerve.

What to Do When Pain Is Poorly Controlled

When a medical professional tells a patient a procedure "might cause some discomfort," that's often hospital-speak for "It can hurt like hell." What one patient describes as "a mild stinging or burning" may feel like a fiery dagger to someone else. Every human body is different, and our individual perception of pain is highly subjective. If the patient says it hurts, it hurts. That's the *only* practical standard.

When discussing pain management for your loved one, ask the doctor about worst-case scenarios. For example: "And what do we do if he finds it more painful than you predict?" Some practitioners tend to minimize pain. "It's not that bad" or "My other patients don't complain this much" are clear tip-offs that you're talking to the wrong person.

Sometimes patients do not complain, or they describe their symptoms in ways that fail to capture the medical team's attention. In order to get the most effective treatment possible, it's essential that patients and caregivers describe pain accurately to the doctor:

- *Ask your patient to rate her pain on a one-to-ten scale*, with one denoting "pain free" and ten "unbearable."
- *Observe if the pain in any way limits normal function.* For instance: "The headache was so bad she stayed in bed all day with the lights out, getting up only long enough to vomit" or "It hurts so much she can't take a deep breath" or "It hurt so badly she couldn't sleep all night."
- *Help loved ones find the words to describe the pain.* A "shooting" pain is different from a "dull ache." Throbbing, stabbing, burning, pressure, vicelike, crampy, radiating, pinching, stinging—each describes a different type of pain, often with a different cause.
- *Be able to tell the doctor when pain occurs.* Is it at different times of the day or night? After eating or exerting himself? Following certain medications or procedures? The medical team needs a clear picture of the type of pain, its intensity, and its patterns in order to formulate adequate treatment.

If your loved one's pain is still not managed adequately, consider calling for a formal consultation with a pain specialist or pain team. Formally organized pain teams are usually found only in medical centers, particularly facilities that specialize in treating cancer or AIDS, or in rehabilitation hospitals and hospices. A pain team usually incorporates professionals from several disciplines in order to make sure every parameter of pain is addressed. These can include an internist, a neurologist, an anesthesiologist, a pharmacist, a nurse, a social worker or psychologist, and a psychiatrist.

If you have little luck locating a pain expert at your local medical center or hospice, request a referral from:

☎ Cancer Information Service, 800-422-6237.

☎ American Pain Society, 4700 West Lake Avenue, Glenview, IL 60025-1485, 847-375-4731.

"Patients should not tolerate being in pain," asserts Matthew Loscalzo, who works exclusively with cancer patients, many of them terminal. Given the many interventions available, he says, "that just should not happen."

Essential Skills for Preventing and Managing Specific Complications

Digestive Complications
Appetite Loss and Anorexia

Johnetta Romanowski: I remember once cooking Dennis twenty-one different meals in one week to get him to eat something. It wasn't a question of not being able to keep things down, it was the smell, because of his chemotherapy. He'd ask me to make him something, and by the time it was ready, he didn't want it anymore.

Causes Include

Nausea • chronic sore mouth or throat • altered sense of taste or smell • dry mouth • pressure of a tumor or enlarged emphysemic lungs pressing against the stomach • indigestion • inability to swallow normally (dysphasia) • bowel obstruction • headaches and other types of pain • fatigue • depression

Sick people have a host of reasons not to feel like eating. For those expected to die imminently, we help them eat whatever they like. If they are not hungry or thirsty, we don't pressure them, for one of the ways the body naturally shuts down is to refuse fuel.

If we're caring for someone who is expected to live, we don't strictly enforce rigid diets if it means he ends up eating too little. After my father's heart surgery, his cardiologist put him on a heart-healthy diet: low salt, low fat, low cholesterol. For Bob, a connoisseur of fried foods, this amounted to a restrictive diet. By the time my teenage niece came to stay with him for the summer, Pop had decided the diet was making him to sick to his stomach, and he went back to eating what he wanted. "Every morning," Lorna recalls, "we had eggs, grits, bacon, and biscuits." My father also used to send her out on burger runs.

The biological process of fighting disease and tolerating treatment demands vast, continuous expenditures of energy, comparable to that of an athlete. This often results in *cachexia*, or wasting, a common but dangerous condition. Once the body has used up all its stored carbohydrates from sugar and starches, and burned up all its remaining fat, it resorts to breaking down muscle and connective tissue to fuel vital functions. Many patients become shockingly gaunt, weak, severely anemic, and extremely vulnerable to deadly secondary infections.

The caregiver's main task is to provide them with any and all nutrition and hydration they can tolerate comfortably. Important exceptions to this general rule of thumb, however, include diabetics and people with impaired kidney function, congestive heart failure, or pulmonary edema. Failure to carefully balance intake of sugars, fluids, sodium, and other vital minerals and nutrients can bring on serious, even life-threatening problems. ▶ *See "Caring for Someone with Diabetes: The Diabetic Diet," page 397; "Caring for Someone with Kidney Disease: The Renal Diet," page 455.*

Tricks for Stimulating Appetite

◆ **Prepare familiar, favorite foods,** as Audree Siden did while trying to entice her terminally ill mother to eat. "At one point I decided to appeal to the old Russian smells in her brain," she recalls. "My grandparents had been in the dairy business, so I went down to the Kiev Restaurant in lower Manhattan and bought her thick lentil soup, kasha varnishkas, and pickled herring. She smiled and ate them."

◆ **Encourage your loved one to take meals at the table with the family whenever she's feeling up to it.** If the person is on a restricted diet, it's sometimes easier for the rest of the family to alter their eating habits, as Gerri Clarke discovered during the thirteen years her husband, Paul, was on dialysis and had to watch his intake of salt, fluids, and various minerals. She and the Clarkes' two young daughters "generally adapted our food to fit his diet," she recalls, "because my life was a little too busy to be able to cook four different meals."

◆ **Set aside plenty of time for meals,** so that you and the sick person do not feel rushed.

◆ **Serve several small meals throughout the day,** instead of three large meals. "A big plate of food seems overwhelming," explains hospice nurse Mary Ann Reeks. Small portions are more appetizing, and less exhausting to swallow and digest.

◆ *To supplement calories,* add whole or powdered milk, cheese, butter, sour cream, yogurt, eggs, nuts, wheat germ, peanut butter, or beans to the fare that is offered.

◆ *Keep plenty of convenient, ready-to-eat, healthy snacks around the house and in the fridge,* such as fresh fruit, sports bars, trail mix, pudding, ice cream, or yogurt.

◆ *For folks who have trouble swallowing or who have sore mouths and throats, cut solid food into bite-sized pieces.* Make food softer by adding sauces, soups, or gravy. Avoid spicy foods and rough textures, like dry crackers. Avoid very hot or very cold foods.

◆ *Pay attention to aesthetics.* "Try to make the food look attractive on the plate," advises Betty Lindstrom, whose husband, Clarence, was severely disabled and bed-bound with advanced Parkinson's disease. "I used to buy parsley and tuck a little green here and there and place a cut-up cherry on top of his pudding." Set a pretty table, turn down the lights and light candles, eliminate noise and play some soothing music—whatever helps to make eating a more pleasant experience.

◆ *Encourage your loved one to get some light exercise or at least do some deep breathing before eating,* both of which aid digestion. Or accompany her on a leisurely walk following meals, if she's up to it.

◆ *Ask the doctor about using liquid nutritional supplements* such as Ensure, Sustacal, Nutren, or Advera. Taste-test several brands before you stock up, though: These products are expensive, and some are easier than others to digest for different people.

Most brands go down better cool or cold. "They don't have to drink the whole can at once," says nurse Jane Pilecki. "Let them sip small amounts through the day."

◆ *Also ask the doctor or hospital dietitian about prescribing an appetite stimulant* such as Marinol, Periactic, or Megace. Many people with cancer and AIDS find that smoking marijuana is also highly effective at stirring appetite, minimizing nausea, and reducing anxiety. Although it's still a misdemeanor in most states, California has legalized medical marijuana use, and similar laws are pending in several other legislatures around the country. ▶ See *"Thoughts on the Medical Use of Marijuana," page 164.*

◆ *When cooking meals, prepare extra food and freeze individual portions for later.* You'll be glad you did the first time your loved one suddenly feels like eating precisely when you have no time to cook.

Complications That Interfere with Eating

Altered Taste

Oral infections as well as many common medications can change or diminish a patient's sense of taste, making it unpleasant if not impossible to enjoy eating. Chemotherapy, radiation, and some diseases can also cause this problem, with many people complaining of a constant bitter or metallic taste in their mouths. Others become hypersensitive to certain tastes and smells.

Here's What You Can Do

◆ *Encourage your loved one to rinse his mouth before meals with a solution of hydrogen peroxide or baking soda and warm water.* (Caution her not to swallow it.) Or use a soft-bristle toothbrush and a good-tasting toothpaste to clean the teeth and tongue. Remind her to take any prescribed antifungal medications regularly.

♦ **Choose and prepare foods that smell appetizing to the patient.**

♦ **Try serving foods at room temperature,** so the flavor is less intense.

♦ **Cold numbs the taste buds:** spoon out ice cream, sherbet, fruit ices, or frozen yogurt.

♦ **Tart foods can mask metallic tastes.** Try serving orange juice or lemonade with meals. Add vinegar, lemon juice, pickles, and relish to food. Marinate meats in wine, salad dressing, soy sauce, vinegar, or fruit juice.

♦ **Experiment with small amounts of flavorful seasonings** such as basil, oregano, rosemary, thyme, or cumin, and season vegetables with small pieces of bacon, ham, or other aromatic meats.

♦ **Vary the texture of food** to make it more interesting. Add chopped nuts or seeds, or puree vegetables into a soup.

Dry Mouth

Certain medications, breathing dehumidified oxygen, breathing through the mouth, diseases of the salivary glands, and general dehydration all contribute to an abnormally dry mouth. Many diabetics also complain of a constantly dry mouth. It makes eating almost anything unpalatable, even painful.

Here's What You Can Do

♦ **Make sure your loved one drinks plenty of fluids,** and consider running a humidifier when he's sleeping.

♦ **Stimulate salivation** by having her suck on sugar-free sour balls, ice pops, ice chips, or chew sugarless gum.

♦ **Moisten food** with butter, yogurt, salad dressing, gravy, soup, or sauces. Dunk bread, crackers, or biscuits in milk, soup, juice, or olive oil.

♦ **Remind your loved one to sip water or another liquid between bites** of food. Suggest he use a straw.

♦ **Keep lips well moisturized** with salve, balm, or petroleum jelly.

♦ **Minimize alcohol and caffeine consumption and smoking,** which exacerbate dehydration. ◄ *See "Oral Hygiene," page 123.*

Sore Mouth or Throat

The throat and esophagus can become extremely sore as a result of local infections or tissue damage from radiation or chemotherapy. Severe acid reflux from the stomach can also irritate the lining of the esophagus and the throat, making swallowing food an ordeal.

Here's What You Can Do

♦ **Remind your loved one to gargle several times a day** with any of the following: a solution of warm salt water, a mixture of baking soda and water, or equal parts water and hydrogen peroxide. Skip the commercial mouthwashes, which are too harsh for tender membranes.

♦ **Dispense antacids** to buffer stomach acid.

♦ **Avoid irritating, spicy, salty, or highly acidic foods** (citrus fruit or juices, for instance). Instead serve bland foods and liquids: rice, chicken stock, baby food.

♦ **Food shouldn't be served hot.** Cold or frozen items such as ice cream, sherbets, and ices are easier to swallow.

♦ **Don't serve coarsely textured foods such as crackers and raw** *vegetables*, which will only irritate the throat. Try soft foods. Examples include milkshakes, bananas, applesauce, oatmeal and other cooked cereals, mashed potatoes, macaroni and cheese, scrambled eggs.

♦ *Moisten food* with butter, yogurt, salad dressing, gravy, soup, or sauces. Dunk bread, crackers, or biscuits in milk, soup, juice, or olive oil.

♦ *Tobacco and alcohol should be avoided.*

♦ *An anesthetic spray or gargle can help soothe the throat.* Examples of each include Chloroseptic and viscous Xylocaine.

♦ *Keep dentures clean* and remove them whenever the patient's gums are sore or irritated.

Special Care: Feeding a Loved One with Physical Impairments

The tremors associated with Parkinson's disease and the declining motor skills from a stroke or amyotrophic lateral sclerosis can make dining an overwhelming physical challenge. There are a wide range of special eating utensils manufactured for folks with unsteady hands or for one-handed eating. These include wide-based cups with lids and large handles; knives and spoons with built-up grips; and guards that clip around plates or bowls. The right tools —and plenty of patience—make all the difference. ► *See Appendix B: "Adaptive Technology," page 504.*

Special Care: Feeding a Loved One with Memory Loss, Confusion, or Intellectual Impairment

People who have trouble concentrating may forget to eat, or lose interest in eating when something distracts them.

Others may not remember having just eaten and gorge themselves throughout the day. Keeping these folks properly nourished requires planning and constant, gentle supervision.

Here's What You Can Do

♦ *Call or stop by* at scheduled meal times.

♦ *Maintain a consistent routine for meals,* and stick to familiar, favorite menus.

♦ *Eliminate unnecessary distractions during meals.* Turn off the TV and avoid cross-talk. Keep the table setting simple and strictly functional.

♦ *Don't rush, and keep instructions simple.* Avoid too many choices. Offer one food or condiment at a time; the same goes with utensils.

♦ *Serve food and beverages in easily managed portions.* Use straws for liquids, or pour drinks into large mugs, filling only halfway. Your best bet for serving solid foods is a heavy bowl with steep sides and a wide base. Also, consider serving finger foods and letting your patient eat with her hands.

♦ *Ignore declining table manners.* Be prepared for spills and drooling, and don't overreact when they inevitably occur. If a meal becomes too stressful or frustrating for your loved one (or for you), let it go until later, when everyone's feeling calmer.

♦ *Store food out of sight between meals* for those who tend to forget they just ate.

Indigestion and Nausea

Debbie Bryant: My mother decided she didn't want to have chemotherapy anymore, because it just made her so sick and nauseous.

Causes Include:

Antibiotics and various other medications • sluggish GI tract (reduced motility) due to illness or immobility • surgery to remove part of the stomach or bowel • obstruction of the digestive tract • overeating • peptic ulcer • gallbladder disease • gastritis • headaches • chemotherapy • radiation therapy • Parkinson's disease, due to the disease affecting the brain's nausea-control center • kidney disease, due to inadequate dialysis treatment • AIDS • and on and on . . .

One of the most physically and psychologically debilitating aspects of serious illness is unremitting queasiness. Upset stomachs can range from mild indigestion, to severe *dyspepsia* that doubles a person over with stabbing pains. And relentless nausea and vomiting can literally drain the life out of a very sick person.

Whatever the cause, there are many things we can do to mitigate the effects of an upset stomach.

Here's What You Can Do

◆ **Try to keep a little food in the stomach at all times** to buffer stomach acid and digestive juices. Small frequent meals or snacks throughout the day are far easier to keep down and to digest than heavy meals. Avoid greasy, fried, or spicy foods.

◆ **Serve cool or cold foods.** Hot food exacerbates the feeling of nausea.

◆ **For persistent indigestion or dyspepsia, ask the doctor about common and wonderfully effective antiulcer drugs** such as Tagamet or Zantac.

◆ **Experiment with over-the-counter antacids** such as Tums, Rolaids, chewable calcium tablets, Pepto-Bismol, and Mylanta.

◆ **Also ask about highly effective antinausea drugs called** antiemetics. Frequently prescribed brands include Compazine, Phenergan, Zofran, and Reglan. They come in a variety of convenient forms, including syrups, pills, skin patches (for continuous delivery), suppositories (for when a patient cannot keep down oral medicines), and injections (for the very worst episodes of vomiting or dry heaves). Medicate patients aggressively for nausea before they miss more meals or lose too much sleep. ◀ *See "Routes of Drug Administration," page 144.*

◆ **Observe the patterns of nausea and indigestion, and medicate patients before symptoms arise.** Like pain, nausea is easier to prevent than to control. My dad had suffered with ulcers all his life. Getting him to eat after he was sick was a daily challenge due to his almost constant nausea and indigestion. We quickly learned to give him a big dose of antacid *before* each meal if he was to have any chance of keeping it down. In addition, the morphine Bob took for pain could always be counted on to make him nauseous. We found that giving him a dose of Compazine half an hour before it was time for his morphine usually enabled him to rest comfortably and even keep down a little food.

◆ **Remember not to serve favorite dishes when someone is feeling queasy.** She may develop an aversion to the one food she would be most likely to eat once she's feeling better.

◆ **Drinking herbal tea with honey or chewing a piece of fresh ginger root** can often settle an upset stomach.

◆ **Reduce external stimulation:** lower the lights, turn down the volume —of conversations as well as radio, TV, and other background noise—and don't jostle the bed!

◆ **Patients should not lie down immediately following a meal.** Encourage them to take a walk instead, or at least to sit up in a chair for an hour or so.

◆ **Cool air helps alleviate nausea.** "I like to use cold air from an air conditioner, or a cold, wet washcloth behind the head or neck," says nurse Mary Ann Reeks. Turn a fan on the person's face or let him suck ice chips.

◆ **The nonpharmaceutical pain-management techniques described earlier** work well to help control nausea, too. Find out more about biofeedback, hypnosis, deep breathing, and progressive-relaxation techniques, meditation, and guided visualization. ◄ See "Nonpharmaceutical Pain Management," page 156. ► See "Feeding, Hydration, and the Dying," page 303.

Thoughts on the Medical Use of Marijuana

Maida Bryant, dying of cancer in 1978, was racked by relentless nausea that would not respond to any of the drugs her doctor prescribed. Her daughter Debbie, then twenty-four, talked her into smoking marijuana. "She did," says Debbie, "and it eased her nausea a lot."

Despite tremendous advances in pharmaceutical research and many highly effective drugs now on the market for controlling nausea, more sick people than ever before are smoking marijuana. Not only is it clinically effective at relieving nausea, but it also stimulates appetite and elevates mood. As a direct result of consumer demand and decades of lobbying from groups such as the National Organization for the Reform of Marijuana Laws (NORML), state prohibitions are changing slowly to recognize the legitimate, medical uses of marijuana. Nonetheless, it's still a crime to buy or sell it most places. Though prosecutions are rare, possession of even a small amount for personal consumption can still get you into trouble with the law in many states.

My father was unconcerned with the legal implications when my brother offered him a joint during one episode of unremitting nausea. The pot worked fine at settling Bob's stomach, but he didn't like the feeling of being "high," and never tried it again. Pop's doctor, like most physicians these days, was willing to see if the marijuana worked, and looked the other way.

Marinol, the prescription form of tetrahydrocannabinol (THC), the main drug in marijuana, can now be ordered by doctors to stimulate appetite. But Marinol lacks the other psychoactive, or mind-altering, ingredients of natural marijuana and doesn't provide the same mildly euphoric sensation that comes from smoking the marijuana plant. It's worth a try—provided your patient and you are comfortable with it—particularly when nothing else is working well.

When a Patient Vomits

Vomiting leaves a person feeling physically out of control, vulnerable, and embarrassed, so let's not get upset when someone throws up. Sometimes it helps to encourage your loved one to go ahead and vomit instead of laboring to repress the urge; she'll feel much better, at least for a little while.

◆ **If the patient is in bed** when he starts to throw up, roll him immediately to one side so he doesn't choke on the vomit.

◆ **Don't let loved ones make a run for the bathroom.** People slip and fall and are seriously injured that way. Instead keep a towel, vomit basin, or plastic-lined trash basket handy for unexpected episodes of vomiting.

◆ **Encourage your patient to take slow, deep breaths** through her mouth when she feels nauseous or during episodes of retching and heaving. The extra oxygen will ease the worst sensations of nausea and even help prevent vomiting.

◆ **The odor of vomit can make someone sick again.** So, too, can the smell of heavily perfumed chemical air fresheners. Open a window or turn on a fan when someone is throwing up. Plenty of fresh air is the answer.

◆ **Remind your loved one to brush his teeth or gargle** after throwing up. The aftertaste can make him sick all over again. What's more, the regurgitated stomach acid seriously damages tooth enamel.

◆ **The only thing worse** than relentless nausea is the "dry heaves." If someone has vomited up everything in her stomach but continues to retch and heave, encourage her to sip a glass of water with a little baking soda in it. The bicarbonate helps buffer the stomach acid, and the water provides some liquid to throw up until the episode passes.

Difficulty Swallowing (Dysphagia)

Betty Lindstrom: Swallowing becomes a problem for many Parkinson's patients. I had to convince the health department that it was all right for me to get a suctioning device so I could clear my husband's throat, without being a registered nurse.

Causes Include

Mechanical difficulties, as may be seen in stroke, traumatic brain injury, Parkinson's disease, amyotrophic lateral sclerosis • forgetting to swallow, due to dementia from stroke, AIDS, Alzheimer's disease • painful swallowing, as results from radiation therapy to the neck • surgical removal of all or part of the tongue • certain chemotherapy agents and other drugs

When a patient has problems swallowing normally, the caregiver has two major concerns. One is that the person won't be able to eat enough to stay adequately nourished. Even more dangerous, however, is the possibility of choking or inadvertently inhaling food or liquid down the windpipe and into the lungs, inducing what is called *aspiration pneumonia*, a potentially deadly complication.

Here's What You Can Do

◆ **Always feed your loved one while he's sitting upright** in a chair. If he's bedridden, elevate the head of the bed and prop him up with pillows until he's as close to a sitting position as you can manage.

◆ **Encourage her to remain sitting upright** for at least twenty or thirty minutes after eating.

◆ **Remind your patient to take a deep breath before swallowing,** and to exhale or cough after each bite. Do not suppress the cough reflex, because coughing is the body's way of keeping the windpipe and airways clear of foreign matter.

◆ **Set aside plenty of time for feedings,** so that you and your loved are not rushed.

◆ **Keep talking to a minimum** while eating. Eliminate other distractions by turning off the TV or feeding young children before or after the patient.

◆ **Encourage her to keep her chin down** at a natural level when swallowing. Tossing back the head increases the possibility of diverting food or liquid into the windpipe.

◆ **If liquids are well tolerated, alternate sips with bites of food.** But be careful with thin liquids! "Water is especially easy to aspirate," points out hospice nurse Ellen Wilson. Sipping from a flexible drinking straw may make liquids easier to swallow.

◆ *Cut food into small pieces* and experiment with pureed dishes of various consistencies. Ask a nutritionist about adding thickeners to liquids. One good product is called Thick-It, but cornstarch works just as well with many common foods.

◆ *Avoid very hot or very cold foods,* which can cause a spasm in the esophagus while swallowing.

What to Do When Someone Is Choking

Keeping a loved one's airway clear is a matter of life and death. Folks who have trouble swallowing are in particular danger, since each bite of food and every sip of water carries the risk of aspiration.

1. Encourage her to spit out whatever food is in her mouth or throat immediately and to cough vigorously, until the airway is clear.
2. With the patient leaning forward (and coughing), cup your hand and thump her on the back (as you would a child) between the shoulder blades to help dislodge or shake loose foreign matter in the windpipe.
3. Use a mechanical suction device to clear liquids, runny foods, and secretions from the airway. Note that suction machines are useless for lifting solid pieces of food.
4. If solid food remains lodged in the airway, administer either the Heimlich maneuver or abdominal thrusts on patients who you cannot position upright. ► *See "Using a Suction Device to Clear the Airway," page 177; "The Heimlich Maneuver," page 182.*

Tube Feedings and Total Parenteral Nutrition (TPN)

Sometimes swallowing problems become so severe that the physician may recommend bypassing the mouth altogether by surgically implanting a feeding tube. The most common types are *gastrostomy* tubes ("G tubes"), inserted into the stomach, and *jejunostomy* tubes ("J tubes"), which deliver nutrition and medications into the small bowel. You may hear the G tube referred to as a PEG, which stands for *percutaneous endoscopic gastrostomy.* Increasingly, the tubes are able to be inserted by way of an endoscope through a small incision barely half an inch long.

Caregivers will receive thorough training and regular supervision by a home-care nurse before being expected to routinely administer tube feedings at home. A few key rules to remember:

◆ *Check the placement of the tube* before each infusion by aspirating the gastric contents the way the nurse showed you.

◆ *Administer tube feedings with your patient sitting or propped upright* and encourage her to remain upright for at least twenty or thirty minutes following the feeding.

◆ *Flush the tube with water* before and after every infusion, just as you were taught, to make sure it does not become clogged.

◆ *Never inject air into the tube,* which can result in bloating, cramps, and gas.

◆ *Conscientiously store and prepare liquid foods for tube feedings according to the instructions.* Administer tube feedings at room temperature.

◆ *Monitor how well your loved one tolerates each tube feeding.* Be vigilant for constipation, diarrhea, nausea, vomiting, excessive gas, belching, flatulence, cramping, and/or bloating. Keep a log of adverse symptoms and consult with the physician or home-care nurse about adjusting the feedings.

◆ *Carefully record the amount of each administration and measure urine output.* Roughly half the volume of the feeding should be excreted as urine.

◆ *Keep a close eye on your loved one for signs of dehydration.* You may need to add water to subsequent feedings along with the liquid nutrition.

◆ *Report any sign of infection to the nurse or doctor immediately,* such as fever or redness, swelling, pain, or foul drainage at the insertion site.

For people who cannot swallow or digest adequate nutrition in their gut, *total parenteral nutrition* is administered. Also called *hyperalimentation,* TPN involves infusing liquid nutrients directly through a central intravenous line. ◄ *See "Central Venous Catheters," page 150.*

Constipation and Gas

Sarah Eilenberg, hospice nurse: Most people don't know it, but constipation can kill you.

Causes Include

Dehydration • fiber-poor diet • immobility • narcotic pain relievers, anticholinergics, and many other medications • bowel obstructions • neuromuscular conditions such as Parkinson's disease and diabetes-related gastroparesis, which slow down the GI tract

As everyone knows, you don't have to be sick to get constipated. But it's a particularly dangerous problem with the very ill and with old people in general, who are five times more likely than young adults to become constipated. Besides the discomfort, constipation can lead to life-threatening conditions such as fecal impactions, perforated intestines, and peritonitis, an inflammation of the membrane that lines the wall of the abdominal cavity.

The caregiver's main task is seeing to it that our loved one never becomes constipated in the first place. The most effective preventive strategy, says nurse Sarah Eilenberg, is to make sure ill people move their bowels regularly "no matter what, even if they're no longer eating." Nurse Ellen Wilson observes that sometimes patients avoid moving their bowels "because it entails using the bedpan or getting to the commode. Down the line, though, it's going to cause serious problems." Eilenberg has cared for patients "who hadn't moved their bowels in a month," she says, "and that becomes very unpleasant for the person."

Here's What You Can Do

◆ *Encourage your loved one to drink plenty of fluids.* In folks whose kidneys are functioning, transparent urine should flow at regular intervals throughout the day. If it does not, they're not drinking enough water. For most adults that means drinking two to three quarts of water per day to keep the body well hydrated.

◆ *Maintain a schedule of regular physical activity.* Long walks are best. Even the bed-bound can help stimulate bowel movement by frequently changing position and breathing deeply.

◆ *Serve plenty of high-fiber foods* such as raw vegetables and bran. If eating enough fiber is a problem, consider adding a fiber supplement such as Metamucil, which doubles as a bulk-forming laxative.

◆ *If constipation persists, consult the nurse or doctor about other laxatives and stool softeners.* Plain glycerin suppositories work well for many people.

◆ *Never administer an enema without first consulting the nurse or doctor.* An occasional case of constipation may be helped along by a warm-water enema or a Fleet enema. However, enemas can seriously injure a person suffering from a bowel impaction, obstruction, or perforation. Frequent enemas also weaken bowel muscle tone and disrupt the bowel's internal chemistry, leaving a person dependent on more enemas in order to have a bowel movement.

◆ **Establish a daily "bowel routine" for folks prone to constipation,** especially those with neurological damage. For example: laxative before bed; suppository first thing in the morning; after breakfast and a hot drink, straight to the toilet. Allow plenty of time for nature to work; that means no rushing or interruptions.

◆ **A bowel routine may need to include manual or digital (with the fingers) stimulation,** particularly in the neurologically impaired and bedbound. This should not be attempted without careful instruction and supervision from a nurse or doctor.

What Is a Fecal Impaction?

When constipation persists for several days, the dehydrated fecal matter in the intestine begins hardening into a stonelike mass that adheres to the wall of the colon. Stool and gas back up behind it, producing abdominal pain, bloating, nausea, and vomiting. Though the impaction is first caused by persistent constipation, your loved one may still experience episodes of explosive diarrhea or flatulence, as backed-up gas and stool squeeze past the impaction under great pressure.

The danger in impactions are many. The patient is unable to eat and digest food. He is unable to absorb water in the intestines normally. The bowel wall becomes ulcerated, and pressure against the impaction can lead to a perforation of the colon. When the contents of the bowel spills into the abdominal cavity, life-threatening peritonitis quickly results.

✝ *Notify the doctor, home-care nurse, or hospice nurse immediately if a constipated person spikes a fever.*

Sometimes impactions can be relieved with a combination of hydration, physical activity, fiber supplements, laxatives, and stool softeners. Enemas—either oil retention, tap water, or hypertonic phosphate—are also used to lubricate the bowel and soften the stool. When all else fails, patients are digitally or manually disimpacted by a nurse or doctor. That's a fancy way of saying they use a gloved hand to pick apart the impaction if they can reach it. It's excruciating and dangerous. *Patients and lay caregivers should not try to relieve an impaction manually themselves.* Impactions too high up in the colon to reach by hand must be removed surgically.

Gas Pains

Gas pains are a common consequence of constipation, as gases in the digestive tract are unable to escape out the anus. Conversely, diarrhea, too, is often accompanied by severe cramps, as gas bubbles expand violently through the colon, leading to explosive episodes of flatulence mixed with liquid stool. Various foods are responsible for gas production. Dairy products, for example, can make life miserable for the lactose intolerant. Antibiotics and other common drugs disrupt the chemistry of the digestive tract, producing severe gas pain. You can have air pumped directly into your intestines during a colonoscopy and other procedures, and many folks will say that postoperative gas pain is the worst imaginable.

Avoiding foods known to cause gas and scrupulously avoiding getting constipated are key. Some drugs like Mylanta and Mylicon help reduce gas (as does Lactaid for the lactose intolerant), but their best effects are in the upper gastrointestinal tract. As with belching, the only relief from gas pains emanating from the lower bowel is to pass gas.

Long walks and warm baths stimulate the intestines, thus helping work the air bubble down and out. A hot-water bottle or heating pad clutched firmly to the belly helps ease the cramps.

Diarrhea

Mary Vitro: By the end of Rick's life, he had no control of his bowels at all. In the hospital they wouldn't even let him wear underwear anymore.

Causes Include

Many drugs, including the popular anticoagulant warfarin (Coumadin) • diabetes • AIDS • radiation therapy to the abdomen or pelvic region • infections and diseases of the colon • food sensitivities such as lactose intolerance

Of all the digestive complications, diarrhea is the most dangerous, because vital nutrients and water speed through the digestive tract without being absorbed. Patients are left severely dehydrated, malnourished, and with serious imbalances of electrolytes such as sodium and potassium, which can lead to muscle cramps and abnormal heart rhythms. In the worst cases, as with the AIDS-related intestinal infection cryptosporidiosis, diarrhea can literally run to several quarts each day, quickly depleting and killing the person.

✚ *Notify the doctor, home-care nurse, or hospice nurse immediately should diarrhea persist for more than twenty-four hours or if it is accompanied by sudden fever.*

Here's What You Can Do

When someone has diarrhea, the caregiver's main tasks are to stem the continued loss of fluids and electrolytes and to replace them quickly.

◆ *Imodium and Lomotil,* available over-the-counter and in stronger doses by prescription, are extremely effective at slowing or arresting most cases of diarrhea. Ask your doctor or pharmacist for more information. Care must be taken with these and similar drugs, since giving too large or too frequent a dose can cause severe constipation.

◆ *Fluids must be replaced* in amounts at least equal to what's lost, and quickly, before serious metabolic complications emerge. Early symptoms of rapid dehydration and electrolyte imbalance include cramps, palpitations, headache, and/or dizziness. Encourage your loved one to drink water, diluted fruit juice, Gatorade, or lactose-reduced milk throughout the day. ◀ *See "Tricks for Getting Patients to Drink," page 104.*

◆ *Switch to a clear liquid diet* (water, herbal tea, apple juice, broth, gelatin) as soon as diarrhea starts.

◆ *Potassium and sodium,* along with other vital minerals, can be quickly replenished by eating bananas, oranges, melons, grapefruit, tomatoes, or potatoes.

◆ *Avoid caffeine and alcohol* completely.

◆ *Fastidious hygiene is crucial.* Liquid stool is highly acidic and can cause the skin to break down. After each bowel movement, wash the anus and perineal area instead of using toilet paper. Dry the skin thoroughly and apply moisturizer. Rub petroleum jelly on the anus before it becomes irritated and sore.

Until the diarrhea starts to improve, stick to low-fiber foods: rice, bread, well-cooked vegetables, cream of wheat, baby food. Avoid high-fiber foods or foods that cause gas, among them raw fruits and vegetables, beans, cabbage, whole-grain breads and cereals, and milk and milk products. "When somebody has really severe diarrhea for days and days, and nothing seems to be helping them," says nurse Sarah Eilenberg, "we put them on what's called the BRAT diet: bananas, rice, apples, and herbal tea, and nothing else. The combination seems to bind things and makes people a lot more comfortable after a few days."

Urinary Tract Complications

Incontinence

Betty Lindstrom: *Clarence became incontinent. At home I sometimes washed sheets three or four times a day. Adult incontinence is one of the main reasons why many caregivers eventually resort to nursing homes. They can handle many things, but this becomes something that many cannot handle.*

Causes Include

Neurologic disorders • spinal-cord injury • surgeries of the prostate, rectum, female reproductive tract • urinary-tract infection • diabetes • vaginal infection/irritation • constipation • various medications • enlarged prostate gland (benign prostatic hyperplasia)

Some loss of bladder control is inevitable as we age. Roughly one in five men and women over the age of sixty-five complains of some degree of urinary incontinence, usually a result of ever-increasing slack in the muscles that control urination. Many other sick or aging people suffer what is called *functional incontinence*, meaning simply that they're too frail or too incapacitated to get to the toilet when they need to.

When the bladder is not regularly emptied, forcing urine to spill out without warning, we refer to it as *overflow incontinence*. Other types include *stress incontinence*—wetting oneself while coughing, sneezing, laughing, or just changing positions in bed or getting up from a chair—and *urge incontinence*, in which the signal to urinate comes on so abruptly that there's no time to make it to the toilet.

For some there are surgical procedures to cinch up sagging muscles, and specific exercises to increase strength and control of the abdominal muscles. For a small percentage of people with limited neurological damage, *bladder training* can be helpful. Bladder training can include anything from a prescheduled daily toilet routine and exercises to biofeedback techniques and careful timing of fluid intake. For most caregivers facing this problem, though, incontinence becomes a chronic nursing challenge to be dealt with repeatedly every day for the rest of the patient's life. Our goals are to make sure our loved one empties his bladder regularly, as well as to minimize the risk of a urinary-tract infection, and, above all, to keep skin exposed to urine meticulously clean. According to Dr. Katherine F. Jeter, retired founder of the patient organization Help for Incontinent People (now the National Association for Continence), "an incontinent, immobile patient is four times more likely to develop skin problems."

Here's What You Can Do

◆ **Establish a toileting routine.** Notice when and how often the person urinates throughout the day and night. Then make sure she goes to the bathroom or gets on the bedpan at regular intervals, well before she wets herself. If accidents have been occurring during the night, wake her for prescheduled pit stops.

◆ **Coordinate the intake of fluids with your patient's toileting routine.** Cut back on fluid intake two or three hours before bedtime, and make sure she always empties her bladder before turning in.

✻ *Keep in mind that foods such as ice cream, Jell-O, and soups contain a great deal of water.*

◆ *Have your loved one dress in easily removable clothing:* for example, loose-fitting skirts, nightgowns, or housedresses, or roomy pants with an elastic waistband or drawstring. Loose clothing not only makes it easier to use the bathroom, it also disguises bulky diapers or panty-liners, essential items for avoiding embarrassing accidents when up and about.

◆ *Place a commode or urinal beside the bed* for folks who have trouble maneuvering to the bathroom.

◆ If your loved one is mobile but easily confused or disoriented, *clearly mark the door to the toilet and remove clutter and distractions from the bathroom.*

◆ *Talk to the medical team about prescribing doses of diuretics so that their peak effect occurs during the day.* Remember that foods and drinks containing caffeine, such as coffee and many sodas, have a profound diuretic effect on most people, too.

◆ *Place absorbent chucks under the patient's midsection* to draw moisture away from her skin, and to prevent the sheets and mattress from getting soiled. For male patients, ask the doctor about *condom catheters*, an apparatus that attaches around the outside of the penis and directs urine into a drainage bag, which is often strapped to the patient's leg.

◆ *Meticulously wash skin exposed to urine as quickly as possible.* Dry it thoroughly and apply a thin layer of moisturizer or ointment recommended by the nurse or doctor. Even regular bath soap may be too harsh for skin that is irritated by frequent contact with urine. Use baking soda and water or a commercial product designed specifically for skin care in the incontinent. Diaper rash is not only painful but can

set the stage for bedsores and leave the body open to deadly infections. ◀ *See "Daily Hygiene," page 110; "Toileting," page 124.*

The graying of America has meant a boon to manufacturers of products for coping with incontinence. Movie stars of yesteryear pitch competing brands of panty-liners and diapers on TV as unselfconsciously as they hawk denture adhesives. Publications targeted to retirees are jammed with advertisements for absorbent pads, catheter-care supplies, as well as special soaps, deodorants, moisturizers, and disinfectants. For more information about the broad array of products and techniques for managing incontinence, contact the following national organizations:

☎ National Association for Continence, P.O. Box 8310, Spartanburg, SC 29305-8310; 800-252-3337/864-579-7900.

☎ The Simon Foundation for Continence, P.O. Box 835, Wilmette, IL 60091; 800-237-4666/847-864-3913.

Urinary Catheters

Many men and women require indwelling catheters during the course of their medical treatment. When a patient is unconscious, as during surgery or a coma, or otherwise gravely ill and receiving intensive care, a flexible catheter is fed through the urethra and into the bladder in order to monitor precisely the output of the kidneys. Catheterization has the added advantage of continually draining the bladder, thus preventing soiled beds and eliminating the need to maneuver the patient onto a toilet or bedpan.

Others are catheterized intermittently, when something is preventing them from urinating normally. Conditions that might call for periodic catheterization include: a swollen prostate pressing against the urethra; urethral infections causing it to swell shut; bladder spasms or loss of control due to brain damage; or tumors or other masses pressing against the urethra, pinching it closed. Patients requiring frequent catheterizations are often taught to do it themselves, or their care partners are. Whatever the reason for the catheter, patients are dangerously susceptible to urinary-tract infections, which can infiltrate the bloodstream. Therefore meticulous hygiene and sterile technique become matters of life and death.

When Changing a Urine Drainage Bag

- Wash your hands and glove up before handling someone's urine-drainage system.
- Empty the drainage bag several times a day before it gets full. Several times a week, replace the drainage bag and connective tubing, or disconnect them and rinse them thoroughly with a solution of chlorine diluted in water.
- Using soap and water, thoroughly wash the area where the catheter enters the body. Do this at least daily.
- Take care to keep the drainage bag below the level of the patient's bladder at all times. Backflow of urine that has been collecting in the bag could introduce a serious infection into the bladder and kidneys.

✚ *Notify the doctor, home-care nurse, or hospice nurse immediately whenever a catheterized person develops a fever.*

Urinary-Tract Infections

Nola Miller: *The last year of Walter's life, his prostate enlarged, closing off his urethra. Until he had a transurethral resection, he had to be catheterized, and he developed urinary-tract infections.*

For healthy people, infections of the urinary tract come and go, often without treatment, the worst part being the twin sensations of burning and con-

stantly feeling the urge to urinate. For a sick or frail person, though, urinary-tract infections can go on to destroy the kidneys and cause overwhelming blood poisoning *(septicemia)*. Bed-bound patients and people with catheters are the most susceptible to these infections, and require especially conscientious bladder care.

Here's What You Can Do

◆ **Make sure your loved one drinks plenty of fluids.** Constantly flushing the system is nature's way of eliminating infectious agents.

◆ **Encourage your loved one to urinate regularly,** not only to flush the system but to empty the bladder so infections are less apt to flourish there.

◆ **Report any episode of fever to the medical team.** Antibiotics may be required to head off an infection.

◆ **Wash your hands and slip on gloves** before tending to a loved one's intimate needs. Likewise, wash and dry his private parts thoroughly following every urination and bowel movement. ◀ *See "Tricks for Getting Patients to Drink," page 104.*

Insomnia and Other Sleep Disorders

Diane Young: *My father would stay up pacing all day and night, on account of his Alzheimer's disease. We were all just exhausted. I had some Benadryl, an antihistamine, with me because I have hayfever. I put it in a glass of root beer. "Daddy," I asked, "would you like something to drink?" "Oh, yeah!"*

I gave it to him, and he drank it down. All of a sudden I became hysterical! I knew I wasn't hurting him, but he was so grateful for the drink, and I was just giving it to him to make him sleep. Still, he did sleep that night, which was wonderful, because then we could all sleep.

Causes Include

Cancer and cancer treatments • medications • depression, anxiety, stress • hyperactivity due to Alzheimer's disease • malnutrition • anemia • Parkinson's disease • difficulty breathing due to chronic obstructive pulmonary disease, congestive heart failure, other causes • pain • indigestion and other digestive symptoms • night sweats

People have trouble falling asleep, staying asleep, or getting back to sleep for a wide variety of reasons. The problem with sleeplessness is twofold: The patient gets progressively weaker, and the caregiver loses sleep, too. Not only does a lack of sleep render everyone irritable, depressed, and fuzzy-headed, it increases the frequency and intensity of pain and nausea, and even leaves people vulnerable to infections. "It is well documented that people who are deprived of sleep have weakened immune functions," notes Dr. Mary Jane Massie, a psychiatrist at Memorial Sloan-Kettering Cancer Center in New York.

Here's What You Can Do

Fifty million adults in the United States suffer from some form of sleep disorder, and experts have devised about that many different ways to cope. Universal do's and don'ts for getting to sleep include:

◆ *Try to go to bed and to get up at approximately the same time each day.* If your loved one prefers to doze well into the morning, let her and plan daily activities for the afternoon. Conversely, if she naturally tends to turn in early and beat the sun up each morning, alter the household schedule accordingly. As much as possible, stick to a routine, but let natural biorhythms dictate sleeping patterns, not the clock on the wall or other people's schedules.

◆ *Establish a bedtime ritual* and follow it each night—caring for skin, hair, and teeth, sipping herbal tea or a beer, watching TV or reading—the same activities in the same order each evening to train body and mind to prepare to sleep.

◆ *Make the most of the sleep they do get.* Cut down on fluids two or three hours before bedtime to minimize waking to urinate. Turn on the answering machine and turn off the ringer on the phone. Hang a DO NOT DISTURB sign on the front door. Draw the curtains or shades when you turn in.

◆ *Avoid caffeine and large meals for several hours before turning in.* Instead, about an hour before bedtime have a snack rich in protein (milk, for example) as part of the nightly ritual.

◆ *Pay attention to whatever makes the patient feel comfortable and relaxed:* a warm (not hot) bath, clean sheets and soft pajamas, room temperature and ventilation, sound and light levels, plenty of pillows and lightweight blankets.

◆ *Get as much exercise during the day as possible,* and keep naps short. But abstain from all exercise for several hours before bed.

◆ *Schedule pain medications or other drugs that cause drowsiness* (such as antihistamines and antiemetics) for half an hour before bedtime.

◆ *Nonprescription pain relievers can help you sleep* more soundly by relieving muscle aches and tension. Many people find that over-the-counter sleeping aids are also highly effective for occasional insomnia.

◆ *Consult the medical team* if your loved one has trouble falling asleep, getting back to sleep, or finds himself waking unusually early more than twice a week. They might recommend trying Benadryl or chloral hydrate. Or a prescription sleeping aid such as Restoril or Halcion may be required to reestablish normal sleeping patterns.

Many times, however, no matter what you do, a sick person's sleep cycle will be disrupted for days or weeks at a time by disease, treatments, and complications. The caregiver's wisest survival strategy then is to adapt her own sleeping schedule to the patient's, grabbing shut-eye whenever the patient does. ▶ See "Tricks for Keeping Your Body Running: Resolve to Rest; Steal Some Sleep," page 248.

Respiratory Complications

Difficulty Breathing (Dyspnea)

Nola Miller: Sometimes Walter simply couldn't catch his breath, especially in the spring. And when he got to where he couldn't breathe, absolute fear would set in, which only made the problem worse.

Causes Include

Pain and weakness following surgery • medications • respiratory infection • chronic obstructive pulmonary disease • impaired ability to expand the chest due to Parkinson's disease, amyotrophic lateral sclerosis, spinal-cord injury • edema of the lungs due to congestive heart failure • radiation therapy to the chest • asthma

There's no more frightening experience than feeling you can't catch your breath, and the sense of panic only compounds the problem. Beyond the psychological terror, however, is the critical need to maintain a steady and adequate supply of oxygen to the brain and other vital organs. The caregiver's tasks are to make the patient as comfortable as possible, to keep the airways clear, and to provide him with additional oxygen when necessary.

Here's What You Can Do

◆ **Elevate your loved one in bed.** Dr. Howard Grossman of St. Luke's-Roosevelt Hospital in New York City advises, "Sit the person up, so that gravity assists the work of breathing." Some patients may be able to sleep only while sitting up in a recliner.

◆ **Medicate for anxiety,** and do whatever you can to help your loved one remain calm. Whenever Dennis Rivera began struggling for breath due to his terminal lung cancer, his fiancée would calm him down by rubbing his back. "I used to cradle his head on my chest or on my stomach and just massage him," Johnetta Romanowski recalls.

◆ **Help keep his airways clear by encouraging him to cough up mucus and saliva,** and by helping remove the thickest secretions with a mechanical suction device. Ask the hospital respiratory therapist or home-care nurse to demonstrate other methods for maintaining open air passages, such as manual chest physiotherapy. ▶ See "Using a Suction Device to Clear the Airway," page 177.

◆ **Ask the medical team about drugs that can ease breathing.** There are *bronchodilators* to open up air passages, *diuretics* to unload excess fluid from the body, *mucolytics* to help expel pulmonary secretions, and *narcotics* to alleviate the worst sensation of suffocation—just to name a few.

◆ **Help allay the sense of panic and air hunger by quietly and calmly coaching your loved one through** *controlled breathing cycles.* Ask the respiratory therapist or home-care nurse to teach you abdominal breathing and pursed-lip breathing techniques.

Administering Supplemental Oxygen

Until the underlying cause of respiratory distress can be reversed, most patients will require a supplemental supply of oxygen. This is most commonly delivered through flexible prongs in each nostril, called a nasal *cannula.* But there are also many other devices, such as *venturi masks,* for delivering specific concentrations of oxygen, and special tubing and attachments to deliver humidified oxygen through a *tracheostomy:* an artificial opening surgically created through the neck and in the trachea (windpipe).

Some patients require oxygen around the clock for the rest of their lives, as with end-stage emphysema or congestive heart failure. Anemic patients depend on supplemental oxygen, too, since they have a shortage of red blood cells that transport oxygen throughout the body. Others require oxygen for only a few minutes each day following an episode of angina, for example, or after a fit of coughing or vomiting that leaves them panting and wheezing.

Patients and their caregivers who will be expected to administer oxygen at home will receive training from the hospital nurses and respiratory therapists prior to discharge, and supervision and emergency assistance later from home-care nurses and technicians. A few rules merit repeating, though:

◆ *Keep flow rates within the range prescribed by the doctor.* When someone can't catch her breath, our first impulse is to turn up the flow rate on the oxygen. But too much oxygen can, ironically, have the opposite effect, dangerously depressing respirations.

◆ *Strictly observe safety precautions.* No smoking within fifty feet of oxygen equipment—whether or not it's in use. Secure tanks firmly to the wall or leave them fastened to the bases they're delivered in. If a tank is dropped or knocked over and the valve breaks off, the cylinder becomes a high-powered projectile. Consider buying or renting an oxygen concentrator. It's portable (even works in the car!), far safer, and less cumbersome than tanks, and cheaper in the long run.

◆ *People breathing supplemental oxygen all day* tend to have dry, cracked sinuses, frequent sore throats, and dry mouth, all prime breeding grounds for infection. Supplemental oxygen should always pass through a humidifier en route to the patient. Humidifiers should never be allowed to run dry, and reservoirs and tubing should be cleaned and sterilized each day according to the nurse's or technician's instructions.

Mechanical Ventilation

Alas, many people are unable to breathe adequately on their own. Head and spinal injuries and strokes, infections of the brain and progressive neurological diseases, heart or kidney failure, and advanced disease of all types can result in an array of conditions in which insufficient oxygen gets to the brain and other vital organs.

Whether breathing stops suddenly, as during a cardiac arrest, or deteriorates gradually with a progressive disease such as emphysema, a tube is inserted into the windpipe and connected to a mechanical ventilator, often called a *respirator.* Ventilators can take over completely for a patient in respiratory failure, controlling the volume, rate, and oxygen concentration of every breath, or they can assist a patient who is still breathing on his own but not able to move enough air by himself. Frequent analysis of arterial blood gases enables the medical team to adjust the respirator precisely to the patient's changing needs.

For someone expected to be dependent on a mechanical ventilator for more than few days, an opening is made surgically into the windpipe, a tracheostomy tube inserted, and the respirator connected there. Even after the patient becomes independent of the ventilator, the "trach" (pronounced "trake") is often left in place and humidified oxygen delivered to it through large-bore plastic tubing.

Intubated patients are at extremely high risk for infections, since a direct path is provided to the fragile membranes of the lungs. Ventilator tubing, humidifiers, and reservoirs must be replaced by sterile ones at least daily. This applies as well to large-bore tubing and connections.

Tracheostomies and oral endotraceal tubes need to be suctioned regularly, and dressings and connections changed daily. Step-by-step trach care initially requires intense training and close supervision by a nurse or respiratory therapist. Family caregivers handily tend to trach patients all the time, but not until mastering the sterile technique explained earlier in this chapter. ◄ *See "Three Steps to Sterile Technique," page 121.* ► *See "Artificial Life Support and Extraordinary Measures," page 294.*

Difficulty Expelling Secretions

Nola Miller: It was so hard for Walter to cough up the sputum that was clogging his airway, especially the last days of his life. He'd been sitting in his recliner chair. When we put him in the hospital bed and he lay back—this was for the first time in months—this thick, ugly garbage just came pouring out of him.

Causes Include

Chronic obstructive pulmonary disease (emphysema) • stroke • amyotrophic lateral sclerosis, multiple sclerosis, and other conditions affecting the muscles and nerves of the chest • pneumonia and other infections of the lungs and upper respiratory tract • pulmonary edema • lung cancer

When sputum in the lungs and upper respiratory tract becomes too thick to cough up, caregivers must constantly assist loved ones in maintaining a clear airway. The same is true for patients who cannot cough efficiently due to weak or uncoordinated muscle contractions in the throat and/or chest, or who are overwhelmed by the sheer volume of secretions.

Here's What You Can Do

◆ ***Position your patient upright,*** at least at a 45-degree angle. "When you're lying flat on your back, you don't ventilate as well, and you accumulate secretions," explains Janelle Fail, a respiratory therapy technician at Springhill Memorial Hospital in Mobile, Alabama. Sitting up also lets gravity aid the work of the diaphragm, easing the effort of breathing and coughing.

◆ ***Keep your loved one well hydrated. Also, consider running a humidifier*** so that membranes and secretions in the lungs stay moist and well lubricated. Be careful not to let the humidity get too high, though. Not only does humid air increase the sensation of difficulty breathing, but as Dr. Norman Edelman, chief of pulmonary medicine at Robert Wood Johnson University Hospital in New Brunswick, New Jersey, reminds us, "it can foster the growth of molds around the house," which further irritate delicate lung tissue.

◆ ***Periodically inhaling an aerosol saline mist*** may help to loosen tenacious secretions. Various drugs can also be delivered through an aerosol spray, or other routes. These include bronchodilators to open air passages, mucolytics and expectorants to thin and lubricate secretions, and steroids to reduce tissue inflammation. Ask the doctor or respiratory therapist to help you develop a regimen tailored to your loved one's individual needs.

◆ ***Drugs such as antihistamines and seasickness patches containing scopolamine*** can help dry up overly runny secretions.

◆ ***Ask the nurse or respiratory therapist to demonstrate mechani-***cal *techniques* for helping move secretions; for example, manual *chest physiotherapy* or *percussion, postural drainage,* and *controlled coughing exercises.*

◆ ***For patients who drool or produce copious secretions*** while sleeping or unconscious, position them on their side to facilitate drainage away from the airway. Hospice nurse Sarah Eilenberg suggests, "Tuck a towel under the person's chin, or tie a washcloth or terry cloth bib around her neck."

Using a Suction Device to Clear the Airway

Choking on secretions can be a horrifying experience, and our keeping the airway clear becomes literally a matter of life and death. End-stage emphysema, pulmonary edema, and progressive neurological diseases present the worst-case scenarios. Caregivers must become adept at suctioning secretions and liquids from the airway, both routinely and in emergencies using a *suction catheter.*

In the hospital there are vacuum lines built into the walls, but at home an electrical pump is used to create a vacuum in a reservoir that can be emptied later. Connective tubing is attached to the reservoir and a sterile, disposable catheter attached each time the patient needs to be suctioned.

A care partner will receive extensive instruction and supervision before being sent home with a patient who requires frequent suctioning. But sometimes folks who need it are discharged without an order for suction equipment, and it falls to the caregiver to act as advocate with the doctor and home-care agency long before emergencies arise. The most crucial rule to remember is to never suction for more than ten seconds at a time, because when you aspirate secretions, you are also sucking oxygen out of the airway. "The proper technique," says Janelle Fail, "is to let them take a couple of breaths, then suction, then let them oxygenate again before suctioning once more." ◄ *See "Administering Supplemental Oxygen," page 175.* ► *See "The Heimlich Maneuver," page 182.*

✱ *Suction catheters are useful only for clearing liquids from the airways. If a loved one is choking on solid matter such as food, administer the Heimlich maneuver.*

Chronic Coughing

Nola Miller: *Sometimes Walter would cough so hard that he'd pass out.*

Causes Include

Emphysema and chronic bronchitis • infections of the lung, such as pneumonia and tuberculosis • excess fluid in the lungs (pulmonary edema and congestive heart failure) • upper respiratory tract infections • radiation to the throat, chest, breast, or lungs

While coughing is essential for clearing the airway, unrelenting coughing can lead to loss of sleep, stress incontinence, a collapsed lung, and render eating impossible. Long fits of coughing can also send heart rates soaring dangerously high, and leave patients gasping for breath.

Here's What You Can Do

◆ *A cough that persists for more than two days* should be called to the attention of the medical team. Also report to the nurse or doctor immediately when someone with a cough spikes a temperature. Antibiotics may need to be ordered and other causes of the cough investigated.

◆ *Make sure your loved one's airway is clear;* help him eliminate secretions such as mucus using the tips listed above, or by using a mechanical suction device.

◆ *Eliminate dust, pollen, and other respiratory irritants* by frequent vacuuming, and change filters in the heating and air-conditioning systems often.

◆ *Ask the doctor about prescribing a cough suppressant,* especially for bedtime. Narcotics used for pain management, most notably codeine, also have an antitussive property.

◆ *Most people don't appreciate how painful a chronic, hacking cough can be.* Folks with brittle bones have even been known to break ribs. Chest and abdominal muscles become very sore and guarded. Aspirin, acetaminophen, or ibuprofen helps relieve the pain. Splinting the sore muscles by holding a pillow or cushion firmly across the abdomen while coughing also helps. Ask a nurse or respiratory therapist to demonstrate this for you.

Circulatory Complications

Edema, Blood Clots, Phlebitis, Orthostatic Hypotension

Betty Lindstrom: *Clarence started to get terrible phlebitis. Every morning I used to exercise and massage his arms, legs, and calves, which made him feel so much better.*

Causes Include

Prolonged bed rest and immobility • congestive heart failure • kidney failure • chemotherapy • various common medications

Lying in bed for extended periods of time can cause fluid to build up in body tissue, particularly in the legs and feet. This is called *peripheral edema* (or *dependent edema*), and it can lead to the breakdown of the blood vessels in the swollen area *(phlebitis).* "Thrombophlebitis is a serious problem," observes Dr. Fletcher McDowell, "because the clots that form in the vein in the leg can break off and move on to block circulation in the lungs." The resulting *pulmonary embolism* can be fatal.

Congestive heart failure and poor kidney function can also cause fluid to accumulate in the bloodstream and in the spaces between tissue cells. When this happens in the cavity separating the two-layer membrane that encases the lungs (the *pleura*), it is called *pleural effusion*. Immobility and weakness can also cause the blood flow to the lower extremities to respond sluggishly, setting the stage for a blood clot to form in a deep vein, and making the heart slow to respond to changes in position or levels of activity.

Orthostatic hypotension is a sudden drop in blood pressure that occurs when rising quickly from a lying or sitting position. The blood pools in the lower extremities instead of making its way back to the heart. Patients can feel dizzy, disoriented, and have blurry vision, which of course can lead to a serious fall.

Medications that treat circulatory problems include diuretics such as Lasix (furosemide) to rid the body of excess fluid, and the anticoagulants Coumadin (warfarin) and heparin to thin the blood and prevent clot formation.

Here's What You Can Do

♦ **Keep the patient's legs elevated** whenever sitting or lying down. Dr. Donald Leslie of the Shepherd Spinal Center in Atlanta recommends keeping the feet "four or five inches above the level of the heart." Similarly, if you notice that a loved one's arm appears swollen, place a pillow under it.

♦ **Those prone to orthostatic hypotension should keep their heads elevated** when sleeping or lying down. They should take care to always rise slowly, and to sit or lie back if they become suddenly dizzy. Hot showers can also trigger sudden drops in blood pressure in people with sluggish circulation.

♦ **Reposition the person in bed every hour.** This not only improves circulation but also serves to prevent pressure ulcers. ◄ See "*How to Prevent Pressure Ulcers*," *page 118.*

♦ **Keep skin clean and well moisturized.** Poor circulation makes wounds heal more slowly, culminating in infections. ◄ See "*Skin Care*," *page 116.*

♦ **Encourage your loved one to stay as physically active as possible, or help her to exercise in bed.** Assist the bed-bound with basic range-of-motion exercises and gentle stretching several times a day. Ask a physical therapist or home-care nurse to demonstrate. ◄ See "*How to Perform Passive Range-of-Motion Exercises*," *page 136.*

♦ **Elastic support hose, also known as antiembolism stockings,** are good for preventing clot formation in the lower legs. Anyone confined to bed for more than a few days, or with a history of clotting disorders, should wear antiembolism hose at all times. Ask the nurse to demonstrate how to put them on, taking care that the elastic bands at the top do not impede circulation in the leg.

♦ **Restrict the intake of dietary sodium** (salt), which makes the body retain fluid. Avoiding large meals and eating smaller, more frequent meals can also help to minimize episodes of hypotension.

Bleeding and Bruising

Anticoagulants, as well as other common drugs, can inhibit the blood from clotting normally, leading to easy bleeding and bruising. Chemotherapy, too, frequently causes the same problem, by diminishing the number of blood platelets, the cells that initiate clotting. Other symptoms of clotting disorders include frequent nosebleeds; vomiting blood or coffee-ground-like material; pink or red streaks in sputum, urine, or stools; and tiny red or purple spots or blood blisters on the skin or in the mouth.

♦ **Report any episodes of unusual bruising or bleeding** to the medical team. They'll need to figure out what's causing the clotting disorder, whether medications or disease, and change course accordingly.

♦ **To control local bleeding, gently press a gauze pad against the site until the bleeding stops.** Squeezing a bleeding nose shut while tilting the head back and applying an ice pack to the face usually works.

♦ **Ice packs slow bleeding and reduce bruising.** Be careful using ice on swollen extremities with sluggish circulation, though. Make sure there's plenty of blood flow to the foot by pressing on a nail bed and releasing it quickly. If it turns pink right away, there's adequate blood flow, and it's safe to use ice for a few minutes.

♦ **Consult with the doctor or nurse before dispensing aspirin or products containing aspirin** like Alka-Seltzer or Excedrin. Instead, use Tylenol, aspirin-free Excedrin, or other acetaminophen pain relievers.

♦ **The patient should use soft-bristle toothbrushes,** and avoid flossing if it makes the gums bleed excessively. Rinse regularly with a solution of equal parts water and hydrogen peroxide.

Basic First Aid

Managing Seizures and Convulsions

Seizures occur when disease or injury scrambles the electrical signals from the brain, causing muscles to contract throughout the body in an uncoordinated manner. Seizures can range from the *petit mal*, which includes twitching of the hands, face, or an extremity, to the *grand mal* seizure, or full convulsion, in which the body flails violently, risking injury to the patient.

Seizures are usually more frightening to the caregiver than they are dangerous to the patient. While it's imperative that the medical team quickly investigates and corrects the cause of seizures, there's little to do to control a seizure while it's happening. A few precautions though:

♦ **Report fevers of greater than 101 °F to the medical team.** To lower the fever until the medical team advises you what to do, administer aspirin or Tylenol and wipe down your loved one with cool water or alcohol. Call 911 if someone with a temperature goes into convulsions.

♦ **Do not try to catch someone who is falling!** You'll both get hurt. Instead guide his head away from walls or furniture, and prevent it from striking the floor. If your patient is in bed, make sure the rails are up so that he doesn't fall to the floor.

♦ **When someone is having a seizure, roll her onto her side** so that vomit and secretions are not aspirated into the lungs. Use a suction device to clear the airway, if necessary. Loosen collars, ties, and other clothing to make sure they do not constrict the throat. ◄ See *"Using a Suction Device to Clear the Airway," page 177.*

♦ **Do not attempt to place anything inside the mouth during the seizure.** In the past, the conventional wisdom called for putting a tongue depressor wrapped in gauze in patients' mouths to prevent them from biting their tongues. "We've stopped using 'bite blades,'" explains hospice nurse Jane Pilecki. "For one thing, once the seizure starts, you usually can't get it in. But, second, sometimes the people inserting the depressor would inadvertently push back the patient's tongue. Nowadays, the general tendency is to discourage the use of bite blades; if the patient bites his tongue, he bites his tongue."

◆ **Do not struggle to restrain someone in the midst of a seizure.** Instead protect her from injury by placing something soft under her head and by gently steering her hands, elbows, feet, and knees away from solid objects that might cause injury.

◆ **Seizure-controlling medications,** such as phenobarbital (Donnatal, Quadrinal, among others), may be prescribed for frequent convulsions.

Cardiopulmonary Resuscitation (CPR)

When someone stops breathing or his heart stops—and one always quickly follows the other—permanent brain damage or death will result if breathing and circulation are not immediately restored. There is no time to wait for the ambulance. Nor will there be any chance of saving the person if the brain and heart go much longer than two or three minutes without sufficient oxygen.

People have all sorts of misconceptions about CPR because actors on TV do it all wrong, pounding the chest with their fists, or what have you. CPR is so simple and straightforward that Girl Scouts and Boy Scouts learn and use it every day. It's truly simple enough for a child to learn, if she's physically large enough for the work.

The best way to learn CPR is by signing up for a course at your local chapter of the American Red Cross. There's no substitute for good training and plenty of experience (if only on the resuscidoll) when someone you love is literally depending on you for every breath and every heartbeat. A few key reminders about basic CPR:

◆ **When someone loses consciousness suddenly or appears to stop breathing, call for help immediately** while checking for a pulse and checking to see whether she's breathing. ◄ *See "How to Take a Pulse," page 139; "How to Monitor Respirations," page 141.*

◆ **Remember the ABC's of CPR:** Airway, Breathing, Circulation. Those are the only things to concentrate on: making sure that air is moving in and out of the lungs, and that oxygenated blood is moving from the lungs to the brain.

CPR, Step-by-Step

If your patient is not breathing, or is breathing so shallowly that you cannot detect whether or not she's breathing:

1. Position her on her back on a firm surface (the floor is best), and tilt her head back to extend the airway open.
2. Use your fingers to clear any food, vomit, or secretions out of her mouth and airway.
3. Pinch her nose closed, take a breath, and cover her mouth with yours.
4. Exhale into her mouth, keeping your mouth sealed around hers to prevent air from escaping. Notice the chest rise as you force air into the lungs. Do this two times in a row.
5. Then check again for a pulse in the neck and for signs of spontaneous breathing.
6. If there is no pulse, initiate chest compressions: Kneeling beside the patient, place the heel of one hand directly over the lower half of the breastbone, and the other hand on top of it. Lock your elbows out straight and, bending from the waist, compress the chest firmly about one and a half to two inches. Repeatedly squeezing the heart muscle between the breastbone or sternum and the

spinal column is what forces blood to circulate. Keep pace by counting out loud, "One and two and three and . . ."

7. Alternate two big breaths with fifteen chest compressions until help arrives, or until the patient resumes breathing and a pulse on her own. It is much easier to perform CPR with two people: One of you gives a breath for every five chest compressions, which is closer to normal rates. If you attempt the one-to-five rhythm solo, though, you'll faint or collapse in short order.

8. Do not initiate CPR on someone who is imminently terminal, or allow someone to be resuscitated when she has expressed her wishes to the contrary. It's one thing to know how to save a loved one during a life-threatening emergency, and another thing altogether to subject her to needless suffering. One of the greatest gifts we can give a dying loved one is to resist the impulse to interfere when death is at hand. ► *See "Artificial Life Support and Extraordinary Measures," page 294;* ► *Appendix B: "CPR (Cardiopulmonary Resuscitation)," page 506.*

The Heimlich Maneuver

If you've never read the poster on restaurant walls, the Heimlich maneuver is a life-saving technique used to dislodge foreign matter from the windpipe. People choking on food or other material are unable to speak, and it falls to the caregiver to recognize when someone is in trouble.

If a choking person is conscious, he usually coughs violently, grabs at his throat, and makes loud, desperate wheezing noises as air is forced past the obstruction under high pressure. If he has lost consciousness due to insufficient oxygen getting to the brain, the only way you'll know that something is stuck in the throat is the fact that the skin turns an eerie blue color, and you're unable to force air into the lungs when you try mouth-to-mouth resuscitation.

The Heimlich Maneuver, Step-by-Step

The Heimlich maneuver is administered with the victim sitting up or standing.

1. Grasp him from behind around the waist. Make a fist with one hand and position the thumb side on the victim's abdomen, halfway between the belly button and the rib cage.

2. Grab the fist with your other hand and thrust forcefully inward and upward. Do this repeatedly, using separate, distinct thrusts each time.

3. If the patient is unconscious, lay him on his back on the floor and straddle him on your knees.

4. Place the heel of one hand against the abdomen halfway between the navel and the ribs, lock the elbows, as with CPR, and thrust upward and inward to try to dislodge the obstruction.

❋ *If the victim is obese or pregnant, multiple thrusts can be applied to the breastbone, or sternum, with the victim sitting, standing, or lying down.*

Choking is a life-and-death emergency that allows no time for hesitation. Use your fingers to aggressively reach down the victim's throat to clear out whatever blockage you can reach. Vigorously pound him on the back with a cupped hand as you would a choking child. Stand behind him and administer the Heimlich maneuver athletically. Your loved one may be sore afterward, but a few bad bruises is a small price to pay to avoid suffocation.

When Should You Call an Ambulance?

As we discuss in chapter 10, "Journey's End," one of the greatest gifts we can give someone expected to die in the next several days or weeks is to restrain the normal urge to dial 911 in the face of a life-threatening medical emergency. However, if we haven't reached that point and have reason to believe our loved one can survive the immediate crisis, each of the circumstances below warrants a trip to the hospital.

Should a severe or unfamiliar symptom crop up suddenly, don't delay in summoning professional help. *Assume the worst.* The chest pain your loved one is complaining about may be nothing more serious than heartburn; in someone with a history of atherosclerosis or blood clotting, it could very well signal an impending heart attack. How quickly medical intervention is begun will influence the outcome enormously.

Sure signs that your loved one needs immediate medical assistance include:

- Unusual difficulty catching one's breath, or breathing has stopped entirely
- Extremely weak or rapid pulse, or no pulse
- Dangerously low or elevated blood pressure
- Fever that exceeds 102 degrees for twenty-four hours
- Worsening chest pain, particularly if accompanied by labored breathing and/or clammy, blue-tinged skin
- Unconsciousness, sudden delirium, or disorientation
- Partial or full paralysis in one or more areas of the body, or a marked decline in motor skills, speech, vision
- Convulsions in a patient who never has suffered seizures before
- Severe allergic reaction to food or medication, the symptoms of which can progress from relatively mild (itching, swelling, hives) to potentially fatal (plummeting blood pressure, abnormally rapid heart rate, difficulty breathing due to airway constriction) ◄ *See "Allergic Reactions and Anaphylactic Shock," page 151.*
- Airway obstruction, due to an allergic reaction or solid matter lodged in the throat ◄ *See "The Heimlich Maneuver," page 182.*
- Cuts, burns, bleeding, fractures, sprains, falls, and any other injuries requiring immediate medical treatment.
- Signs of internal hemorrhaging:
  1. copious amounts of bright red blood in vomit or stool
  2. abdomen hard and distended
  3. profuse perspiration, rapid pulse, and cold, wet skin

Merely straining to pass a large, hard stool can ulcerate the anal canal, leaving the toilet brimming with bright red blood. Pretty scary stuff, but hardly grounds for dialing 911. Call the doctor. A number of conditions that are in no way life threatening can produce an alarming amount of bleeding from the stomach or the intestines. But here the bleeding is usually chronic. The characteristics of internal hemorrhaging are uncontrolled bursts of fresh blood that come on suddenly. Seeing blood in the urine also tends to send patients and care partners into a panic. It, too, is a symptom common to many diseases, and a side effect of certain chemotherapy agents, as well as other medications. Again, call this to the physician's attention. But EMS? No.

Whom Do You Call?

When symptoms come on rapidly, or you can't determine how serious the person's condition is: Call the local emergency number, with the understanding that Emergency Medical Services policies around the country usually require their ambulances to deliver patients to the nearest hospital— one where your loved one's primary doctor might not have privileges. In this instance, an emergency room physician assumes the role of attending doctor temporarily, and if the person has to be admitted as an inpatient, a house staff physician will oversee his care. We always feel most confident when a doctor comes recommended by a physician we trust. Call your patient's regular doctor from the hospital; perhaps he can refer you to a colleague who practices there.

* *If 911 (or whatever the local emergency number may be) is busy or does not answer, phone the fire department or the local police precinct and state, "I have a medical emergency."*

When symptoms seem to come on slowly: Call the doctor, who will direct you to a hospital. She'll either meet you in the emergency room or phone ahead to alert the ER staff or house staff M.D. you're on your way. If no one can drive the patient, use a private ambulance service. Hopefully you've thought ahead and already asked your doctor to recommend a reliable company. Unlike EMS, these vehicles will transport a patient to his local hospital of choice, so long as the patient is not in any immediate danger.

* *Wait up to two hours for the doctor's callback, unless your loved one's condition appears to worsen. If that's the case, use 911.*

Personal Emergency Response Systems

For a loved one who is healthy enough to continue living by himself, it is advisable to invest in a personal emergency response system. A fall could leave a person lying helplessly on the floor, unable to reach a telephone for hours. The American Red Cross, in partnership with a Massachusetts company called Lifeline Systems, offers an emergency-response service for $35 or $45 a month, plus a one-time $50 connection charge. Patients wear a lightweight pendant or wristband bearing a waterproof button, which they press in the event of an emergency any time of day. A communicator device transmits a signal to a Lifeline operator, who speaks to the patient over the device's two-way speaker phone and promptly summons assistance.

Injury from falls is the fifth leading cause of death in the elderly. Another benefit of Lifeline is that the communicator enables users to access incoming phone calls from across the room, so that they don't have to get up and answer the phone every time it rings.

At the very least, an ill person living alone should be wearing a Medic Alert bracelet or necklace. The engraved emblem apprises paramedics of a patient's medical conditions, medications, and any drug allergies. EMS personnel can call a twenty-four-hour Medic Alert hot line for further details from the person's confidential computerized record, including her physician, pharmacist, emergency contacts, and whether she has executed an advance directive pertaining to life support. The basic stainless-steel emblem costs $35 and can be updated anytime by phone or mail for a $7 fee.

☎ American Red Cross Lifeline, 800-959-6989

☎ Medic Alert, 800-432-5378

☎ The National Kidney Foundation issues Medic Alert jewelry and cards free to kidney patients. For more information, call the NKF at 800-622-9010.

—4—

Matters of the Heart

Confidence in your proficiency as a nurse frees you to focus on the most essential skill of all: tending to your loved one's emotional needs. For some caregivers this poses their most formidable challenge. This chapter will help you speak from the heart and listen empathetically, skills that all of us need brushing up on from time to time. If you tend to shy away from emotional intensity and intimacy, you owe it to your loved one, as well as yourself, to work at overcoming barriers to communication. Doing so will enrich your relationship not only with that person but with others in your life. I know many men and women who say the experience of caring for an ailing loved one transformed them, awakening a caring, compassionate side they had come to neglect or never realized they possessed.

The So-Called Five Stages of Coping

Most of us have heard of the five stages of coping made famous by the legendary hospice pioneer Dr. Elisabeth Kübler-Ross through her best-selling books and public appearances: *denial, anger, bargaining, depression,* and *acceptance.* These common and highly effective adaptations to fear and loss provide extremely useful landmarks for anyone trying to understand what a sick person is thinking and feeling. One popular misconception among novice caregivers, however, is that sick folks progress neatly through each stage in discrete phases and in a predictable sequence. Nothing could be further from the truth.

People with a life-threatening illness are prone to a complex array of powerful emotions and intrusive thoughts that overlap and change daily—even hourly —with their circumstances. The young

VOICE OF EXPERIENCE

"My daughter acted as if her hepatitis was no big deal. It was very hard for me to go along with that and not show her how scared I was. But you have to do that, because you don't want them *to become scared."—Naomi Black*

mother recently diagnosed with breast cancer might be deeply depressed following surgery and chemotherapy. During a period of uninterrupted good health, she goes about life as though nothing were wrong, only to find herself enraged upon learning that her tumor markers are alarmingly elevated at the next doctor's visit. Others, however are spared this hellish roller-coaster ride, progressing through an illness with remarkable equanimity.

Caregivers are just as susceptible as patients to these wide-ranging reactions. When someone we love might be dying, it's only human to act out our own versions of denial, anger, bargaining, depression, and acceptance. While you're comforting a sick person, it's important to keep in mind that the two of you might not be on the same page that day. Just because you are projecting great hope and resolve this week, don't assume that Mom isn't feeling bitterly angry right now. Conversely, once you've finally accepted that a loved one's death is inevitable, don't be surprised to find him talking excitedly about a new treatment the next morning. Further clouding the mix is the fact that thoughts, feelings, and behavior don't always operate in agreement.

Learning to listen carefully and compassionately, and building honesty with ourselves and empathy with the patient's situation are essential skills if you're going to be able to stay with your loved one through all this turmoil.

Denial

Most of us think of denial in terms of the desperately deluded terminal patient who acts as if nothing is wrong or seems convinced that he and he alone

will be the first ever to beat his disease through some yet unproven treatment. In fact, denial is a miraculous trick our subconscious brain plays to protect us from overwhelming fear and the initially unbearable pain of profound loss until we can mobilize all our other defenses and adjust to bad news.

What's more, a reasonable amount of denial is precisely what enables all of us, sick or not, to get through each day. If we woke up every morning thinking *I'm going to die*, even getting out of bed would seem pointless. Instead, we push intensely uncomfortable thoughts and feelings to the back of our minds just long enough to be able to get about the daily business of life. It's even more important that sick people be given latitude to set aside their worst fears temporarily, through what's called *adaptive denial*.

When to Question Denial

Over the years I've known too many men and women who postponed follow-up biopsies or stopped taking critical medications when they started feeling better. I've watched otherwise rational people, frustrated with their progress on standard treatments, turn their backs on Western medicine entirely, opting for fad diets, new-age gurus, or quack "cures" rather than acknowledge a dire situation. I've seen grieving children land in foster care because a dying parent had failed to make appropriate arrangements.

When a person's denial threatens to cause him or someone else irreparable harm, it's time for us to speak up, preferably *before* it's too late to solve the most pressing problems. Rather than refute a sick person's beliefs directly, we encourage him to ponder the practical implications of his actions or failure to take action. The most effective way to do this is to ask open-ended questions: "So, how do you see the next few months going?"

My friend George Kingsley had been running a fever and losing weight for months. Fearing he had AIDS, he avoided going to the doctor. George threw himself into work as if he were fine when in fact he felt terrible and was literally killing himself trying to keep up. He might well have improved his prognosis at the time by taking drugs to prevent deadly infections.

When George finally got under the care of a good doctor and was feeling less fragile, I asked him, "What if all this doesn't go well, George?" Such discussions not only allowed the two of us some deeply intimate exchanges but also prompted him to write a will, execute a medical power of attorney, speak more frankly and assertively with his medical team and his employer, and start talking with other friends and his family about assisting in his care. Even toward the end when George signed out of the hospital in the middle of the night, slightly demented and convinced he didn't need to be there, I helped steer him back on track simply by asking, "So, George, what happens now?" The mere act of contemplating the immediate, practical consequences of leaving the hospital diffused the denial that was preventing him from getting the level of nursing care he needed.

Sometimes we're forced to accept the fact that a loved one will die in deep denial, in which case we must set aside our ideas about how others "ought" to die and remind ourselves that everyone dies *in his or her own way.* Try to anticipate the worst consequences and prepare the survivors for the fallout. If your constant reassurances and most thoughtful attempts to help a sick person face a bad situation fail, let it go. Wait for him to come around on his own, or try again later. What he's telling you is that he cannot deal with the circumstances any other way right now. The progression of disease can usually be depended on to yank a patient ruthlessly back into reality. Hammering away at denial out of our own frustration only renders a loved one defenseless and terrified.

So when your ailing loved one says "I just know I'm going to beat this!," in your own words say "I'm going to be by your side every step of the way."

Anger

Anger is a normal, *healthy* reaction to any perceived threat. Part of this is man's instinctive biological response to danger. More insidious, however, is the infuriating relentlessness with which disease robs a sick person of control: over her body, her mind, her emotions, her time. Beneath the helplessness and frustration, a profound sense of personal loss can lead to bitterness or rage.

"My husband was furious about his lung cancer and dying," recalls Audree Siden. "He'd say, 'I'm only forty-seven years old! What the hell is going on here?' Ron was outraged over the complete loss of control over his life, plus his business had gone bankrupt—he was a mess. He was on steroids and bloated, he would cough and cough and cough, and then the oxygen tanks . . . He didn't want his parents in from Chicago; he didn't want people seeing him in this deteriorated state. He was embarrassed and humiliated, *and* he was dreadfully depressed." The morning Ron Siden died, in New York's Mount Sinai Medical Center, "he smashed the hospital tray with his hand and wrote to me on a napkin, *What's happening?*"

Caregivers are frequently knocked off kilter when an ailing parent, spouse, or sibling lashes out with uncharacteristic venom. Dr. Donald Leslie, medical director of the Shepherd Spinal Center in Atlanta, observes, "Patients can get very demanding. Because they've lost so much control, they try to control other people, and that oftentimes causes real conflict within families."

Dealing with a
Loved One's Anger

Very few people handle anger calmly and thoughtfully, whether their own or someone else's. Most of us simply stifle the emotion until the indignation becomes unbearable. Then we explode, often saying things we don't mean or behaving in ways that unfairly punish those closest to us. It's no different for sick folks; if anything, it's much worse. The balance of power is forever tilted against them. The caregiver's two main tasks, then, are to help a loved one find effective outlets for righteous rage and to learn how to cope with unreasonable outbursts.

Listen carefully to what he's saying. Even though his angry behavior might seem inordinate, often a sick person has been provoked by something we can fix: The doctor ignored a specific request. A closely guarded secret was betrayed. Someone made a thoughtless remark.

Hear him out until he's finished venting, then encourage him to tell the transgressor exactly what he thinks. Offer to set things right yourself. If you're partially to blame, own up to it. You might say, "You're right. I'm sorry. I'll never let that happen again." Then see to it that you keep your promise.

Encourage appropriate expressions of anger. Sometimes all a person needs is an empathetic ear. Let him have his say without always feeling compelled to try to make the situation better right then. Conversely, some people are overwhelmed by the intensity of their emotions and are profoundly reluctant to express the real depths of their frustration. By suppressing their anger, they risk turning it on themselves by giving up or by shutting out the people they need.

Give them "permission" by telling them how *you* feel: "I'm amazed you've held your tongue this long. I'd be furious if that happened to me." Peer support groups are also an especially useful means for getting a patient to unload. ◀ *See "National Support Groups," page 34.*

Never tell a sick person how she "ought" to feel. Sometimes we're so uncomfortable ourselves in the face of unbridled anger that we inadvertently minimize what a loved one is telling us: "I wouldn't let that bother me" or "You shouldn't let him get to you" or "What's done is done." Such statements telegraph to a frustrated person that we're not listening, that what she feels is unimportant. Simply listen quietly or say "I can see how that would make you mad."

Be a safe target. One reason patients lash out at loved ones may be that they know their behavior won't drive us away. Subconsciously, they might even be testing our staying power. Johnetta Romanowski's fiancé, a cancer patient, "would go through bouts where *nothing* I did was right," she says. "You have to understand where the anger comes from. He was angry at the situation. I think you just have to ride it out and not get angry in return—which," she admits, "was very hard for me to do."

Be efficient. It's easy to understand why a sick person becomes impossibly impatient. Sometimes, no matter how fast you're working, it isn't enough to please them. "Would you hurry up!" or "Now look what you've done!" can rattle even the most experienced caregiver. Stoic efficiency on your part will always see you through, at least for the time being. Think through the steps of the tasks at hand, take a slow, deep breath, then get done quickly. The best nurses in the world go about their business with stony aplomb, especially in the face of gratuitous abuse. Take a lesson.

Enforce appropriate boundaries. Protect yourself. Because we are a safe target, angry patients can become shockingly abusive. Behind your back and to your face they criticize you and others, hurling personal invective and cruel recriminations. People curse, throw things, even deliberately soil themselves, just to name a few of the most taxing antics. Obviously, you won't be able to care for them very long if your own physical and mental health are at risk.

In your most even voice, tell them when they've gone too far, then walk away until everyone calms down, as Nola Miller did when her husband, Walter, "got a little strong-armed. It was out of sheer frustration. I just said to him, 'I have been good to you, and I am going to continue to be good to you, but you are *not* going to behave that way.' "

Don't take it personally. Get off the defensive. With the loss of inhibition that comes with frayed nerves, mood-altering medications, or progressive dementia, sick people can dish out some choice insults. Sometimes it becomes extremely difficult to figure out how much of the deep-seated hostility is symptomatic of the disease and how much is genuine. While it may be difficult to dismiss the hurt, arguing with them is pointless. You can't win with logic, and often you'll only agitate them further. To the extent that you can, distract them for the moment or absent yourself until everyone can cool off. Most important, find a place to vent your own pain, frustration, and resentment before you start taking it out on loved ones or yourself. Seek solace with a friend, family member, minister, or support group.

Recognize the subtle signs of anger. When Bob got home following his heart surgery, wasted and gaunt from months of illness, getting him to eat was a constant challenge. After weeks of my slavish catering to Pop's pickiest culinary whim, one evening a visitor presented him with a greasy casserole. As my father proceeded to wolf down a heaping portion, he enthused, "Damn, that's good! I haven't had a decent meal in a week." His old friend wagged a finger at me and admonished, "You need to feed your daddy, boy! He's losing weight!"

I wanted to scream, but I held my tongue, realizing just then how frustrated and desperate Pop must have been feeling. His ongoing dependence on me probably rankled him. I did, however, take some perverse satisfaction in the knowledge that five minutes after the company left, Bob would throw it all up. Which he did.

Passive-aggressive behavior can test a caregiver's stamina worse than the most histrionic shouting matches. Excessive dependence, needling remarks, indecision, forgetfulness, ignoring doctors' orders, and chronically overextending themselves are just a few of the nerve-racking tricks at the disposal of sick people, who are not always conscious that they're angry about something. Encourage them to directly express whatever's bugging them by calmly stating how *you* feel. Choose a quiet moment later and confide, "You know, when you do that, it makes me feel _____. You hurt my feelings when you said _____."

Aggressively medicate anxiety, sleep disturbance, pain, and depression. All of us have short fuses when we're feeling lousy. Sleep deprivation and pain—even minor, nagging pain—quickly render even the hardiest folks irritable. A short temper is often the first sign of inadequately managed anxiety and incipient depression, too. Rarely do sick people consciously choose to feel miserable. *These are medical symptoms that can be treated.* Talk it over with your patient and his doctor, and get the right meds on board before things get worse. ◀ *See chapter 3, "The Everyday Angel's Cram Course in Essential Nursing Skills."*

Bargaining

Bargaining is another brilliant maneuver the subconscious mind employs to protect us from the full brunt of traumatic news. Sick people buy emotional breathing room precisely by setting goals for themselves and by making promises—often unspoken—to God and loved ones. Occupying time and energy with unfinished business fends off their worst fantasies about the future, even for months at a time. Not only does this delay the most intense feelings of impending loss, but for many it provides a reason to live.

When Diane Desiderio was first diagnosed with liver cancer several years ago, she reacted with an almost comic obsession over work. Diane is an ace microbiologist at Bellevue Hospital Center in New York, the people to whom infectious disease specialists always turn to identify a rare bug or to figure out the best combination of drugs to kill a new resistant strain. At the time of her biopsy, her own lab was in the middle of several large-scale experiments that had taken years to prepare. I'm sure she does not believe that her life has been extended because she kept a promise to publish the results herself, but having a specific objective definitely enabled her to face years of treatment and partial disability with far greater resolve.

Caregivers make bargains, too. Through the long ordeal of Uncle Billy's Alzheimer's disease, my aunt Kitty set aside worries about her own precarious health by promising God each evening at mass, "I'll faithfully care for Billy every day until he dies if You'll just keep *me* well until then." To some it might sound medically irrational, but her oath to that celestial pact was all that got her through the worst days.

Rules of the Bargaining Table

Bargains cause problems only when folks have made commitments they can't keep. Just as denial can masquerade as false hope, unrealistic goals can cloud medical judgment, place unnecessary strain on loved ones, and set the stage for bitter disappointment at the end of life.

I've known dozens of people with cancer who threw themselves into a newfound "healthy" lifestyle when they were first diagnosed. With the passion of a religious convert, they vowed celibacy; stopped smoking and drinking and staying up all night; started obsessively exercising, meditating, and attending church; and radically altered their eating habits with complicated diets. There's certainly no harm in cleaning up your act, but a few of them also postponed surgery or delayed starting chemotherapy and grew much, much sicker.

As with denial, direct confrontation doesn't usually work and might even leave your loved one despondent. Anyway, the progression of an illness will ultimately dictate which business actually gets finished and which goes undone—with or without our meddling. The caregiver's job becomes helping sick folks fulfill realistic commitments and consoling them in the face of grave disappointment.

Help him achieve his goals. Encourage your loved one to tackle whatever objectives he tells you are important to him. A sick person who's engaged in meaningful day-to-day activity has little need for pie-in-the-sky rationalizations. Undertaking new projects, doing good deeds or plotting revenge, social obligations, pilgrimages—just about any activity is preferable to the grim pastime of lying around waiting to die.

Suggest he set his sights on short-term goals. Most often disease gradually erodes a sick person's psychic and physical energy. He naturally adapts over time by lowering his expectations little by little. Sometimes, though, as when health takes an unexpected turn for the worse, the guilt and shame of broken deals and unkept promises can catch a person off guard. We can buffer the immediate impact in a sudden crisis by setting new goals temporarily. Statements like "Let's just make it through today" or "Let's just concentrate on getting you home from the hospital" can make a bad situation seem much more manageable for the moment. Propose one simple goal you can reliably achieve right then.

Make promises you *can keep.* Sometimes, no matter how carefully we try to keep unrealistic expectations in check, disappointments are inevitable. When a sick person is feeling disillusioned, listen quietly as she catalogs her regrets —and resist the impulse to try to cheer her up. Remind her of the things she *can* depend on: "I'll stand up for you at Johnny's wedding." "I'll look out for the kids if anything happens to you."

Arguing with seemingly irrational promises only further strips a sick person of defenses. On the other hand, if all the wheeling and dealing becomes an excuse to ignore medical advice or pressing responsibilities, we gently step in.

Depression

It's amazing how many families and medical professionals are more than willing to confront denial, anger, and bargaining, yet stand by helplessly in the face of obvious depression. You can probably chalk this up to the value that our culture places on maintaining a stiff upper lip, but I can't tell you how often otherwise conscientious caregivers drop the ball when someone is clearly in deep psychic pain. Most of the time we either put on a brave front and say nothing, or, worse, act as sadistic cheerleaders—as though our loved one could choose not to feel so awful.

To understand some of the confusion about clinical depression (defined as depression that produces plainly visible symptoms), it helps to divide it into two types: *reactive* depression and *major* depression.

Reactive depression includes all the normal feelings of sadness associated with bad news. Whether the source is illness, divorce, losing one's job, or any other situation that threatens plans for the future, people get the blues and lose confidence and motivation—the basic emotional tools needed to get through a very tough time. Although reactive depression can go on to cause severe psychological and physical problems requiring treatment, this dark cloud lifts when the circumstances improve.

When major depression is left untreated, its grip only tightens. People shut down completely or become utterly inconsolable. They lose all interest in life and develop all sorts of serious medical complications.

In an all-too-common scenario, family members will observe an ailing loved one clearly mired in depression. But rather than report this to the doctor, they assume the patient is merely "down in the dumps" over his situation. Who wouldn't be? According to Dr. Mary Jane Massie, when she began practicing psychiatry at New York's Memorial Sloan-Kettering Cancer Center in 1977, "That was one of the many myths we heard about people with cancer and depressive illness: 'Everybody with cancer is depressed'; 'Lord knows *I'd* be depressed if I had cancer'—or you can substitute any other severe illness.

"What we know now," she continues, "is that depression is an illness," one that often has such organic roots as

- chemical changes in the body, which can exacerbate the predictably sad feelings that come with failing health;
- metabolic imbalances triggered by disease or treatment;
- kidney failure, stroke, brain tumors, severe head injury, certain thyroid conditions, AIDS dementia, Alzheimer's disease, cancer, Parkinson's

disease—which disrupt a body's fragile molecular biology.

Many commonly prescribed drugs, too, can bring on severe depression, mood swings, and changes in personality. Culprits include blood pressure medications, some antibiotics, many heart drugs, sleeping pills, tranquilizers, narcotics, chemotherapy agents, hormones, and steroids.

Naomi Black: To help Nancy's liver heal, the doctors put her on prednisone [a widely prescribed steroid], which has many not-so-wonderful side effects, like mood swings. You're happy, then you're crabby. My daughter could be very ornery and get very upset with the family. I think that probably affected us more than anything else we ever went through with her. For two or three days she'd be fine, then there'd be three or four days of emotional outbursts. Then she would be fine again for a few days.

Being depressed is not only psychologically debilitating, but it can make sick folks even sicker. As Dr. Howard Grossman points out, "People who are depressed do worse, whether it's because the depression suppresses their immune system or maybe because they don't take their medications or eat properly as a result of being depressed." According to a study conducted at Albert Einstein College of Medicine in the Bronx, New York, deepening depression may actually signal an impending medical crisis. Of the people studied, survivors of strokes, heart attacks, and cancer who grew depressed were 60 percent more likely to suffer another stroke or heart attack or cancer progression than those who did not become depressed. They were also 80 percent more likely to die.

"To disregard the presence of an illness like depression in someone who has cancer or heart disease, or any other disease," remarks Dr. Massie, "is really missing half the problem."

Recognizing the Signs of Depression

People who are depressed are not crazy, weak, feeling sorry for themselves, or simply in a bad mood. While part of our job as caregivers is to quietly comfort a seriously ill loved one through the inevitable sadness, we have to stay alert for the signs of depression

CHECKLIST
Common Signs of Depression

- ❑ Chronic sadness, anxiety, complaints of feeling "empty"
- ❑ Tiredness, lack of energy
- ❑ Loss of interest or pleasure in ordinary activities, including sex
- ❑ Difficulty falling asleep or getting back to sleep, waking up early in the morning; or the reverse, excessive sleeping
- ❑ Loss of appetite or overeating
- ❑ Frequent crying
- ❑ Unexplained aches and pains
- ❑ Difficulty concentrating, paying attention, remembering, or making decisions
- ❑ Increased irritability
- ❑ Disinterest in routine grooming or hygiene
- ❑ Expressions of guilt, helplessness, hopelessness, worthlessness
- ❑ Uncharacteristic withdrawal from other people
- ❑ Sudden manic activity
- ❑ Increased alcohol consumption or drug use (including prescriptions)
- ❑ Thoughts of suicide; a suicide attempt

✚ *Notify the doctor, home-care nurse, or hospice nurse should two or more of these symptoms persist for more than two weeks.*

—and when we recognize it, call in the experts. If you can't put your finger on the exact behavior that concerns you, Dr. Massie advises, "let the primary physician know that this person has changed, that he's not the same way he used to be."

Sadly, most depressed people resist asking for help. To some, acknowledging that they're having trouble coping is akin to an admission of character deficiency, a sign of weakness. Others believe that you have to be mentally ill— as in "crazy"—to see a mental health professional. Like people who needlessly suffer physical pain due to the misguided fear that they'll become addicted to medication or that the side effects will leave them zombielike, we tend to romanticize the so-called rugged individuals who "bite the bullet," "hang tough," or "buck up" during hard times. Just the lingering stigma of having "psychological problems" can prevent a loved one from seeking the treatment needed for the *medical condition* called depression. If the people around them harbor the same antiquated notions, the illness goes undiagnosed.

"The unfortunate thing about missing a diagnosis of depression," Dr. Massie notes, "is that today we have very effective treatments." Nine in ten people who receive therapy for depression or other mental health disorders improve or recover completely.

How Depression Is Treated

Clinical depression is usually managed quickly and effectively with antidepressant medication, which in the last ten years has come a long way in terms of breakthroughs in pharmaceutical research as well as refinements in dosage. "The good news about today's antidepressants," explains Dr. Massie, "is that whereas the older ones had side effects that were difficult for many patients to adjust to, the newer drugs on the market are very easily tolerated by most patients. They won't mess with your mind

and won't make you feel sicker." For those willing and able, talk therapy with a mental health professional can also be helpful, either one-on-one or in a group setting with other patients.

Since many sick people are inclined to put on a happy face for others, it often falls to us to call their depression to the medical team's attention and get the ball rolling. The home-care nurse, hospice nurse, or physician will almost always know what to do or whom to call. They've seen this problem many times before. A psychiatrist, clinical psychologist, or medical social worker will diagnose the depression and, if necessary, prescribe the appropriate medication or recommend that the patient's own doctor do so. Many internists and family practitioners are well equipped to diagnose routine cases of depression themselves.

If for any reason your health care team fails to follow up on persistent symptoms of depression, consider booking a mental health consultation yourself. For referrals to professionals skilled at recognizing and treating depression, try contacting

- any hospital's department of social work, psychiatry, or psychology;
- the patient's state or county department of mental health;
- the patient's Area Agency on Aging;
- local chapters of disease-related organizations;
- United Way of America;
- other caregivers and patients;
- one or more of the following:

☎ American Psychiatric Association, 202-682-6000.

☎ American Medical Association, 312-464-5000.

☎ American Psychological Association, 202-336-5500.

☎ National Association of Social Workers, 800-638-8799/202-408-8600.

Expect a depressed loved one to initially recoil at the idea of seeing a psychotherapist or attending a support group. But once the right medications are on board and the patient's outlook improves, it's still important to get him to talk about what's happening. Regular face-to-face assessments allow the team to adjust the medication dosage, watch out for drug interactions, and keep an eye peeled for new symptoms as they crop up. Your loved one might also find fresh perspective from others who have been down the same road, learn all sorts of new coping skills, and even make friends and find renewed purpose in life. ◄ See "National Support Groups," page 34. ► See "Patient Support Groups," page 199.

But Is It Covered?

Medicare helps pay for outpatient mental health treatment at hospitals and community mental health centers. The federal health insurance program also covers hospitalization in a Medicare-participating psychiatric hospital. Private insurers place a cap on ongoing psychotherapy but usually cover a psychiatric consultation ordered by the primary care physician of a hospitalized or terminal patient. Antidepressant medications are included in policies with pharmacy benefits.

Part and parcel with depression in sick folks is what's called anticipatory grief. A person with a life-threatening illness has much to mourn, and caregivers often find themselves at a loss for things to say. Just as frequently we find that our attempts to comfort a loved one backfire, causing him to lash out or withdraw even further. When a person is despondent, don't try to continually cheer him up. See to it that his physical pain is well controlled and that his anxiety and sleep disturbances are adequately managed. You can encourage him to set simple goals each morning and try to make as many decisions for himself as he can throughout the day. But after that, accept the fact that you can't make the situation better for him. When someone is feeling helpless or hopeless, the only real tonic is often our calm and continued presence.

✽ When someone you love says "I'm not going to make it, am I?," take her hand, look her in the eye, and reassure her, "Whatever happens, I'll be right here with you."

Acceptance

Does anyone ever truly accept death's inevitability? Some people may be more resolved to their fate than others or express fewer regrets, but human beings are hardwired not to give in until we give out. Acceptance is the measure of how well we all cope with actual circumstances, not compliance with fantasies about how seriously ill patients and their families "should" behave.

Overly romanticized sickbed scenes foisted on the public psyche by movies such as Philadelphia, Camille, or Love Story lead inexperienced caregivers to expect Hollywood story lines. Folks face sickness just the way they are no matter what we may want. Real people have regrets; real people get too sick to cope; real people suffer and die.

Sometimes behavior that passes for acceptance is actually a mask for terror. There are such things as "premature" and "false" acceptance—a recently widowed aunt, told she has a treatable form of cancer, goes home to die. Or a young man diagnosed with AIDS disappears alone into his apartment to await death. At the other extreme is the Super Patient whose seeming clear grip on reality is really the prelude to a big crash.

The Fundamentals of Caregiving

If there's a caregiver's credo worth immortalizing on a bumper sticker, it is this: Be where the patient is. To wit, put yourself in that person's place and take your cues from him. Is he having a good day or a bad day? Does he seem talkative or introspective? Reflect what *he* is feeling. "I bet you hated to see Dave go home, huh, Pop?" If you can't gauge the patient's mood, don't be afraid to ask him what's on his mind: "Hey, Lynn, you want to sit out here on the porch and talk, or would you rather just watch the news?"

In order for us to be in tune with our loved one, though, we need to have some understanding of the whirlpool of emotions she may be experiencing. Losing one's health often sets in motion a string of losses, with the elements that give life meaning and bolster self-esteem toppling like dominoes:

- Loss of status if the person can no longer work or do the things that brought him satisfaction or contributed to his self-esteem
- Altered body image or feelings of sexuality if the person's appearance has changed or she is not able to function normally
- Shifting balance in a relationship; for example, where both partners had previously shared responsibilities equally and cared for each other, but now one is fully dependent on the other
- Most of all, a surrendering of control over one's destiny—over *everything*, it seems

"The losses keep compounding and the person's world shrinks," observes Louise Fradkin, cofounder of the caregiver's support organization Children of Aging Parents (CAPS). "That's very hard."

How to Be Supportive (Without Becoming a Pain in the Neck)

Treat the person just as you did before, to let him know that your relationship is still the same. If you've always valued your father's advice about money, solicit his opinions as you normally would. Act naturally around him

—don't pretend as if nothing unusual is going on—but *be yourself.*

Try not to objectify "patients." Whether "patients," "victims," or "cases," sick *people* are bombarded with stereotypes. Everyone they encounter has some preconceived notion about how sick folks ought to act or feel or look. "Well, you know how they get with Alzheimer's . . ." "Cancer— what a terrible way to go!" Keep it personal. Use real names, not categories, when speaking to or about sick folks.

Don't assume a false cheerfulness. Sick people will see through you every time. In the film *Terms of Endearment,* when the dying Debra Winger sees her mother and best friend shuffle into her hospital room wearing forced smiles, her immediate reaction is "What's wrong now?"

Allow your loved one every opportunity to make decisions, no matter how seemingly inconsequential, from choices about medical treatment to selecting which clothes to wear. "Let me know when you're ready for your eyedrops, Rita." "Hey, Bob, you want to wear those jeans you had on yesterday?" Not "It's time for your medicine, Ma." Not "Just put on what you wore yesterday, Pop." However, too many decisions can confuse and annoy people with cognitive impairment or problems with speech and language. ▶ *See "When a Loved One Has Impaired Communications Skills," page 208.*

Don't take offense if the person doesn't follow your advice or resists your offers to handle personal matters. What's really at work here is an attempt to retain independence and preserve the dynamic of the relationship. "A lot of times older parents haven't been able to view their children as adults," observes Fradkin, who cared for her own elderly mother for eighteen years. "It can be difficult for them to accept that although they've been independent all their lives, now they can't take care of themselves. So you have to be very diplomatic when you approach 'taking over' for an adult."

Help him stay connected to the outside world by assisting him with writing letters, making phone calls, and arranging visits with friends and family, each of whom is a unique asset in the patient's care. Keep him up to date on current events, goings-on in the community, the latest gossip. Discuss her interests with her or read aloud from newspapers and magazines.

Include him in family life. Too often families exclude ailing loved ones from family discussions and activities or speak through them as if they were invisible. Even my aunt Kitty, the most sensitive of all caregivers, would say to me right in front of Bob, "Do you think your daddy would like to try some shrimp tonight?" Bob and Kitty's other sibling, our beloved uncle Howard, would turn to me with Pop sitting three feet away and earnestly ask, "So how's he been doing?" I'd say, "Hey, Bob, talk to your baby brother"—then get up and leave them alone together.

Choose your words carefully when speaking of the past. Toward the end of his life, when a maudlin colleague was struggling to thank Bob for his guidance over the years, Pop leaned over and whispered to me, *"Nice eulogy."*

Consider moving her bed into a room that's more centrally located —for instance, near the kitchen, living room, or den. Even the sickest folks can often rest comfortably for hours in a recliner or propped up on a sofa. Or roll her wheelchair out on the patio. Deliberately draw her into the hub of family life.

"Instead of focusing on what patients can't do anymore, relish what they can do and make the most of it," advises Diane Young, who watched Alzheimer's disease mentally incapacitate both her father and her father-in-law. "You can still do things together as a family. Just because a patient is having a bad day today, don't assume tomorrow is going to be as bad."

Encourage youngsters to read to the ill person or play games with him. For Bob, patiently baiting hooks or sprinkling bread crumbs in the canal so kids could marvel at the swamp critters did wonders for his spirits. Keep the visits short, though. Sick people are not baby-sitters. Kids can quickly exhaust even the hardiest adult.

Have some fun with the person yourself. My fondest memories of my stepmom Lynn are the long afternoons she and I spent playing cutthroat canasta around the kitchen table with her old girlfriend Oklas Lambert. I cherish those extended cocktail hours and the easy company of those two shameless cheats. All of us knew at the time that Lynn was not long for this world, but in the meantime we had a *ball.*

Make the most of good days. During the last six months that Mary Vitro's husband, Rick, suffered from AIDS, the Florida couple practiced a morning ritual to determine what the day might bring. "Every day we would get up," she recalls, "and I would sit on the edge of the bed and ask, 'Okay, how are we feeling this morning? *What* are we feeling?' If we didn't need to go to the doctor, Rick would lie on the couch in the living room and watch TV. If he felt good, maybe we'd go over to his mother's house for dinner." Good days are times to invite visitors over or take a short excursion.

Help him to lead as normal a life as possible. As often as you can, encourage your loved one to

- get out of bed, bathe, dress in street clothes;
- eat meals at the table;

- pick up the newspaper and sort the mail;
- do some household chores;
- take a nap;
- read books and magazines (or package inserts on medications);
- get on the phone;
- rent videos or listen to music;
- go for a walk or sit outside.

Help your loved one find meaningful activities and short-term goals. Suggest she arrange photo albums or scrapbooks, or start a family tree. Some sick people find it cathartic to keep a journal, to write that children's book they've always talked about, or to conduct a "life review" by starting their memoirs. Dying folks have far fewer regrets when they've wrung the life out of every minute. So do we.

* *It's up to us to do everything in our power to assure the ill or dying that their lives are still precious.*

Learning to Listen

It was from working alongside a perceptive social worker named Dixie Beckham that I first learned that "uh-huh . . ." can be a complete sentence—"uh-huh" as in "I hear what you're saying."

As director of Chelsea Psychotherapy Associates in Manhattan and for a number of years the clinical coordinator of the AIDS Support Program at Memorial Sloan-Kettering Cancer Center, Beckham has counseled hundreds of terminal patients and their families. She taught me the magical healing powers of the unadorned "yes" or "no," and how a well-timed nod, wink, or smile, a knowing glance, or a pregnant silence can communicate volumes more than most elaborate speeches.

Relentless intimate probing, like incessant chatter, is generally a sign that *the caregiver* is feeling unbearably powerless to make things better for the patient. Listening quietly and calmly is a discipline acquired only with experi-

ence. The greatest insights, for us and for our loved one, come during thoughtful reflection.

Let the person know that it's okay to talk to you. Maybe he's afraid of upsetting you. Maybe he feels he's already too much of a burden. Nervous chitchat or his spending more time than normal with family members may be a tip-off that he is anxious to discuss what is happening. Keep your antenna up for these and other subtle signals.

Ask a leading question: "What's on your mind, Pop?" Or try drawing him out by succinctly telling him how *you* feel: "I can't quit thinking about what that doctor said. What do you make of all that, Bob?" On the other hand, disease consumes so much of a patient's time and energy that sometimes it's all we ever seem to talk about. If someone is evasive or changes the subject, take the hint and go along with him.

Five words to avoid: "I know how you feel." We can't ever really know someone else's pain. The most you can honestly say is "I can only imagine what must be going through your mind right now."

Don't shy away from talking bluntly about the person's condition or prognosis. After my father learned he had terminal cancer, it irritated him no end whenever someone would mince words in discussing his disease. If Dad was scared, he never let on. Many times in his final months he said, "I've had a fine life; I'm just lucky to have had the good years I've had." One time a young bank employee, trying to be polite, said unctuously, "Well, Mr. McFarlane, in *your situation* . . ." Dad leaned forward and propped his elbows on the woman's desk. "Listen," he said firmly, "I'm *dying*, and I know it. And it doesn't hurt me for you to say that."

Tolerate the silences. Many people, men especially, feel compelled to solve

Some Common Fears and Our Responses

Common Fears	Our Responses
"I'm afraid of dying."	"Me, too. What worries you the most?"
"I'm afraid of dying alone."	"I will stay by your side every step of the way. I will make sure you're not left alone."
"I'm afraid of dying in unbearable pain."	"We can make sure that doesn't happen. Let's talk to the doctor now so it never comes to that."
"I don't want to die disabled and dependent."	"I will always be here for you. I will see to it that you're well cared for, come what may."
"I'm afraid of being a burden and that you'll start to resent me."	"I am here by choice. I will not abandon you."
Fear of the unknown: "What's going to happen to me now?"	"Whatever happens, we'll take it one step at a time together. What worries you the most?"
"I don't want to be kept alive on artificial life support."	"We can take care of that now." Help him discuss the matter frankly with the doctor and loved ones, then execute a living will and medical power of attorney. ► See "Advance Medical Directives," page 298.
"What's going to become of my family if I die?"	"What worries you the most?" Help her execute a will, arrange custody for children, settle financial affairs, plan a funeral, and say her piece with loved ones. ► See chapter 9, "Preparing for the Worst."
"My life has been a waste; I am a failure."	Tell him what he means to you. Let him mourn.
"I feel as if I'm being punished for something I did."	Confess your own regrets and forgive her for any past wrongs to you. Remind her that bad things happen to good people, too.
"What will happen to me after I die?"	"I don't know. What do you believe?" Suggest discussing it with a trusted loved one, minister, or spiritual guide who is experienced with the seriously ill.

every problem put before them. When patients express anger, frustration, or sadness, they're looking to us not necessarily for a solution but for a sounding board. Try saying *nothing*. The person isn't inclined to open up? Respect that and shush. True intimacy cannot be forced. Don't feel that you have to entertain the person perpetually, settle arguments, or see to it that every moment is loaded with meaning. You'll exhaust yourself and your patient. Use silence like rest.

Fewer words, more touching. A quick hug, squeezing a hand, mopping a sweaty brow, smoothing a cowlick, a pat on the rear, fluffing a pillow, and throwing a blanket over bare feet are just a few of countless ways we can reassure patients they are not alone— without ever opening our mouths.

✳ *Bear in mind that not everyone is comfortable with or comforted by physical contact. Respect your patient's boundaries.*

Other Sources of Patient Support

Patient Support Groups

Whoever said "I wept because I had no shoes until I met a man who had no feet" must have just come from a support group meeting. Perspective can sure come in handy when things look bleak. It helps to know that someone else has traveled the same road, that everything about to happen to us has already happened to somebody else, that we don't have to make the same mistakes. The real lowdown, the skinny, the tricks of the trade can come only from folks who can look us in the eye and say, "Been there, done that."

For a long time I questioned the value of support groups. But when the AIDS epidemic struck in the early 1980s, thousands of desperately ill young people suddenly had no place to turn for advice. Medical knowledge was sketchy, and there were no organizations that knew what to do. People with AIDS turned to each other.

Borrowing the "psychoeducational" group model from cancer patients—traditionally led by a nurse or hospital social worker—and co-opting the self-

help model of peer support groups like Alcoholics Anonymous, a vast network of all sorts of patient support programs exploded across the country. Right away hospitals, mental health agencies, and other disease groups followed suit.

While there's much comradeship and solace to be found in a group of similarly situated individuals, most often it's about survival and a shared enemy. Patients sort through medical information together, compare notes, debunk statistics, help one another avoid common pitfalls, and focus their collective wisdom on recurring problems. They provide one another with living, breathing reminders that they're not finished yet.

Patient support groups can also provide a constructive, welcome outlet for folks debilitated by illness to exercise their social skills or, in Walter Miller's case, a talent for organization. For Miller, whose chronic emphysema forced him into early retirement from the Union Pacific Railroad, founding the Better Breathers of Utah evolved into a part-time second career.

"My husband had been depressed," says his widow, Nola. "I told him, 'You have a choice: You can either see a psychiatrist, or you can start doing something for people who have lung problems.' Walt was really dedicated to this group. He would print out all the mailings himself and pick up the refreshments and line up the speakers for the monthly meetings. This was his baby. It was great." Her husband died of his disease in 1992, but, she says, "I still have contact with some of the people we met there."

Support groups can range from highly structured meetings supervised by a nurse, social worker, psychologist, or psychiatrist to three elderly men sitting on the porch swapping prostate cancer stories. It helps to think of attending a support group like a military reconnaissance mission. There's vital information out there, but there's also risk involved. I've seen a few newly diagnosed people who were unnerved at the sight of someone in the advanced stages of their own disease or who grew depressed as member after member dropped out and died. Groups can occasionally dissolve into directionless free-for-alls, or, conversely, one person can monopolize the conversation for an hour. Don't be put off. Attend another group or start your own.

One-on-one visitation from someone with the same illness may be preferable for those who don't feel comfortable making themselves heard in a group. A church member or another of their own doctors' patients might fit the bill. The American Cancer Society's Reach to Recovery program matches women newly diagnosed with breast cancer with survivors. The American Heart Association's Mended Hearts program performs a similar service for people with heart disease. Local affiliates of the National Kidney Foundation, too, will hook up patients for one-on-one conversation. ▶ *See Appendix A, "Recommended Resources," page 489.*

Finding Hope and Comfort in Faith

Most sick people and their loved ones will never attend a support group meeting. Likewise, hospital social workers, psychologists, and psychiatrists are usually far too overloaded with cases to counsel patients for more than a few minutes at a time. Instead, many ill folks and their families find their greatest solace in familiar religious rituals and active spiritual faith. Even when Uncle Billy was thoroughly demented from end-stage Alzheimer's disease, attending mass seemed to bring him a measure of inner calm. "To the very end, no matter how upset he was," my aunt recalls, "I could take him to church, and he would sit there like a mouse."

Many patients derive great comfort from going to church and practicing their faith during a time of sickness. Others suddenly discover religion and

spirituality once they become ill. The opposite may also be true, in that serious illness can severely test or shatter a seemingly unshakable faith. The challenge is to find a minister, priest, rabbi, or chaplain experienced with and comfortable around seriously ill people. Not all clergy know what to say around the sick, especially in reply to the inevitable question: How can God allow this? Talk to ministers recommended by close friends or fellow patients and caregivers. Ask them directly what training and experience they have had with the seriously ill before putting your loved one in touch.

A common mistake is to assume that someone is in need of spiritual aid simply because he's sick. Hospitalized myself for bacterial pneumonia one time, an aged nun would approach me daily to offer communion. Frankly, I was in no mood to start confessing my sins, but I feared terrible retribution if I refused the sacrament. It often falls to caregivers both to protect loved ones from heavy-handed zealots and help them find a dependable spiritual companion.

Increasingly, hospitals are hiring chaplains with special training in ministering to the sick and dying. Christine Swift, a staff chaplain at Georgetown University Medical Center in Washington, D.C., studied bereavement counseling and hospice care before entering seminary school for clinical pastoral education. Forty years old at the time, and a mother of six, she had decided to become a hospital chaplain after a sister died of cancer in a medical center that offered little counseling, spiritual or otherwise.

"I see my function as being a companion along the journey, as someone who's invited in to share an experience with those who are in difficulty, in pain, and who are trying to discover the meaning of their life," Chaplain Swift explains. "Basically I think of myself as a listener, to help get them in touch with themselves, with God, with what their values are." The visits, she emphasizes, do not have to touch on spirituality at all. Although a Catholic chaplain, "I visit all patients, not just Catholics. I just try to meet people where they are and let it happen, whatever 'it' is. It may never evolve into some deep, spiritual conversation. But, then, it may."

Long-Standing Conflicts

A loved one's health crisis doesn't take place in a vacuum. Pat Still, an everyday angel from New York City, observes frankly, "I used to say that my husband wasn't a very nice person to begin with, and getting ill certainly didn't change his character."

Still, now executive director of the Well Spouse Foundation, a national caregiver's support organization, nursed her husband at home for six years following a stroke. "When you're a caregiver," she points out, "you're not necessarily caring for someone that you're madly in love with." Family conflicts or personal problems that existed prior to an illness don't magically resolve themselves. A loved one's serious illness may be set against the backdrop of a loveless marriage, abuse, or addiction.

Baseball Hall of Fame sportscaster Walter Lanier "Red" Barber, best remembered as the voice of the Brooklyn Dodgers and later of their perennial World Series rivals, the New York Yankees, died in 1992 at age eighty-four. His wife, Lylah, had been suffering from Alzheimer's disease for several years; she was also a chronic alcoholic. The couple's care fell to their only daughter, Sarah Lanier Barber, a retired English professor living in Santa Fe, New Mexico. The Barbers lived in Tallahassee, Florida. "Both my parents had problems with alcohol," she says. "My mother consistently, and my father kind of on and off."

Several times a year Sarah would visit her parents "for three or four days," she says, "which was about all that the three of us could tolerate." Much to Sarah's distress, her father regularly fed Lylah martinis—perhaps, she conjectures, as a way to "medicate" his volatile wife, who between her dementia and her drinking was prone to frequent tirades. But whenever Sarah tried broaching the subject with her father, who was hard of hearing, "he would take his earpiece out of his ear, which pretty well put an end to the conversation."

Sometimes sickness provides an opportunity for growth and forgiveness. But sometimes, when someone is seriously ill and long-term survival seems unlikely, we're beyond the point of trying to patch things up or make amends. Our focus becomes self-preservation, in which event you should keep your visits brief, spread the work around to siblings and relatives from the get-go, and, most important, seek solace for your own pain with family, friends, clergy, or support groups. ▶ *See chapter 5, "Mustering the Troops"; chapter 7, "Care for the Caregivers."*

Caring for People with Special Needs

When a Loved One Is Not Conscious

A person can be unconscious and still retain fragments of conversation. ICU nurses can tell you stories of people who emerged from deep comas able to recount entire discussions that took place around them. That is why you'll see the staff in an intensive care unit or hospice carry on one-sided conversations with their comatose patients as if they were awake: "Okay, I'm going to roll you over on your side, Mrs. Chase."

Many caregivers find talking to a comatose loved one extremely comforting. As my father lay unconscious at the end, each of us sat with him for hours, saying things like "I'm right here, Pop," and "I'm just going to pull the covers up a little." Remember that some of what we say may reach the person's subconscious. Take your arguments outdoors and don't discuss your fears at the bedside.

✽ *Every time you enter or leave the patient's room, tell him so in a normal voice even if he appears unconscious. Likewise, announce your intentions before you touch an unconscious person.*

When a Loved One Suffers from Brain Function Impairment

Much of the foregoing advice in this chapter flies right out the window when you're unable to communicate normally with sick people. Whether it's because they can't process incoming information or because they're unable to express their own thoughts effectively, patients with neurologic problems become progressively more isolated, even from those who are closest.

The signs of dementia—or what used to be referred to as "senility"—include short-term memory loss, confusion, agitation, an inability to concentrate or reason, and diminished personality. According to the Family Caregiver Alliance, a support organization that serves men and women caring for brain-damaged adults, roughly one in five

American families is caring for someone who is cognitively impaired.

Many medical conditions also mimic dementia. These "pseudo dementias," as they are called, are usually reversible. For instance, a patient may become confused and disoriented as a result of severe depression or lack of oxygen, or as a side effect of many medications. Metabolic disturbances caused by kidney failure, liver disease, and several other conditions can also cloud consciousness. True dementia, defined as an organic disorder of the brain, is usually irreversible and often progressive.

Few situations can test the stamina of a caregiver as severely as progressive deterioration of the nervous system. People suffering from dementia don't lose their sensitivity. Our frustration and tension only makes them more upset. It becomes an Olympian exercise in patience, reminding ourselves constantly that the person is not deliberately acting this way.

There are many things we can do to mitigate the symptoms of dementia. What follows are some tips for dealing with short-term memory loss; delusions; agitated, paranoid, and combative behavior; wandering; and problems with speech and language. ◀ *See chapter 3 for tips on bathing, dressing, and feeding loved ones suffering from dementia.*

Causes of Dementia

- Cerebral degenerative diseases such as Alzheimer's disease, Parkinson's disease, Huntington's chorea, and multiple sclerosis
- Cerebrovascular stroke or a series of small strokes
- Traumatic brain injury
- Brain tumor
- HIV encephalopathy
- Loss of oxygen to the brain, or anoxia
- Encephalitis and meningitis, two infections of the brain
- Hydrocephalus, a buildup of fluid within the brain, or an increase in pressure on the brain due to swelling

Memory Loss

It helps to think of the central nervous system as a home computer. A malfunction in any part cripples the rest. Software is useless if the memory bank is wiped out. Even if all the data remain intact, one loose connection can make it impossible to retrieve. As caregiver, our goals are threefold: to feed information to our loved one in a way he can understand and use; to help him make the most of his remaining powers; and to protect him and others from danger.

Some degree of memory loss is one of the tradeoffs of living to a ripe old age. All of us have walked into a room and suddenly been unable to remember why, or started to tell a story and then forgotten the point. Have you ever referred to your nephew by his father's name? Caught yourself rereading the same paragraph three times? Awakened in a darkened hotel room and felt that fleeting rush of panic because you momentarily couldn't recall where you were? Now imagine all of these things happening at the same time all the time, and you can appreciate what life is like for someone with severe memory loss.

Truly dangerous situations arise during ordinary daily activities—often before family and friends recognize the pattern of forgetfulness. Mom can't remember where she parked the car, runs out of gas on a back road after dark, or misplaces her keys and purse. She grabs a hot copper skillet without a potholder, sticks an aluminum pan in the microwave, or leaves the iron on all day. Many otherwise functional folks forget to eat or take their medicine. As memory deteriorates, often slowly over several years, it falls to the caregiver to ensure home safety and to supervise medical care and activities of daily living.

Complicating our tasks is the fact that patients don't necessarily notice right away that they're having trouble remembering things. If they are aware of it, they may avoid mentioning anything, to the extent of concealing the problem as long as they can. Most often we discover it for ourselves when a loved one's memory loss begins to cause undeniable problems. Once the situation becomes clear, organization, routine, and gentle, diplomatic reminders go a long way toward preventing serious mishaps.

Alert the medical team if the person becomes noticeably more forgetful or confused. Drug interactions or a treatable medical condition may be the cause.

Keep distractions such as TV, music, and cross-talk to a minimum. In conversation, stick to one train of thought at a time.

Regularly orient the person to time and place. Place digital or large-face clocks and calendars in easy-to-spot locations around the house. Let him know what's happening now by "thinking out loud" to yourself: "Today's Wednesday. We need to go to the market this morning." Maintain familiar surroundings by keeping furniture and objects around the house and yard in the same place. Turn on a night-light. Use the same route when traveling to everyday destinations around home and the neighborhood.

Maintain a regular schedule. Keep a calendar with reminders of daily tasks. Keep a shopping list in the kitchen. Write down appointments and important messages and post them plainly in sight on the bathroom mirror, the kitchen table, or the refrigerator door.

Choose a permanent place to keep important items. Make it clear that no one is to deviate from returning objects to their designated spots. Place a big bowl in a central location for house and car keys, wallet or purse. (Buy a key chain that attaches to his belt, or one of those electronic gadgets that locates her keys when she claps.) Stash a spare set of eyeglasses in a drawer and tie her favorite pair to a string around her neck. Keep dentures in a brightly colored container next to the bed or the bathroom sink.

Clearly mark all medications with basic instructions. Unless it seems more confusing, consider purchasing a plastic pill organizer at the drugstore and sort each dose in an individual compartment. Either way, carefully inventory all medications at each visit so that you can tell whether he's forgotten to take something.

Phone or show up at planned mealtimes and remind your loved one to eat. Ditto for crucial medications. Review the instructions and safety precautions *each time.*

When giving instructions, break down each task into simple steps. Slow down and make sure the person understands you before moving on. Use simple sentences. Pause often and give him plenty of time to respond. Keep unnecessary choices and long explanations to a minimum. If he doesn't seem to follow you, rephrase statements rather than repeat yourself endlessly.

If you can avoid it, don't correct the person or give her instructions in front of others. *Never* mock or tease even if you're just trying to make light of an awkward moment. You embarrass her by calling attention to her memory deficit, and self-consciousness or anxiety only heightens the confusion. Don't condescend or let impatience creep into your voice. If a task becomes too frustrating to finish, let it go until later.

Anticipate other potential headaches:

- Set up one central file exclusively for bills and other important correspondence.

- Arrange for the mail to be picked up or forwarded to you, and for someone trustworthy to pay the bills—or arrange for creditors and the phone, utility, and cable companies to call you if payments are not made on time.
- Consider ordering a checkbook that makes carbon copies of every entry.
- Encourage your loved one to leave his credit cards at home or bring along only one at a time when setting out to make a specific purchase.
- Write down bank and credit card account numbers and pertinent "800" telephone numbers.
- Photocopy any hard-to-replace documents such as a driver's license, passport, insurance, and Social Security card before they get lost.
- Leave a spare set of house and car keys with someone living close by.

▶ *See "Declaring Someone Incompetent," page 292; chapter 20, "Caring for Someone with a Progressive Neurological Disease."*

Delusional or Hallucinatory Behavior

Rick Vitro, in the throes of AIDS-related dementia, drifted in and out of objective reality the last weeks of his life. One morning he shook his wife awake.

"We've got to warn the government!" he blurted. "It's urgent!"

"What?" Mary asked sleepily. Her husband explained excitedly that during the night he'd been riding an elephant in India and overheard terrorists conspiring to drop an atomic bomb on the United States. He insisted that Mary drive him to the nearest military base.

"I thought he was joking at first and began laughing," she recalls. "Then I realized he was completely serious." She defused Rick's agitation by assuring him that they would warn the government after breakfast, by which time he'd forgotten all about the foreign plot, as she knew he would.

Delusions are the intellectual equivalent of hallucinations. Instead of seeing things that aren't there because the circuitry is defective, our loved one entertains thoughts that don't jibe with reality. Although they may sound bonkers, they're not necessarily crazy. They're simply laboring under a different set of assumptions.

The "good" news about delusional folks is that many of them are quite weak physically by the time their mind is far gone. Their ability to concentrate is often impaired, too, so they find it difficult to sustain a jag and are often unable to act directly on their impulses. We quietly reassure them that *the situation is under control* and, most important, that *they are safe.*

Others have innocuous delusions that don't require action on our part. Dad wakes up thinking someone is coming over who is not. Mom shows up for church or a doctor's appointment on the wrong day. It's agonizing to witness, but there's no real harm done.

If a deluded person's confusion persists, don't argue with him or constantly try to correct him. Maintain his trust by accepting his reality at face value. Go along until you can distract him, as you do with a young child, taking care not to condescend or became impatient.

You can also take these steps:

- Check to see if he has an obvious fever, indicating a possible infection of the brain.
- Make sure he is not in pain, short of breath, nauseated, tired, hungry, lost, frightened by something specific, or needing to go to the bathroom.
- Notify the medical team of frank delusions. Medications may need to be adjusted or new symptoms investigated.

Agitated or Paranoid Behavior

Depending on which parts of the brain are injured, a loved one's personality may seem to change dramatically. He may make thoughtless or hurtful remarks or unreasonable demands; over-

react with laughter, tears, or anger at the slightest provocation; treat us and others with surprising suspicion, mistrust, or contempt. It's important to remember that his personality has not truly changed, but, rather, his ability to express himself. Speech tumbles out uncensored, thoughts get distorted— and tension mounts.

Abstract concepts like morality and conscience become all but useless when impulse control starts to diminish and higher reasoning begins to fail. It becomes extremely difficult to discern which statements and actions are intentional and which can't be helped, as Sarah Barber discovered during visits with her verbally abusive mother.

"My father and I had a relatively good relationship, and I think he found my presence comforting. But I had an extremely tense, strained relationship with my mother. Even before she got ill, after about two or three days, there would be a lot of tension in the house. I think part of it came from my lifestyle, which my parents never made peace with." Freed of inhibitions by the Alzheimer's and the alcohol, Lylah Barber "really let Sarah have it with both barrels," observes Sarah's longtime lover Gloria Donnadello.

"There were just no restraints. Sarah struggled very hard to understand that this was partly the illness, but also partly what her mother was really like —and how her mother felt, at least partly, toward her." Gloria, a seasoned psychotherapist and retired professor of social work, offered Sarah a piece of advice that she had shared with patients who were embroiled in conflicts with their elderly parents: "People don't always grow out of their problems; they grow *into* them."

Suggestions for handling agitated or paranoid behavior:

- Reduce external stimulation, including noise, clutter, bright lights, excess movement, and the number of people in the room. Remove your loved one from stressful situations.

- Speak calmly and maintain eye contact. Do not surprise or provoke a confused or agitated loved one with sudden movement. Approach him from the front. Don't whisper. Don't talk about him in his presence. Assure him that he is safe.
- Help orient him to time and place. Identify yourself—"It's me, Uncle Billy, *David*"—and state your intentions: "I'm just going to hang up your coat right here." Leave on a night-light to reduce disorientation in the dark.
- Eliminate obvious causes of agitation. Make sure the person is not hungry or thirsty, too hot or cold, short of breath, nauseated, tired, in pain, bursting to go to the bathroom, or frightened of something specific. And don't serve him caffeinated coffee next time.
- Try to calm her down. Listen attentively to her complaints and don't argue or directly contradict faulty logic. Quietly encourage her to continue talking. Take a walk together or sit in a rocker holding hands and listening to soothing music—whatever has worked in the past.
- Keep choices to a minimum and instructions simple.
- Explain to family members and other care providers that the person's behavior is a result of her illness.
- Do not hesitate to leave and summon help if at any time you believe your own safety is in jeopardy. If you have to call for outside assistance, make it abundantly clear that your loved one is extremely ill and confused.
- Consider storing sharp knives, cigarette lighters, matches, household chemicals, and guns in a locked cabinet.
- Have the medical team evaluate patterns of sudden mood swings, extreme reactions to everyday situations, or expressions of *unfounded* fears. Medications may be causing side effects. New medications may need to be ordered to control severe agitation or high anxiety.

Combative Behavior

All of us have literally kicked the dog or a loved one out of bed when we weren't quite awake. Whenever a loved one pushes us away, throws or breaks something, or flails at someone, it's usually because he's frightened or confused. Don't take it personally. The caregiver's main job here is to deescalate the situation so that no one gets hurt. Remember that many of the worst episodes can be avoided altogether by paying careful attention to what upsets your loved one and eliminating the cause before things get out of hand.

Suggestions for handling combativeness:

- Remain calm. Take a few steps back and give the person plenty of room.
- Agree with her. Tell her that she is safe. *Do not argue or struggle with her!*
- Try to identify what's upsetting him: Is he overstimulated by people, noise, or clutter? Is he disoriented, or does he think he's been abandoned? Is something specific hurting or frightening him? Is he frustrated with a task, or are you asking too many questions or giving too many instructions at once?
- Assess the level of danger. Unless the person represents an immediate physical threat to herself or to someone who can't get out of her way, stand by quietly until she runs out of steam. If someone is about to get hurt, step in and simply say *"Stop"* or *"No"* in a calm but firm voice. Gently restrain the offending limb at close range with an affectionate embrace.

❋ *Always stay within an arm's reach of "runners" when you're outside.*

- If you have any doubt about your safety or that of others, don't hesitate to clear out immediately and call for help. Make sure that whoever you call understands that your loved one is sick and badly confused.

- Alert the medical team to episodes of uncontrolled rage or violence, no matter how mild, or any dangerously impulsive behavior. Medication side effects or another medical condition could be the problem. New combinations of *antipsychotic* drugs, tranquilizers, or medications to reduce anxiety, depression, pain, or sleep disturbances may also be in order.

Restraints

Rarely is it necessary to resort to physical restraint, which should be used strictly for safety's sake, not convenience. In their confusion, demented patients have been known to yank out IV lines, urinary catheters, and breathing or feeding tubes, and to pick repeatedly at their skin, dressings, or drainage bags. In these common situations, *passive* restraints are sufficient. Simply wrap thick, soft rolls of cotton gauze around each hand and secure each "mitt" with lightweight paper tape.

Some folks struggle so aggressively that they tumble out of bed and hurt themselves. Others jump up and head off on irrational missions. Rick Vitro died in a St. Petersburg, Florida, medical center. A few days before the end, he had to be physically restrained in bed "because the nurses found him wandering around the halls, stealing other patients' urinals," his wife recalls. "I didn't want him to be tied down, so I hired round-the-clock nursing."

Wandering

The first year following Duane Travers's car accident, before he entered a rehabilitation facility, he used to disappear impulsively from his mother's home at all hours. "She used to call me in the middle of the night to say 'Duane's gone,'" recalls his sister Roslyn. "We would have to look for him in clubs we knew he used to frequent. One time we found him in a pool hall."

Without keeping a patient captive in the house or treating him like a child, there's much we can do to protect a loved one who tends to wander off. Our tasks are to minimize his confusion, set up safe boundaries and buffer zones, and make him easy to find if he should get lost.

Look for reasons for the person's wandering. Has he lost something? Is he trying to find someone? Is he overstimulated, frightened, disoriented, anxious, or uncomfortable? Report episodes of wandering to the medical team; drug interactions or another medical condition may be the cause.

Schedule regular exercise to reduce restlessness and dissipate nervous energy. Take frequent walks together. Have the person sweep around the house or rake the yard.

Schedule regular rest periods. Confused people often sleep only fitfully night after night; they become cranky and agitated when they're tired. Turn down the lights and background noise for short, frequent naps or quiet times throughout the day.

Stick to a daily routine and avoid situations known to upset or confuse your loved one. Place your phone number in his pocket so he can call you if he ever gets lost.

Complicate the task of his leaving the house without your knowledge or assistance. Slip child-safe plastic covers over doorknobs or install a sliding bolt or trip latch. Place a stop sign on ground-floor doors or attach a bell or chime. Stow out of sight essential escape tools such as keys, coats, or glasses. Keep the garage door locked or have a coded electronic lock installed on the car's ignition. Consider fencing the yard.

Review home safety and personal security precautions. Upgrade them

---

Safe Return Program

Consider enrolling a loved one who wanders in the Safe Return program sponsored by the Alzheimer's Disease and Related Disorders Association. For $25, your loved one is registered in a nationwide database. Should he ever wander away from home, you call a special toll-free number to report him missing. Safe Return then alerts a network of 17,000 local law enforcement agencies across the country in an effort to get him home safely. You'll receive a wallet ID, clothing labels, and a bracelet or necklace for the person to wear.

☎ For more information call Safe Return at 800-272-3900.

---

if need be. Wandering may be a symptom of deteriorating memory or increasing confusion. Make sure the person doesn't cause an injury accidentally.

Alert family, friends, and neighbors about your loved one's tendency to wander. See to it that they all know how to reach you. If he has a favorite destination, make sure the folks there are aware of the situation. (Tip them lavishly or come bearing gifts.) Make friends with beat cops, community watch patrols, roving security personnel, crossing guards, mail carriers, newspaper carriers, doormen, store clerks, and neighborhood busybodies.

Have the person wear a Medic Alert or similar ID bracelet or necklace. Or have dog tags made up. With a laundry marker or sew-on labels, place identifying information and emergency contact numbers in all her favorite garments. As much as you can, keep her well groomed and neatly dressed so that she's not ignored on the street or shooed away like a homeless person. Keep a recent photograph of the person

on hand. ◄ See *"Personal Emergency Response Systems," page 184.* ► See *"Caring for Someone with Alzheimer's Disease: Hyperactivity," page 473.*

When a Loved One Has Impaired Communications Skills

Debra Bulkeley: *My father was always a talker. Whenever we had family holiday dinners, he would always tell jokes and be the center of the conversation. But Lou Gehrig's disease eventually made it too exhausting for him to talk.*

This really struck me the Thanksgiving before he died. I thought, This isn't fun anymore. Dad doesn't talk or tell jokes. *A few weeks later I said to him,* "Gee, Dad, you've just got to tell a joke at Christmas dinner." "Okay," he said. "I think I can still do that." *I didn't bring it up again.*

During our Christmas dinner, just before dessert, my father said, "Debra asked me . . . to tell a joke at dinner . . . and so I'm . . . going to tell . . . a joke." *It took so much effort for him to tell that joke, but he did it, which was really touching for all of us.*

The term *aphasia* is used to describe an assortment of communication impairments that can arise as a result of Alzheimer's disease, stroke, traumatic brain injury, Parkinson's disease, amyotrophic lateral sclerosis, and other conditions. Aphasia encompasses difficulties with speech, listening, reading, and/or writing. The problems may be mechanical in nature, cognitive, or both. For instance, a stroke survivor might have trouble making himself understood because his injured brain can't supply the appropriate words. Another patient might have the cognitive ability to compose eloquent statements, but damage to the neurofibers that activate the muscles around the mouth or tongue prevent him from enunciating the words he wants to say. Dementia's impairment of short-term memory and concentration can interfere with listening. "Obviously," points out Dr. Fletcher McDowell, executive director of the Burke Rehabilitation Hospital in White Plains, New York, "when patients are unable to communicate what their needs are or can't understand what you're saying, it can make caring for them very difficult."

Ways to make ourselves better understood to our patient:

- Eliminate distractions: Turn off the TV or radio while talking to your loved one.
- Stand in front of him so that he can see your lips move and read your facial expressions.
- Make eye contact. Emphasize nonverbal cues such as smiling or nodding your head at the end of sentences, or raising your eyebrows to indicate a question has been asked.
- Condense what you want to say into short, simple sentences. Avoid negative phrasing like "Don't stay outside." Instead use the directive: "Come inside." Simple hand gestures help, too.
- Word questions so that they elicit a yes or no answer: "Would you like to go outside?" rather than "Would you like to go out or stay inside?"
- When describing a task—getting dressed, stepping into the bathtub— do so in the exact sequence in which it should be done. Give only one instruction at a time.
- Speak slowly and clearly, but monitor your tone of voice. Make sure you don't sound condescending or impatient. Don't speak louder than normal unless the person is hard of hearing.

- You may have to repeat yourself more than once. Rephrase your statement choosing different words if he still doesn't appear to understand you after a couple of tries.
- If the person is better able to comprehend the written word, write down what you want to tell him.

✴ *When with a group of people, make it a point to include the person in the conversation even if he cannot respond. Make eye contact and acknowledge his presence so he doesn't feel left out.*

Ways to help the patient express himself more clearly:

- If she can communicate better through writing, let her, even though this may be more time consuming.
- Study your loved one's facial expressions and gestures as he speaks.
- Establish simple codes for expressing yes or no. Have her point to objects to communicate straightforward needs.
- If you don't understand something, ask her to repeat it.
- Be a patient listener. Resist the temptation to speak for the person or to finish his sentences.

Communication Aids

As long as a loved one can still indicate yes and no—even with a mere nod of the head, movement of the eyes, or by squeezing a finger—we can still get through to each other. It just takes patience and persistence. With experimentation and experience, caregivers and their patients quickly work out their own shorthand, codes, signals, and abbreviations.

People with mechanical problems of

the throat or mouth tend to speak softly. AT&T leases a telephone amplification device for less than $1 a month. There are also sophisticated amplifiers available through catalogs and specialty stores.

For folks who can't speak at all, try a simple variation on grade school flash cards. Remember flash cards? Using a grease pencil or erasable marker, write commonly used words and phrases around the perimeter of a washable laminated drawing board, which you should be able to find in any toy store or art supply store. Then either you or the patient can simply point to PAIN, WATER, BEDPAN, CHOKE, and so on until you figure out the problem through process of elimination. You can also leave room in the middle of the page for scrawling missing phrases. (Think of it as a cross between Scrabble and Charades.) ► *See "Speech/Language Loss (Aphasia): Telephone Amplification Devices, Computer Technology for ALS Patients," page 483; Appendix B: "Adaptive Technology," page 504.*

☎ To rent a telephone amplification device from AT&T, call 800-555-8111. To buy one, call 800-222-3111.

☎ To learn about the extraordinary gamut of communication aids on the market, call Abledata (800-227-0216; 301-608-8998), a free service of the National Rehabilitation Information Center in Silver Spring, Maryland.

—5—

Mustering the Troops

Four weeks after Dad's emergency heart surgery, we all were beginning to think something was wrong. He had survived the bypass, his lungs were clear, and the incisions were healing nicely. He was up and around under his own steam, even taking short walks alone outside. But my father had suddenly begun to look frail, losing weight and getting weaker.

I kept telling myself, "He's an old man. He's been sick for nearly a year. He just had major heart surgery. It's just taking longer than we thought." I had done what I could for the time being. I'd been away from home a month by this time and needed to get back to work. Somehow, we were going to have to keep a close eye on Pop.

All the way to the airport I thought to myself, *This is not a good recovery. This is not good.*

I barely had my feet on the ground in New York before the mystery of Pop's lingering ailments unraveled.

"Rodger, it's David. Bob's got cancer. It's advanced lymphoma."

Aunt Kitty had been trimming my father's hair when she discovered a painful bump behind his left ear. My aunt called her friend Dr. Wiley Justice, a local ear, nose, and throat specialist. Pop also knew him well, having overseen a renovation at Dr. Justice's home the year before.

It was Wiley Justice who finally figured out what was wrong. After putting Bob on antibiotics for a week, he took a sample of the lump for biopsy and told Kitty to bring him back two days later. "When we got to the office," she recalls, "Wiley said he wanted to speak to Bob alone. I knew right then it was bad." Over the wall divider (leave it to Kitty) "I heard him tell Bob it was time to start putting his ducks in a row."

"Okay, Wiley," my father said. "Just tell me how it's gonna be."

The doctor laid out Bob's options: Chemotherapy for stage III non-

Hodgkin's lymphoma could *possibly* prolong his life another year or two. That is, *if* he responded to the therapy and *if* he didn't die of complications in the process—a not unlikely prospect for a sick and emaciated seventy-three-year-old man.

"And if I don't go for the treatment?"

"You have maybe two months."

Bob's reply: "I'll take it." In his mind, the chemo wasn't likely to alter the outcome (he was probably right), so why put himself through needless torment?

Just like that, our care plan changed course radically: from tag-team nursing Dad through a few weeks of postsurgical recovery to terminal care for—who knew how long? It also had to be managed with Bob at his own home, if he was to have his way.

As it turned out, Pop's condition remained stable over the summer. He was to live four months beyond the two-month prognosis, for the most part in surprisingly good health. With Mary Foster, Dad's wife, debilitated by heart problems and caring for a daughter dying of breast cancer at her own house, my brothers and I set about pulling together a network of family and friends to cover the next few months.

At Dad's request, our brother John and his family immediately drove down from Fort Riley, Kansas, to settle the sale of his beloved house to the next-door neighbors and arranged for him to live there until he died. When it was time for John to report back for Army duty, our brother Bobby's two teenagers trooped in from Shreveport, Louisiana. Mary would sit with Bob for a few hours several times a week, too, and occasionally spent the night. Around Labor Day, David made it a point to swing through Mobile to assess Bob's situation.

Throughout, Aunt Kitty checked up on Dad several times a day. His brother Howard and his sister-in-law, our dear aunt Virginia, stopped by often, brought food, and ran errands. Our late stepmother Lynn's former cleaning lady gave the house a good once-over every couple of weeks. There was a steady stream of old friends, colleagues, and church folks through Bob's place. Darlene and Ron Twilley, his wonderful young neighbors, couldn't seem to do enough for "Mr. Mac." All of us stayed in touch by phone with Pop and with one another every few days—several times a day during transitions or when there were problems.

Spreading the Work Around

Gerri Clarke: For the first five years I was dialyzing my husband at home, three times a week, I liked to have somebody in the house with me. Both our daughters were babies, and there was always the concern that if something went wrong with the kidney dialysis machine, I needed to be able to concentrate completely on helping Paul.

My mother would come over one night, my mother-in-law another night. My sister was here whenever I needed her. And our friends were absolutely wonderful. When Paul was in the hospital, they had my kids over for dinner almost every night. So I received an enormous amount of support. I never felt totally out there by myself.

Fully half the primary care partners in America tend an ailing loved one with no outside assistance at all. Certainly in many cases circumstances have left these folks with little choice but to go it alone. They may not have any surviving family, or their family lives far away or is just plain unsupportive. They may have just moved to a new area and haven't yet established social contacts. They may live in a small, isolated community that offers few support services.

But others suffer in silence unnecessarily because they don't ask the people around them for help and don't investigate whatever practical assistance they may be able to receive from social service agencies and organizations that serve patients and families affected by a particular illness. Louise Fradkin, co-founder of the caregivers' support organization Children of Aging Parents, observes, "One of the most important lessons for caregivers is to learn how to ask for help. They don't have to do it all themselves."

Caring for a seriously ill or dying loved one often calls for sacrificial efforts on our part, but it demands as well a brutally frank assessment of our limitations. Superhuman investment in another person's life is possible only a limited number of times. Sooner or later you're bound to crack. And if you do, everyone suffers. You drop the ball when you're needed most. The care plan falls to pieces at the worst possible moment. Instead of looking back with pride and resolution, you live to regret the experience and to resent bitterly those who didn't do enough to help. Remember, you have to spread the work around in order to survive.

If there is one essential rule of thumb for primary caregivers, it's this: *Don't do anything someone else can do.* It's our task to make sure things get done and done well, but trying to take on all the major responsibilities singlehandedly is a formula for failure.

We take-charge and caregiving types are naturally inclined to think that it's simpler to handle everything ourselves, that we'll do a better job, that it's not worth upsetting or bothering others, or that it would be easier if everyone just did what they were told. We probably wouldn't adopt that attitude at work, given a complicated, open-ended project to oversee, but when it comes to protecting our own, it's easy to fall instinctively into a siege mentality.

Like sick folks, family members respond in character to illness. The Super Moms will know more than the doctors about a loved one's disease inside of two weeks, while the passive-aggressive types and perennial "victims" will instantly take to wringing their hands—with every variation in between.

First, foremost, and always, talk to your ailing loved one. Her cooperation is critical for any of your plans to work. She can also do some of the asking for herself.

She's often the person most able to comfort and encourage those who are hesitant, frightened, or just don't know what to do.

She's in the best position to speak to those who aren't pulling their share of the load.

She probably has ideas and angles you might not have considered.

She might not be as worried as you are about certain things. She can set her own priorities or help adjust yours.

✱ *Leave as much responsibility in her lap as she can reasonably manage.*

Discuss your own availability and limits frankly with her. In order to minimize unrealistic expectations, miscommunication, and lingering resentment, tell your loved one specifically what you are willing and able to do under the circumstances. This is not to suggest that sick folks deliberately take advantage of caregivers, but it's easy to sit by passively when a highly competent person is anticipating your every need.

Two months after getting home from the hospital following bowel surgery and a badly complicated recovery, Rita Richardson was still languishing in bed watching TV all day. Her grown daughters were knocking themselves out caring for her night after night, week after week—and spending a small fortune on home health aides to keep an eye on their mother while they went off to their own highly demanding day jobs.

Susan and Barbara finally told Rita point-blank that she had to do more for herself. They taught Rita to empty her ileostomy bag, brought in a physical therapist for a few sessions, and kept encouraging her to get up and around

---

VOICE OF EXPERIENCE

"My father-in-law had Alzheimer's disease and couldn't be left alone at night. There were four grown children, including my husband. Each of us would take a weekend and either stay with him or bring him to our house. We had a sitter and some of the teenage grandchildren to stay with him, too."—Diane Young

---

until she was fit enough to feed herself, take her medications, use the telephone, and get to the bathroom under her own steam. Within two weeks they were finally getting a decent night's sleep, while still making sure Rita was safe and well cared for. Rita felt much better, less dependent, and more confident, too.

Extend yourself only when necessary. Save your energy for the inevitable crunch times. As a loved one's health deteriorates or as medical crises come and go, a caregiver can quickly overextend herself. If you rush to his side at every twist in the trail, you'll neglect your own job, family, and health, and find yourself exhausted or unavailable when it matters most.

Unless you know someone is dying imminently—or that this might be your last chance to see him conscious or spend quality time together—as much as possible recruit others to do the in-person comforting and to manage his activities of daily living. Remind yourself that the sick person in bed may be your father, but he's also somebody's brother, grandfather, uncle, husband, colleague, neighbor, and friend. Dole out your time, trips, and emotional reserves judiciously.

Discuss your availability and limits with the rest of the care team. It's easy for others to step back when you appear to have everything under control. Don't wait until you're out on a limb to start sharing the burden.

The Family Conference

Families have different styles and different dynamics. You may be able to coordinate everyone's schedules informally by way of daily telephone updates, as my brothers and I did. For other families, periodically sitting down face-to-face may be more effective. Either way, by having the whole gang lay out a care plan, each player becomes accountable to the group instead of to an individual she may or may not get along with. You'll find surprising sources of support, practical assistance, and insight, plus you'll quickly figure out who can truly be depended on and who to write off from the get-go.

Strategy sessions, no matter how informal, should always be undertaken with the prior knowledge and direct participation of the sick person whenever possible or practical. Whether it's at the bedside, around the dining room table, in a hospital waiting room, or by way of a conference call, let her know who has been invited and exactly what you plan to discuss. If she's unable to attend, report back to her immediately about the meeting and any follow-up conversations. This keeps all of us on our best behavior. Most important, it keeps the locus of control precisely where it belongs, for ultimately it is *her* life, not ours.

Calmly and frankly explain the diagnosis and prognosis as the medical team has presented it, as well as the patient's stated wishes concerning which treatments he wishes to undertake or refuse, how

---

INSIDE INFORMATION

"It's very tiring having to relay the same information over and over," remarks Debbie Bryant, an everyday angel from Gulf Shores, Alabama. "Sometimes you just wish people would leave you alone." To avoid having to recite the patient's medical history interminably, record a daily update on your phone machine: "Hi. It's Tuesday, July 10. Jane is home from the hospital and doing well. The doctor expects her to be feeling better in a few days. Right now she's too tired to receive visitors, but we appreciate your call and your concern. We hope you'll understand if we're not able to get back to you for a little while. Thanks again!" You can also send updates via the mail or E-mail.

---

he prefers to be cared for, and so on. If the sick person isn't up to this himself, then whoever is most familiar with his needs and the particulars of the illness should take the lead. Everyone should be given the same information so that they can thoughtfully consider all the implications for the others involved. Recount a typical day step-by-step, describing explicitly what caring for the sick person entails. This is an ideal opportunity for family and close friends to ask questions, raise specific concerns, and compare notes on availability.

Review a checklist of specific responsibilities. Read it aloud or, better yet, pass around copies and wait for folks to volunteer their time and talents. If you're not getting any feedback, ask the sick person, "So, Mom, how would you like us to handle this?" Try to get things rolling by simply stating what you're able and willing to do yourself and those areas where you could use some help.

Don't let slackers off the hook, but take them to task behind closed doors, not in front of the group.

When divvying up jobs, ask yourself, What are this person's strengths? What is he most comfortable doing? What is convenient for him? Distance, work, dependents at home, and other factors will automatically limit some people's involvement. Chances are, you already know the top three names on your roster of care team

members. Your assertive sister, the corporate attorney, is the natural choice to write a letter protesting the HMO's decision to deny payment for a particular drug, while your quiet and loving brother contributes by cooking, cleaning, and sitting with Mom three evenings a week.

Begin with the absolute basics—activities of daily living, home safety, and medical care—and then work back from there.

Don't let others fall into a pattern of watching from the sidelines. From the outset make sure that everybody can be depended on for at least one task. Ask a reticent family member to take charge of something you know he can master easily. If a person can't manage a task on his own, give him the responsibility of seeing to it that it gets done, either by paying someone else to do it or by mobilizing his own friends and family.

Establish a communication protocol. Put one person in charge of tracking schedules and keeping everyone informed and up to date. Set up a telephone tree and agree on call-back procedures.

Make sure everyone knows how to reach one another at all hours and who to call if they have problems or need to swap assignments. Photocopy and circulate contact information to everyone on the team, then post your copy on the fridge or by the phone.

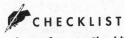

CHECKLIST

Family Conference Checklist

What family, friends, and neighbors can do to help.

Personal Care
- ❑ Provide hands-on nursing care or serve as a daily companion
- ❑ Assist with turning and lifting, bathing, or moving patient around the house
- ❑ Assist regularly with daily meals, dressing, and routine medications
- ❑ Look in regularly on patients who live alone for safety, daily symptom updates, and friendly support
- ❑ Baby-sit or feed primary caregiver's children or elderly relatives
- ❑ Give patient a regular shave, shampoo, haircut or styling, manicure, pedicure, or massage
- ❑ Track down information requested by patient or caregiver regarding anything from treatment options to mail-order buyer's clubs that deliver medications and medical supplies at a discount

Transportation
- ❑ Drive patient to and from doctor and hospital visits
- ❑ Chauffeur children and elderly relatives to and from daily activities
- ❑ Take car in for seasonal maintenance and inspections before problems arise
- ❑ Gas up, wash, and vacuum car
- ❑ Clean out garage

Errands
- ❑ Shop for groceries, especially perishables and bulky or heavy items
- ❑ Have prescriptions filled and pick up medical supplies
- ❑ Get the mail and accept hand deliveries
- ❑ Drop off and pick up dry cleaning
- ❑ Obtain cash or make deposits

"If There's Anything I Can Do ..."

This will be a constant refrain from family, friends, and neighbors. Most of the time they sincerely mean it, but unless you come back at them with a specific request, the offer benefits no one and isn't likely to be made again.

Don't be reluctant to specify what you need: "Would you be able to sit with Pop for three hours Thursday morning? I have an appointment at his lawyer's office." You'll find that most people *appreciate* being given concrete tasks to carry out. When they say, "Call me if you need something," they're usually just sounding you out for clues—not suggesting that you can't manage on your own. Without personal experience caring for this particular person, few folks have any idea what your needs are.

The assumption is that a crisis calls for some sort of extraordinary commitment, a daunting if not paralyzing thought. In reality, everyday acts of kindness—driving the kids to soccer practice, mowing the lawn, anything that eases stress for the caregiver—are profoundly helpful.

Help Around the Home

❑ Prepare meals in advance or while visiting
❑ Make sure laundry gets done regularly and garbage is put out on time
❑ Mow the lawn, shovel snow, clean out gutters, fire up the boiler—any routine yard care and strenuous or time-consuming household chores
❑ Care for pets and houseplants
❑ Reinforce banisters and handrails
❑ Install grab bars in the shower and nonskid liners under rugs
❑ Lift and move furniture that needs rearranging
❑ Install perimeter lights, night-lights, and smoke and carbon monoxide detectors
❑ Hire electricians, plumbers, and others for necessary repairs

Bills and Personal Affairs

❑ Handle patient's monthly bills and banking
❑ File insurance claims and track down payments
❑ File legal documents and tax forms
❑ Assist financially: assume a car or house note temporarily or make the minimum payments on the person's credit cards; pay for extra private-duty nursing; hire a cleaning service; pick up the primary caregiver's phone bill
❑ Find out about specific services or aid, such as home-care agencies and government entitlements
❑ Pick up paperwork, make copies, send faxes, run to the post office, and arrange for messengers and hand deliveries
❑ Help out with correspondence and telephone messages

It's also smart to accept help occasionally from peripheral caregivers. Audree Siden recalls that the day before her husband died of lung cancer, "a close friend called and said, 'I'm coming over. What would you like?' I don't know why, but I said, 'Fresh flowers and oranges.' And she brought them! She looked around the house and told me, 'I'm not leaving,' and she stayed in one of the bunk beds and helped me."

Suzanne Mintz, who cares for her husband, stricken with multiple sclerosis, cofounded the National Family Caregivers Association in 1993. "We suggest that caregivers make a list of all the things they do and keep it by the phone," she says. "When somebody calls and asks, 'Is there anything I can do?,' they have a ready answer." As needs arise—you just ran out of toilet paper or garbage bags—speak up. Don't make the extra trip yourself.

Getting Men Involved

Seven in ten primary caregivers in America are women. According to a report issued by the Older Women's League (OWL), a national advocacy organization specifically for middle-aged and older women, a woman can expect to spend eighteen years of her life help-ing an aging parent.

Part of the disproportionate burden on women is simple demographics. Sta-tistically, women currently outlive men by more than seven years. By the year 2000, the ratio of women to men sev-enty-five and older will be five to two. Although women worldwide have tradi-tionally been the caretakers, nowadays nine in ten American women who are tending a sick or aged person also have a job that accounts for half the house-hold income (in many cases, all of it) or have children to care for, or they suffer from health problems of their own.

So, where are the guys? To be sure, there are good soldiers out there who faithfully nurse a dying wife, parent, sib-ling, or grown child. However, it's more typical for men to stand uncomfortably on the sidelines, perhaps at best helping with tasks that don't require hands-on contact with the sick.

Lou Glasse, president emerita of OWL, attributes this reluctance to get involved to "our early socialization of boys and girls and men and women. We grow up expecting women to take re-sponsibility for providing the compas-sion and care, especially in the home." Many women would probably agree with the blanket generalization that the male of the species tends to exhibit a profound aversion to facing, or even ad-mitting to, the intense emotions a loved one's life-threatening illness kindles.

"My two brothers just could not face our daddy's illness," reflects Diane Young, whose father died of complica-tions from Alzheimer's disease. "One used to say to me, 'I hate to see Daddy like that.' The other was working in a hospital in Saudi Arabia at the time, and when he'd call, he wouldn't want to hear about Daddy."

What can women do to counteract the withdrawal, disappearance, and distanc-ing behavior men often fall into and in-stead draw them into the caregiver fold?

Ask the patient to do the asking first. Instead of constantly badgering your slippery brother to lend a hand, turn to Mom and say, "It would really help a lot if Charles could do your gro-cery shopping this weekend. Would you mind asking him today?" The patient may also be the person best able to en-courage or reassure men who are intim-idated or incapacitated by grief. "I think Charles is nervous about coming over here, Mom. I know he'd feel so much better if you talked to him first."

Save the guilt trips for later and don't assume the worst right away. Maybe he's thinking, *Nobody asked me to help*, while you're thinking, *I shouldn't have to ask*. He may presume you have everything under control. Or he may not know what to do or how to go about it.

Lavish him with positive reinforce-ment. Reward compliance and initia-tive, and don't criticize him if he doesn't get the job right the first time. "I can't tell you what it means to me to know that I can depend on you right now." "Thank you. I love you."

Don't let him off the hook. Some-times it just seems more efficient to let Mom or Sis do most of the grunt work. That might be fine for a short-term cri-sis, but she can't carry all the weight forever. With every new task, ask your-self, "Is this something one of the guys can help with?"

Your husband is squeamish? Put him in charge of keeping up the house, car, and yard. Hand him specific financial or business transactions. Let him go shop-ping and run errands. Lay every practi-cal task you can at his feet. You'll frequently find that the more competent and comfortable he begins to feel, the more he's able to tackle harder assign-ments. Reel him in gradually.

Steal breaks every chance you get. Several men devoted to my father never would have volunteered to care for him directly. Every time one of these friends or former business partners showed up

I'd say, "Sit right there for a few minutes, would you? I need to hop in the shower" or "I just need to run up to the store." I'd disappear and take my time, secure in the knowledge that no matter how uncomfortable the men felt, they had sense enough not to leave Bob alone and to call for help in an emergency.

Get resentments off your chest. Nothing wears down a caregiver like walking around angry and feeling put-upon. Susan Richardson and her sister Barbara uprooted their own lives to care continuously for their ailing mother at home. Their younger brother, a successful business executive with no children and living less than an hour away, offered no practical help and showed up unannounced only on random Sunday afternoons. When his behavior failed to improve in response to a heartfelt letter from Susan, she was able to write him out of her plans with a clean conscience and never look back.

The Ready Reserves: Teenagers and Children

Come July, my brothers and I were in a jam. John and his family were getting ready to leave; Bobby had just started a new job in Savannah, Georgia; and Dave and I both knew we had to ration our own trips judiciously, anticipating the day Pop would require round-the-clock nursing. None of us felt that our father should stay alone.

We got lucky. It was summer and school was out. Without hesitation, Bobby's sixteen-year-old daughter and fourteen-year-old son volunteered to move in with their grandfather temporarily. Lorna and Aaron wound up staying until Labor Day. As my niece recalls, "When I got there, Papa wasn't really, really sick, but he couldn't get out of the house much. I'd go to the store, get his prescriptions filled, and just try to keep up with the normal household chores: washing the clothes, cleaning,

cooking—whatever he needed." Aaron was her man Friday.

Obviously, not all young people are prepared for the weighty responsibilities of caregiving. It is not fair to expect children to rise to the occasion, and it can scar them for life. While it can be healthy, even desirable, to demystify illness and death by carefully exposing young people at an early age, it's up to the grown-ups to make sure they're not in over their heads.

Tell the kids what's going on. Children have amazing capabilities when they understand a situation. Keep them in the dark, however, and they can imagine things to be far worse than they are. Don't tell a child that Grandma is going to get better if she's not. If he wants to see her or participate in her care, tell him that Gran might look different and that she might be feeling tired. Before involving him, make sure he understands that in no way did he cause the illness.

Take your lead from the youngster. Some kids, younger ones especially, jump right in when the adults around them are coping well. Others, particularly adolescents, pull back. Don't try to force a young person to accept any more responsibility for a sick person than she has asked for and you're positive she can handle.

Examine their motives for wanting to help. A number of subconscious impulses may be at work here: to feel useful or grown-up; for girls especially, to follow in the footsteps of their role model, Mom; to receive praise. Perhaps they're seeking the love and attention they've been missing since all the grown-ups became preoccupied with the sick person. Kids sometimes do what they think adults expect from them without fully understanding the implications. There is no such thing as informed consent in this situation.

Assign tasks they can master easily. Stick to duties you know kids can manage, like social interaction (reading, going for walks, playing games) or routine activities (assisting with eating, running errands, housekeeping). Intimate physical care and nursing should be left to adults unless a young person has demonstrated exceptional skill and maturity—and has *freely* volunteered for the job.

Long-Distance Angels

Geography may prevent us from tending a loved one in person, but it's no excuse to stand by idly. As long as you can pay the phone bill, you're still in business.

Louse Fradkin: *I live in Pennsylvania and my sister lives in Atlanta, so when it came to taking care of my mother, I was an only child as far as I was concerned. Finally I decided that I wanted her to help. My mother had lost her short-term memory. When she was still living in her own apartment, I would have to call her on the phone in the morning and talk her through getting dressed, then talk her through getting undressed in the evening. My sister and I worked out a system where she took over the weekend shifts. I wrote out a script for her, timed it for her, and worked out all the pitfalls.*

Fully half the jobs on the Family Conference Checklist (pages 216–217) can be managed over the phone or through the post office, E-mail, fax, or messengers and overnight couriers. Granted, it's easier face-to-face, but out-of-town relatives and friends can provide all sorts of practical and emotional support to ailing loved ones and their caregivers. ▶ *See "Working the Phones," page 226.*

When Friends and Family Disappoint

You can't always predict how the people in your life will respond to a loved one's illness. Some transcend expectations, while others you thought you could rely on may disappoint bitterly.

Walter Miller, suffering from end-stage emphysema, wanted to die at home. "We had the most wonderful people around us," recalls his wife, Nola. "Every Tuesday morning one of our neighbors would sit with Walt so that I could get my hair done." Her husband's condition had deteriorated to the point that "he could have died while they were here," she says, "yet they never rejected us.

"Walt's feet were swollen with edema. One dear neighbor used to come over and rub his feet, saying, 'Walter, I love you.' Another neighbor, a doctor, would help carry him in his wheelchair up and down the stairs. People would just come."

Sadly, the opposite is also true. A 1983 car accident left Duane Travers permanently brain damaged. His older sister, Roslyn, has borne most of the responsibility for Duane, who can no longer work and requires regular supervision. Their father has refused to be involved in Duane's care because Duane had been drinking the night his friend's car veered off the road and into a tree. Duane, then twenty-five, spent several days comatose on a respirator.

"Daddy went to the hospital to identify Duane," says Roslyn. "Then he left town on business for a week, not knowing whether his son was going to live or die. Ever since, Daddy won't have anything to do with Duane. My father is financially very comfortable, yet do you know that he will not help Duane financially in any way? It just kills me. Mother always told me Daddy had a selfish side to him; I guess I realized then that she'd been right."

Pat Still, executive director of the Well Spouse Foundation, a national support organization, observes, "Almost every 'well spouse' discovers that once it becomes clear the patient is not going to get better, eventually most people disappear. Either it's too frightening for them, or they don't want to see the patient the way he is now. We hear that over and over again in our meetings." She, too, had been a "well spouse," caring for her husband, a stroke survivor, until his death from a second, fatal cerebral hemorrhage nine years later.

Betty Lindstrom: For many reasons, you find that friends stop visiting. They never knew if maybe I was trying to catch a few winks of sleep. Then once my husband's Parkinson's disease made it extremely difficult for him to talk, his old buddies and friends didn't want to see him in that condition and didn't know what to say to him. They didn't like to call on the phone because they were afraid that would discourage him.

I felt sorry for the fellows that came over. They loved Clarence and were friends, but eventually they knew they wouldn't come back. And Clarence knew, too.

When friends and family vanish, take the initiative to get in touch. They may be concerned that to call or visit would be an intrusion on you or the patient, and are awaiting your cue.

Also be honest with yourself: Have your friends abandoned you, or have you been forced to abandon them? Priorities change; you get busy with more pressing matters. You'll renew the friendship later—or not.

If all else fails, accept the legitimate limitations, reservations, and even the character flaws of others, and try to move on. "It's hard when you feel all the responsibility is on your back," says Diane Young. While her husband's siblings mobilized to care for her father-in-law, when her own father also developed Alzheimer's disease, "we were not as successful," she admits.

"My husband used to get angry with me and say, 'You've got to get your brothers and sister on the phone. You've got to get them over here.' I'd try, and they would do what they could. But some people can't handle it, and you have to accept that."

Resentment can fester until it poisons relationships, often permanently. "Many primary caregivers become very bitter," comments Louise Fradkin of Children of Aging Parents. "They'll say, 'After Mother or Dad dies, I'm never going to speak to my brothers and sisters again.'"

Nothing tests the bonds of family as sorely as serious illness and death. It shows you exactly what the people around you are made of. Long after the crisis is over, you'll remember who was there when it mattered and who wasn't. Make sure your own conscience is clear, and leave others to live with the ramifications of their own decisions.

How to Handle Weepers and Wailers

Hysterics, weepers, and handwringers, as well as people who constantly criticize and undermine us, need our help finding more productive ways to express their concern. Keep them busy and distracted, and they'll feel useful and behave better.

Sometimes patients lap it up from

others and dish it out themselves. Needling and suspicion are taken for protective concern; histrionics or Sturm und Drang pass for love and heartfelt grief. Outrageous behavior on the sick person's part can be chalked up to his feelings of loss of control over his life. As we pointed out in chapter 4, "Matters of the Heart," the balance of power is dead-set against them. We hold healthy people who just need to get a grip to a very different standard.

After an acquaintance with AIDS lapsed into a sudden coma, I contacted his family, who lived out of state. His mother and two brothers rushed straight from the airport to the hospital at two in the morning exhausted, hungry, dehydrated, agitated—and it was clear they had been drinking. Mom "fell out" on top of her comatose son twice while the two men argued at the top of their lungs over some ancient family conflict. I gently steered them out of the room and calmed them down. I instructed the brothers to take their mother to their hotel, shower, eat something, grab some sleep, pick up the mail, bring their ailing brother fresh socks and underwear in the morning, and make an appointment to meet with his doctor. It doesn't sound like much, but it sure did work. As long as they were busy and distracted, they felt useful and were well behaved.

Suzanne Mintz of the National Family Caregivers Association points out, "Most caregivers work, so a lot of them have business or professional skills, but they forget them when it comes to caregiving. There are things that we let happen in caregiving situations that we would never tolerate at work, such as unfair criticism, lack of recognition, and, most of all, lack of help." When behavior works at cross purposes with the care plan—and that includes interfering with the caregivers' attention to the patient—it's time to take action:

Direct people who act out in destructive ways; give them constructive tasks. Stay two steps ahead of them. Send them off on frequent errands and heap tedious chores on them *before* they get on your nerves or upset the patient. Try putting one high-maintenance visitor in charge of another: "Uncle Avery's just beside himself, Nell. Would you please look after him until I can get finished here? What would I ever do without you?"

Give him the bum's rush. While it's helpful to understand the psychology behind people's dysfunctional behavior, you do not have to tolerate it. And you probably don't have the emotional reserve to deal with it. You are well within your rights to ask the person to leave. Choose your tactics from the caregiver's arsenal: a big smile and a white lie for a gentle sendoff or the honest, direct approach to clear the room of any visitor whose presence is upsetting you or the sick person.

Cheap Shots and Target Practice

Just as sick people can lash out or unreasonably criticize caregivers, sometimes we also find ourselves the target of others' denial, guilt, or frustration. I've witnessed situations where one family member has tried to manage all the responsibilities, leaving him a physical and emotional wreck, and inciting the resentment of family and friends who want to help but feel displaced. Likewise, folks you haven't seen or heard from for weeks will breeze in volunteering all sorts of backhanded "advice" about what you should have done or ought to be doing differently.

Johnetta Romanowski: Dennis's younger brother David was in total denial about how sick Dennis was with lung cancer. He wouldn't visit because he didn't want to see his brother die. One day in the hospital Dennis told him that he knew he wasn't going to make it. When David heard that, he stormed out of the room. Dennis got very upset. I went after David, and we had a huge fight. He accused me of never telling him that Dennis could die, when I had been updating him consistently about everything that was going on.

Finally, I said to him, "Listen, enough of this. We can't be fighting over Dennis's bed. If you want to walk out, don't come back. Don't blame me because you've stayed away from your brother, for whatever reason." We talked for two hours and kind of resolved things. He said to me, "I don't want my brother to die."

Normal friction among the team is handled differently from friction with folks you don't really need. When my brothers and I would occasionally butt heads, we had an unspoken agreement to take it outside. We never disagreed in front of Pop, other family members, or the medical team, always presenting a united front. We didn't avoid discussing our conflicts, for that creates even worse problems. We'd sit on the porch and talk it out or go for a drive if we needed to yell at each other.

When your motives are questioned or your character is impugned, ignore the charges or confront them directly. Judicious investment in power struggles is essential here. As long as *you* know that your loved one is well cared for, opinions to the contrary can be safely disregarded. In deciding how to best handle the situation, ask yourself this: Will your words or actions upset the patient or make life more difficult for the team? Or will it get a heckler out of your hair and send an important message to everyone else to pull their weight or keep quiet?

Caregivers who spread the work around from the very beginning are best positioned to receive plenty of positive reinforcement. Those who don't substantially involve other people from day one run the risk of being abandoned.

A Memo to Family and Friends Who Want to Help . . .

Unless you've experienced it personally, it's hard for anyone to appreciate the magnitude of stress caused by caring for a seriously ill person. Caregivers don't always get the thanks they deserve from patients or other beleaguered loved ones. Similarly, some caregivers feel too guilty to complain or to ventilate mounting frustration and sadness. Besides providing practical help to the patient, there's much friends and family can do to ease the caregiver's burden.

Just be there. Listen. Allow caregivers to unload their anger, resentment, and grief. Offer to run interference for them with folks who work at cross purposes.

Show your appreciation and offer praise. "If the family lives a distance and there's only one person doing the caregiving," says Louise Fradkin, "one of the things others can do is send thank-you notes or say, 'I appreciate what you're doing.' "

Make yourself easy to find. Stay in touch regularly, let family and friends know where they can reach you at any time, and urge them not to hesitate to call. Don't force them to play telephone tag just to make a simple request or to find a friendly ear when they need it most.

Don't offer advice unless you're asked. Remember that most caregivers need a sounding board more than another critical opinion. Hear them out and hold your tongue until your personal judgment has been solicited.

Community Support Services

If you have little or no backup, accessing local resources becomes a necessity. Even if you're surrounded by competent, helpful people, it's worth your while to find out about support services available in your area through government and private agencies. (Better still, give the assignment to a friend or relative.)

"Community services" encompasses an array of helpful programs, including adult day care, meals delivered to the home, and transportation to and from medical appointments. Yet only about one in fifteen family caregivers avails himself of these services. To be sure, not all areas have the resources to offer the full spectrum of programs, and a person who lives in a remote burg may be out of luck entirely. But that low figure also reflects the public's lack of awareness. Louise Fradkin of Children of Aging Parents remarks, "I'm amazed at how many of the caregivers who call our organization have no knowledge of the social service structure or how to access it."

Support services for patients, other ill or elderly dependents, and children include:

- Transportation to and from medical appointments, day programs, and other services provided by volunteer or professional drivers, by bus, taxi, or ambulette (a specially equipped van).
- Meals and nutritional programs provided in a group setting at a central location such as a church, synagogue, senior center, or school, or delivered to the home by local meals-on-wheels or food-bank programs.
- Homemaker services from nonmedical personnel who assist with light chores and housework, shopping, errands, and routine food preparation.
- Home health care and home hospice care provided by nurses, trained home health aides, physical therapists, nutritionists, and other professional services, including medical equipment for the home.
- Respite care, relief for family and friends so they can take a break, either through adult day care or home-care programs, or an overnight stay for the patient in a residential nursing facility.
- Adult day care for ambulatory patients or other dependent adults. These programs offer supervision and organized group activities at a central location for a few hours per week; some provide basic nursing assistance as well.
- Child care or after-school programs for youngsters of primary caregivers.
- Friendly visiting by volunteer groups, including home visits or telephone contact to provide social support and to keep tabs on changes in the patient's condition or new problems as they arise.
- Expert advice on legal affairs, insurance disputes, government entitlements, debtor-creditor and landlord-tenant relations, and the like.
- Nursing home placement for patients who require skilled nursing care that can't be managed at home.
- Mental health services that include individual or family counseling and support groups for bereavement, depression, addiction treatment, or any other social or psychological concerns of the patient and caregivers.

BUT WHAT DOES IT COST?

Many of these services are free. Sometimes donations are requested or the fee is on a sliding scale, based on a person's ability to pay.

- Professional assistance for developing a comprehensive care plan and arranging required medical and social services.

We don't want to give the impression that you merely pick up the phone and order a free car ride. Even when these services exist, it's not always possible to coordinate the logistics. For example, many chapters of the American Cancer Society offer transportation to and from chemotherapy or radiotherapy treatments—provided that a volunteer driver is available the same time as your loved one's appointment, which is not always going to be the case.

Quality and availability of community support services vary widely around the country. Depending on state and county budgets, local charitable contributions, and community involvement in church and volunteer programs, there may be little or no help available beyond family and friends. Even large, well-funded programs may have long waiting lists or highly restrictive eligibility criteria—all the more reason to thoroughly investigate what's out there long before you need it.

How to Find Support Services in Your Area

Government Agencies

A good place to start is the Area Agency on Aging serving your loved one's locality. Created in 1973 as part of the Older Americans Act, AAAs arrange services for senior citizens either directly or through contractors. Programs vary, but all of the more than 650 AAAs nationwide render most if not all of the services described above. They can refer you to services they do not provide di-

rectly or through cooperating agencies, and by law they're supposed to follow up to make sure you got what you needed.

☎ For the number of the Area Agency on Aging serving your patient's community, call Eldercare Locator (800-677-1116), a free referral service administered by the National Association of Area Agencies on Aging.

✳ *AAAs sometimes go under different names, such as Administration on Aging or Senior Citizen's Division.*

Private Agencies

The vast majority of medical and social services in America are provided by not-for-profit organizations, religious denominations, and voluntary civic groups. Get started by calling your local affiliate.

Catholic Charities USA, the country's largest private social service network, serves over 10 million people of all religious and ethnic backgrounds through its more than fourteen hundred local agencies and institutions.

☎ Check the white pages for the Catholic Charities nearest you or call the organization's Virginia headquarters, 703-549-1390.

United Way of America has more than twelve hundred offices throughout the United States. Primarily a fundraising foundation, United Way is a terrific source of information and referrals to community care programs.

☎ Check the white pages for the United Way in your area or call its Virginia headquarters, 703-836-7100.

Others Who May Be Able to Help

- A church, synagogue, or other house of worship to which you or your loved one belongs
- Civic organizations such as the Elks, Kiwanis, Rotary, B'nai B'rith, Sons of Italy
- Local chapters of disease-related organizations
- The county department of social services
- Community Chest organizations
- Union clubs

Transportation services:

☎ American Cancer Society, 800-227-2345/404-320-3333.

☎ Amyotrophic Lateral Sclerosis Association, 800-782-4747/818-340-7500.

* *Airlines rarely publicize the fact that many of them offer what are called "compassion and bereavement fares": reduced rates for people who need to travel by plane to receive medical care or to attend a funeral. Reservation clerks generally aren't able to arrange this service (if they're even aware it exists). Direct your call to the carrier's corporate headquarters or public affairs office.*

Meals programs:

☎ National Meals on Wheels Foundation, 616-531-9909.

Assistance with legal or insurance matters:

☎ American Association of Retired Persons, 202-434-2277.

☎ American Cancer Society, 800-227-2345/404-320-3333.

Others who may know about local support services:

- Social workers at hospitals, dialysis centers, nursing homes, and hospices
- Area churches and synagogues
- The staff at area senior centers
- Physicians and nurses

- Other caregivers and patients you meet at the doctor's office, support group meeting, and so forth.
- National Self-Help Clearinghouse, 25 West 43rd Street, Room 620, New York, NY 10036; 212-354-8525. ▶ *See Appendix B: "Community Services," page 502.*

Working the Phones

We caregivers spend much of our time with the telephone receiver pressed against one ear, foot tapping impatiently, whether it's to line up community services, to inquire into our patient's eligibility for Medicaid, or to question a charge on the hospital bill. Obtaining the information and cooperation you need requires the courteous but assertive phone manner of a telemarketer and the news-gathering skills of a reporter. The tricks below will help you come across more effectively.

Still, brace yourself for frustration. As when dealing with any bureaucracy, at times you'll be tempted to heave the phone out a window. But even when your patience is wearing thin, try to show a little sympathy for social service agency workers, many of whom are underpaid, undertrained, and overburdened with ridiculously large caseloads.

Tips for networking by phone:

- The best time to call is usually in the morning, before the day's phone messages begin piling up.
- Set aside ample time for making important calls.
- Don't take an impatient or angry tone. No matter how frustrated you're feeling, remind yourself, "I can't be the first person to ask this question or have this problem. Let me try another approach." Save your complaints until you've got what you need or until you can get a senior worker on the line.
- Sit down with a pen and a loose-leaf binder or legal pad for taking notes.

INSIDE INFORMATION

If you are orchestrating a loved one's care from afar, order the white pages and Yellow Pages directories for the person's area. You'll recoup the cost by not having to call long-distance information.

- Be concise yet thorough. Organize your thoughts before dialing. Jot down specific questions you have, then cross them off as each is answered. Avoid long harangues, lengthy explanations, and rambling stories. State your business!
- Write down the name of each person you speak to so that when you speak to the next person you can say, "Yes, hello. Janice Jeffries in the billing department suggested you were the person who could help me. My father . . ."
- When the voice at the other end says, "Hold on, I'll transfer you," ask for the extension number in the event you get disconnected. This also allows you to bypass the main switchboard or electronic triage the next time you call.
- After you've written down a name, phone number, or extension, repeat it back to the person; people transpose numbers and misunderstand names all the time.
- Repeat any instructions before you hang up: "Okay, so I have to get the doctor to sign form M11Q, then send it to Regina Law at the Visiting Nurse Service at 555-5000. Is that correct?"
- If your note-taking skills leave something to be desired, consider purchasing an inexpensive telephone recording device so you can tape the conversation and listen to it afterward. Check the instruction booklet for your answering machine; most models have a feature that allows you to record short conversations on the line.
- When those automated electronic voices answer, offering various options that don't clearly meet your needs, remember that you can almost always get a human being on the line by pressing "0" at any time. When you reach a real person, try asking, "Who is the person I should talk to about ———?" They'll say either "I can take care of that" or "You need to call so-and-so at extension ———."
- When waiting for callbacks from service providers, make sure you're available at the number you left. Don't expect them to track you down.
- Be persistent. If you don't find the information you need by following instructions, do not hesitate to ask to speak to a supervisor, unit director, or the agency's public affairs office. Likewise, ask about formal grievance procedures. Sometimes you'll find a decision more forthcoming when you lay out the case to someone in a position to rule on eligibility on the spot.

Professional Case Management

Although the hospital social worker can set the process of accessing community services in motion, the phone work, paperwork, and legwork soon fall to us. For people who live a distance away and have the money, hiring a professional case manager may be a desirable option.

Case managers are usually social workers or nurses who can help assess a patient's needs, identify available services, and help the family maneuver through all the various eligibility requirements and paperwork. They can also work with families to resolve conflicts over the treatment plan or a patient's resistance to new options. They're not cheap, though; professional case managers can charge $75 per hour or more just for an initial evaluation. But it's worth every penny if you can afford it and don't have the time or availability to make up your own plan from scratch.

Resources for Finding a Professional Case Manager

☎ Area Agency on Aging, 800-677-1116.

☎ National Association of Professional Geriatric Care Managers, 1604 North Country Club Road, Tucson, AZ 85716-3195; 520-881-8008.

Social workers, nurses, and psychologists who belong to NAPGCM, founded in 1986, act as private consultants. Depending on the patient's and caregivers' needs, they offer a wide range of services, including screening, arranging, and monitoring in-home help; assisting with financial, legal, or medical issues; and providing counseling and support. A list of members costs $25 (payable by credit card over the phone).

—6—

The Caregiver as Consumer Activist

As fall rolled around, Dave made it a point to visit Pop while heading back east to begin his busy season. "Old man," he teased affectionately, "you're gonna have to hang on past New Year's 'cause I'm on the road until the day after Christmas." Bob laughed and retorted, "I'll see what I can do, son."

Mercifully, although advanced-stage lymphoma commonly spreads to the liver, brain, and lungs, my father never developed symptoms attributable to these particular complications. Still, he was visibly frail and fatigued, often racked by nausea, and steadily losing ground.

Had Bob not decided from the outset to forgo therapeutic treatment, this would have been a time to look into experimental therapies, or *clinical trials*, or to investigate treatments outside the medical mainstream. David and I would have tracked down the necessary information and helped him make sense of it all—as we had done for many friends before.

What Are Clinical Trials?

"Clinical trials" is a broad term used to describe the complicated process of testing new drugs—or new applications of existing medications—in human volunteers. Once approved by the Food and Drug Administration (FDA) for commercial use, a treatment may be officially prescribed as standard therapy and is recognized by insurance companies.

When existing regimens are of limited effectiveness—as with many types of cancer, particularly advanced malignancies—experimental therapies are often used as front-line treatment. In AIDS, none of the FDA-approved antiviral agents and protease inhibitors can claim to subdue HIV permanently. Many thousands of people with AIDS and other severe conditions come to depend on clinical trials for virtually all their medications—and hope.

There are also investigational studies under way around the country to find drugs to improve the quality of life for such presently incurable neurologic conditions as Parkinson's disease, Alzheimer's disease, and amyotrophic lateral sclerosis (ALS). New drugs and procedures for treating heart disease, high blood pressure, liver disease, and kidney failure frequently offer the only chance for survival to folks who are beyond the help of conventional therapy.

Who Pays for Clinical Trials?

The federal government is the single largest source of funding for biomedical research in this country. For every known disease, a corresponding office at the National Institutes of Health oversees science in the field. The NIH, a division of the U.S. Department of Health and Human Services, receives billions of dollars in appropriations from Congress annually, to be divided among the various institutes. Some research is carried out in laboratories and clinics on the NIH campus in Bethesda, Maryland, but the majority of work is contracted out to universities, medical centers, and private labs through fiercely competitive grant applications.

Pharmaceutical manufacturers and biotechnology companies also spend billions on research and development (R&D) of new treatments. Like studies underwritten by the government, corporations contract out human trials to academic medical centers and hospitals nationwide. A few well-endowed private laboratories, too, sponsor original biomedical research. It's hard to imagine where medicine would be today without the likes of the Salk Institute, Rockefeller University, the Mayo Clinic, Memorial Sloan-Kettering Cancer Center, the Aaron Diamond Foundation, and many, many others.

Fair warning: Clinical trials are no bargain. Health care plans rarely pay for experimental treatments. Should you require hospitalization, home care, diagnostic tests, or other drugs to manage side effects and complications, you must submit all claims to the insurer just as if your family doctor had ordered them. You also waive your right to hold the manufacturer and the medical center liable for adverse outcomes, including premature death.

From Laboratory to Marketplace

For every five compounds pronounced safe enough *to test* in humans—after two or more years of laboratory study and animal experiments—*four thousand* others were judged unsafe or ineffective, and abandoned. Of those five that make it to human trials, only one will go on to receive the FDA's blessing. Until very recently, every patient who enrolled in a formal drug protocol at a medical center was randomly assigned to a *control* group or a *study* group. Members of control groups receive the standard form of approved treatment, while study group participants are given the new treatment. During the earliest phases of drug testing, the control group may sometimes receive what's called a *placebo*, or an inactive medication. Patients are told they have the right to drop out of a study at any time and receive the standard treatment, if one exists.

Phase I studies principally measure the *toxicology* of a new drug, or how dangerous it is to humans. They are usually "open-label," meaning that the patient and doctors know precisely what's being given. Phase II and III studies, also known as *efficacy* trials, are often "single-blind": The patient doesn't know whether he's receiving standard or experimental treatment. In "double-blind" trials, neither the patient nor the investigators know which combinations or doses are administered.

When volunteers have terminal diseases, though, the rules are far less restrictive. For people who would likely die without further treatment or for whom standard treatment has failed,

TABLE 6
The Development and Approval Process

Objective	Number of Volunteers	Approximate Length of Time
Phase I		
Determining safety and dosage	20 to 80 healthy people and patients considered incurable	1 year
Phase II		
Evaluating effectiveness and severity of side effects	100 to 300 patients	2 years
Phase III		
Further evaluating effectiveness and long-term side effects	1,000 to 3,000 patients	3 years

the FDA routinely allows them access to (1) new, unapproved drugs and (2) "off-label" drugs that have been approved for other purposes. This practice, known officially as "compassionate use," often provides quick knowledge about the effectiveness and shortcomings of investigational new drugs for AIDS, cancer, and many other incurable diseases. A patient must be advised of possible known risks and must give *informed consent* in writing to receive such treatment.

In another effort to speed up the drug development-and-approval process, since 1989 the FDA has allowed researchers to combine Phases II and III if a new medication is intended to fight a life-threatening condition. New community-based research models—in which dozens of physicians around the country simultaneously compare notes on the use of a new drug on many patients at various stages of disease—are quickly replacing double-blind, placebo-controlled studies.

For diseases in which *every* treatment option is experimental, studies have begun that simultaneously compare the performance of multiple new drugs against one another. These trials don't involve placebos and, thanks to new statistical models, allow far more hard data to be collected over a much shorter period. Doctors and patients can also decide for themselves which doses and combinations to attempt.

When a given trial has yielded sufficient data, the findings are presented to the FDA. Although by law the FDA is supposed to complete its review within six months, the process may stretch to two years. Still, a 1995 report showed the FDA approved drugs twice as fast as it did just half a decade before, when ten years was the average. Once approved, the new drug takes its place among licensed therapies, and the long process of teaching doctors to use it begins.

How Do You Find Out About Clinical Trials?

Start by asking the doctor if he knows of any local trials accepting patients that might benefit your loved one. If so, he can directly contact the investigators running the study and see if the person meets the eligibility requirements, which can be highly restrictive for scientific reasons. For example, a new combination chemotherapy protocol for metastatic breast cancer may require that a patient have already failed to respond to two or three other drugs; or a trial testing a new protease inhibitor may be limited to AIDS patients who are not taking other protease inhibitors.

According to the Center for Medical Consumers in New York, "Studies have shown that fewer than half, and sometimes fewer than one-third, of physicians are aware of important new medical information even years after it has been published." Consequently, it often falls to us as the patient's advocate to unearth what's available and where, and contact the investigators ourselves.

Call around to teaching hospitals. Ask for the medical department concerned with your loved one's disease. Tell the receptionist, "My mother has _____, and I need information about standard and experimental treatments. Who is the person I should talk to there?"

Expect to reach a research nurse or a postdoctoral fellow in charge of recruiting volunteers for various protocols. Make an appointment to see them or ask them to mail you information. With a little coaxing they'll even help you find out what is available elsewhere, if only by sending you copies of medical journal articles and newsletters. Check the footnotes for more citations that you can look up yourself at the library or order reprints of material that's of interest.

Also, many hospitals, especially large medical centers, have established community affairs offices and patient information services for just this purpose. Ask the switchboard operator to connect you.

Call the government-run information lines and patient-support or-ganizations listed below. While they usually can inform you of all studies being sponsored by government agencies, not all may be aware of the many privately funded trials. This requires a little more legwork.

Call the pharmaceutical manufacturers themselves. For numbers of drug companies, consult the *Physicians' Desk Reference* at your local library or bookstore. The hefty reference book includes an index of drug manufacturers, most of which have toll-free numbers. Ask them about their experimental products you've read about in articles or heard mentioned by doctors or other patients and caregivers.

Hop on the Internet with the help of a computer-literate friend or family member. Visit the CenterWatch Clinical Trials Listing Service at http://www.centerwatch.com/LISTING.HTM or drop into any of the various chat groups for diabetics, people with HIV, cancer, heart disease, and other groups of patients.

The Pros and Cons of Participating in a Clinical Trial

For a few exceptionally altruistic or desperate souls, trying new treatments may bring satisfaction just in knowing the results may yield vital information that will benefit other patients in the future. But deep down most of us are naturally predisposed to want to know what's in it for us. With good reason, a seriously ill patient is scared for his life and, understandably, susceptible to hopeful claims.

Research protocols, though conducted by legitimate institutions and distinguished individuals, need to be investigated carefully. Doctors have their own biases and will tend to present studies in their rosiest light, but our loved one has nothing to compare them to and in general has no basis on which

Whom to Call to Learn About Clinical Trials

AIDS/HIV
AIDS Clinical Trials Information Service
  800-874-2572
AIDS Treatment Data Network
  800-734-7104
American Foundation for AIDS Research
  800-392-6327
Gay Men's Health Crisis Hotline
  212-807-6655
People with AIDS Coalition of New York
  800-828-3280
Project Inform Treatment Hotline
  800-822-7422

Alzheimer's Disease
Alzheimer's Disease and Related
  Disorders Association
  800-272-3900
Alzheimer's Disease Education and
  Referral Center
  800-438-4380

Amyotrophic Lateral Sclerosis
The Amyotrophic Lateral Sclerosis
  Association
  800-782-4747
Les Turner Amyotrophic Lateral Sclerosis
  Foundation
  847-679-3311

Cancer
American Brain Tumor Association
  800-886-2282
American Cancer Society
  800-227-2345
Cancer Information Service
  800-422-6237
International Myeloma Foundation
  800-452-2873
National Brain Tumor Foundation
  800-934-2873

Cardiovascular Disease
American Heart Association
  800-242-8721

Cerebrovascular Stroke
National Stroke Association
  800-787-6537
Stroke Connection of the American Heart
  Association
  800-553-6321

Diabetes
American Diabetes Association
  800-342-2383
National Diabetes Information
  Clearinghouse
  301-654-3327

Head Injury
Brain Injury Association
  800-444-6443

Liver Disease
American Liver Foundation
  800-223-0179

Parkinson's Disease
The American Parkinson's Disease
  Association
  800-223-2732
National Parkinson Foundation
  800-327-4545
  800-433-7022 in Florida
Parkinson's Disease Foundation
  800-457-6676
United Parkinson Foundation
  312-733-1893

Rare Disorders
National Organization for Rare Disorders
  800-999-6673

to make a truly informed decision. Before signing the consent form, patients need to consider carefully all possible outcomes, such as:

What if the side effects are unbearable? Discuss this up front with the medical team. If a terminal patient is racked with pain or nausea, we can keep loading narcotics and antiemetic drugs until he's essentially unconscious. However, this is neither practical nor safe in conjunction with receiving ongoing treatment.

Bank on the fact that all powerful treatments will cause side effects and that complications will inevitably arise in every major disease. It is essential that we and the medical team agree from the start on the parameters of symptom control. Discuss both best-case and worst-case scenarios explicitly. If at any point side effects and complications threaten to outweigh the benefits of continued therapy—or if the patient simply cannot tolerate the treatment—consider alternatives: Find out in advance whether the patient can switch to another trial, if such a thing exists, and what the eligibility requirements and restrictions are. Can he choose to return to a standard treatment again, if one exists, with heightened attention to symptom management? Can your loved one refuse further therapeutic treatment and opt for *palliative* medical care to control symptoms?

What if the treatment proves too risky? Death and disability are possibilities that must be explored explicitly with the doctor before starting. Chances are, if a patient responds poorly in a protocol, we'll see the decline come gradually. But during treatment some people suffer sudden, severe drug reactions or organ failures; others develop overwhelming infections and life-threatening blood disorders.

This is why it is so important that the decision to participate in a trial be an informed one, based on reasonable hope rather than desperation or fear. While it's essential to think positively when undertaking new treatment, the stakes are too high to indulge in wishful thinking.

Questions to Ask the Physician When Considering Participation in a Clinical Trial

- What is the purpose of the study?
- What tests and treatments are involved: what is done, where is it done, how is it done, and by whom?
- What will likely happen to me with and without this new treatment?
- What effects will the new medication or procedure likely have on the disease and on me?
- What are my other choices, and what are their advantages and disadvantages?
- Are there standard treatments for my disease, and how do they compare to the investigational treatment?
- Are there other experimental studies being conducted elsewhere?
- How will this affect my daily life?
- What side effects can I anticipate, and what can be done to manage them?
- How long will the study last?
- What medical options will I have after the study is over?
- Will I have to be hospitalized? If so, how often and for how long?
- How frequently will I have to travel to the hospital, doctor's office, or clinic for treatment and tests?
- How long does each trip really take?
- What kind of delays typically crop up during routine visits?
- What are the actual financial costs to me? (You'll need to know exactly, because many of them will fall to you and your insurer.)
- If the experimental treatment harms me, to what medical treatment would I be entitled?

• What kind of long-term follow-up care is part of the study?

"Also ask if there have been any preliminary results from earlier phases of the trial," suggests Dr. Jack Lord of the American Hospital Association. In what ways is the patient similar to subjects who responded well to the new treatment? How does his case differ?

Most important of all, ask the doctor conducting the study or a research nurse to put you in touch with someone who dropped out of the trial previously. (Many times people discontinue experimental treatments due to straightforward medical reasons and opt for another treatment under the same doctor's care.) The person's case might not be comparable to your loved one's, but you'll pick up inside information about pitfalls that were overlooked or underestimated, or that have been glossed over or minimized by the medical staff. Talking to people currently in the trial can also provide practical tips about managing symptoms and negotiating institutional hurdles.

The big question few people ask is "Will it make a difference?" Point-blank. "My father has lymphoma. Do you have any treatment that's going to save his life? Yes or no. Or, more likely, is it going to buy him a few weeks or months, in which case, what will his quality of life be like?" Answering questions such as that honestly and directly is one of the kindest and most helpful things a health care professional can offer, as much as we might hate to hear it.

A Rational Approach to Unconventional Treatments

Out of necessity or frustration, both patients and those around them may be tempted to try treatments outside the medical mainstream. A survey published in the *New England Journal of Medicine* estimated that Americans now spend billions of dollars on socalled alternative therapies annually.

Biofeedback and acupuncture are just two nontraditional therapies that have found places as valuable *complements* to traditional treatment, to help combat symptoms or side effects such as high blood pressure, pain, nausea, and anxiety. In 1991 the NIH established an office of alternative medicine—a welcome sign that Western medicine had finally begun to consider unconventional treatments seriously.

This is a path to proceed down cautiously, however. Peruse health newsletters or web sites on the Internet, and you'll come across practitioners of dubious qualification claiming to have cured cancer through macrobiotics or vitamin therapy.

"What's the harm of trying them?" In many instances, there is none as long as the patient doesn't ignore her regular doctor. In fact, anything that doesn't cause further harm is worth a try if it makes a sick person feel better. On the other hand, a few patients have starved to death following unsupervised lowprotein macrobiotic diets when they were already dangerously wasted from cancer or AIDS, and excessive doses of various vitamins frequently produce highly toxic reactions.

While many proponents of unconventional therapies claim that their treatment produces minimal side effects or none at all, a 1991 study conducted at the University of North Carolina offered contradictory evidence. The terminal cancer patients who subjected themselves to several extreme "cures" endured harsher side effects than those who accepted chemotherapy and radiation. Nor did they live any longer than the men and women treated conventionally.

"When dealing with any terminal illness, particularly cancer and AIDS, there are a lot of charlatans out there who are out to make money," warns Dr.

Howard Grossman, an internist and AIDS specialist at St. Luke's–Roosevelt Hospital in New York City. "It's important for patients to read a lot about what's going on in alternative medicine, and also to have a doctor they can trust."

Certainly not all practitioners of alternative medicine are charlatans—far from it. For example, pain teams at the most sophisticated medical centers in the world routinely use hypnosis and massage to augment their narcotic cabinets. Nutritionists, psychiatrists, and chiropractors have been the close allies of heart surgeons, oncologists, and neurologists for decades now.

When researching scientifically unproven treatments or so-called cures, bear in mind that patients and care partners alike are dangerously vulnerable to fanciful claims. The sensible guidelines below will help you avoid potentially grievous mistakes:

- *Exercise healthy skepticism* when considering practitioners who boast degrees unrecognized by accredited or well-known academic institutions or professional associations, such as a doctor of naturopathy or doctor of metaphysics granted by a mail-order university.

  ✳ But also keep in mind that impressive advanced degrees from a prestigious school don't guarantee that a doctor isn't a mercenary healer providing window dressing for a pharmaceutical manufacturer or product promoter.

- *Question practitioners who cry persecution* by the Western medical establishment or U.S. regulatory agencies . . .

  ✳ . . . though this happens to a few exceptionally rare scientists who are truly ahead of their times. For proprietary reasons alone, pharmaceutical executives and government scientists have also been known to deliberately delay releasing into the American marketplace new drugs or techniques already approved in Europe or Japan.

- *Think twice about practitioners who do not report their findings* in professional journals, reputable health newsletters, or science magazines but only in promotional materials intended for laymen's eyes.

- *Steer clear of practitioners who distort facts* or offer flimsy scientific proof of their successes. For instance, inflated accounts of patients restored to health by way of alternative means often neglect to mention that these folks were receiving standard treatment at the same time. Others tell outright lies.

  ✳ The doctor's promotional brochure boasts of curing fifty people suffering from Lou Gehrig's disease? Don't be swayed by claims that sound too good to be true.

- *Carefully investigate practitioners who are not licensed and registered* by the state or not working in an institution where their peers regularly review their work. However, many helpful practitioners often work independently of medical centers and hospitals. Ask for and thoroughly check their references. If they refuse your request, beat a hasty retreat.

- *Avoid practitioners who claim* their product is effective at treating a wide range of ailments, although some tried-and-true ancient techniques, such as Chinese herbs or meditation, may have broad applications when it comes to symptom control.

- *Avoid practitioners who fail to disclose* the specific treatment methods used, including substances, devices, vitamins, serums, and so forth.

- *Avoid practitioners who promise* a quick and painless cure in exchange for money.

If more than a couple of these general warnings hold true, you should probably consider other options. Above all, disregard any treatment which promises that it alone can cure a disease, that advocates abandoning conventional Western medical care, or that attempts to blame sickness or disease on the patient or some "conspiracy" to conceal cures from the public.

✱ *Should a loved one decide to try an unorthodox therapy, be sure to inform her primary physician.*

How Do You Find Out About Alternative Therapies?

Other patients and caregivers, newsletters, journals and magazines, information lines, and medical professionals can be valuable resources. The Internet, too, is a vast repository of information —and, unfortunately, misinformation. Because many health forums, news groups, and web sites go unedited by informed medical professionals, cyberspace is littered with mistakes or outright fabrications. The FDA investigates unfounded claims only *after* unsuspecting consumers have been duped.

✱ *Report suspected instances of fraudulent drug offerings on the Internet by E-mailing otcfraud@cder.fda.gov.*

Your patient's physician should always treat your questions seriously, no matter how ostensibly preposterous. His response should be along the lines of "I don't know about that, but if you'll give me a copy of the article, I'll look it over, and we can discuss whether this might be something worth trying."

If instead the doctor's reaction is profoundly negative, ask him what experience he has with the technique and how he came to such an unequivocal conclusion. Thoughtfully consider the physician's advice before trying anything new and ask him if he would still be willing to follow the patient if the unconventional route were taken despite his reservations.

When Is Enough Enough? Changing Course from Cure to Comfort

Whether investigating standard, experimental, or alternative treatments, patients and caregivers have to ask themselves honestly if they're being realistic in chasing after a cure. As long as a sick person is determined to persevere with treatment no matter the outcome, it's our job to help him do so. On the other hand, inevitably there comes a time to turn our attention from therapeutic treatment to supportive care.

Sometimes you have no choice: Your loved one takes a sudden turn for the worse as a result of complications of the disease or treatments. More often, when treatments plainly fail and no other reasonable options remain, folks switch to palliative care—in which symptom control and patient comfort take medical priority. Others, like my dad, make a conscious choice. Either way, a sick person has to stare down death; our preeminent task as caregivers is to reassure our loved one constantly by word and deed that we can be depended on no matter what path he chooses.

Any decision to terminate treatment needs to be examined carefully. Is the patient temporarily depressed, momentarily overwhelmed by side effects, and simply feeling hopeless? Are the caregivers utterly exhausted, stressed-out, bankrupt, and heartbroken? These are some of the toughest judgment calls we will ever make.

Take your lead from the patient. It's her life; it's her death. Whether she declares she's through or that she'll never give up, tell her you'll be by her side every step of the way.

Discuss all possible outcomes with the doctor before stopping or continuing therapy. The idea of going home to die peacefully surrounded by loved ones may sound very appealing to someone who has just endured a terrible and ineffective round of chemotherapy, without realizing what dying at home from cancer actually entails. Likewise, a patient or caregiver may have sadly naive notions of what's to come when he vows, "I'll do whatever it takes. No matter how bad it gets, I'm going to keep fighting."

Discuss the patient's wishes and rationale with the entire care team. To avoid unrealistic expectations, mixed signals, and later recriminations, keep friends and family abreast of decision-making criteria and time lines.

Discuss your own feelings and preferences explicitly with the patient. Maybe she's afraid of becoming an even greater burden, whether she chooses to keep fighting or to go home and die. Neither decision should be clouded by guilt. Make sure she knows you're with her either way.

When Bob told David he was considering skipping chemo, he admitted to one reservation: "I don't want to cop out or anything."

David assured him, "If it were me, I wouldn't do anything, either." To hear that from his son who had been living courageously with the HIV virus for more than ten years meant an awful lot.

Making Other Arrangements: Home Care, Hospice Care, and Nursing Home Care

Louise Fradkin: In 1973 my seventy-seven-year-old mother went in for an operation perfectly alert, healthy, and active. During the surgery, there was a lack of oxygen to her brain, and she lost all of her long-term memory. It was as if nothing had ever happened to her in her life before that point.

She functioned all right in her apartment for a while. Eventually, I got a home health aide to monitor her, because her short-term memory started to fail, and then her mental faculties. For the next seven years she lived with me and my husband.

Finally, I had to put my mother in a nursing home. She was incontinent and by this time had forgotten how to walk. I have a bad back and could not physically transport her anymore. Plus, I was just worn out. We kept her in her apartment longer than we should have, because we felt her independence was important to her. We refused to look at the situation realistically. It's very hard to accept the fact that the person you love is different and is slipping.

It's the rare adult who grapples ahead of time with the medical, emotional, financial, and logistical implications of caring for sick folks at home or in a nursing home. Caregivers and patients alike frequently make hurried decisions in mid-crisis, only to regret them later. In order to formulate a care plan that will hold up, come what may, we need to know exactly what resources are available, then make the most of them.

Why Home Care?

The advantages of home care are obvious in many cases. The patient enjoys the comfort, privacy, and security of home. For caregivers it can be far more convenient than institutional alternatives, and we can personally supervise the nursing care and our patient's activities of daily living. What's more, professional advice—from a doctor or home-care agency—is just a phone call away.

Home care is infinitely less expensive, too. For example, daily hospital costs for an AIDS or cancer patient total about $800, and exponentially more if the patient is critically ill or dying. Decent nursing homes, if you can even find a bed, cost upward of $400 a day just for minimal services. A day of home care, on the other hand, costs less than $100 on average.

Improved medical technology has made many treatments possible outside a medical institution. IV infusions, sophisticated pain management protocols, dialysis, tube feelings, and mechanical ventilation are all routinely administered at home. And with the rapid escalation of health care costs, insurance companies and large employers have come to encourage hospitals to discharge patients as quickly as possible, often before they've recuperated sufficiently to care for themselves. Whether we choose it or are forced to accept it, home care often provides the most humane and cost-effective way to care for the sick.

The downside? You receive only a few hours of outside help a day; you pay out of pocket for any extra shifts. Medicare and private insurers also enforce strict time limits for ongoing home services. Even more significant than cost, however, is the practical impact of home care on family life. Strangers troop through your home, an unnerving experience for novice caregivers. And when they go, you're left to nurse a seriously ill person around the clock essentially alone—a daunting prospect, to say the least.

Home Health Care Personnel

The most important members of a home-care team are the spouse, children, other family, and close friends who in fact provide most of the care. But there's a wide array of health care personnel and services to back you up.

Professional Nurses

The first person you meet from a home-care agency is usually a registered nurse. She reviews the medical orders, examines the patient, consults with the physician if necessary, draws up a list of home-care duties, and helps arrange all other essential services. The nurse becomes the medical case manager for the patient, scheduling home health aides, looking in on the patient periodically, and responding to medical questions or emergency calls.

During subsequent visits she provides skilled nursing services such as IV therapy, injections, wound management, ostomy care, catheter care, and the like. The nurse also instructs family members how to perform all the various medical tasks, keeps tabs on medications, tracks new symptoms, and communicates with the doctor as problems arise.

Home Health Aides and Homemakers

Day-to-day care of the patient falls essentially to *home health aides* or *nursing assistants*, trained to provide routine help with bathing and toileting, feeding, dressing, turning and bed changing, and just getting around the house. They monitor vital signs, measure fluid intake and output, and perform any other duties assigned by the nurse. They do not administer medications.

Homemakers assist with household chores such as light cleaning, shopping, and basic food preparation but not nursing care.

Therapists and Dietitians

Physical therapists and *occupational therapists* help patients and families develop essential skills for daily life, such as teaching someone to use crutches, a cane, walker, or wheelchair; helping patients learn to dress, eat, sit, stand, and walk after a brain injury; or just showing family members simple range-of-motion exercises to prevent painful muscle contractures in a bedridden patient.

Speech and language pathologists help folks who have trouble talking or swallowing; *respiratory therapy technicians* treat breathing difficulties. *Di-*

etitians help families develop palatable menus for medically restricted diets. They also make sure the patient stays adequately nourished in spite of symptoms like nausea and diarrhea by prescribing nutritional supplements.

Social Workers

Although they're trained counselors, *social workers* at home-care agencies are principally occupied with administrative case management. They sort through the patient's eligibility for government entitlements—especially Medicare, Medicaid, and Social Security benefits—and arrange other services available in the community such as meals and transportation.

Many hospitals, nursing homes, and hospice programs run their own certified home-care agencies. Large nonprofit organizations such as the Visiting Nurse Association, as well as many independent operators, provide excellent home care, too.

Home Hospice Care

Home health care and home hospice care really need to be discussed in tandem. Many folks think of a hospice as a *place;* to be sure, many hospitals and nursing homes do have inpatient units that are especially for dying patients who can't be managed at home. More often, however, hospice is a philosophy. It is simply conscientious home care without the expectation of the patient's recovering. As hospice nurse Ellen Wilson explains, "What we try to do is use some of the technologies we have available so a person can die in comfort, whether physically, emotionally, or spiritually."

Hospice programs offer palliative care, which includes controlling pain and managing other adverse symptoms such as nausea, anxiety, and shortness of breath. Particular attention is paid to the practical and emotional needs of the patient and family. Hospice programs were extremely rare in America until the mid-1960s, but more than two thousand exist today. The number of people dying in hospice care has risen 13 percent annually over the last ten years, a trend that only promises to accelerate as the population ages and more programs are established around the country.

How to Locate Home Health Care and Hospice Care

Besides talking to the physician and the hospital discharge planner, contact any of the following national organizations for referrals to reputable home-care agencies and hospice programs in the patient's area:

☎ Catholic Charities USA, 703-549-1390.

☎ Hospicelink, 800-331-1620.

☎ National Association for Home Care, 202-547-7424.

☎ National Hospice Organization, 800-658-8898.

☎ United Way of America, 703-836-7100.

☎ Visiting Nurse Associations of America, 888-866-8773.

► *See Appendix C, page 515.*

Making Home Care Work

Unless you're financially well off enough to hire live-in staff or a paid companion, rarely are caregivers in a position to select the specific individuals who will provide home care. Instead we hire an agency, usually the one recommended by the hospital discharge planner or the doctor's office, and the agency assigns the necessary personnel to our case. Many areas have only one or two local providers (both probably understaffed to begin with), which means that the caregiver's job is less about shopping around than about knowing how to get what you need from the agency.

The advantages of working with a certified home-care agency are twenty-four-hour backup, a pool of trained personnel to call on, and reimbursement from third-party payers like Medicare and private insurers. You also have a place to complain about lapses in care, a source to turn to for logistical glitches, and expert assistance when creating or modifying the treatment plan as new medical problems develop.

Make sure the home-care agency is Medicare certified. Certification or lack of certification is not an indication of quality; it simply means that the agency accepts reimbursement from third-party payers, a necessity for most of us.

Make sure the agency is licensed by the state and accredited by its professional association. Licensure is a *minimum* standard set by the state department of health and therefore no real indication of quality. However, accreditation does at least signify that the agency is periodically inspected by other professionals in the field for compliance with industry standards. Check with one of the following groups if you have any doubt about the status of an agency:

☎ Community Health Accreditation Program, 800-669-1656.

☎ Foundation for Hospice and Homecare, 202-547-7424.

☎ Joint Commission on Accreditation of Healthcare Organizations, Department of Home Care Accreditation Services, 630-792-3004.
► *For more information about these organizations, see Appendix C, page 515.*

Find out whether an individual is currently licensed and registered. To do this, check with the department of health, board of regents, or department of education listed in the directory of your state capital. You need only sup-ply the person's name, although a license number or Social Security number speeds the search. Never hesitate to ask anyone you're considering hiring for their license number—it's public information—and be wary of anyone who resists giving it to you. Just because an agency is Medicare certified, state licensed, and fully accredited does not mean that your home-care experience will be free of problems. Further checking will alert you to common complaints and drawbacks, and perhaps save you some time and grief.

Check references. Ask your doctor or hospital discharge planner if he regularly makes referrals to the agency and his impressions of the services. Inquire among friends, family, and fellow patients who have used the group before. Ask the agency to give you a list of people familiar with its reputation, then call them.

✳ *When hiring individuals to provide home care, check their references thoroughly yourself. There's simply no other way to screen for dependability.*

Outline a job description. Sit down with the visiting nurse and make a comprehensive list of the daily duties to be carried out by home-care personnel. Review the list at the beginning of each shift with every worker. Don't presume that they've been adequately briefed on your patient. Tell them exactly what you need and respond to any questions or reservations they may have. Inspect their work regularly and call any oversights to the attention of the nurse or worker immediately.

Define unacceptable behavior explicitly. Diplomatically but emphatically make it clear to the supervising nurse and to each worker what you expect up front. You don't have to like a home-care worker; as long as she's competent and kind to your loved one, you're darn lucky to have her. On the other hand, when people are in your home to do a job, they need to know the ground rules.

Reasonable demands include consistent punctuality, advance notice of schedule changes or cancellations, rules about smoking or swearing around the patient, limiting personal phone calls to two or three minutes, not admitting anyone into the house you haven't specifically authorized, and so on. Ask the nurse to explain procedures for terminating a worker *before* problems crop up. Don't hesitate to complain to the agency's chief administrator or clinical supervisor.

Agree on billing and payment procedures before hiring an agency or individual. Make sure you get a separate written statement that explains all costs that appear on the bill. Maintain your own up-to-date records of the specific hours worked by all agency personnel as well as the purpose of each visit. Don't be a miser, though. It doesn't hurt to tip or bestow thoughtful gifts or favors on especially helpful home-care workers who make your life easier. Be as flexible and accommodating with their schedule as you possibly can.

Make sure workers know what to do and whom to call in an emergency. Remind each worker at the beginning of each shift how to reach you at all times. Make sure the nurse has briefed workers on special requests, such as *not* calling 911 should the patient stop breathing. Reiterate all special instructions at the beginning of each shift.

As with members of the hospital staff, developing a rapport with the people from a home-care agency is essential. There's no substitute for knowing what's going on yourself and whom to call to keep things running smoothly. Regular inspections and constant communication with the nurses and home-care workers is the only way to make sure that your loved one's care is up to snuff.

In those rare circumstances where you suspect dishonesty, abuse, or neglect, take up the matter with the nurse or agency administrator immediately. Act on your instincts and ban any worker who makes you or the patient uncomfortable. It may mean more work for you temporarily, but it's a small price to pay for the safety and peace of mind of your loved one—and you.

When Cultures Collide: Building Rapport Across Class, Race, and Gender

More than nine in ten home-care aides and nursing assistants are women. Most earn minimum wage, and less than half have health insurance. According to the Older Women's League, a Washington-based education-and-advocacy group, "The women who bathe, feed, dress, and care for our parents and children earn less than parking lot attendants."

Needless to say, there is great difficulty recruiting and retaining well-trained and experienced people for such thankless work. Home care is one of the few alternatives for entry-level employment outside the fast-food industry. Recent immigrants, unskilled young people just joining the workforce, retirees and moms looking for part-time work are often the best and only takers. Those who do persevere and manage to eke out a living are stretched to the limit. You can bet your loved one is not the only seriously ill person your aide is tending. Workers are always on their way to or from another patient's house, and delays crop up routinely. Aides get stuck at other jobs; nurses get sidetracked and reschedule with little notice as often as not. At any point a perfect stranger is likely to be assigned to your case temporarily.

It's natural to feel uneasy when someone you've just met is given free rein in your home. But mix in even the slightest suggestion of racial bias, chauvinism, or arrogance on the part of the patient or caregiver, and instead of working together as a team, a counter-productive working relationship develops. Some address aides and nursing assistants condescendingly or disrespectfully, or are overly critical. Others keep looking over the shoulders of dependable workers, long after they've proved their competence. We're not suggesting that caregivers and sick people suddenly start worrying about acting politically correct in their own homes. It's just that common social prejudices, sexually suggestive remarks, simple faux pas, and perceived slights frequently sabotage the best-laid home-care plans and leave you without the help you so urgently need.

Shortly after Bob's diagnosis of lymphoma, he signed up with the same home-care program that had cared for our stepmother Lynn. My dad was earnestly respectful of and sincerely interested in every man and woman he met, no matter their age or race. That was part of his charm. Yet he was a son of the Old South and still given to occasional use of the n word. Each morning before the home-care worker arrived, David and I would threaten to drown Pop in the canal if he didn't watch his mouth.

We also warned the aides that Dad and some of his friends would inevitably slip up and say something offensive. We implored each of the women who cared for Bob to give us a chance to speak to him before they quit in a huff. Our dependence on the solid team we had assembled and organized far outweighed any discomfort Bob felt being censored by his sons. All in all, he did behave like a gentleman most of the time.

When someone you've never met is on her way over from the agency, pause for a moment and put yourself in her shoes. Make it your business to get off to a good start by treating her as you would expect to be treated if the tables were turned.

Eliminate awkward social exchanges by taking the initiative. Greet new arrivals at the door, look them in the eye, and offer a firm handshake. Introduce yourself and tell them outright how to address you and the patient. "Hi, I'm Mr. McFarlane's son. Please call me Rodger. This is my father, Mr. McFarlane." If you can't be there in person, phone her at the beginning of the shift.

Until she tells you otherwise, refer to and address her by her surname, preceded by "Ms." Make it a point to introduce her formally to everyone else who is present. Say "please" and "thank you." Answer with "yes, ma'am" and "no, ma'am" if she's obviously older than you, until she volunteers that there's no need.

Start establishing a rapport by striking up a conversation. Break the ice and get to know a little about her. Ask her how long she's been with the agency or if she's cared for someone in your loved one's condition before. Give her a tour of the house. Show some interest in her work and help out all you can, especially in the beginning. Explain a little about your own circumstances.

Make requests instead of giving orders. It's easy to sound condescending when you use the imperative voice. Ask people to do things instead of telling them. Demonstrate the way you like things done and offer suggestions rather constant criticism.

Get out of her way! None of us does our best work with someone hovering over us. Offer to pitch in with jobs made easier by an extra set of hands, such as turning or lifting. Otherwise, leave her to her tasks unfettered and inspect the work when she has finished.

Don't let others boss her around. This includes the patient. The aide is there to complete specific nursing duties, not to be a general helper to other family members or visitors.

Take your criticisms and suggestions to her before reporting them to the nurse or other agency officials. Nothing breeds mistrust like going over somebody's head. Give workers a fair chance to correct their mistakes before resorting to telling the boss.

Nursing Homes and Residential Care

Diane Young: Putting Dad in a nursing home was a horrible decision to make. My grandmother was ninety-two when she died, but my father would never let Mother put her in a nursing home. When Dad was sick with Alzheimer's disease, my mother would say, "Your daddy was so good to Grandma. I'm never going to put him in a nursing home."

I have a sister and two brothers, and we finally had to tell our mother, "Look, we're losing Daddy to something we have no control over. But we're losing you, too." She was fading right before our eyes. So we just made the decision ourselves.

My mother and I did go around and look at nursing homes, with a very heavy heart. Most of them were pretty bad, and they all had waiting lists. I called around until I found a bed. Actually, I couldn't find a nursing home bed; we put Dad in the geriatric unit of a psychiatric hospital, and he stayed there about a month.

The morning he was to be transferred to the nursing home, I made him a sandwich, and I knew that was going to be the last lunch I'd ever fix him.

Studies have found that just as many elderly people are placed in institutional care due to relatives' burnout as on account of any sudden decline in their medical condition. Whether it's because a family is taxed beyond endurance or because a loved one's medical care is too complicated to manage at home, nursing homes for most people are a last resort.

Many folks avoid admitting patients to a residential nursing facility until long after they probably should have. For some it's a sign of failure or excessive guilt. For others there's simply not an empty bed to be found when they need it.

Many struggle alone at home because of the staggering cost of institutional care: $36,000 a year, on average. Since Medicare pays only for short stays—no more than 150 days in most cases—under rigidly defined medical restrictions, most people have to exhaust all their savings and "spend down" to Medicaid eligibility. Even the most expensive supplemental insurance policies pay for only a few weeks. Many elderly people end up selling their home, if they're lucky enough to own one, in order to afford a decent nursing facility.

The reason most people resist, however, are legitimate concerns about the quality of care. Though federal and state regulation of nursing homes and residential facilities have improved substantially in the 1990s, we've all heard the horror stories.

Even in the best units, with dozens or hundreds of very sick old people to care for, a few will end up lingering in soiled pants or enduring frequent delays with bathing, medications, meals, or therapy. Except in the most exclusive private rest homes, I've rarely heard a caregiver express complete satisfaction. It's simply not possible for a patient to receive the same level of care we would give them at home if we could. In that regard, our concerns (and some of our guilt) are justified.

When a loved one moves to a nursing home, whether by choice or sheer necessity, it falls to the caregiver to make sure he's well cared for. Although shopping around to avoid the worst facilities is essential, there is no replacement for our constant attention. Most of the time we end up choosing the one nursing home in the area that had a bed available. Inspecting the quality of care with our own eyes several times a week, if not daily, is the only way to make the most of residential care, and building a rapport with the staff and scheduling a constant stream of visitors through the room become more important than ever.

Tips on Finding a Nursing Home

The umbrella term *nursing home* encompasses several kinds of facilities offering different levels of care:

* *Residential care facilities* board people who are unable to live alone but don't warrant skilled nursing services.
* *Intermediate care facilities* accept folks who are relatively independent but need assistance with activities of daily living and minimal nursing assistance, such as routine medications. They are not licensed to accept incontinent or bedridden (*nonambulatory*) patients.
* *Skilled nursing facilities* are usually called nursing homes, convalescent hospitals, or rest homes. They provide continuous nursing services under a registered nurse or licensed practical nurse in addition to assistance with activities of daily living.

The best way to find a nursing home is to ask the patient's doctor, hospital discharge planner, or social worker. Recommendations from experienced friends or family, fellow support group members and patients, and local chapters of disease-related organizations are good, too. To obtain a list of facilities in the patient's area, contact the Area Agency on Aging or call:

☎ American Health Care Association, 202-842-4444.

☎ Nursing Home Information Service, 301-578-8938.
► *For more information about these organizations, see Appendix C, page 515.*

Four Steps to Ensuring Quality Nursing Home Care

1. *Choose a facility that is licensed and accredited.* As with home-care agencies, this is no indication of quality, but insurance companies won't pay unless a nursing facility is state licensed and meets the standards set by the government and professional associations. Check them out by calling:

☎ Community Health Accreditation Program, 800-669-1656.

☎ Joint Commission on Accreditation of Healthcare Organizations Accreditation Services, 630-792-3004.
► *For more information about these organizations, see Appendix C, page 515.*

2. *Inspect the facility personally—several times, if possible—and interview the administrator or head nurse.* To get an accurate sense of how a nursing home is run, the Nursing Home Information Service in Silver Spring, Maryland, recommends visiting during mealtimes, on weekends, or between the hours of 4:00 P.M. and 8:00 P.M.

3. *Ask for and check references.* Speak to social workers, discharge planners, and doctors who regularly refer patients to the facility. Ask to speak to family members of other residents.

4. *Read the contract closely.* Make sure you know what extra costs are incurred above room and board and how they're calculated. What would happen should your loved one run out of money? The law says nursing homes can't transfer patients who become impoverished enough to qualify for Medicaid, but it happens all the time. Ask them to explain their policy and practices under those circumstances.

Another question to ask: Will it be necessary to move from the facility should the sick person require more intensive or less intensive care in the future?

Never sign a contract that holds you personally responsible for the patient's bill.

✎ CHECKLIST

Points to Consider When Inspecting a Nursing Home

❑ Are the patients clean, well groomed, and neatly dressed?

❑ Is the facility sanitary and well maintained? Take note of any foul odors, especially those of urine, or food and garbage lying around.

❑ Are staff members friendly and helpful?

❑ Are staff members neat, clean, and well groomed?

❑ Are any clients being physically restrained? Ask about house guidelines for employing restraints. Too many drowsy and listless patients may indicate excessive use of tranquilizers for the staff's convenience.

❑ Are there organized activities for the residents, and services such as physical therapy?

❑ How many patients is each nurse responsible for?

❑ How many assistants does each nurse have on each shift?

❑ Do the meals look appetizing? Are they served on china or on paper plates?

❑ Are fresh fruits and vegetables served?

❑ Does there appear to be sufficient staff to assist patients who can't feed themselves?

❑ Are you allowed to chat with the current residents? If not, why?

❑ Is there a residents' council? Ask to speak to the president.

Rectifying Problems Encountered in Nursing Homes

Many nursing home residents spend all their days confined to bed due to physical frailty. Others are chemically or physically restrained whether or not they need to be. Three hundred thousand develop bedsores each year. Many others simply languish alone, isolated and hopeless until they die.

Even though Susan Richardson and her sister Barbara had placed their mother in a reputable private nursing home, they were shocked to encounter problems during every daily visit: Rita's ostomy bag was leaking; she hadn't been bathed or turned; she was dangerously dehydrated. Only by working closely with the staff and supervising Rita's care directly could they make sure their mom received the care she needed.

If you can't correct problems internally by working with the nursing director and administrator, it helps to know that each state is federally mandated to appoint a long-term-care ombudsman. These may be listed under the state department of health or department of aging in the Government Listings section of the white pages. The National Citizens Coalition for Nursing Home Reform in Washington, D.C. (202-332-2275), can refer you to the state agency responsible for investigating and resolving such matters. The NCCNHR, a consumer advocacy organization, also has experienced staff members on hand to advise callers on quality-of-care and quality-of-life issues.

—7—

Care for the Caregivers

It's the catch-22 of caregiving that everyone you meet and every book you read—this one included—tells you the same thing: *Take good care of yourself!* No argument there—except you're stretched to the max already. How and when are you supposed to find the time and summon the energy to tend to your physical and emotional needs?

To be sure, there are people who persevere with little or no relief. But caring for the seriously ill is often a protracted process, and even the strongest individuals are bound to fall apart somewhere along the way. Caregivers wreck their own health or in exhaustion say and do things they come to regret. They neglect the kids; they become careless at work; they allow their marriages to crumble.

Ironically, overextending ourselves can ultimately harm the patient. You drop him in the bathtub, throwing out your back in the process. After too many sleepless nights, you nod off on duty, medications are missed, doses mismeasured, or new symptoms overlooked.

In order to make it through these difficult weeks, months, or years, it's critical to recognize our limitations. We offer commonsense strategies for preserving your stamina and your sanity—with the understanding that you may be able to incorporate only a few into your daily routine.

Maintaining Your Physical Stamina

More than one-third of all primary care partners are contending with their own major medical condition at the same time. Even if you're healthy to begin with, erratic eating habits, dehydration, fatigue, sleep deprivation, and chronic stress conspire to make you a magnet for every bug that comes along as well as a host of orthopedic problems, chief among them disabling back injuries. Without adding hours to your day, there are several straightforward things you

247

can do to take care of your body. In fact, some of these tactics will save you time and money while making you feel better, too.

Tricks for Keeping Your Body Running

Resolve to Rest; Steal Some Sleep

Rather than approach caring for the sick like the physical and emotional marathon it is, novice caregivers sometimes behave as if they're in a contest to prove who is the most concerned. But savvy runners sprint only at the end of a race. Except for a death watch or a bona fide medical emergency, going without uninterrupted sleep for more than a day is not an indication of commitment, it's a disaster in the making.

To the extent that you can, schedule sleep around your patient's sleeping habits. If your loved one's sleep patterns are erratic, take catnaps whenever he sleeps. "I had a schedule where I had to be up every two hours throughout the night to give my husband fluids," says Betty Lindstrom, an elderly caregiver from Columbus, Ohio. "So during the day I would try to catch up on my sleep by dozing off in a chair at ten in the morning and again at noon." Even if it's midday, leave your chores for later, click on the answering machine, draw the blinds, turn off the lights, and lie down or kick back in a recliner until your loved one needs you again.

Schedule some "catch-up" every week. If you're going to be up and down all night for several days in a row, schedule someone to relieve you to let you get eight hours of uninterrupted shut-eye as often as possible. (This is an ideal assignment for teenagers and the elderly.) Ask a family member or friend to spend a weeknight with you or spell you for a long weekend afternoon. All you need is a dependable person who can fetch things for the patient, an-swer the phone, and wake you if a problem arises.

Make the most of the sleep you do get. Turn off the ringer on the phone and hang a DO NOT DISTURB sign on the front door. Put clean sheets on the bed, take a shower or bath, sip herbal tea, or drink a beer—whatever helps you relax before turning in.

Other tips: Reduce the volume of fluid you drink a couple of hours before bedtime to avoid late-night trips to the bathroom. Stay away from caffeine after dark. Experiment with over-the-counter pain relievers such as acet-aminophen, aspirin, and nonsteroidal anti-inflammatory drugs (NSAIDs)—whatever is easiest on your stomach. You'll fall asleep sooner and relax more thoroughly if nagging aches, pains, sore muscles, and tension spots are soothed, but you'll wake up alert when you need to.

When our loved one doesn't sleep, neither do we. If you're losing sleep night after night because your patient is sleeping fitfully, talk to the medical team about prescribing a sleeping aid for her. ◄ *See "Insomnia and Other Sleep Disorders," page 172.*

Eat and Drink Sensibly and Conscientiously

Just feeling tense, angry, sad, or belea-guered is enough to sour the hardiest appetites. When we finally do feel faint with hunger, we're too busy or tired to shop and cook something nutritious. We grab whatever is easiest, whether it's McDonald's or snacks from a vending machine. That's fine in a pinch, but it's no way to live when others are depending on us. Our bodies need quality fuel and plenty of water every day.

Weigh yourself at the same time each day using the same scale. To many Americans, losing three or more pounds in one week sounds like a dieter's dream come true. But dropping weight when you're not trying to—even if you were overweight to start with—is a potentially dangerous medical symptom that demands daily attention for two reasons. First, a stressed-out caregiver may not notice the trend and become sick before realizing she has a problem. Severe fluctuations in blood pressure, fierce swings in blood sugar, and electrolyte imbalances not only can knock a caregiver out of commission but can be life threatening. Second, if weight loss continues for a month or more, we need to see the doctor to rule out other causative medical conditions.

Don't let yourself become dehydrated. Keep small bottles of water handy: next to the bed, by your favorite chair, in your coat pocket or purse, in the car, and so on. Start drinking when you first get up and sip water all day—instead of more coffee, tea, or caffeine-laced soda, which are strong diuretics. Order juice spritzers or mineral water with meals, and chew sugarless gum between meals to keep your mouth fresh and moist. Don't wait until you're thirsty to drink more water. By then you're already dehydrated.

✻ *You're not drinking enough water unless your urine is transparent and flowing at regular intervals throughout the day.*

If you drink liquor, which is extremely dehydrating, compensate by downing at least five times as much water as booze per sitting. Chase beer or wine with an equal amount of water or seltzer. Fill up on water, fruit, or unsalted vegetable juices immediately before cocktail hour, and you'll imbibe less of the hard stuff. And *never* drink alcohol on an empty stomach.

Memo to cigarette smokers: You need to drink at least 30 percent more water than nonsmokers to stay thoroughly hydrated throughout the day.

Start each day with a substantial meal. At the very least, an instant breakfast drink, fresh fruit, and toast or cereal. Science has proved our moms right about the importance of breakfast. Our stomachs are empty of everything but gastric juices when we wake, and our blood sugar is at its lowest. If you skip breakfast or just chug coffee, the acid and bile concentrations in your stomach intensify, and you feel even less like eating. Then when you finally do eat, you frequently get indigestion or even severe reflux that persists for hours—which leads to skipping subsequent meals. Unless we constantly keep a little something in our stomachs to buffer the acid, these symptoms cascade, and we begin a vicious cycle of induced anorexia, or a version to eating, setting the stage for serious ulcers in the esophagus, stomach, and intestines.

Also, when we experience that inevitable midmorning "sugar crash" (acute hypoglycemia), we tend to reach for something sweet, loading up on empty calories like refined sugar and saturated fat instead of the complex carbohydrates and high-quality protein our bodies desperately need.

✻ *If you are skipping meals because of persistent indigestion, ask your doctor about preemptive doses of Zantac or Tagamet, commonly prescribed and highly effective antiulcer medications usually taken once a day before bedtime.*

Stock up on healthy snacks. On your next trip to the supermarket, buy baked goods, fresh fruit, and vegetables that can be enjoyed without cooking. (Wash, peel, or chop them for eating before placing them in the fridge or on the table, and you'll be more apt to eat them.) Toss a bagel, a banana, or a couple of apples in your coat pocket or purse. Keep peanut butter, cereals, milk, cheese, whole-grain bread or crackers, and dried fruit or trail mix around the house for easy-access munching. Eat a little throughout the day instead of waiting until you're famished and gorging on junk.

* *If overeating is your problem, remember that several small meals throughout the day will make you less likely to binge. Don't wait until you're hungry, tired, or upset to eat.*

Experiment with commercial nutritional supplements. For anyone skipping meals, instant breakfast drinks that you mix with milk or juice can be a lifesaver. Also, stop by the health food store and sample the various prepackaged snacks.

Stash a couple of sports bars in your desk, glove compartment, bedside table drawer, and so forth. A brand called PowerBar is the best-seller among endurance athletes and often rated tops in consumer surveys for taste and digestibility. Keep something nutritious at your fingertips at all times.

Ask your doctor about canned supplements such as Ensure, Advera, and Sustacal. We suggest you taste-test them first, however. The concentrated protein slush sits heavy on the stomach for hours. It's a small price to pay when you're medically undernourished, but hardly appetizing.

Add a multivitamin and mineral supplement to your morning ritual. But don't take them on an empty stomach; they'll ruin your appetite.

When shopping and cooking, prepare extra portions for freezing. Lots of sensible small meals beat the heck out of starving or living on fast food, but they are no substitute for three squares. You're much more apt to eat something nutritious and satisfying if you've prepared it yourself and merely have to warm it up.

* *When making rice or pasta dishes for freezing, it's best to undercook them slightly. Before reheating them, add a little liquid, and they'll turn out great.*

Accept other folks' offers to cook or shop for you. Their home-cooked meals can be frozen and served later when you're pressed for time. Soups, sauces, and casseroles are best because they're easy to prepare, transport, and serve. Also keep a shopping list near the phone, and don't be shy about telling visitors and well-wishers specifically what you need.

Don't turn eating into a chore. Serve food in the same dish you heated or cooked it. Use paper plates and disposable cups. Leave dirty pots and pans to soak for faster cleaning later.

Take Steps to Prevent Infection

Pay special attention to skin care. Like patients, cracks in our skin leave us wide open to viruses and bacteria. Since we're also likely dehydrated, malnourished, and under constant stress, our immune systems are not at peak performance, either. What's more, not bathing regularly or spending too much time in sweaty clothes (particularly synthetic fabrics) breeds all sorts of irritating fungi. Personal hygiene is not simply a matter of comfort and appearance; it's fundamental to good health.

Moisturize, moisturize, moisturize. This is not just a beauty tip, and it goes for men, too. Bathing strips our skin of its natural emollients. Help maintain the skin's elasticity and integrity by rubbing a thin layer of lotion over your whole body immediately after a shower or bath. Pay particular attention to hands and cuticles, lower legs and feet, elbows and face—any area prone to dryness, cracking, or edema. Keep a pump dispenser of your favorite hand cream next to each sink and smooth on a little each time you wash your hands. Always keep lip balm handy in your pocket or purse.

Wash your hands compulsively. The single most important infection control policy of hospitals and sick rooms is fastidious hand washing. Always wash before entering a sick person's room and when leaving. Wash your hands after handling money, before and after preparing food, eating or touching door-knobs or bathroom surfaces such as a spigot and toilet handles, and after touching children or their toys. Wash your hands every chance you get; use paper towels whenever possible; wipe up behind yourself; and remember to moisturize. Send germs down the drain before they stake a claim in someone's body and you find yourself with two or more patients.

Exercise

Pat Still: During the years I cared for my husband at home, I did high-impact aerobics fives days a week. Though I was doing it mostly for my head, my body looked great!

If you're a former athlete or inveterate health club denizen, you know there's nothing like regular exercise to keep fit, control weight and blood pressure, promote healing, clear your head, dissipate nervous energy, banish depression, and jump-start libido. Even if you haven't set foot in a gym since high school, there's a lot you can do to improve or maintain your stamina, to strengthen muscles and sinew to avoid orthopedic injuries, and to shake out kinks and sore spots. But before you begin any exercise regimen, however informal, discuss it with your physician first.

Schedule exercise two or three days a week. Take long, brisk walks as often as you can. Work your way up gradually until you're engaged in some form of physical activity for at least twenty minutes per session several times a week. Consider buying or borrowing a treadmill or stationary bike, but only if you're likely to use it. Set it up near your loved one's bed and work out while you watch the news together. Join the "Y" or local recreation center and put in some laps at the pool, by far the safest and most effective exercise for folks of all ages and fitness levels.

> Should an exercise ever cause a sudden or sharp pain, stop immediately and gently stretch. Consult your doctor if it persists.

You'll find right away that regularly pumping up your heart rate and breaking a sweat makes you feel much better, partly due to the natural rush of *endorphins*. These chemicals, released by the brain during exercise, blunt pain and induce mild euphoria. More important, however, are the lasting benefits of aerobic exercise: You don't tire as quickly, your blood pressure settles down, your appetite improves, and you sleep more restfully.

✻ *Keep workouts as simple and convenient as possible so that you're more apt to do them.*

Coddle your lower back. Nothing knocks caregivers out of the saddle faster than pinched nerves or pulled back muscles. The pain is excruciating, you're useless to others, and it can take years to recover completely.

The following simple stretching exercises for the lower back, hamstring muscles, and abdominal muscles will help prevent most common problems.

Gently stretch out your lower back muscles each morning after you've been up and around and gotten your blood circulating—and always before and after strenuous activity:

1. Lie prone on the floor or on a very firm mattress, with your knees bent and the soles of your feet on the floor. For comfort, place a folded towel or thin cushion under your hips.
2. Place your hands on your knees and slowly draw them toward your chest, exhaling steadily the entire time. Repeat the motion six or eight times at least once a day, and more often whenever your back starts feeling a little tight or tired.

The worst injuries can usually be avoided by pausing to remember to bend your knees and exhale whenever lifting, turning, pushing, or pulling.
◀ See "Turning, Maneuvering, and Lifting," page 132.

To stretch your hamstrings, the long muscles in the backs of your thighs:

1. Sit on the floor with your back flush against a wall and your legs extended, the knees bent slightly.
2. S-l-o-w-l-y lean forward from your hips as far as you comfortably can, hands resting on shins or knees, exhaling deliberately and continuously through your mouth. Don't bounce or pull yourself downward with your hands. Just concentrate on relaxing your butt and lower back, while passively letting the weight of your upper body stretch those hamstrings.

If you try this standing (like old-fashioned toe touches), remember to bend your knees slightly and keep the feet about shoulder-width apart. Do not bounce, hold your breath, or stand upright suddenly. You can also stretch your hamstrings by sitting on the edge of a sturdy chair with the backs of your heels resting on the floor just far enough in front of you that when you bend forward from the hips, you feel a gentle stretching sensation up the backs of your thighs.

To strengthen your legs, practice the "up one/down two" rule at home, the hospital, the office: Every chance you get, skip the elevator and take the stairs up a minimum of one flight or walk down at least two flights.

Strong abdominal muscles shore up and splint the lower back, and keep our hips, torso, and legs stable when lifting and turning. Most chronic back ailments are due at least in part to lower abdominal weakness.

To strengthen abdominal muscles, forget sit-ups; they're murder on

middle-aged backs. Try a few sets of these simple exercises:

1. Lie on your back, knees bent and soles of the feet flat against the floor.
2. Support the back of your head with your hands or drape your arms across your chest and *slowly* raise your shoulders off the floor just a few inches by squeezing with your gut.
3. Exhale through your mouth continuously as you squeeze, while steadily pressing your lower back into the floor. Begin with two or three sets of six or eight gentle crunches. Take your time and work up slowly to more repetitions over the course of several weeks.

Isometric abdominal exercises work well, too. Using only your abdominal muscles, press your bellybutton firmly against your belt or the edge of your desk for a count of ten while exhaling slowly through your mouth. Or try holding a coin or sheet of paper between your knees while sitting up straight in a chair, then tightly squeeze your abdominal muscles and exhale while you count to ten. Do this several times throughout the day.

Don't Postpone Your Own Doctor and Dental Appointments

Preventive medicine works on caregivers, too. Keep your blood pressure and blood sugar in check by visiting your doctor regularly. If you're feeling run-down, ask her about seasonal flu shots and vitamin B_{12} injections. Inquire whether you need a hepatitis vaccine.

When you're under the gun, it may seem like too much trouble to go to the dentist for routine hygiene appointments and exams. But it's better if you find a cavity or cracked crown before you suffer the pain and fever of an abscess—and end up with a time-consuming and expensive root canal or gum routing instead of a simple cleaning or filling.

Don't Try Doing It All

You can't do it all—not indefinitely, at any rate. "I believe there are a lot of times when caregivers are reluctant to share the caregiving," says Lou Glasse, president emerita of the Older Women's League. "They convince themselves that only they can care for the ill person and that no one else can do it as well, which is a disservice both to the ailing loved one and to the rest of the family. If that occurs, we need to reevaluate whether we are protecting our own self-image rather than doing what is best for the ill one."

One common manifestation of this behavior is the caregiver who becomes a "squatter" at the hospital, refusing to go home. Unless your loved one is on the brink of death, when the hospital nurses suggest you go home, listen to them; they're trying to tell you something. Sitting up all night in a waiting room or dozing fitfully in a chair does not lessen your anxiety about your loved one's current crisis. If you can help, stay. But if you can't do anything practical, go get some rest. You'll need it later.

"A caregiver, like any other worker, has to be given a break," says Dr. Donald Leslie, medical director of the Shepherd Spinal Center in Atlanta. "You can't take care of a patient twenty-four hours a day, seven days a week. You've got to have backup, somebody to relieve you."

Consider Respite Care and Adult Day Care Services

Respite care, arranged through agencies such as the Area Agency on Aging and United Way of America, sends a trained volunteer, home health aide, or nursing assistant to the patient's home to give the caregiver a break for several hours. In adult day care, patients or other dependent adults enjoy group activities and a meal at a senior center or other central location, also for a few hours. Before you get your hopes too high, we should warn you that these

---

For Referrals to Respite Care (RC) and Adult Day Care (ADC)

American Health Care Association
☎ 202-842-4444 (ADC)

Area Agency on Aging/Eldercare Locator
☎ 800-677-1116 (RC/ADC)

Catholic Charities
☎ 703-549-1390 (RC/ADA)

National Institute on Adult Day Care
☎ 202-479-1200 (ADC)

Nursing Home Information Service
☎ 301-578-8938 (ADC)

United Way of America
☎ 703-836-7100 (RC/ADC)

Visiting Nurse Associations of America
☎ 888-866-8773 (RC)

---

services are extraordinarily difficult to pull together—if they're even available. Still, it's certainly worth inquiring to the agencies in the sidebar.

Poor Aunt Kitty couldn't find adult day care *or* respite care in Mobile while caring for Uncle Billy. So she improvised, taking him along with her on her outings to Little Sisters of the Poor, the nursing home where she volunteered as an arts and crafts supervisor several times a week. It was the only break she ever got. ◄ *See chapter 5, "Mustering the Troops."* ► *See Appendix B: "Community Services," page 502; Appendix C, page 515.*

Slow Down

Relax household routines and take frequent breaks. For the time being use paper plates. Sweep or vacuum instead of mopping and waxing. Ask someone else to do the laundry. Pay a kid to cut the grass. (And ask a good friend to rub your neck, shoulders, and feet!)

Pace Yourself

If we don't have a sound knowledge of the disease process and a close rapport with the medical team, we overextend and wear ourselves out too soon. Then when the patient needs us the most, we have nothing left in reserve. Save your greatest efforts for true crises.

Finding the Emotional Strength

While our bodies take a beating in the process of caring for a seriously ill loved one, it's more often the emotional challenges that threaten to overwhelm us completely. Our ability to recognize and effectively defuse high anxiety will determine how well we cope not only during the illness but also long after our loved one is gone.

Sometimes caregivers get so caught up worrying about the patient and other family members that they try to ignore their own emotional suffering. Big mistake. Stoicism may carry you through a temporary crisis, but when stress is relentless, even the strongest people start to crack. We have to be scrupulously honest with ourselves about what we're feeling—and what is making us feel that way—and find ways to get a grip on the most disturbing emotions, enforcing what psychologists and social workers call "appropriate boundaries."

Emotions Common to Caregivers

"I Feel as if I'm in a State of Shock"

Roslyn Travers: It took me a good while to accept that my brother was brain damaged from his car accident. Emotionally I was just absolutely drained. I honestly thought I was going to have a nervous breakdown.

When the combination of bad news, confusion, and overwhelming demands descends on a caregiver at the same time, shock is a common reaction. Shock immobilizes us temporarily and makes concentration and listening to what the medical team and others are saying next to impossible. Emotionally we're like a flag at the mercy of the wind, flapping this way and that. Or, conversely, we shut down completely, seeming to feel nothing and utterly unable to organize our thoughts.

Skills for Coping

- *Talk about your feelings with someone who is more level-headed or has a calmer perspective at the moment.* Once you've found a good listener, keep talking every day until you begin to sort out what is required of you. Don't try to hold it all in.
- *As much as possible, allow yourself to experience the entire range of emotions before taking action or making decisions.* Sometimes medical circumstances demand that certain decisions be made on the spot. More often, though, big decisions can be postponed until you've had time to talk things through and stabilize your emotions. You'll be less likely to make decisions you later regret.
- *Remember that feelings are not necessarily facts.* Just because it *feels* as if life as you knew it is over doesn't mean you're not going to survive—and perhaps even thrive—once the crisis passes.

"I Feel So Angry and Resentful"

Nola Miller: One of the things I resented was having my life in slow motion. My husband would want me to sit with him at night, which I found extremely difficult. I don't know why. Perhaps it was because I was fighting really hard to hold on to the fact that I was still alive, whereas for all intents and purposes he was not.

Anger is inevitable for a caregiver whose life has been disrupted by a loved one's illness. The patient may be excessively dependent or demanding, or aim his own frustration at those he knows will not return it. Family, friends, and the medical team may not be as helpful or understanding as you expect. Some people feel betrayed by God or let down by their faith. These are normal—even healthy—reactions to loss, disappointment, and injustice. But if we walk around constantly fuming, we turn anger inward and punish ourselves by neglecting our own health, giving up entirely, or lashing out at others.

Skills for Coping

- *Get resentment off your chest. Express your anger long before you blow your top.* When someone ticks you off, tell the person right then while you're still able to do so calmly. Folks often think that by suppressing their anger over "little things" they can avoid confrontations or unpleasant scenes. What's more likely is that we store up resentment until we explode, overreacting and then saying too much. Relationships are destroyed or permanently damaged, and recriminations linger long after the patient has died.
- *Avoid people who will definitely make you angry. Step away from frustrating situations until you can cool off.* In the heat of the moment, our own reactions can make others angry, upset the patient, or inflame an already bad situation. Steer clear of annoying people or stay one step ahead of them by keeping them busy and *away from you.* If you feel your face flush or your blood pressure rising, drop what you're doing and go for a walk. Wait until you've composed yourself before confronting infuriating people or problems.
- *Find other ways to express your anger.* Yell and scream in a car or alone in the basement, pound a pillow, or exercise furiously. Some people cook or clean obsessively or weed a flower bed violently until the most intense feelings pass. Do whatever has worked for you in the past. Blow off some steam before you lose your temper with others.
- *Talk to a close friend or family member about why you feel anger.* Explaining how you feel to someone who will not judge you can help you gain perspective and understand your reactions. It may help just to vent, and you might come up with better ways to cope or to recognize and express your frustration more effectively in the future.
- *Remember that others are stressed out, too.* Some people are better than others at dealing with anxiety. Recognize that family, friends, and the medical team may also be on edge. Try to see things from their points of view. If you express empathy instead of impatience ("I can see that this has upset you, too"), you'll probably find it returned in abundance.

"I Feel So Guilty"

Diane Young: *My father was in the nursing home at Christmas time. During the holidays, whenever I'd find myself laughing about something, I'd immediately think,* Oh, I shouldn't be laughing; Daddy's lying in that bed alone, not knowing where he is.

Maybe you blew your stack with a loved one or harbored murderous thoughts in a moment of frustration. Maybe you feel as if you should be able to do more to help the ill person, whether or not you can. Maybe at some point during this ordeal you wished it would all be over. Maybe you did something in the past that hurt a loved one, and you've never owned up to it or made amends. Guilt haunts us all, with or without justification.

When we're caring for the sick, though, guilt can cloud judgment. Instead of recognizing our limitations or the harsh reality of a terminal diagnosis, we try to do more than we can and overextend ourselves. We lay blame and put undue pressure on others—not because the patient needs us to but to make ourselves feel better, to "prove" how much we care or that we're not bad people.

On the other hand, guilt can cause such shame that a caregiver avoids the sick person or other family members altogether, compounding the problem and setting the stage for even more bitter regrets later on. Whatever its origins, guilt needs to be recognized and redirected before it starts interfering with the care plan.

Skills for Coping

- *Try your best to avoid doing the things that make you feel guilty!* Nothing trumps guilt like righteousness and a clear conscience. Do the right thing, as they say, and you'll always feel better. Be nice to people. Take good care of yourself. Help others. Deal honestly and directly with everyone around you. Go the extra mile whenever possible and practical. You'll never regret it.
- *Confess real transgressions, make amends, and offer forgiveness for old hurts.* As with anger, ignoring guilt doesn't make it go away. Make the most of your time together and take every opportunity to speak from the heart.
- *Don't dwell on your mistakes. Nobody's perfect.* Admit when you make a mistake. Apologize if necessary, see to it that you don't repeat the error (though you'll certainly make others), and keep moving. There's no better tonic for guilt than knowing in your heart you did the best you could.

"I Feel So Isolated and Alone"

Sarah Lanier Barber: *I frequently felt very alone with this dual responsibility for both parents and the fact that there really were no family members involved. We were a very closed three-*

some. *Plus, my father wouldn't tell anybody—not even his sister!—about my mother's Alzheimer's disease.*

When you're running back and forth to the hospital or nursing a loved one at home, there's not much time or energy to spare for a social life. Friends and family may not know what to say or do, or they feel as if they're in the way, so they call and visit less often. Even when plenty of loving and supportive folks surround us, lying awake at night wondering what the future holds can be a suffocating exercise in solitude.

Skills for Coping

- *Pick up the phone!* Call friends you haven't heard from lately. Invite someone over just to chat while you cook or clean. Ask a colleague to join you on your lunch hour. You don't have to utter a word about sickness or death unless you want to. You're just looking for a simple human connection and companionship during hard times.
- *Make new friends, especially those who understand what you're going through.* Caregivers must reach out to others before they find themselves facing a crisis alone. Join a support group. Visit with other sick folks and their caregivers or invite them over for a short visit. Attend educational and social activities organized by local chapters of disease-related organizations. Surf the net for chat groups. Renew your ties with a church, synagogue, or other place of worship. Find someone who can bring perspective to your situation, suggest ways to cope better, or just lend a friendly ear or share a laugh.

"I Worry All the Time"

Mary Vitro: *When I crawled into bed late at night, that's when everything would hit me. What's going to happen tomorrow? What's it going to be like when Rick dies? What's going to hap-*

pen to Dougie and me? I would lie there and repeat to myself, "Everything's going to be okay, everything's going to be okay."

When we're frightened, tired, and heartbroken, it's natural to fret. But when obsessively ruminative thinking, intrusive negative thoughts, or just plain practical concerns start disrupting sleep and eating habits or leaving us constantly on edge, it's time to take action. Excessive worry and constant anxiety are symptoms of poorly managed stress.

Skills for Coping

- *Learn all you can about your patient's disease and the disease process, and cultivate a close rapport with the medical team.* When you know what to expect and approximately when, you can at least prepare yourself. Talk to other caregivers and patients, too. They'll alert you to pitfalls you hadn't anticipated and solutions you never thought of.
- *Break down big problems into small, manageable tasks.* When we receive bad news, it's natural for our fantasies to race ahead to the worst-case scenarios. Sometimes the news is truly dire. We get stuck at the point where we obsessively wonder "What am I going to do now?" Or we become paralyzed at the realization, "Oh my God, he's going to die!" Reframe your concerns into specific tasks you know you can carry out. Just take things one day at a time or even one hour at a time until you feel your equilibrium returning. ▶ *See "Techniques for Managing Stress and Anxiety," page 258.*

"I Feel So Helpless"

Debra Bulkeley: *I went through tremendous frustration over not being able to do enough for my parents because there's no treatment for Lou Gehrig's disease.*

Watching someone we love deteriorate before our eyes and being powerless to stop it is often the first step down the road to major depression. The challenge is to take control of the things we can while working toward some degree of acceptance of the things we can't change. It's the ultimate test of emotional maturity.

Skills for Coping

- *Set realistic goals such as concentrating on symptom management and quality of life.* Instead of feeling helpless to change the course of the disease, focus on what you *can* do: keeping your patient as comfortable as possible and making his remaining days full and rich. The only way to survive the overwhelming sadness and frustration of watching someone inexorably slip away is to know we did everything in our power to prevent them from suffering needlessly.

"I Feel as if He's Already Gone"

Louise Fradkin: *Many of us who cared for our parents for many years did our grieving before they died. I didn't cry at my mother's funeral because mentally I'd already buried her. It was the only way I could cope. I told myself, "I'm going to take care of this lady who* looks *like my mother; the mother I knew is gone."*

Grief is our basic emotional reaction to loss. When someone is seriously ill, the losses begin compounding not at the time of death but at the onset of symptoms. Whether it's the loss of one's status as husband, wife, parent, sibling, provider, protector, or romantic partner, or the loss of a social life and hopes and dreams shared together, we feel disoriented and betrayed by fate.

"One of the wonderful things in a marriage is to sit down and say, 'By the way, did I tell you such-and-such happened today?' " reflects Betty Lindstrom, who was married to her husband, a Parkinson's patient, for forty-five years. "Eventually I realized that Clarence no longer understood what I was talking about. So you grieve at losing that part of them, and you lose more every day."

It's hard to imagine our future so fundamentally changed until we have passed through much of the inevitable sadness. You should experience and express grief without treating the patient as if he's already dead and before you're mired in hopelessness or major depression.

Skills for Coping

- *Make the most of the time you have together and concentrate on the things you can share instead of the things you've lost.* As the everyday angels in this book demonstrate time and again, caring for a seriously ill or dying person can provide new opportunities for growth and profound intimacy. While without question it is a very sad time, nothing can bring two people together quite as closely as facing a crisis side by side. Cherish your time together; the good memories will sustain you through many of the darkest moments.
- *Tell your loved one how you feel.* Share your fears and sense of loss with your patient. You'll often find he's thinking the same thing and is grateful and relieved to talk about it. Say something like "This is breaking my heart. I don't know what I'm going to do without you." When you send the signal that it's okay for him to open up with you, opportunities are created for supporting each other.
- *Allow yourself to grieve.* Sometimes we feel guilty, fearing that we're giving up prematurely. Or we're afraid our obvious sadness will depress our patient. Sometimes we think that if we open the floodgates of grief, we'll never be able to shut them. More often, if you have a good cry or confide your sadness to someone, you'll feel stronger and better able to cope a little longer.

Techniques for Managing Stress and Anxiety

Mary Vitro: I was under so much stress, my neck would get all knotted up and I'd have a migraine headache every day. The first thing I did every morning was take two Tylenols; I lived on Tylenol.

Many different definitions of "stress" are used by psychologists in clinical and academic settings. What they all have in common, however, is a disparity between the demands placed on us by our environment and our perception of our ability to respond effectively. Beyond the familiar feelings of frustration and tension, *stress is anything that requires us to make changes in our life in order to cope with circumstances.*

Just the emotional fallout—what's commonly called "anxiety"—from relentless stress is obvious to any adult who is overworked, heartbroken, financially troubled, or frightened. When you're caring for a seriously ill loved one, stress is unavoidable and potentially debilitating. We know from research that long-term physical and psychological tension impairs different components of the immune system. One study conducted at Ohio State University compared the healing of minor skin wounds in women who were caring for a relative with Alzheimer's disease versus those who were not under that kind of chronic strain. The stressed-out group took nine days longer to heal.

Set aside time for yourself whenever possible. Take a break from caregiving at least once a day. You don't have to leave the house or take much time. "Whatever makes you happy, comfortable, or more relaxed," advises Louise Fradkin of Children of Aging Parents, "whether it's having your hair done or just sitting down and staring off into space. You have to figure out what little moments you can take that will give you some relief."

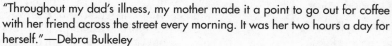

Enjoy a leisurely bubble bath, sit on the porch and read, watch your favorite TV show or rent a video (preferably a comedy)—anything that temporarily takes your mind off sickness. Go shopping or simply wander around the mall. If you're holding vigil at the hospital, don't eat every meal in the cafeteria. Take a walk outside or meet a friend for a quick lunch or supper.

Pamper yourself! Spring for a facial or massage. Dress up and go to a favorite restaurant, or dress down and have a picnic at the park or beach. Attend a cultural or sporting event, or hit the track or a casino with friends. You deserve it and need the break.

Don't let a loved one's illness totally consume your life. Sometimes we're focused so intensely on caring for the sick person that it becomes all we can talk about even when we're off duty. Change the subject to common interests—kids, work, gossip—whatever you used to talk about before the current crisis. It's healthy to take an emotional break when you need to.

Cherish your sense of humor. Sometimes it's the only thing that gets you through. "I remember one time when Rick was lying on the sofa, so sick he could hardly stand up," says Mary Vitro. "My son, who was two, came up to me and said, 'Mommy, I colored the "chitchen."'

" 'What do you mean you colored the chitchen?'

"I followed him to the kitchen, and I realized what he meant: He'd taken a crayon and colored all over the tile floor. Was this funny? Yes! It was *so* funny. This was *life*. While one life was going away, this other one was just starting, and Dougie was such a happy baby. After being at the hospital and dealing with Rick all day, Dougie was my sunshine, my anchor."

Talk to folks who have been through this themselves, be it family, friends, or members of a caregivers' support group. "It gives caregivers an opportunity to either express themselves, just sit and listen, or cry," says Louise Fradkin who cofounded Children of Aging Parents in 1977.

Other family and friends may be supportive and sympathetic, but there are things you can say in a group you'd rarely share at home. Pat Still, executive director of the Well Spouse Foundation, a national organization headquartered in New York, tells of a phone call from a fellow member who had been up day and night caring for a husband with end-stage Parkinson's disease.

"I think it's time for a pillow party," the exhausted woman remarked caustically. Whereas a relative probably would have taken offense at such black humor, Pat laughed along. "This woman adores her husband and would never do anything like that," she explains. Like any caregiver, the caller simply needed to vent her frustration. Pat also notes that when her own husband, a stroke victim, was hospitalized with pneumonia, she found herself surrounded by concerned members of her local group.

What's the best way to locate a caregivers' support group? Start by contacting the nearest hospital's department of social work or psychiatry, or call one of the organizations listed in the sidebar. The Internet is full of on-line

---

Support Organizations Specifically for Caregivers

Children of Aging Parents
1609 Woodbourne Road,
Suite 302-A
Levittown, PA 19057-1511
800-227-7294

National Family Caregivers
Association
9621 East Bexhill Drive
Kensington, MD 20895-3104
301-942-6430

Well Spouse Foundation
601 Lexington Avenue, Suite 814
New York, NY 10022-6005
800-838-0879

---

groups, too. For some folks it is less intimidating to wander into a chat room on-line, for all intents anonymously, than attend a meeting in person. ▶ *See Appendix A, "Recommended Resources," page 489; Appendix B: "Support Groups," page 512.*

Consider talking with a professional counselor, be it a social worker, psychologist, other mental health practitioner, or a clergyman. They can help immeasurably by showing you more effective ways to cope with your emotions.

Seek comfort in God, religion, and spirituality. Asked what his ordeal with his wife Jackie's stroke-induced coma taught him about faith, religion, and God, the Reverend Harry Cole replies thoughtfully, "Ultimately, what I know now and what got me through this was not so much what I learned in seminaries or what I've written about or talked about, it's what I learned in Sunday school: that God loves, God hears prayers, and God answers prayers. And that was what I came to realize: that my prayers for resolution, for deliverance, were answered. They

weren't answered in the way that I had asked, and they certainly weren't answered in a way I had anticipated. But I did get what I needed out of this."

For the more secular minded, don't dismiss out of hand the notion of calling on a clergyman. Many have extensive experience in family counseling and grief counseling. What's more, people are far more likely to attend church than a support group, and ritual and prayer have the same tonic effects as meditation and psychotherapy. Speak to a hospital chaplain or local clergyman to help find your way along the *spiritual* journey that is caring for a sick or dying loved one.

Learn new stress-reduction techniques. Play, total relaxation, shopping, good food, wine, and sex are the old reliables for fighting high anxiety. But there are many more tricks for handling stress. Exercise, meditation, hypnosis, biofeedback, tai chi, yoga, and acupuncture are all highly effective at lowering blood pressure and resting heart rate while significantly reducing anxiety. Try some of the progressive-relaxation and deep-breathing exercises recommended for patients in chapter 3. Ask your family doctor or the hospital social worker how to find out more about specific stress-management techniques. ▶ *See "Acupuncture," "Biofeedback," and "Hypnotherapy," in Appendix B, pages 503, 505, and 507.*

Talk to your doctor about his possibly prescribing medications for sleep disturbance, chronic anxiety, and ulcer prevention. These are medical symptoms of overwhelming stress and are highly treatable. If you're lying awake with worry at night, it might be time to consider taking an over-the-counter sleeping aid or a prescription sedative. Ask the doctor about a mild tranquilizer such as alprazolam (brand name: Xanax) for allaying daytime anxiety. Skipping meals? You probably need an antacid and an ulcer-prevention medication as well. Whatever the symptom, get a handle on it now using everything at your disposal.

When Depression Strikes

Fully half of all caregivers suffer from depression, and as many as four in five of those tending to patients with Alzheimer's disease. Statistically, caregivers use prescription drugs for depression, anxiety, and insomnia two to three times as often as the rest of the population. But that still means millions of others don't reach out for help at all.

As we discussed in chapter 4, depression is a medical symptom that only gets worse without treatment. See "Common Signs of Depression" on page 192. If you have any of the symptoms listed for more than two weeks, call them to the attention of your doctor as you would a physical problem.

Your patient's own doctors and nurses are valuable sources of advice, too, but bear in mind that your health and happiness are not their responsibility. They are not therapists, dumping grounds, or whipping posts for your angst. Ask them to refer you to reliable professionals for your needs. ◄ *See "How Depression Is Treated," page 193.*

Sources of Referrals to Mental Health Professionals

American Psychiatric Association
☎ 202-682-6000

American Medical Association
☎ 312-464-5000

American Psychological Association
☎ 202-336-5500

National Association of Social Workers
☎ 800-638-8799

Plus any hospital's department of social work, psychiatry, or psychology, and your state or county department of mental health

---

Caring for the Other Loved Ones in Your Life

Your Romantic Partner

"I don't think that honoring your father and mother means you destroy your own life," observes Louise Fradkin. "Caregivers have to learn to balance their lives, and that's a very difficult thing." In devoting our time and energy to a sick person, we have to be careful not to let other meaningful relationships unravel. Even with the best intentions in the world, dedicated caregivers can neglect their wives, husbands, and lovers.

When Roslyn Travers's brother Duane sustained permanent brain damage in a car accident, "I got overinvolved and forgot everything else around me," she admits. Her marriage, already on shaky ground, collapsed as a result. Roslyn learned her lesson well, though. Today she and her second husband share responsibility equally in caring for both his elderly mother and Duane.

The most profound conflicts arise when burdens are not shared equally or spouses have radically different assessments of the situation: one optimistic, the other pessimistic (and only time will tell who is the more realistic). During the two years that Eileen and Neil Mitzman's daughter was mortally ill with AIDS, Eileen recalls, "I was totally convinced that we were going to save Marni. It never once entered my mind that she was going to die from this, whereas Neil felt, and he said this to me, 'I'm being more realistic than you.' And I took terrible offense at that."

Tips for Marital Maintenance

Communicate with your spouse. During a protracted medical ordeal, partners can become virtual strangers. In order to avoid misunderstandings, mixed signals, and later recriminations, regularly discuss with your spouse ex-

---

✒ CHECKLIST

The Caregiver Maintenance Checklist

If you answer "Not True" to more than three of these each week, it's time to make some changes before stress gets the upper hand.

Generally True	Not True	
☐	☐	I get out of the house at least once a day.
☐	☐	I get a break from caregiving for several consecutive hours at least once a week.
☐	☐	I get at least 6 to 8 hours of uninterrupted sleep every 24 hours.
☐	☐	I get at least 20 minutes of exercise twice a week.
☐	☐	I eat breakfast every day.
☐	☐	I eat at least 3 meals every day.
☐	☐	I weigh myself every day.
☐	☐	I drink more than enough water every day.
☐	☐	I'm fastidious about infection control, particularly hand washing and my own skin care.
☐	☐	I talk or visit with supportive friends and family at least once a day.
☐	☐	My own symptoms, such as insomnia, indigestion, and anxiety, are well managed.
☐	☐	I assess myself for signs of depression every week.
☐	☐	I keep appointments with my own doctor and dentist.

---

actly what you're doing and why, how much time and energy it involves, and how he or she can help you maintain your other family and professional obligations in the process. If you tell your spouse what you're thinking and feeling and what you need, you'll be more apt to find sympathy and practical support instead of fostering resentment.

As we've advocated throughout, spread the work around. Even if you're doing all the nursing or supervising, make sure your partner helps out by tending the kids, getting dinner on the table, paying the bills, taking care of the house, car, and yard—and providing an empathetic ear for you. Don't fall into the harmful habit of doing everything yourself.

Deliberately schedule "quality time" for just the two of you. Go out to dinner, see a movie, check into a hotel, have some laughs together. Talk about shared interests and good times instead of sickness and death.

Also, don't let illness become an excuse for avoiding physical intimacy. A couple's sexual desire may not always be in harmony, but the anxieties of being a caregiver can occupy one's mind so much that all interest in sex is lost. *Loss of libido is almost always a symptom of poorly managed stress or depression.* Lovemaking is also a wonderful way to release tension and to show how much you care. Make time for romance regularly or find professional counseling if you can't seem to get together.

Children

As many as 40 percent of caregivers have children under eighteen to care for in addition to an ailing relative. "It's hard," says Gerri Clarke, a caregiver to her husband and a mother of two, "the sense of feeling conflicted and being pulled between the different needy members of your family." In the tumult of looking after someone who is seriously ill, it's sometimes easy to overlook kids' emotional needs, especially since youngsters may react to what is going on in ways most adults would never imagine. For example, a child may believe that something he once said or thought has caused the person's illness or that parents have "allowed" the loved one to get sick. Others, particularly adolescents and teenagers, may be embarrassed by the sick person's appearance or the chaos at home and stay away, making it harder still to keep tabs on their feelings.

A traumatic encounter with sickness or death can scar children for life. Many grow into adults who cope poorly with medical crises and grief or, like children of divorce, have more problems than usual developing confidence in themselves and forming new relationships.

Audree Siden honored her terminally ill husband's wish to be nursed in their Manhattan apartment. It wasn't until years later that she realized how traumatizing it had been for the couple's three teenage sons to see their forty-seven-year-old father dying of lung cancer. "My husband wanted it this way, and I believe in the dying person's right, you see. It was a choice I made. But," she adds frankly, "one ought to think about the other people living in the midst of that scene because it may not be *their* choice.

"My children, who loved their father so much, were mortified by the experience, and all of them are still struggling with what went on, in that they feel guilty because they were frightened. This was happening in the middle of the living room, and they could not handle it. They would come in and walk around him." Almost classically, the three boys, all in high school, spent increasing amounts of time at friends' houses.

"For a lot of years," she continues, "my children were angry with me about this. There is indelible damage in their lives. They're heartbroken."

Audree's voice is tinged with sadness, though not regret. "I will never regret caring for anyone at home," she says resolutely. "So I would do it all over again, although I would have more psychological support services for my children."

Helping Kids Through the Crisis

Tell them what's going on. Obviously, you have to modify the message according to a child's age and ability to comprehend, but kids, like adults, will cope better if they understand the situation and how they can help. If you don't know what to say or how to broach the subject without frightening a child, get some expert help or talk to another parent who has been through it. Speak to a hospital social worker, family counselor, or pastor who has experience talking to children about sickness and death.

Be mindful of silent cries for attention. On the surface your child may appear to be "doing fine" when inside she's churning with emotions she can't define or express. Look for

- complaints of psychosomatic symptoms;
- regressive behavior, such as thumb sucking or bed-wetting;
- undereating or overeating;
- sleeplessness or oversleeping;
- aggressive, defiant, or argumentative behavior;
- "perfect" behavior;
- refusal to attend school;
- decline in school performance.

Alert teachers, coaches, school counselors, baby-sitters, and child-care workers to the situation at home. They can keep an eye out for any problems your child has coping and provide additional reassurance and support during the time you're apart.

Make kids' lives as normal as possible. Because you're busy and distracted, it's more important than ever to maintain a schedule. Sticking to a routine for having family meals, attending to homework and studies, participating in extracurricular activities, and playing with friends all help kids find their bearings and maintain an even keel.

Mary Vitro recalls, "When I was fourteen and my mother was dying, no one took time for my two sisters and me. So it was important that my son Dougie have some consistency in his life. I tried to maintain a balance and to keep things as upbeat as possible at home. My husband and I agreed that I would leave the hospital every day by six so that I could be home with Dougie and put him to bed."

Schedule regular quality time with kids and teenagers. Spend time with youngsters individually. When things are tough, they need your undivided attention more than ever, and you need their love and life-focused perspective. Listen attentively to their fears, worries, hopes, and dreams, and respond thoughtfully. Be generous with hugs and praise. Do everything in your power to make sure a kid knows that he is loved.

Reassure youngsters that they did nothing to cause this crisis and are not to blame for your sadness, anxiety, or short fuse. For grown-ups who have known each other intimately over decades, eruptions of temper can be chalked up to experience; they're water under the bridge. It's very different for children or adolescents, however, because they might not fully comprehend what's going on and imagine themselves somehow at fault.

During Paul Clarke's twelve years on home kidney dialysis, the New York attorney occasionally became irritable or depressed, as would almost anyone forced to be hooked up to a machine five hours a day, three days a week. "As an adult," says his wife, "you can turn off your emotional response until the depression or anger clears itself up. It's much harder with children, to explain to them that the short temper, the lashing out, doesn't relate to them. When our daughters were old enough—maybe seven or eight—I explained that there were times when Daddy just became frustrated and that it didn't have anything to do with them. I said, 'When it happens, give me a look, and we'll leave the room and talk about it outside.' At times they understood, and at times they didn't. They're not saints, either. When my daughters got a little older, they would walk out and look at me and say, 'Oh-oh, it's one of those days. Let's stay away from Dad today.' "

Involve youngsters in patient care if they're able and willing. Kids are frustrated by impotence just like adults. They can help by providing companionship to the sick person and by assisting with household chores. By your making them an essential part of the team, young people are better able to cope—and it's great preparation for life. ◄ *See "The Ready Reserves: Teenagers and Children," page 219.*

8

Paying the Bills

My father was extremely lucky. Over the summer we helped arrange for his next-door neighbors Ron and Darlene Twilley to purchase his house on the river. It was an idea that Aunt Kitty, Dave, and I had been after Bob to consider since his heart surgery.

Before he got sick, Pop was by no means poor. His car, truck, RV, and home were paid off. He had his Social Security, a handful of old stocks, a little savings in the bank, and a wad of cash under a floorboard in his closet—which he subsidized with occasional freelance carpentry while he was healthy. But after just a few months of sickness, between his regular monthly expenses and dropping hundreds of dollars at a clip for essential medications and services, Dad's cash flow had slowed to a trickle. We had no idea how long his illness would last or how much care he would require.

As part of the deal for the house, the Twilleys gladly agreed to let Bob stay on as a tenant. Thanks to the quick and friendly sale, which he negotiated himself and my brother John closed, Pop was able to live out his life in the riverfront home he loved, essentially free of day-to-day money worries. I'll repeat: My father was extremely lucky.

For most sick people, their caregivers, and their families, anxiety over dwindling finances adds immeasurably to the daily emotional strain. What's more, millions of Americans are forced to choose their medical care based on what they can afford rather than on what they need. Prescriptions alone can routinely cost someone with cancer, heart disease, or AIDS hundreds and even thousands of dollars per month.

Nearly 40 million Americans have no health coverage at all. But even those who do have insurance are often lulled into a false sense of financial security. Dad's heart surgery, for example, cost over $95,000. His Medicare covered the standard 80 percent of that but left an unpaid balance of roughly $19,000. In addition to his hospital bill, his pre-

265

scriptions and medical supplies cost nearly $1,800 his first month home. Had Pop not been carrying supplemental Medigap coverage, he would have been wiped out.

Not only can a life-threatening illness devastate a patient financially, it can drain a care partner's bank account as well. "The moment my husband had his stroke, our family income was 35 percent of what it had been," says caregiver Pat Still. Looking after an ailing family member forces one in two caregivers to lose time at work, and one in five have to quit their jobs altogether. What's more, it's the caregiver who often absorbs the preponderance of "hidden" health care costs: the out-of-pocket expenses for everything from travel to long-distance phone bills to baby-sitters to parking fees at the hospital garage.

The purpose of this chapter is to show you sensible ways to conserve cash, to get the most out of benefits the ill person is entitled to, and to use *all* available assets to get by.

Bookkeeping 101

The reluctance of many people to discuss money matters frankly and explicitly further complicates the task of managing the financial affairs of a sick person. For many, discussion of finances is a stark reminder of their vulnerability and dependence. If they've been a parent and provider most of their lives, their natural impulse is to try to reassure us that everything is under control rather than admit they're overcome by worry.

It takes diplomacy and finesse to encourage a previously independent adult to tell you his money woes. Unless you routinely discussed financial affairs long before the illness, there's no easy way to broach the subject. (One trick is to express *your* concern, something on the order of "I'm worried about money. How are we going to pay for all this?" Put the person in the position of show-

ing you his plan.) The challenge for a caregiver is to form a clear picture of the patient's assets and liabilities without making him feel like a child or prompting him to question our motives.

Obviously, if our ailing loved one is able to manage her own affairs, all we need do is help with record-keeping, correspondence, and banking. If she's incapacitated, we can simply step in and organize everything ourselves. More often, though, the subject comes up following a medical crisis when seemingly insurmountable bills start piling up. Whatever the case, we have to start with an accurate understanding of the situation in order to formulate a realistic plan.

Writing things down helps reduce these delicate conversations to sheer numbers. Rather than rely on memory, impressions, denial, or wishful thinking, sit down with your loved one at the kitchen table or bedside and make a list of everything coming in and everything going out. Then vow to update it at least monthly. You'll need to create four separate files:

1. *A financial resources file.* List all the person's bank accounts and current balances, including checking, savings, money-market funds, and CDs. Add up the monthly income: take-home pay from work; Social Security and other public entitlements; disability payments and pensions; annuities and stock dividends; and any other income from rental properties, royalties, individual retirement accounts, bonds, or mutual funds.

Once you know exactly how much money he has, write down all predictable monthly expenses: rent or mortgage payments; utilities and phone; car payments; gas, maintenance, and public transportation costs; insurance premiums; food and clothing; child-care or elder-care expenses; unreimbursed medical expenses, especially prescriptions and medical supplies; monthly loan payments; taxes; miscellaneous household expenses; tuition; legal and accounting fees; and any other monthly payables.

Once we know how much is left over each month (or how quickly we're falling behind), we can set about figuring out how to juggle the new bills.

2. *An unpaid-bills file.* Start a flow sheet or use a loose-leaf notebook to list the name of the provider, company, or institution that sent the bill; the invoice, account, and patient identification numbers; the specific item or service provided; the amount of the bill; any amount paid out of pocket; and the amount of any reimbursement that arrived from Medicare or other insurance. Leave some room on each page for making notes.

3. *A medical insurance file.* When calling or writing to insurance companies, local Social Security or Medicare representatives, hospital, home-care and doctors' business offices, you'll need all the latest information about your loved one's case right at your fingertips.

In one central file, keep statements, letters, notifications, and adjustments from the insurance company or Medicare; copies of claim forms and applications you've submitted and letters you've written; proof of payments already made; and any certificates of eligibility and disability determinations.

Before anyone can help you, you'll need to refer to the tracking codes on each letter or statement or form, the patient identification and customer account numbers, exact dates of each piece of correspondence, the names and telephone extensions of the specific individuals you've been in touch with, and the dates of those calls.

Make sure you carefully read and save everything that comes in the mail from service providers, insurers, government and social service offices, creditors, and banks. In addition, faithfully and accurately maintain records of insurance premium payments.

4. *A legal affairs file.* If you haven't done it already, now is the time to sit down with the sick person and discuss the possibility of his granting a financial power of attorney or a springing power of attorney to you, another family member, or a trusted friend or colleague. Bank and credit union accounts should be placed in trust, and up-to-date signature cards and power of attorney placed on file with the financial institution.

You'll also need copies of the medical power of attorney or health care proxy; guardianship appointment; mortgages and deeds; insurance and loan contracts; tax returns; pertinent birth, marriage, and death certificates; and divorce decrees. Make sure you know where the will and life insurance or burial policies are kept, too. ▶ *See chapter 9, "Preparing for the Worst."*

Tricks for Maintaining Cash Flow

Despite crushing bills and limited income, there are many things we can do to get by for months and even years: juggling creditors, negotiating payment plans, using all the assets at our disposal (including credit lines and home equity), and seeing to it that our loved one receives everything he's entitled to from insurers, government agencies, and private organizations. Just like old people on fixed incomes and working folks with young families, the sick survive by using these tried-and-true tactics every day.

Obviously, the person handling money-related matters in this situation could be overseeing the patient's finances or joint finances (in the case of a spouse or romantic partner), or footing many of the expenses himself. For the sake of consistency we refer throughout to *"your* finances," *"your* credit rating," and so on.

Hold off paying the biggest bills. Most of us can't pay monstrous medical bills or large credit card balances the day the invoice lands in the mailbox—

nor should we. In managing money, first and foremost we have to make sure we hang on to enough cash for food, shelter, and medicine.

With medical bills you'll find that the balance due fluctuates as insurance and Medicare reimbursements get sorted out. It can take two months or more just for all the charges and claims to catch up. Many times you can sit on big bills for sixty to ninety days before creditors start complaining in earnest. And as many as six months can go by before a bill is sent out for collection or reported to the credit bureau. Meanwhile, you keep receiving bills and past-due notices—an unnerving experience for people who have always prided themselves on honoring their debts promptly. But once the dust settles, you will work out a payment plan you can afford.

✳ *Important: Don't think you can get away with ignoring bills and collection notices over the long run. Creditors will report you to the credit bureaus and eventually slap a lien on your bank account, house, or paycheck.*

Negotiate with creditors. Most creditors will dicker if you explain the situation and make a reasonable offer before the debt snowballs into a huge problem and damages your credit rating. Get on the phone to the business office preferably before the account is sent out for collection. Collection agencies and lawyers will also often negotiate an extended payment plan or reduced cash settlement; they're paid a percentage of whatever they collect, and it costs them more time and money to sue you.

Apply for several credit cards. First of all, you can pay most bills (including the hospital, doctor, diagnostic center, pharmacy, and supermarket) with a major credit card or take a cash advance in a pinch. If it's a matter of survival or getting the medical care your

loved one needs, make minimum payments on the cards until finances improve.

Given the exorbitant interest rates on unpaid credit card balances, though, this can quickly escalate into a long-term financial burden. Shop around for credit cards that offer the lowest interest rates and consider transferring balances from other cards to these accounts.

The reduced rates are often as much as 10 percent lower and usually remain in effect for about six months—at which point you can most likely transfer the balance to yet another, lower interest card. These offers come in the mail all the time. Tip: Transfer the entire balance on card A to card B, and in no time card A will attempt to woo you back with its own special low rate. Apply for as much credit as you can get just in case you need it down the road.

Consider applying for a second mortgage or home-equity loan, or renegotiating your current mortgage. The interest rates are far lower than credit cards, and the interest you pay is tax deductible. The monthly payments can be adjusted to something affordable by extending the term of the loan.

Each year tens of thousands of older Americans are forced to sell the farm to be able to afford a nursing home or even just to meet monthly household expenses throughout a protracted illness. But putting your home on the market is a risky proposition that's subject to the whims of the marketplace and taxes. It also depletes the estate, a tremendous disappointment to folks who wanted to help provide for their family after death—not to mention the headaches and heartaches of uprooting your life in the middle of an illness.

Even if you're fortunate enough to own a home in the first place, for most folks it's usually their single largest asset and represents an entire life's savings. Think about borrowing against your equity before selling out. Also ask your banker about the advantages and drawbacks of a *home-equity conversion*, or *reverse mortgage*. In this relatively new form of financing, the bank pays the homeowners a monthly income while they continue to live in the home. The catch: The bank gradually acquires a lien against the home. After one of the homeowners dies, the survivor must repay the loan or forfeit the property.

Consider cashing in life insurance policies or selling a policy to a viatical company. Read your life insurance policy or talk to the broker. Most mature policies can be converted to cash prior to the customer's death, albeit at a significant loss.

Higher payouts are often available through *viatical* companies, which emerged in 1988 in response to the AIDS epidemic. (*Viaticum* is the Latin word for "money or necessities for a journey.") These are groups of investors who speculate on "death futures": Depending on how long a patient with a confirmed terminal illness is expected to live, viators pay him a large portion of the insurance policy's face value—typically between 50 percent and 80 percent—and assume all future premium payments in return for collecting the benefits of the policy when the person dies. It may seem a bit ghoulish, but for patients desperately strapped for cash, the lump-sum settlement may allow them to live out their lives in relative comfort, while the alternative is perhaps to lose their home or be forced to go without medications that could ease their suffering.

A fair warning: Viatical settlements are taxable and still unregulated in most states. It pays to shop around and get offers from several companies before cashing in someone's death benefits.

☎ To receive a list of viatical settlement companies, call the National Viatical Association in Washington, D.C., at 202-347-7361.

Keep receipts for cash outlays. The Internal Revenue Service allows you to deduct itemized costs of equipment, furnishings, and permanent changes for access to a home as medical expenses. Even prostheses like artificial limbs and colostomy bags are deductible if they exceed 7.5 percent of a patient's adjusted gross income.

Another good reason to hold on to receipts is to avoid conflicts over financial matters with other family members or heirs to the estate. When Bob was sick, Dave and I used to routinely pay for his household expenses or medicine out of our own pockets. Dad would reimburse us later when he had the cash. Our flawless record-keeping of these transactions eliminated any arguments about money.

Liquidate IRAs or SEP-IRAs for up to two months. If your cash crunch is temporary, you can redeem the money from an individual retirement account or self-employed pension IRA without incurring a penalty as long as you replace it within sixty days, in what is called a *rollover*, and not touch it again for twelve months. You won't accrue any interest during this period, but you can lay your hands on some much needed cash in the meantime.

Take advantage of special payment programs at utility companies. Phone and power companies will almost always work out an affordable payment plan for sick or elderly people if you talk to the business office before the account falls too far in arrears.

If you can't get the help you need that way, contact your local *Community Action Agency*. Established under the Economic Opportunity Act of 1964, CAAs receive federal block grants to help Americans in financial need through a variety of programs, including Low Income Weatherization, which can intervene to stop someone's electricity from being cut off. Some CAAs can also refer you to other community services such as financial counseling or legal assistance for landlord-tenant or debtor-creditor problems.

☎ For a referral to your local CAA, call the National Association of Community Action Agencies in Washington, D.C., at 202-265-7546.

Know your rights! If you are having problems paying creditors, you have four options:

1. If you can afford to make lower payments on your debts, negotiate an extended schedule before the collection notices start piling up.
2. If you have assets or income that bill collectors could conceivably attach, consult an attorney or consumer counseling agency about filing bankruptcy. Don't let false pride get in your way. Bankruptcy is *a right.* Billion-dollar corporations protect themselves this way every day. So can you.
3. If you or your loved one is disabled, living on public entitlements, and have no other income or assets, let your creditors know that you're "judgment proof"—in other words, if they sue you, there'll be nothing to collect.
4. If bill collectors are harassing you, in a phone call or letter demand they stop phoning you at home or at the office. You are under no legal obligation to talk directly to them.

☎ For assistance negotiating payment plans with creditors, stopping harassment, or formulating a workable budget when you're in debt, locate a consumer credit counseling service in your area by contacting the National Foundation for Consumer Credit at 800-388-2227 or 301-589-5600. Make an appointment at your local agency long before you're facing a lawsuit, lien, garnishment, repossession, foreclosure, or eviction.

Financial-Assistance Programs

Government-Funded Programs

Most federally funded financial benefits for retired or disabled Americans are administered by the Social Security Administration. The largest programs include (1) standard Social Security retirement benefits, (2) Supplemental Security Disability Income (SSDI), and (3) Supplemental Security Income (SSI).

Hospital social workers and case managers at social service agencies are particularly adept at helping you find your way through this daunting bureaucratic maze, but the paperwork and legwork inevitably fall to the family caregivers.

☎ To find out the programs for which your patient is eligible, or for a referral to your local office, call the Social Security Administration's information line at 800-772-1213. Request the free booklet "Understanding Social Security."

Social Security Retirement Benefits

Men and women age sixty-five and older are entitled to a monthly retirement check depending on how much and how long they paid into Social Security while they were working. To give you a rough idea of how much Social Security recipients can expect to receive, a sixty-five-year-old retiree who had steady earnings throughout his lifetime and earned $30,000 his last working year would collect about $12,000 a year in retirement benefits, or $18,000 if his spouse does not qualify for her own retirement benefits. At $50,000 the annual benefit would amount to approximately $13,000, or $20,000. Taking early Social Security at age sixty-two results in a lower monthly payment.

Supplemental Security Disability Income (SSDI)

Social Security also makes monthly payments to people under sixty-five should they become disabled through illness or injury. Eligibility for SSDI begins only after six full months of disability and continues as long as the person remains disabled. If your loved one is sixty-five or older *and* disabled, her disability benefits and retirement benefits will be formulated into one monthly payment.

The benefits scale for SSDI is comparable to that for retirement. Again, two examples: If a man had worked steadily until becoming disabled at age thirty-five and he was earning $30,000 a year, he would collect about $12,500 annually, or $19,000 if he has a family. Earning $50,000 a year upon becoming disabled at age fifty-five would bring annual benefits of $14,500, or $21,500 for a family.

It's important to get this process rolling as early as you can. Disability determinations can take months, sometimes years, to gain official approval, especially for folks with chronic or recurring conditions. It's a little easier for patients with a clear-cut, life-threatening diagnosis such as advanced cancer, stroke, or AIDS. The rules change constantly, and the restrictions get tougher each year. You'll need access to all your patient's medical records.

* *After two years on disability, patients become eligible to sign up for Medicare regardless of their age—and sooner if they're on kidney dialysis.*

▶ *See* "*Medicare,*" *page 278.* ◀ *See* "*Obtaining Medical Records,*" *page 87.*

Other Family Members Who Qualify for Social Security and Disability Benefits

- The retiree's or disabled person's spouse, beginning at age sixty-two; he or she may collect a higher Social Security benefit on his or her own record

---

> **Uncle Sam's Definition of Disability**
>
> The Social Security Administration considers a person disabled if "you are unable to do any kind of work for which you are suited, and your disability is expected to last for at least a year or to result in death."

- The retiree's or disabled person's spouse at any age if he or she cares for the retiree's or disabled person's child (who must be under sixteen or disabled and receiving Social Security benefits)
- The retiree's or disabled person's children if they are unmarried and under eighteen or under nineteen but a full-time student in elementary or secondary school, or eighteen or older and severely disabled since before age twenty-two
- The retiree's or disabled person's ex-spouse (or ex-spouses), beginning at sixty-two, if he or she was married to the retiree or disabled person for at least ten years, is currently unmarried, and is not eligible for Social Security either personally or on someone else's Social Security record

Generally, eligible family members collect a monthly benefit of up to 50 percent of the retiree's or disabled person's rate. There is, however, a family cap of roughly 150 to 180 percent of the main beneficiary's payment. Should the sum of the benefits on the account exceed the family limit, family members' benefits are reduced proportionately; the retiree's or disabled person's monthly check goes untouched.

We should point out that a fifty-five-year-old widow who never worked outside the home and has no dependents would not qualify for Social Security for another ten years, at which point she would receive survivor's benefits. Tragically, our society's harshest burden falls on the survivor who finds

Survivors Benefits

When a man or woman who has worked and paid into Social Security dies, certain family members are entitled to survivors benefits: the widow or widower, unmarried children under eighteen (or up to age nineteen if they are attending high school full time), dependent parents at age fifty-two or older, and divorced spouses, provided the marriage lasted at least ten years.

The surviving spouse may collect full benefits beginning at age sixty-five, or beginning at age fifty if he or she is disabled; reduced benefits of 71 to 94 percent beginning at age sixty, or 75 percent benefits at any age if he or she cares for a child of the deceased's who is less than sixteen or disabled. Disabled children are also eligible, as long as they were disabled before age twenty-two.

---

herself in this situation after having endured a partner's death.

❋ *The Social Security Administration does not recognize unmarried partners such as common-law husbands and wives or same-sex couples no matter how long they've lived together.*

Supplemental Security Income (SSI)

People who are disabled or blind or over sixty-five with *extremely* limited income and no significant assets except for a home may be eligible for Supplemental Security Income in addition to their other Social Security benefits. Although the amount of the basic monthly SSI check is standard nationwide, some states supplement it with money of their own.

❋ *If your loved one meets the eligibility requirements for SSI, he's likely eligi-*ble for state-run programs like food stamps and Medicaid, too. Consult a hospital social worker or a case manager at a social service agency for the latest qualification guidelines.*

Aid to Families with Dependent Children (AFDC)

A similar national program, Aid to Families with Dependent Children (AFDC), combines federal aid and state funds to help the poorest Americans survive. Ever since the so-called war on poverty of the 1960s and 1970s, each state administers vast financial assistance programs, commonly referred to as welfare or public assistance.

If you or the sick person has a dependent child under eighteen, you may receive some additional help through AFDC. Keep in mind, though, that available funds are subject to the political vagaries of annual state budgets and federal cutbacks. The restrictions can be severe (Texas and Mississippi are notorious examples), with payments often amounting to as little as $100 per month.

Food Stamps

Food stamps is another federally funded program carried out by the states. Eligibility requirements vary, and the political pressure is on to further restrict access to this vital program that helps feed millions of elderly Americans and young children.

To find out what's available in your locale, check with your state department of social services. Better yet, make an appointment with a social worker or case manager at a hospital or social service agency.

Privately Funded Programs

A few civic and religious groups offer extremely limited financial assistance to the sick and elderly. A rare few dispense small cash grants to reimburse patients for transportation to and from treatment. Some make modest onetime emergency assistance loans to families in dire need. Others lend or help pay for medical equipment and supplies.

Hospital social workers and counselors at patient-support organizations often know what's available—if anything. It doesn't hurt to appeal to local chapters of fraternal organizations and civic groups like the Lion's Club, Kiwanis, American Legion, Disabled Vets, Elks, Jaycees, Shriners, Salvation Army, Catholic and Jewish orders, and the community trust. ► *See Appendix A, "Recommended Resources," page 489.*

A Warning About Pensions

Many newly widowed women are shocked to discover that pension payments often stop when their husband dies. Generally speaking, employees are offered the option of collecting benefits during their lifetime or accepting a lower monthly payment plus a survivor's benefit for their spouse after they die. In the past, married folks weren't required to inform their spouse that they had signed away their survivor's benefits, but federal law now mandates that the partner give prior written consent.

Even though it means receiving a smaller monthly payment during the retiree's lifetime, couples should consider choosing the survivor's benefit, for if the surviving spouse is under sixty-two

and in good health, it might be her only source of income until she reaches Social Security retirement age unless she has a job or substantial savings. Keep in mind that you cannot reverse your decision once pension payments have begun.

Other points about pensions that spouses should be aware of:

- If an employee becomes disabled before retirement, there's a good chance he will have to forfeit his pension.
- Should a husband become disabled and then die before retirement age, his widow might still be able to collect—but not until the date her late husband would have reached retirement age and only if he had belonged to the plan more than ten years.
- The survivor benefits of your spouse's pension plan should be reviewed *before* he gets sick or starts collecting monthly retirement payments.

☎ For information on pensions paid to military retirees or veterans with service-related disabilities, check with the Department of Veterans Affairs at 800-827-1000.

Saving Money on Prescription Drugs

For most seriously ill people, prescription drugs quickly become their single largest monthly expense. Medicare pays *nothing* for outpatient medications, and

TABLE 8
Financial Aid, Equipment Loans, and Cost-Free Medical Care

For People With; Organization	Financial Aid	Lends or Donates Medical Equipment	Free Medical Care
AIDS			
Catholic Charities USA 703-549-1390	✔		
Amyotrophic Lateral Sclerosis			
The Amyotrophic Lateral Sclerosis Association 800-782-4747		✔	
Cancer			
American Cancer Society 800-227-2345	✔	✔	
Leukemia Society of America 800-955-4572	✔		
Kidney Disease			
American Kidney Fund 800-638-8299	✔		
The National Kidney Foundation 800-622-9010	✔	✔	
Lung Disease			
American Lung Association 800-586-4872		✔	
Parkinson's Disease			
National Parkinson Foundation 800-327-4545 In Florida: 800-433-7022		✔	✔
Has designated 13 U.S. Centers of Excellence to treat indigent Parkinson's patients free of charge			

many private insurance policies have extremely limited pharmacy benefits. Medicaid does pay for drugs—but the patient has to be living well below the poverty line to qualify in the first place.

One of the best arguments for buying a Medigap policy or joining a health maintenance organization (HMO) "managed care" plan is the prescription drug benefits. Most Americans, though, are

---

VOICE OF EXPERIENCE

"Toward the end when my husband was really sick with AIDS, I'd go to the pharmacy to pick up Rick's medications, and the cashier would whisper, 'That's $499.' She didn't want to say it out loud. Our insurance reimbursed us, but we had to lay out the cash; some months it came to $1,500. His pentamidine alone was $300 a pop.

"A lot of times the drugs would make Rick sick, and he couldn't take them anymore. In the meantime, we'd paid for eighty pills. I threw out drugs like you wouldn't believe."
—Mary Vitro

---

stuck paying for their medicines out of pocket or laying out hundreds of dollars in cash each month and waiting for reimbursement. It places a stranglehold on cash flow, forcing many people—especially senior citizens on fixed incomes or working folks with young families—to choose between food and shelter and essential lifesaving medicines.

Buyers' Clubs

Keeping costs down as much as possible becomes a matter of survival. You can save some money by asking your doctor or pharmacist to dispense generic formulations of common drugs, but many of the most expensive medications aren't available that way or the generic formulation doesn't work as well for some people as the premium brand. The greatest savings for most people with large monthly drug bills can be found through buyers' clubs.

Buyers' clubs are nothing more than cooperatives. Like farm co-ops or grocery co-ops, members join together to buy products in large volume. By combining their purchasing power, the group pays wholesale prices to the manufacturers and passes along the savings to its members. Depending on the prescription, buyers' clubs can beat retail prices by as much as 30 to 50 percent.

If you're over age fifty, your best bet is the American Association of Retired Persons. The AARP Pharmacy Service offers prompt service and considerable savings on drugs and medical supplies anywhere in the United States. National pharmacy chains like Stadtlanders have also established mail-order buyers' clubs. Buyers' clubs for people with AIDS have also sprung up in nearly every major city, and there are also national suppliers like the Community Prescription Service.

Order membership information from one of the co-ops listed below or contact your local chapter of one of the disease-related patient organizations listed in Appendix A for referrals to buyers' clubs in your area.

☎ American Association of Retired Persons (AARP) Pharmacy Service, 800-456-2277.

☎ American Preferred Prescription, 800-227-1195.

☎ Community Prescription Service, 800-842-0502.

☎ Medi-Mail, Inc., 800-793-3548.

☎ Preferred Rx, 800-843-7038.

☎ Stadtlanders Pharmacy, 800-238-7828.

Prescription Drug Patient-Assistance Programs

Most pharmaceutical manufacturers have extremely limited programs that offer their drugs to indigent patients at no cost. The eligibility criteria vary widely from company to company, and your loved one's physician usually has to make the request for you.

The Pharmaceutical Research and Manufacturers of America in Washington, D.C., publishes a free directory of its members that provide prescription drugs for people who cannot afford them. The booklet lists the name, address, and phone number of each manufacturer as well as the products covered by each program and its eligibility requirements.

☎ To request a free copy of the "Directory of Prescription Drug Patient Assistance Programs," call PhRMA at 202-835-3400.

* *To find out about other programs not listed in the directory, ask the doctor or nurse, check with the information hot line of a patient service organization, or contact manufacturers directly. Addresses and phone numbers of pharmaceutical companies can be found in the* Physicians' Desk Reference, *available in most libraries and large bookstores.*

AIDS Drug Assistance Programs

People with AIDS may also be eligible for the federally funded AIDS Drug Assistance Program. Each state receives money to help those who can't afford critical medications but aren't poor enough to qualify for Medicaid.

☎ For more information on this program, contact your state department of health or your local AIDS service organization. If you can't find its number, call the CDC National HIV/AIDS Hotline at 800-342-2437. ► *See Appendix A: "AIDS/HIV," page 489.*

Paying for Medical Care

Despite money-saving reforms over the last quarter century—including the pro-

liferation of managed-care organizations, utilization review to determine whether medical care is appropriate and necessary, and the development of uniform standards of practice among physicians and hospitals, quality-assurance programs, and tougher audits of hospitals and nursing homes—the cost of health care in America rises year after year. As a nation we spend more money per capita on medical services and drugs than any other.

The good news is that thousands of medical centers, university hospitals, and medical practices offer the finest health care available on the planet. The bad news is that millions of people are forced to choose their treatments based on what they can afford. Working the system effectively—getting your loved one what she needs from insurance companies and government programs such as Medicare and Medicaid—can literally be a matter of life and death.

Private Health Insurance

Most Americans who are covered by private health insurance policies belong to large group plans purchased by employers or labor organizations. The insurance company collects premiums from the group (in many cases, employees have part of the premium deducted from their paychecks), then invests the money aggressively. Many of the largest employers and unions are self-insured, meaning that they set aside money to pay employee medical expenses directly.

By dividing the financial risk among a large group of people, the insurance company or self-insured group can pay the bills for the employees who get sick, yet still show a profit at year's end. The insurer is literally betting money that most plan members won't become ill in any given year. That's important to understand, because it explains why individual policies are so expensive and why it's almost impossible to buy one for somebody who is already seriously ill. For a company to have to pay out more than it takes in is bad business.

That's also why you hear so much about "portability" in the debates on health care reform. As it stands now, if you get too sick to work or get laid off, you lose your group health insurance benefits.

COBRA

The federal Consolidated Omnibus Budget Reconciliation Act (COBRA), passed in 1986, mandates that companies with twenty or more workers allow their employees to continue their company medical coverage after they leave the job. But you have to pay a higher premium yourself—often with fewer benefits, too—and the insurance company is not obligated to cover you after eighteen months. Once the COBRA option expires, finding an insurer that will sell an individual policy at all proves difficult for most, and it is prohibitively expensive for those living on disability or unemployment.

If your ailing loved one is insured through your job's health insurance plan, do not leave the company for any reason until you've asked the benefits manager or insurance company representative to explain your options under COBRA. In 1989 the law was expanded to allow employees to extend their coverage for the full eighteen months even if they find a new insurer, but the policy does not immediately cover any pre-existing conditions—a not-uncommon scenario.

Two important things patients and caregivers should know about COBRA:

1. Though the federal act does not apply to companies with fewer than twenty employees, many states have enacted similar laws. The State Department of Insurance (known in some states by a different name, such as Commissioner of Insurance) can tell you about a state's insurance laws; the best way to find its telephone number is through information assistance.

2. This conversion does not occur automatically. Should you fail to exercise your option at the time of separation, the insurer is under no obligation to continue your coverage.

Consider Open Enrollment

If you're having trouble getting family coverage because of your age or that of a family member or your medical history, scout around for open-enrollment offers. Each state has some form of high-risk insurance pool available, often from companies such as Blue Cross/ Blue Shield that are required to offer coverage periodically to anyone who signs up. There may be a waiting period before coverage kicks in for preexisting conditions—as there are with most policies—but this is often the only way to get insurance. Managed-care groups or HMOs typically offer open enrollment when they're expanding into new markets.

✳ *Ask an insurance broker about open enrollment or check the mail, magazines, health newsletters, and TV for offers. Ask hospital social workers, counselors at social service agencies, senior centers, and disease-related organizations, or the business departments at your patient's hospital and doctor's office.*

Types of Private Insurance

Whether you're covered under a group plan or an individual policy, there are basically two forms of private health insurance: fee for service and managed care.

Fee for service is traditional coverage where you pay premiums and a deductible, then get reimbursed for the cost of your care. (Many hospitals, diagnostic centers, and doctors' offices file claims directly with the insurance company.) Depending on the policy, you will pay about 20 percent of the costs out of pocket up to a certain point. Most policies have annual and lifetime limits on how much they will pay.

Fee-for-service insurance comes in two basic forms: *hospitalization* and *major medical* coverage. "Hospitalization" refers to the cost of institutional care. "Major medical" policies cover doctors' bills and outpatient diagnostic tests and treatments. All but the most expensive private insurance policies pay extremely limited benefits for prescription drugs, home-care services, and nursing homes.

Managed care—HMOs and PPOs (Preferred Provider Organizations)— are groups of health care providers such as hospitals, doctors, pharmacies, diagnostic facilities, and labs that band together to offer comprehensive medical services to members in return for premium payments and a nominal charge at each visit. There's usually no deductible, but there are strict limits on available services. While prescription drugs, visits to primary physicians and specialists, and hospitalization are covered, your loved one has to get permission from the group before undertaking major treatment such as chemotherapy or surgery, or even before visiting the emergency room. Home-care and nursing home benefits are meager.

The obvious advantage to an HMO is its comprehensive benefits. The disadvantage is that it covers costs only within the network. If your patient requires highly specialized treatment or needs to shop around for experts or hospitals, the choices are extremely limited. And should he require medical care when he's out of town, he's on his own except in dire emergencies.

* *If your loved one belongs to an HMO, make sure you understand the contractual requirements for prior notification or precertification before scheduling medical appointments or trips to the hospital.*

Government-Funded Health Insurance

Medicare

People over sixty-five who are eligible for Social Security retirement benefits are also eligible for the federal health insurance program Medicare. Anyone under sixty-five who has been receiving Social Security disability payments for two years also qualifies. (The two-year wait is waived for patients on kidney dialysis.)

Like private insurance, Medicare "Part A" covers institutional care while "Part B" covers major medical expenses such as doctor's bills, outpatient tests, physical therapy, and hospice care. The program pays 80 percent of your loved one's covered health care costs; the rest is left to the patient and any private co-insurance he might have. Medicare does not pay for outpatient prescriptions, and nursing home and home-care benefits are strictly limited.

For more information about Medicare or to resolve a complaint, contact

☎ Health Care Financing Administration Medicare Hotline, 800-638-6833.

☎ Social Security Administration Toll-Free Information Line, 800-772-1213.

You can also contact your local Social Security office, hospital social workers, or case managers at a local social service organization.

Medigap

Medigap is a *private* insurance policy used to supplement coverage under Medicare. It provides additional payments for hospital stays, home care, and nursing home services, and reduces the deductible for other major medical expenses.

Anyone eligible for Medicare is allowed to purchase Medigap coverage, regardless of any preexisting medical conditions. Since Medicare pays just 80 percent of hospitalization and major medical expenses, Medigap insurance can help prevent the financial devastation of a seriously ill person.

There are ten basic Medigap plans (A, B, C, and so on), each with different benefit packages. Only plans H, I, and J provide coverage for prescription medications. Most Medigap policies are administered like standard fee-for-service insurance. Some states are experimenting with Medigap coverage provided by managed-care organizations such as HMOs. This can all get pretty confusing, so it's vital to shop around and gather all the information you can before assisting your loved one in purchasing a policy.

For more information about Medigap insurance, contact

☎ American Association of Retired Persons (AARP), 800-424-3410.

You can also contact the State Department of Insurance or a local insurance broker.

Medicaid

If your loved one has minimal income and few remaining assets, she may be able to qualify for Medicaid. Each state funds its own program in conjunction with the federal Health Care Financing Administration, with the state department of social services administering Medicaid locally.

Eligibility requirements and benefits vary widely from state to state. To qualify, a person must be poor enough to be receiving SSI, welfare, or public assistance. Not only are restrictions stringent and benefits in some states meager, but few hospitals and doctors' offices accept Medicaid in any given locale. Recipients can expect few choices among physicians; they are frequently forced to seek care at public hospitals and clinics. However, some states are now experimenting with allowing Medicaid beneficiaries to join managed-care groups such as HMOs. One bright spot: Prescription drugs are covered.

Fully 40 percent of Medicaid benefits are paid to nursing homes. After using up their benefits under Medicare and any private insurance, folks who need continued care in a skilled nursing facility must "spend down" all their remaining assets until they are sufficiently impoverished to qualify. The healthy spouse often suffers the most. Since many assets are held jointly, and total household income is considered in determining Medicaid eligibility, caregivers are frequently forced into poverty themselves just to get their loved ones the medical care they need.

The Spousal Impoverishment Act

Recent changes in federal law now provide for healthy spouses to hang on to some of their assets and income without disqualifying the ailing person from Medicaid coverage for nursing home care. Instead of both partners spending down to Medicaid eligibility levels, you can keep your home and its contents, your car, burial plot, funeral plan, and up to approximately $1,200 of income per month. Life insurance policies are not exempt from "spend-down" requirements, however; you'll have to cash them out.

For more information on the Spousal Impoverishment Act, contact your local Area Agency on Aging, state department of social services or Medicaid office, a hospital social worker or case manager at a local social service agency, or an elder care attorney.

☎ For more information about Medicaid or to resolve a complaint, contact the state department of social services or the department of welfare; check the white pages for listings. Or call HCFA's Baltimore headquarters (410-786-3000) for a referral to your state Medicaid agency. Hospital social workers and case managers in social service agencies are also adept at navigating the Medicaid bureaucracy.

Veterans and Military Dependents

If your patient was honorably discharged or retired from military service, he might be eligible to receive medical care at a local veterans hospital, clinic, or rehabilitation facility. There's also the *Civilian Health and Medical Program* (CHAMPVA), a health benefits program for dependents of veterans who sustained a permanently disabling injury or became ill while on active military duty. *The Civilian Health and Medical Program of the Department of the Uniformed Services* (CHAMPUS), administered by the Department of Defense, covers military retirees and their dependents as well as families of deceased servicemen or those still on active military duty.

For more information or to resolve a complaint, contact

☎ Department of Veterans Affairs, 800-827-1000.

☎ CHAMPVA, 800-733-8387.

☎ CHAMPUS, 303-361-1126.

How to Get the Most out of Health Insurance

Whether your loved one's medical care is paid for by private insurance, Medicare, Medicaid, or veterans benefits, there are a few tried-and-true techniques to make sure she gets everything she's entitled to:

Read the contract carefully. Novice caregivers have all sorts of misconceptions about insurance. You have to know exactly what services the plan pays for and what it does not pay for in order to formulate a realistic financial survival plan. Don't get caught unaware. Maintain reliable records of your premium payments, too.

✳ *Pay careful attention to requirements for second opinions or prior notification before you schedule consultations or treatment.*

Check each bill for accuracy. Very often you'll find yourself charged for services you did not receive. Either the hospital or doctor's office made a clerical error, or you were charged for a test or treatment that was ordered by the doctor but never carried out. Make sure you're billed only for services rendered.

Submit claims promptly after receiving your bill. When someone is seriously ill and the bills are piling up, the natural inclination is to put off completing all the paperwork. Bad idea. It increases the possibility of mistakes being made either on your end or at the insurance company. File photocopies of all bills and claims that have been submitted, stubs from payments received, explanations of benefits, and rulings from the insurance company.

Resubmit denied claims. Simple clerical errors or inadequate supporting documentation results in millions of claims being denied each year. Maybe the policy or patient ID number was recorded incorrectly. Maybe the diagnosis or medical justification was incomplete. Maybe the dates were wrong or medical orders were not legible or were punched into the computer incorrectly. Get out a new envelope and stamp, and send it again.

Don't take no for an answer. A few years ago my insurance carrier rejected a claim for my unusually lengthy physical therapy following knee surgery. I asked my doctor to write a letter stating that the additional therapy was medically necessary—and the company paid up. A friend was denied coverage for a glucose tolerance blood test when she had breast cancer. A letter from her doctor explaining that he'd ordered the diagnostic procedure in order to rule out diabetes was enough to settle the matter. Sometimes all it takes is a different claims adjuster at the insurance company reviewing the file for a payment to be reconsidered in the patient's favor.

Be persistent! If you're still not satisfied, ask your insurance company about its official procedure for resolving disputed claims. Closer examination of the case can often result in additional payment. If you've exhausted your appeal with the company, talk to a disease-related patient service organization, consult an attorney, or complain to your state insurance regulator.

—9—

Preparing for the Worst

When Bob was first told he had terminal cancer back in June, he immediately called my brother John in Fort Riley, Kansas. "I need you to come home and help me put my affairs in order," he said calmly. Over the next week, John drove Dad around town, making arrangements for us to handle his banking and bills if he became incapacitated, putting the title of the car in his wife Mary's name, and finalizing the sale of the house to the Twilleys next door. Dad, who already owned a cemetery plot next to our mother's and a small burial policy, even had John contact the preacher and the pallbearers for the funeral. "The only thing Pop wouldn't let me do," John recalls, "was buy a casket. That he wouldn't hear of."

Bob planned for the end of his life so matter-of-factly that one night he asked my brother and his wife, Sheri, if they wanted anything in particular from the house. John said that he'd always coveted Dad's brass bed, to which my father replied "Okay!" and disappeared

into his room and began dismantling it. John recalls with a laugh, "I had to tell him, 'No, Pop! You can keep the bed until you die, okay?' He got a big kick out of that."

Bob's candor was an exception. In our culture, most people don't plan ahead for death. We don't even like to talk about it. That's why although numerous polls show nine in ten Americans do not want extraordinary measures taken to prolong their lives should they become terminally ill, only one in five has put that wish in writing. Sick people may avoid planning for their death because they view the discussion as frightening, depressing, or a sign they've given up, while caregivers often avoid it out of their own denial, false hope, or fear of sounding morbid or self-serving.

Time and again I've seen well-educated, articulate men and women—usually savvy when it comes to financial and legal matters—agonize over how and when to broach the subject of wills, living wills, and so on with the seriously ill, repeatedly putting it off until it's too late. That's a shame because messy legal affairs can interfere with medical care, wreak financial havoc, and cause untold grief for caregivers and survivors:

Without a health care proxy or medical power of attorney, caregivers may find themselves with no legal standing to advocate on the patient's behalf. At best, the medical team is forced to figure out which family member to listen to. Without something in writing, who is "next of kin"? And who has the patient's best interests at heart?

Without an advance directive or living will, the medical team and the family must guess (or argue about) what an unconscious or mentally incapacitated patient would want under critical medical circumstances. Even if you know in your heart what your loved one would want you to do, how do you get the doctor and hospital to comply?

Without a financial power of attorney and signatory powers at the bank, how do the patient's bills get paid? Who negotiates with creditors and makes sure the doctor, hospital, and home-care company don't discontinue services? Who can endorse checks and make deposits, file insurance claims, apply for benefits, take out a mortgage or loan, sell a house, or cash out an insurance policy?

When custody of surviving children has not been arranged legally, kids may land in foster care or become pawns in court battles between grandparents, aunts and uncles, stepparents, and so on. Not only is the legal wrangling expensive and time-consuming, but it can cause irreparable emotional damage in children.

Someone who dies without a will— even if the person had few worldly possessions—lays the groundwork for acrimonious and costly fights among survivors. Fees for professional arbitration that should have been avoided eat up the estate, and bitter recriminations linger long after the legal dust has settled.

Getting Started

The truth of the matter is that the moment to discuss crucial issues will *never* seem quite right. But they affect too many people beyond the patient to let our social discomfort get in the way. Naturally, the best advice is to tend to legal matters before anyone gets sick. Long before Mom or Dad becomes debilitated, order living will forms for them *as well as for yourself, your spouse, your in-laws, your brothers and sisters, and your grown children.* Routinely review insurance coverage and periodically update wills, especially during family transitions—marriages, divorces, births, retirements—or when buying or selling a home or business. Designate a trustee for your own bank accounts and appoint a springing power of attorney. Make it a family affair: While you're tending to your business, ask your loved ones if they've taken care of theirs.

If, on the other hand, you suddenly find yourself thrust into the affairs of a loved one in the midst of a medical crisis, it's time for some straight talk. A little diplomacy goes a long way.

Take your lead from the patient. If she's able to manage her affairs with just your clerical assistance, let her. Don't assume that someone is incompetent simply because she's sick or bedridden. She's likely just as concerned as you are about paying the bills and is already thinking about what would happen if she became totally dependent or died.

Help out instead of taking over. The best place to start is with monthly bills or insurance claims. Just by playing secretary while she sorts the bills and bank statements, you quickly get a picture of her current financial situation—what she has and what she owes—and the cash flow she has to live on. Filling out insurance claims or Medicare and Social Security forms provides similar background on her medical coverage.

INSIDE INFORMATION

Try these techniques to get a grip on your loved one's legal and financial matters and to help discussion flow more naturally:

- Bring up the subject of health care proxies and advance directives when someone you and the patient both know is preparing to check into the hospital or sign up for home care.
- Pick up blank signature cards on your next trip to the bank.
- Note the title of the car when you're renewing the person's license plates; review deeds and the title to the house or other real estate while paying her property taxes.
- Help organize receipts or do the photocopying when filing income tax returns.

Most important, these routine bookkeeping tasks give you the opportunity to earn your loved one's confidence in business dealings.

Take it one step at a time. Don't try to tackle everything at once. Break down legal affairs into small, manageable tasks and spread them out over the weeks—or months, if need be.

Involve the medical team. Don't bear the burden for bringing up loaded topics all by yourself. You're well within your rights to ask the doctor to initially broach the subject of living wills and advance medical directives with the sick person. These matters directly and profoundly affect medical care, and the physician's life is made much simpler when they're sorted out early rather than during a crisis. ► *See "Advance Medical Directives," page 298.*

Visit a lawyer. It's an attorney's professional duty to point out risks to clients. Instead of your having to pester your spouse or parent about powers of attorney, advance directives, health care proxies, wills, child custody provisions, and the like, schedule a consultation with a family practice or elder-law attorney. Let the lawyer ask the tough questions. ► *See "How to Find a Good Lawyer," page 286.*

The Paper Trail

In the same way that meticulous bookkeeping is essential to formulating a financial survival plan, up-to-date legal files eliminate the worst misunderstandings between families and the medical team, and help us avoid costly oversights and hassles. Without the requisite paperwork, no doctor will let you dictate Mom's medical care. You can't even write a check, make a deposit, sign an insurance claim, or apply for Social Security. Everything has to be in writing, legally binding, and right at your fingertips when you need it.

By the time this journey is over, you'll need to know the name and address of everyone appointed to act on the patient's behalf as well as all the pertinent professionals: lawyers, bankers, insurance and investment brokers, accountants, bookkeepers, business managers or tax preparers, and former employers. Phew! Start assembling your loved one's legal portfolio today.

Store important documents at home in a fireproof pouch or box. (Office-supply stores and catalogs carry dozens of models.) Or leave the originals on file with the lawyer and take clean copies of everything with you.

✱ *If you need ready access to a document, do not keep it in your loved one's safe-deposit box because when he dies, the bank will most likely seal the box*

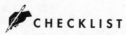

CHECKLIST

A Personal Legal Inventory

❑ Advance medical directives and living wills

❑ Health care proxy or medical power of attorney

❑ Conservatorship or guardianship decree

❑ Health insurance policies, statements of benefits, and proof-of-premium payments

❑ Life insurance policies and proof-of-premium payments, viatical settlements, or buy-out agreements

❑ Disability policies, proof-of-premium payments, and official determinations of disability

❑ Pension and retirement plan contracts, statements of benefits, and eligibility certification

❑ Birth and death certificates of the patient, his spouse, and dependents

❑ Marriage certificates, adoption certificates, divorce and custody decrees, and legal name changes

❑ Proof of citizenship or legal residency such as passport, voter registration card, visa, or green card

❑ Proof of current residence (phone bill, electric bill, rent receipts, etc.)

❑ Mortgage and proof-of-note payments

❑ Deeds to the house and other real estate

❑ Property tax assessments and payment records

❑ Leases and rental agreements

❑ Title and registration for automobiles, recreational vehicles, farm equipment, and any other expensive property

❑ Loan or finance agreements, statements from credit card accounts and any other creditors, and proof of payments

❑ Financial power of attorney or springing power of attorney

❑ Financial records from banks, savings and loans, credit unions, investment houses, and other institutions for checking, savings, money market, CD, and IRA accounts; stocks, bonds, and mutual funds; income from any royalties, annuities, dividends, trusts, or bequests

   ✳ *Be sure to record all account numbers and balances.*

❑ Income tax returns for the last six years as well as supporting documentation for earnings and itemized deductions

❑ Business partnership agreements, employment or union contracts, termination settlements, and buyout agreements

❑ Bankruptcy declarations and court rulings

❑ Any pending lawsuits and past judgments including current liens, defaults, repossessions, garnishments, foreclosures, or evictions *pending probate of the will. That could take months, if not years.*

Items to keep on hand at all times:

- The patient's medical insurance identification card, be it from Medicare, Medicaid, or a private insurer
- At least two forms of photo ID, such as the person's passport, driver's license, photo credit card, or employee ID
- You'll also need to know the whereabouts of your loved one's will, safety deposit box, cemetery plot, and burial policy.

How to Find a Good Lawyer

Elder-law or family practice attorneys are experienced in matters that commonly confront the aging or seriously ill, from executing advance directives to appealing denied insurance claims. They may work solo or as part of a group practice or clinic. Pat Still, a caregiver from New York, sought the help of an elder-law attorney when trying to qualify for federal assistance following her husband's stroke. "I found an elder-law attorney through the department of aging," she recalls. "He knew about recent changes in the Medicaid law that enabled my husband to qualify. The paperwork was incredible; that's why you need a lawyer. He handled the power of attorney and the health care proxy, too."

Areas of specialization of elder-law and family practice attorneys include the following:

- Living wills and advance medical directives
- Durable power of attorney for asset management
- Conservatorships
- Estate planning, including management of assets during life and disposition after death by using trusts, wills, and other documents
- Probate

- Management of trusts and estates
- Claims and appeals for Social Security, disability, Medicare, and Medicaid
- Hospitalization, major medical, and Medigap insurance issues
- Spousal impoverishment laws
- Rights and regulations pertaining to placement in nursing homes and other long-term-care facilities
- Elder abuse and fraud recovery cases
- Housing issues such as discrimination and home-equity conversions
- Employment discrimination based on age or disability
- Retirement and pension benefits
- Health and mental health laws

Finding a reliable elder-law or family-practice attorney is like finding a good doctor. You can start with the state bar association's referral service listed in the phone book. "Many state bar associations have sections on elder law," explains Dan Fish, president of the National Academy of Elder Law Attorneys. "So I would suggest that people call their state bar, ask if they have an elder-law section, and if so, who is on that section."

Better yet, ask for recommendations from social workers at hospitals, dialysis centers, nursing homes, and hospices, and from counselors at social service agencies. Or visit legal clinics sponsored by local chapters of disease-related organizations or senior centers.

✻ *If you or your loved one cannot afford a private attorney, both the American Association of Retired Persons and many Area Agencies on Aging provide free legal information, assistance, and referrals:*

☎ AARP Legal Hotline, 800-424-3410.

☎ Area Agencies on Aging/Eldercare Locator, 800-677-1116.

Last Will and Testament

Fewer than one-third of Americans have wills. Those who do are mostly

---

Legal Ease: Terms You Should Know

Bequest: the disposition of personal property by way of a will

Codicil: an amendment to an existing will

Executor/executrix: the person named in a will to carry out the provisions in that will

Intestate: "not having made a will," as in "He died intestate."

Probate: Before the estate is distributed among any heirs, the will must be probated—officially approved as authentic—in court.

Testator: the person who draws up the will

---

men. Unless you've seen a bereaved family torn apart by battles over money or personal possessions—or a child handed over to an undesirable court-appointed guardian—it's hard to imagine the pain a person's dying without a will can inflict on loved ones. Most folks think, "My children would never sue each other!" or "I don't own anything of much value," but making out a will is one of the few ways we have to exercise some control over what happens to our loved ones after we're gone.

Believe me, it's worth spending the money on an experienced elder-law or family practice attorney rather than trying to write the will yourself (even with the aid of how-to books and computer programs), for there are simply too many mistakes to be made. Every omission, oversight, turn of phrase, and clerical detail is open to interpretation when a person is no longer around to speak for himself.

✳ *Make sure you know where your loved one keeps his will, as well as the name and address of the attorney or executor.*

When helping a loved one make out a will:

Choose the executor carefully. Some people name their lawyer as executor, to spare their families the heartache, strife, and tedious details of carving up an estate. Incidentally, when a person dies intestate, the probate court appoints a lawyer, who then deducts his percentage before any heirs get their due.

Of course, ongoing legal services cost serious money, which is why most folks name a family member or close colleague to tend to business after their death. Bear in mind that an executor needs to have not only the personal integrity to reliably carry out the deceased's wishes but the strength and stamina to face off with creditors and disagreeable family members and business partners.

✳ *It's a good idea to name a backup executor. What if something happened to choice number one before the testator died?*

Arrange for custody of minor children. Making out a will is one of the best ways for parents to leave clear, enforceable instructions about who will raise their children, and how. Should they fail to legally appoint a *guardian*, the kids are going to be sent to their surviving biological parent—even if he long ago relinquished visitation rights and skipped out on child support. To keep kids out of court, out of foster care, or out of the hands of an unfit parent or relative, parents must have a binding will when they die.

✳ *In addition to making their wishes clear in the will, couples should consult a lawyer about appointing a legal guardian or adoptive parent to care for their children should they become incapacitated by illness or an accident.*

This is the other good argument for hiring a lawyer or visiting a legal clinic when drawing up a will.

Make sure the will complies with the civil laws where the testator lives. If a will violates any other legal obligations, such as child support decrees, divorce settlements, or prenuptial agreements, the entire document is invalid.

If the ailing loved one is not married to the person he lives with, a will is the only way to protect his or her interests. Unless specified otherwise, decisions about the deceased's affairs and assets will go straight to his next of kin by blood or marriage. I've seen situations where one partner of an unmarried couple dies, and before the mate of twenty years can arrange the memorial service, the disapproving parents fly in from out of town, clean out the bank account and the apartment, and whisk the body back home for a private funeral. Legally, she has no legal recourse whatsoever.

Don't forget creditors. When helping the sick person structure his will, remember that heirs cannot inherit any money, property, or possessions until all legitimate debts are repaid. Anything left in the estate when the patient dies must first go to pay off hospital and doctor bills, mortgages, loans, credit cards, and tax debts.

Suggest that the ill person consider distributing important assets while he's alive. Instead of Grandpa bequeathing that gold watch of sentimental value to his youngest grandson, perhaps he would derive greater pleasure from personally handing it to him and watching the youngster's excitement. An individual may give away a total of $10,000 in gifts per year, tax free; a couple, $20,000.

There are other ways to see to it that loved ones receive assets sooner rather than later. For example:

- Real estate and cash investments can be transferred into *living trusts* (explained later in this chapter).
- Individuals can be designated as beneficiaries of life insurance policies in- stead of leaving the proceeds to the estate. By doing so, the money bypasses probate and goes directly to the loved ones.

Other benefits of divvying up some of the estate now: Not only does it reduce the potential for bickering among heirs after the person is gone, but assets that do not go through the estate are not subject to estate taxes or legal fees.

✳ *When "gifting" to a beneficiary of the will, it should be specified that the gift is not an* advancement, *so that the amount isn't later deducted from the survivor's inheritance.*

Pay careful attention to details. States require that two, sometimes three, witnesses cosign the will in the presence of a *notary public.* Make sure that none of the participants is a beneficiary or related to one. While not illegal, should the will be contested, the fact that a beneficiary served as a witness would be open to interpretation. Was the patient coerced? Are the witnesses in collusion with other beneficiaries? Having disinterested third parties witness the document eliminates any appearance of conflict of interest. Let the lawyer's staff witness the signing or ask colleagues, neighbors, or clergy—anyone who doesn't stand to gain anything in the execution of the will.

Check dates, spellings of names and current addresses. Uncorrected clerical errors make it appear as if the testator didn't read the will carefully or understand it thoroughly.

Be specific; for example, don't refer to "my son, his wife and children," which assumes the son will always be married to the same woman or never father another brood. Name names.

If you're deliberately leaving someone out, state so and why; otherwise, it looks like an oversight.

The key is to eliminate as many chances for misinterpretation as possible.

Include funeral and burial instructions. No one should ever leave his final arrangements to chance.

Prearranging the Funeral

Many of us learn the hard way that the days following a loved one's death are no time to be making funeral arrangements. Exhausted, our defenses down, we're easy prey for smooth sales pitches, guilt trips, and our own flights of maudlin sentiment. Normally, most folks comparison-shop before plunking down several thousand dollars for merchandise and professional services—but not when it comes to funerals.

While it's important for survivors to feel they gave their dear departed a respectful sendoff, we don't need to risk buying on impulse or unnecessarily burdening the immediate family with weighty decisions when they're submerged in grief. If funeral and burial arrangements are made long before death, the family can concentrate on the social and spiritual rituals of grieving and remembering, instead of haggling and organizing.

Besides giving clear instructions in the will, there are several things patients can do to keep costs in check and to make sure they receive the kind of memorial they want:

Join a funeral and memorial society. Over 500,000 Americans belong to memorial societies, the main goal of which is to help members plan ahead for simple, dignified, and affordable funerals. Some societies survey area funeral homes and distribute price lists to members; others have contracts with one or more funeral homes, enabling members to purchase services at a substantial discount. Expect to pay a one-time enrollment fee of $10 to $30. Some charge annual dues, usually no higher than $10.

☎ To contact one of the approximately 150 societies located across forty states, call the Funeral and Memorial Societies of America, P.O. Box 10, Hinesburg, VT 05461, at 800-765-0107.

Shop around for goods and services. Many funeral directors will visit patients at home or in the hospital. But if the ailing person has asked you to make the arrangements for her, take a hard-bitten friend or relative with you and visit more than one funeral director. The Federal Trade Commission requires that funeral homes have printed price lists on hand for consumers. Never accept verbal quotes: Get itemized, written estimates before making any decisions.

Separate charges may be incurred for each of the following goods and services:

- Body pickup from the place of death; escort and transportation costs
- Embalming fees and supplies
  ✻ *Don't pay for embalming unless it is aesthetically necessary or required by civil or religious law, particularly if the remains are to be cremated or interred immediately.*
- Preparing the body for public viewing, including bathing and disinfecting, sealing and reconstruction, refrigeration, makeup, hair, manicure, dressing, dry cleaning, laundry, even shoeshine
- Caskets
  ✻ *These big-ticket items are not required by law for anyone who chooses cremation. Rent a display casket for viewing the body.*
- Use of the funeral home facilities during visiting hours, including the viewing parlor, bathrooms, lobby, guest lounges, parking lot, telephone, and message service
- Assistance of additional funeral home staff, including the director's associates, receptionists, porters, ushers, bathroom attendants, doormen, security guards, and parking valets
- House music, flowers, candles and incense, guest registry, prayer cards,

printed programs for the memorial service, and thank-you notes

- Use of hearses, limos, vans, and drivers to transport the body, the family, and the flowers to the church, cemetery, and home
- Fees for using the chapel, church, or meeting hall
- Honoraria for clergy and musicians
- Traffic permits and police escort fees for the funeral procession
- Cemetery fees for opening and closing the grave or tomb
- Burial vaults, where required by law or individual preference
- Cremation costs
- Urns for ashes
- Shipping containers, body preparation, biohazard permits, escort fees, and transportation costs for moving the remains out of state
- Obituary announcements
- Filing fees for death certificates and certified copies
  * *You will need at least five.*

Buy a cemetery plot or a burial policy. Funeral directors and memorial societies can also help you shop around for a plot or space in a mausoleum, headstones or memorial plaques, and perpetual maintenance services for the interment site. If your loved one finds this all too morbid to contemplate, suggest he talk to the funeral director or his insurance broker about buying a policy to help cover these costs when he dies.

Consider prepaying funeral and burial costs. There are several affordable plans for prepaying funerals, such as the standard burial policy (in actuality just a life insurance policy designated to cover funeral and burial costs) or a specially structured savings account or bank trust held jointly with the funeral home into which payments are deposited. Before your loved one signs up, though, find out if the money is refundable in part or in full should she change her mind.

* *Taxes must be paid on any interest earned.*

Other questions to ask before buying:

- What happens if by the time the person dies prices change or the funeral home no longer carries the model casket or urn she ordered?
- What happens if the sick person moves away?
- What happens if the funeral home is sold or goes out of business?
- What happens if there's money left over from the funeral and burial? What if there's not enough?

Know your rights! If at any point you feel you've been taken advantage of or

---

treated unfairly, complain to the Funeral Service Consumer Assistance Program, a free service of the National Research and Information Center, at 800-662-7666.

Legal and Financial Power of Attorney

Upon discovering that he had AIDS, a friend and colleague named George Kingsley asked if I would agree to become his *attorney-in-fact*, a legally appointed surrogate charged with making financial transactions on his behalf should he become physically or mentally incapacitated. George, who was forty-seven, lived alone, thousands of miles from his immediate family. Before he died fourteen months later, he endured several lengthy hospitalizations and episodes of profound dementia. At one point he lapsed into a weeklong coma. Had I not been legally authorized to open George's mail, sign his checks, and submit claim forms, his rent, medical bills, credit card bills, and insurance premiums would have gone unpaid. Before he even realized it, George would have been evicted, a lien slapped on his bank account, the phone and power cut off, and his health and life insurance policies canceled.

If the prospect of handing financial control to someone else makes your loved one uneasy, assure him that there are several ways to tend to business without granting any more authority than he wishes:

He can sign a *durable power of attorney* (DPA) authorizing his lawyer, spouse, or anyone else he trusts to act on his behalf at any time.

Or he can execute a *springing power of attorney* that kicks in only if a doctor or a judge declares him mentally incompetent.

Or he can customize a power of attorney, limiting the authority however he sees fit. For example, he might authorize a loved one to handle banking and bill paying, but prohibit the *attorney-in-fact* from purchasing or selling major property, incurring debt on his behalf, altering his insurance coverage, or touching his investments.

✽ *If you have been chosen to be a loved one's financial proxy, as long as you make it clear that you are acting on the patient's behalf, creditors cannot hold you personally liable for his debts.*

Other Legal Instruments

Depending on the situation, your loved one might wish to put other legal instruments in place, such as:

Living Trust. This is an arrangement whereby one person (the *settlor* or *trustor*) transfers ownership of her assets to someone else (the *trustee*) should she become disabled, with written instructions about how she wishes her assets to be managed. The trust may be permanent (*irrevocable*) or subject to amendment or termination (*revocable*). For all intents, living trusts are more complicated versions of durable power of attorney.

Joint Tenancy. Placing assets in joint tenancy—with a spouse, say—allows the other person to oversee whatever is in the account. This could include bank accounts, stocks, bonds, mutual funds, cars, homes, and businesses. While the assets go directly to the surviving tenant upon the other tenant's death, avoiding probate, this setup has its disadvantages, not the least of which is that one joint owner could conceivably liquidate the account and run off with the money. The other owner would have no recourse other than to sue. What's more, one party's debts may become the other party's responsibility.

While it's simple enough to add a friend or family member's name to a bank account (a seemingly minor decision that should be considered judiciously, for obvious reasons), there's no getting around talking to a lawyer about who will manage your affairs when you're unable to do so yourself.

* *As with estate executors, it's wise to appoint a backup attorney-in-fact.*

Declaring Someone Incompetent

My uncle Billy's mental deterioration from Alzheimer's disease began while he was still a busy banker and real estate investor. "First I noticed he was getting careless with his driving, not recognizing stop signs," recalls Aunt Kitty. "Next he began losing his handwriting; he'd always had such beautiful handwriting. Then he started paying bills two, three times. I just had to stop him from making business decisions."

Billy eventually recognized that he was slipping. With Kitty's encouragement and the help of a trusted lawyer, he granted her a broad power of attorney and named her as a joint tenant of all his property. If he hadn't, Kitty would have been forced to ask a judge to declare Billy legally incompetent and then try to convince the court to appoint her as *conservator*—instead of another of Billy's relatives or a business partner or anyone else who claimed to have Billy's best interests at heart. A conservator is allowed to handle an incompetent person's finances, whereas a court-appointed *guardian* has the power to make health care decisions for that person.

When a court is petitioned to declare someone incompetent, the judge immediately chooses a lawyer to act as temporary guardian. This attorney oversees the affairs of the sick person until the matter is settled. Much like determining child custody, the court ultimately awards guardianship to whoever it believes will act in the patient's best interest. That might not necessarily be someone you approve of or even know.

If someone you love is unquestion-ably declining mentally, it's important to know that you can intercede legally if need be. We don't have to remind you that the sick and elderly are frequently taken advantage of by unscrupulous individuals. Unconscious or badly confused people can't make responsible medical decisions. Others simply can't feed themselves or walk safely across the street. It's sad but it happens. The only way to avoid having a court decide your loved one's fate is to encourage him to sign a power of attorney and health care proxy long before a crisis arises.

Discrimination Against the Sick and Disabled

While many employers are models of corporate responsibility, people with cancer, AIDS, heart disease, end-stage renal disease, paraplegia, and other conditions routinely run into serious problems at work. Discrimination is impossible to ignore precisely because layoffs and demotions fundamentally affect the patient's insurance coverage and cash flow—literally, his ability to survive and to provide for his family.

The problem with federal Equal Employment Opportunity Commission (EEOC) actions, as well as complaints filed with city or state human-rights offices, is the tremendous backlog of cases. Investigations, hearings, and court rulings, not to mention enforcement, often take several years to conclude and therefore might have little practical benefit while the patient is alive. They also gobble up vast amounts of time and psychic energy, two resources that are already in short supply.

On the other hand, civil suits filed directly against an employer by a patient's attorney often proceed much faster than EEOC actions, particularly if you have a clear-cut case. Sometimes all it takes is a phone call or visit from your loved one's lawyer to set things right.

If illegal discrimination is plainly evident, the employer's lawyer will likely offer to settle the complaint out of court in order to avoid the expense of a trial, negative publicity, and the risk of being ordered to pay an even higher award. Company lawyers and personnel directors are usually quick to recognize when employers and their staffs have broken the law. Caught in an indefensible position, many will forgo officially contesting the charge and encourage their client to settle quickly.

If the complaint is not that simple—and most are not—prepare to do battle. To discourage others from filing suits in the future, the company is likely to come after your loved one with its big guns. A platoon of lawyers and liability risk managers will dedicate themselves to smearing his professional reputation and discrediting his claims. They will countersue, lock him out, cut off his pay and benefits, refuse to authorize unemployment checks, and drag their feet on disability and pension claims until a judge orders them to do otherwise. They will badger his colleagues and former allies at work. They will swamp his attorney with paperwork, burying her in motions, continuances, and appeals while effectively keeping the plaintive tied up in court until he dies or drops the charges.

For a strong case, the boss has to fire the ailing employee, demote him, or ask him to quit or cut back on his hours, while stating outright or clearly implying in front of witnesses or in writing that his decision is motivated at least in part by the illness or injury. This happens every day because some supervisors lack good business sense (they're dumping a productive team member and squandering other valuable corporate resources), are insensitive (it's terrible for morale and public relations to abandon sick workers, and probably immoral), or are arrogant (they think they know what's best or that these decisions are up to them). Many managers are simply oblivious to or uninformed about the law and explicit personnel directives to the contrary.

Bosses frequently make mistakes—even big, costly ones. Some examples:

"You know we're here for you . . . but maybe it's time to start thinking about clearing off your desk."

"Wouldn't this be easier on you if you just went out on disability?"

"Are you sure you feel up to taking on this project? How can I be sure you're going to see this job through?"

Short of firing, demoting, or forcing an ill employee to resign, discrimination also includes a boss singling out that person for harsher treatment than other workers. Let's say your fifty-two-year-old mother, a three-time Employee of the Month at the office where she has worked for the past seven years, is diagnosed with ovarian cancer. Her recovery from major abdominal surgery alone sidelines her for two months. For the next six months she misses days here and there when the side effects of chemotherapy leave her feeling too sick to get out of bed. The quality of her work never suffers. Nevertheless, all of a sudden a supervisor starts giving her unusually poor evaluations or promoting less-qualified, less-senior candidates over her.

Employees who previously interacted directly with the public or important clients can also find themselves reassigned to back-room duties—in the process losing valuable commissions and opportunities for advancement—or laid off for trumped-up or capricious reasons when in reality it's because the worker's appearance, speech, or mobility changed as a result of chemotherapy, surgery, paralysis, or the like. Whether it's a misdirected cost-cutting measure or simply irrational prejudice, these practices are clear violations of the federal Americans with Disabilities Act of 1990 (ADA) and many state statutes as well.

As long as someone is able and willing to carry out the essential tasks of his job, employers of more than fifteen workers are bound by law to provide "reasonable accommodation" in the workplace, such as modifying work schedules or assignments, and altering equipment or providing handicap access to the facility and work stations. While employers may argue over exactly what comprises reasonable accommodation, people with illnesses or disabilities always have a fundamental, constitutional right to hang on to their job or a comparable one within the company.

Should your loved one sue her employer and win, she will be awarded back wages, including any promotions and benefits she forfeited. She's entitled to her old job—or, far more commonly, to accept a negotiated or court-ordered cash settlement to compensate for unfair treatment. Out-of-court settlements often include a gag order, which prohibits both the employee and the employer from discussing the case publicly. Those considering a lawsuit should never overlook the fact that their lawyer will receive a hefty percentage of any money collected.

If your loved one loses in civil court, she must pick up the pieces of her life and personally pay off thousands of dollars in legal fees and court costs; this is reason enough not to move forward with complaints that seem anything less than sure bets. Although the plaintiff's lawyer usually works on a contingency basis, she will have incurred all sorts of legitimate expenses, including hours of expensive staff time for taking depositions and researching case law. There are also hard costs for mailing, telephone, fax, messenger, photocopying, and filing fees. It all adds up staggeringly fast. ◀ See "How to Find a Good Lawyer," page 286.

Job Discrimination and the Caregiver

The Americans with Disabilities Act also addresses discrimination based on one's relationship to or association with a disabled person. Spouses of the seriously ill and workers with aged parents are sometimes refused hiring, promotion, or choice assignments based on the employer's assumption that they will file large claims under the company medical benefits plan or miss a lot of work. Spouses, children, and roommates of people with infectious diseases like hepatitis, tuberculosis, or AIDS get fired because of misplaced fear of contagion. These practices, too, are illegal.

☎ If you have questions about patients' and caregivers' rights under the Americans with Disabilities Act, call the federal Equal Employment Opportunity Commission at 800-669-4000. The EEOC will not dole out legal advice or opinions about the merits of a specific case over the phone; however, it can help you figure out avenues of redress and show you how to initiate a complaint.

☎ Another valuable source of information or support is your local human rights commission; its number is in the white pages under "Government Listings."

✳ Union members should contact their local representative.

Artificial Life Support and Extraordinary Measures

Techniques used to help keep critically ill people alive improve daily. Cardiopulmonary resuscitation (CPR) successfully revives thousands of clinically dead Americans every year. Respirators breathe for us during and after surgery or keep us plugging until our brain, heart, and lungs can recover from a severe illness or injury. Dialysis keeps folks living for a long time after disease has destroyed their kidneys.

The problem is that too often doctors use these and other miraculous procedures, drugs, and equipment to sustain life long after they probably should stop trying. Many terminally ill people suffer painful, protracted deaths tethered to machines, surrounded by strangers, isolated in high-tech intensive care units or languishing on hospital wards simply because we have the technology to keep them "alive."

Public awareness of these risks has increased over the past twenty-five years, and we've made great strides in legally guaranteeing each of us the right to refuse or discontinue any treatment we see fit, even when it might prolong life. On the other hand, the medical profession has not kept pace, particularly when it comes to initiating discussions of end-of-life health care decisions with their seriously ill patients as well as carrying out patients' wishes. In order to formulate clear instructions for our doctor and family, it's crucial to understand the broad range of life-sustaining measures at the medical team's disposal:

Cardiopulmonary Resuscitation. When someone's heart suddenly stops beating or she suddenly stops breathing (one always quickly follows the other), CPR can keep vital oxygen moving to the brain while the medical team tries to correct whatever caused the arrest— that is, if CPR is begun soon enough and is well executed.

During CPR, air is forced into the lungs through mouth-to-mouth respirations, or a tube is inserted down the windpipe and oxygen is pumped through it. Compressing the chest keeps blood circulating by literally squeezing the heart muscle repeatedly between the breastbone and spine. Mechanical ventilators, electrical shocks to the chest *(cardioversion)*, and rapid IV infusions of powerful drugs to stimulate the heart are also administered aggressively during CPR.

If the brain and other vital organs are deprived of oxygen for more than a few minutes, permanent damage or death results. The longer it takes to restart the heart and breathing, the bleaker the prospects. The vast majority of resuscitations *(codes,* in hospital vernacular, as in "code blue" heard over the public address system) end with the patient's death, usually due to the underlying problem that caused the arrest in the first place. But outcomes vary widely.

When a Do Not Resuscitate order or No Code order is written, it means that CPR is not supposed to be initiated when the patient has stopped breathing or his heart has stopped pumping. The idea is to spare a dying person the violence of a futile resuscitation and to avoid altogether the possibility of inflicting additional suffering by needlessly protracting a person's death.

People with DNR orders are frequently resuscitated against their wills, often ending up comatose on a respirator. Maybe the first nurse or doctor on the scene isn't aware of the order. If the patient is picked up by an Emergency Medical Service (EMS) ambulance, the paramedics have no choice but to perform CPR until a physician tells them otherwise.

✳ *Doctors or medical proxies can decide to stop or to continue CPR during the procedure or elect to disconnect or leave in place life-sustaining equipment once the patient is stabilized.*

◄ *See "Cardiopulmonary Resuscitation (CPR)," page 181.* ► *See "Enforcing Advance Directives," page 301.*

Intubation, Artificial Respiration, and Mechanical Ventilation. When a patient has trouble breathing adequately on his own or is not breathing at all, a plastic *endotracheal tube* is inserted through the mouth or nose and into the windpipe *(trachea)*. Once the patient is intubated properly, the medical team can force air into the lungs, either by manually squeezing a flexible bladder called an *ambu bag* or by connecting the endotracheal tube to a mechanical ventilator, commonly called a respirator.

Blood is repeatedly drawn directly from arteries to measure various gas concentrations (like O_2, CO_2, and blood pH) so the ventilator can be adjusted accordingly. If the endotracheal tube is likely to be required for more than a week or so, it is replaced with a *trache-ostomy tube*, which is inserted surgically into the windpipe.

Cardioversion and Defibrillation.

Life-threatening cardiac or respiratory problems are very often caused by or lead to irregular heart rhythms. Even minor arrhythmias can quickly deteriorate into deadly ones. If the heartbeat is disrupted sufficiently, the muscle just quivers uncontrollably without pumping blood to the brain. This is called *fibrillation.*

Dangerous arrhythmias can often be reversed by applying a strong electrical charge across the chest, called, as you might have guessed, *de*fibrillation. Defibrillation is also commonly used to jump-start a heart that has stopped altogether *(asystole)*. Some arrhythmias can be reversed by special cardiac drugs or by overriding the heart's faulty electrical signals with a *pacemaker.*

Pharmaceutical Life Support. These

days there are hundreds of powerful drugs available to pump up the heart's muscle tone and to stabilize its electrical rhythm. There are medicines that raise blood pressure and others that lower it. There are potions to speed up the heart and to slow it down. Some, like *epinephrine*, can even be injected directly into the heart muscle to jolt it back into action. Others, like *intracoronary thrombolysis therapy*, are injected into the blood vessels supplying the heart muscle to break up blood clots and to allow oxygen-rich blood to reach the muscle tissue. Think of ITT as Liquid Plumber for the heart.

Strong diuretics are given to force the kidneys into overdrive, reducing the fluid load on a weak heart *(congestive heart failure)* or water-logged lungs *(pulmonary edema)*. Plain old *sodium bicarbonate* is injected to adjust the acid-base balance (pH) of the blood. Steroids and other powerful drugs are infused to reduce the swelling of an injured brain. Thanks to breakthroughs in pharmaceutical research, the list gets longer every day.

Dialysis. Most of us think of dialysis

as the routine procedure that purifies the blood of people with chronically damaged kidneys, like many diabetics. But dialysis is also used to keep critically ill people alive in ICU after their blood pressure has fallen so low that their kidneys fail *(shock* or *vascular collapse)* or when disease or infections outpace renal function *(toxemia* or *septicemia)*.

Transfusions. When patients have lost

a lot of blood *(hypovolemia)*, whole human blood and volume-expanding fluids are administered intravenously. If their bodies fail to manufacture enough of a particular type of blood cell, blood products such as packed red cells or concentrated clotting factors can also be infused.

IV Hydration/Nutrition and Feeding Tubes. For people who can't drink

or eat, vital hydration and nutrients are administered by the medical team directly. Water, glucose, saline, electrolytes, and vitamins are infused continuously through an IV. After a few days or weeks, depending on the condition of the patient, he will eventually starve unless he receives more nourishment than the IV alone can provide.

Specially formulated liquid nutrition can be poured into the stomach by way of a *nasogastric* feeding tube. NG tubes are inserted in the nose, then fed down the throat and esophagus and into the stomach. For long-term artificial feeding, a surgical opening is made and an indwelling tube implanted directly into the digestive tract. This is called *gastrostomy* or *jejunostomy.*

Emergency Surgical Procedures and Tests. Many patients and families

find themselves forced to decide quickly whether or not to consent to potentially lifesaving operations. Some examples:

- Opening up the chest or skull to clamp an aneurysm that's about to burst or to tie off a blood vessel that's hemorrhaging internally or to remove a dangerous clot
- Operations to drain and repair life-threatening abdominal abscesses caused by infection *(peritonitis)*
- Drilling holes in the skull to relieve pressure on a swelling brain *(cerebral edema)*
- Insertion of a cardiac pacemaker
- Surgically creating a tracheostomy

With the patient's or health care proxy's permission, many other surgical procedures and invasive diagnostic tests (cardiac catheterizations, arteriograms, spinal taps, just to name a few) may also be performed by the medical team.

Pain Management and Antibiotic Therapy. Sometimes the doses required to relieve severe pain are high enough to induce coma and even hasten death. Many folks prefer to be pain-free whatever the cost, whereas others will tolerate extreme suffering if it means staying lucid and being able to communicate. Antibiotics routinely prescribed to fight life-threatening infections can also prolong the life of a dying person. Sick people have the right to take or refuse *any* type of medication.

You can see why it's not so simple to say, "I never want to be hooked up to all those machines." Each person has highly subjective definitions of what constitutes "extraordinary measures," particularly in reference to personal life-and-death decisions. And those definitions may change along the way as death draws nearer.

If a loved one's medical crisis is temporary, she might agree to one or more lifesaving procedures, depending on the circumstances. Those who prefer not to risk ending up dependent on these various forms of artificial life support must take specific legal steps to ensure that the interventions they do not want are not performed. ▶ *See "Living Wills and Medical Proxies," page 299.*

Coma, Persistent Vegetative State, and Dementia

There are various levels of consciousness, ranging from being fully awake and alert all the way down the scale to death. A *coma* is an abnormal period of unconsciousness in which the person exhibits no meaningful response to external stimulation. The eyes may be open and unfocused but are usually closed. And while a comatose patient may go through detectable sleep-and-wake cycles, there is no coherent speech.

A coma can be chemically induced by, say, general anesthesia or heavy doses of pain medications such as morphine *(narcosis)*. A brain injury stemming from a blow to the head, intracranial bleeding, or a stroke can plunge a person into a deep coma. Frequently, loss of oxygen to the brain during cardiac or respiratory arrest, or as a result of an obstructed airway, leads to coma. Comas can be temporary while the brain mends itself, or permanent if the damage is beyond repair.

Persistent vegetative state (PVS) refers to a protracted coma, one from which it is unlikely the patient will recover. "In PVS," explains Dr. Jam Ghajar, a neurosurgeon, "there are no signs that the person is aware. Patients still have sleep-wake cycles, but there's no purposeful interaction with their environment." An estimated five thousand Americans are kept alive in this state by ventilators and feeding tubes.

Dementia refers to cognitive brain impairment. To varying degrees, patients suffer from memory loss and an inability to concentrate; they appear confused and disoriented. The same conditions that can trigger a coma can also bring about dementia. A person may experience temporary dementia due to an infection of the central nervous system or a drug reaction. Or this mental state may be permanent and progressive, as with Alzheimer's disease.

Regardless of their causes, coma, PVS, and dementia all leave patients unable to understand what is going on and therefore incapable of rendering medical decisions for themselves. If they haven't appointed someone to make these choices on their behalf or do not have a living will containing explicit instructions, they're almost certain to end up on artificial life support whether they want it or not.

Advance Medical Directives

Dr. Thomas G. Rainey: *I once heard a British lecturer joke that Americans think death is somehow optional. And I had to laugh because I've been struck by the same thought. You'll see patients with cancer that is clearly advancing, and neither they nor their physicians have addressed the issue of death and the patient's desires.*

A 1995 study—the largest ever to examine death and dying in U.S. hospitals—documented just how difficult it is to die according to one's wishes. Researchers at the Robert Wood Johnson Foundation monitored the medical care afforded more than 9,000 critically ill men and women at five major medical centers. Of the 4,300 patients who participated in the study's first phase:

- Seven in ten patients were never asked their preferences at all.
- Fifty-one percent of the patients who requested a Do Not Resuscitate order from their doctor never received it. Those who did often had to wait three to ten *weeks* for the order to be written. About half the time, the DNR wasn't entered into the medical chart until the person was within forty-eight hours of death.
- About four in ten of the patients who died spent at least ten days in ICU, kept alive by a mechanical respirator.
- Three in ten patients said they did not want to be revived with CPR, but four in five of the doctors either misunderstood or ignored those wishes.
- Of those patients who remained conscious, about half were forced to endure moderate to severe pain, according to family members.

For phase two of the study, begun shortly after passage of the 1990 Federal Patient Self-Determination Act, 4,800 critically ill men and women were treated under a program specifically designed to provide more humane care. Specially trained nurses assisted patients and families with executing advance directives. Nevertheless, these patients fared just as poorly as those in the first group. They were equally likely to have their advance directives ignored and to wither away in the critical care unit, racked with pain.

The study pointed up what many of us have known for some time: Many physicians are clearly uncomfortable, reluctant, or inept at discussing dying and death with their patients. Although things appear to be changing for the better—albeit slowly—medical schools have programmed doctors to do battle with disease at all costs, even unto the patient's dying breath. Dr. Howard Spiro, director of the Program for Humanities in Medicine at Yale University School of Medicine, observes, "We've trained two generations of physicians that if they look far enough and deep enough, they can find the answers to everything." Fear of medical malpractice suits and pressure from colleagues only reinforce this deeply ingrained ideology so that too few physicians will sit down with a terminally ill patient, hold her hand, and concede, "We're not going to beat this. But I will stay by your side and keep you as comfortable as possible."

Dr. Richard Gan, director of the ALS Clinic at Boston University Medical Center, remarks, "Sometimes the message conveyed to patients and families is, 'We've got life support, wonderful machines, gastrostomy feeding tubes. We'll keep you alive forever!' At times I think to myself, *Are these clinicians treating the patient? Or themselves?*"

To be fair, patients and families are often willing partners in our culture's dance around end-of-life issues. "This isn't just a problem of the big, bad medical profession not listening to patients," says Dr. Christine Cassel, chairwoman of the department of geriatrics and adult development at Mount Sinai Medical Center in New York City. "People don't like to talk about these things. They aren't explicit about their needs or expectations; most don't even really know what to expect."

Dr. Tom Rainey spent twenty years as director of critical care at Fairfax Hospital in Falls Church, Virginia. "Patients and their caregivers should feel empowered to speak up about what they want and refuse to be put off," he advises. "And the time to decide is long before admission to the intensive care unit." The most effective way for patients to spell out their wishes is through *advance directives:* a *living will* or a *durable power of attorney for health care* —preferably both.

Living Wills and Medical Proxies

A living will is a document that instructs loved ones and the medical team how to make medical decisions for the patient in the event that he is unable to speak for himself. A *medical proxy* is the person the patient chooses to render medical decisions on her behalf. Proxies are appointed by signing a durable power of attorney for health care. Most states recognize both living wills and health care proxies, a few just one or the other, but all fifty have laws that provide methods for us to choose

and refuse medical treatments when we're unconscious or confused.

Under the federal Patient Self-Determination Act of 1990, all health care facilities that receive Medicare or Medicaid funds are required to inform patients about their rights to refuse medical treatment and to sign advance directives. That essentially encompasses all facilities. Many hospitals, nursing homes, and home-care agencies —and all hospices—hand you the forms at admission. But as Mary Ann Wanucha, manager of the patient and family service department at Bayfront Medical Center in St. Petersburg, Florida, points out, "Often, when people are admitted, they're not up to answering those questions."

Rather than wait until a hospitalization, we suggest you call Choice in Dying (800-989-9455), which annually distributes more than 250,000 preprinted forms for establishing a living will and for appointing a durable power of attorney for health care. The organization charges a nominal fee for each set of documents. Another advantage of obtaining the forms through Choice in Dying is that doing so places you in its database. "If a person's state law changes," explains spokesperson Deborah Kaufman, "we notify them by mail that they must update their forms."

Remind your loved one to consider the following points when making out a living will or appointing a medical proxy:

Carefully select the person who will make medical decisions for you. The medical proxy, called the *attorney-in-fact* or *agent*, must possess the personal integrity to reliably carry out the sick person's instructions, as well as the wisdom and courage to make and enforce life-and-death decisions. He also needs the availability and the skills to deal effectively with contentious family members and the medical team.

As with wills and financial powers of attorney, it's smart to name a backup proxy in case something happens to the patient's first choice. By law, members of the medical team or employees of institutions providing medical services are prohibited from serving as health care agents or attorneys-in-fact.

✻ *A patient should make sure her agent thoroughly understands her instructions, is fully briefed on her medical history and current situation, and knows the members of the medical team.*

A living will should contain guidelines for making critical medical decisions. We can't anticipate every possible medical situation that might arise. It's not enough for a patient to declare, "I don't want to be kept alive on a respirator." What if he's undergoing surgery and merely needs a ventilator temporarily in the recovery room? Or what if he's experiencing a drug reaction and momentarily is having trouble breathing? A living will should advise the proxy and the medical team on *how* to make decisions rather than what to do in every circumstance.

My own reads like this:

I do not want efforts made to prolong my life, and I do not want life-sustaining treatment to be provided or continued: (1) if I am in an irreversible coma or persistent vegetative state; or (2) if I am terminally ill and the use of life-sustaining procedures would serve only to artificially delay the moment of my death; or (3) under any other circumstances where the burdens of the treatment outweigh the expected benefits. In making decisions about life-sustaining treatment under provision (3) above, I want my agent to consider the relief of suffering and the quality of my life, as well as the extent of the possible prolongation of my life.

It also spells out my own personal definition of "life-sustaining treatment," which includes everything from CPR to routine antibiotics.

If your loved one prefers to be kept alive at all costs, the advance directive should state so. The point is to get into writing what's important to her, who will make the decisions, and how they'll decide when the time comes.

Pay attention to the details. As with wills, clerical errors, omissions, and oversights lead to misinterpretation or invalidation. Check the dates and make sure all names and addresses are correct. Here, too, the witnesses and the notary should not be close relatives or anyone who could conceivably stand to gain from the patient's death.

Consult a lawyer when drawing up a living will or medical proxy. There's no substitute for expert legal advice when the stakes are this high. Not only do state laws change constantly, but subtleties and distinctions in medical language and legal jargon have implications the patient never imagined—especially when she's unable to explain what she meant. ◀ *See "How to Find a Good Lawyer," page 286.*

Review all instructions with the doctor and the medical team. A patient should discuss her specific concerns, fears, wishes, and preferences with her physician and *continue* talking and negotiating until both agree on which life-sustaining treatments will and will not be attempted under the various circumstances. Advance directives are much more likely to be carried out if a doctor clearly understands and concurs with the patient's wishes.

✻ *A patient should ask her doctor point-blank if he will abide by her living will and respect the decisions of her proxy. If not, it's time to find a different primary physician.*

Discuss your wishes with family and loved ones. A patient should never presume that family members in-

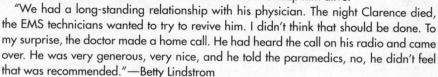

VOICE OF EXPERIENCE

"We didn't have a living will. But my husband had always told me that he didn't want a lot of tubes and artificial devices used to keep him alive.

"We had a long-standing relationship with his physician. The night Clarence died, the EMS technicians wanted to try to revive him. I didn't think that should be done. To my surprise, the doctor made a home call. He had heard the call on his radio and came over. He was very generous, very nice, and he told the paramedics, no, he didn't feel that was recommended."—Betty Lindstrom

tuitively know what he would want done medically should he lapse into a coma or become cognitively impaired. In several studies where family members were asked to guess which treatment choice a patient would make, they were wrong 30 percent of the time.

"People should think about critical and terminal illness as a family matter, just as we do when a baby is being born," advises Dr. Cassel, who chaired an Institute of Medicine panel that in 1997 issued a major report on death and dying, *Approaching Death: Improving Care at the End of Life.* "And in our modern society, we have to think of family in absolutely the broadest terms, too. These are the people who matter to the patient."

If spouses, children, or siblings disagree over the patient's advance directives, the doctor will do whatever he thinks best. Needless to say, that may not coincide with the patient's wishes. All too often an unconscious patient ends up on a respirator solely because the physician is afraid that letting the person die might invite a lawsuit from the "next of kin."

Doctors shouldn't be expected to referee family conflicts. It's up to the patient to enlist the family's support and cooperation while he's still well. Anyone close to him—spouse, relatives, friends—should be made aware that he has drawn up a living will and be informed of its content and the identity of the person legally appointed to make his medical decisions.

Enforcing Advance Directives

Once the patient's advance directive is completed:

1. Give the primary physician a copy of the living will and medical power of attorney, along with phone numbers for reaching the attorney-in-fact.

2. Anytime the patient checks into the hospital or nursing home or signs up for home care or hospice services, see to it that copies of the advance directives are placed in his chart.

3. Do Not Resuscitate orders should be prominently noted throughout the chart for all the medical staff to see.

Never is it more important to promote a rapport and open communication with the medical team as when it comes to exercising your authority as guardian or attorney-in-fact. No matter how conscientiously living wills and medical proxies are drawn up and communicated, they're useless if the physician does not carry them out.

The primary physician can be your greatest ally at this time or your biggest problem. You're going to need the doctor's cooperation no matter what you decide. The patient's doctor is in the best position to convey your instructions to the rest of the medical staff and to advocate for you within the institution when problems crop up. You're going to need him to certify the patient for hospice care, home care, or nursing home placement as well as write prescriptions for symptom control and attend to your loved one's medical needs until death. The primary physician would also have to personally write any DNR orders and transmit them to the rest of the team. You're going to need his concurrence to forgo or disconnect a respirator, feeding tube, or IV, or to halt dialysis.

There's no problem if the family is unanimous and the doctor agrees with them. But there can be serious disagreement between physicians and families —and among family members—about how to proceed medically in any given case. In order to resolve conflicts over the medical care of an unconscious or otherwise incompetent person, consider the following:

Call a family conference. Sit down with close family and friends and discuss the situation frankly. Consult the patient's lawyer and pastor as well. If you can reach some consensus, the attorney-in-fact or next of kin can make a more compelling case to the doctor.

Make an appointment to meet with the doctor formally. Whether it's your longtime family physician or a member of the hospital staff you've just met in the ICU or ER, the health care agent has a better chance of securing the doctor's cooperation when he can present the family's concerns and wishes calmly and cogently. Rather than putting the physician on the spot in the middle of a crisis, sit down together and talk things over. *Be sure to have a copy of the living will and medical power of attorney in hand.*

A physician's unilateral refusal to honor a legal advance directive is grounds for firing him. It's one thing to disagree about what's best for the patient, but something else entirely to ignore the patient's explicit instructions or those of his agent. Don't do anything rash; make sure you have another physician lined up before making any changes in the team. ◄ *See "When Is It*

Appropriate to Change Doctors?" page 98.

Schedule a case conference with the entire medical team. The social worker or head nurse assigned to your patient's unit can get all the key players on the phone or around a table together for a powwow. Put the whole team to work on resolving the conflict. This brings in some alternate points of view and keeps the conversation focused on the patient's medical situation instead of on all the drama and emotion of the moment. Be sure to include the primary physician, the social worker, the nursing director, the patient's attorney or health care proxy, and key family members.

Be persistent. If there's still no consensus or the doctor refuses to comply with your instructions on behalf of the patient, work your way through the institutional hierarchy:

1. If it's during business hours, have your patient's attorney or health care proxy call or fax the chief administrator of the hospital or the legal department, or make an appointment in person. Don't be dissuaded.

2. Make formal appeals to the chairman of the institution's ethics committee, the chief of medicine, and the director of professional affairs.

3. If it's the middle of the night and you need an immediate resolution, contact the hospital nursing supervisor or the senior administrator on duty. She and the physician will settle on a temporary solution with you until a case conference or ethics review can be arranged the following day.

Most complaints will be resolved long before you go to these extremes. If you've exhausted all recourse within the hospital but you and the doctor are still at loggerheads, there are three choices left:

1. If the patient is medically stable and you're able to manage her care at home, the attorney-in-fact can refuse further treatment on the patient's behalf and have her discharged from the hos-

pital "AMA"—against medical advice. This is not a sound idea unless you have another physician who you know will oversee the patient's home care or admit him to a nursing home or hospice.

2. You can complain to the state department of health. Patients (or their health care proxies) have a legal right to refuse treatment and to choose who makes medical decisions for them.

3. Your loved one's lawyer can petition a civil court judge to order a medical institution to abide by a legally binding advance directive or to appoint a guardian if no medical power of attorney exists.

Resisting the Impulse to "Do Something"

Bystanders, in their helplessness or frustration, sometimes make decisions they quickly come to regret—giving in to pressure from the hospital staff to prolong a loved one's life or summoning EMS to the bedside of a dying person. Do you consent to emergency treatment or not? It's hard to know at the time whether we're doing the right thing.

"Usually," comments Dr. Richard Gan, "fifty years of family issues have preceded this event. Things that perhaps weren't said in a whole lifetime are now being said in the final, terminal phase. A lot of guilty feelings come out, and sometimes people try to 'make it up' to the ill person by making sure they get put on a ventilator, for example." Dr. Howard Grossman has seen "over and over where family and friends won't allow the patient to take off his oxygen mask." Out of guilt or mistrust of doctors and institutions, I've heard distraught family members demand, "Do everything in your power to save my father!" without stopping to think what's best for Dad or what he might want.

Even if we're confident of our decisions, have legal advance directives in hand, and enjoy a close rapport with a trusted physician, all sorts of things can go wrong, such as:

Eighty-two-year-old Rita Richardson had to be transferred from her nursing home to the hospital in the middle of the night due to kidney failure. By the time her two grown daughters made it to the emergency room, an ER physician was conscientiously preparing to put Rita on kidney dialysis, a procedure she had decided to forgo weeks earlier. After Susan and Barbara sat down with the doctor and calmly outlined their mother's recent tortured medical history—the surgery, the month spent in a coma—he agreed that it would be cruel to place her on a dialyzer. Had the sisters arrived just an hour later, though, that's exactly where they would have found Rita.

Feeding, Hydration, and the Dying

It's not just in these plainly evident life-and-death decisions that we can inadvertently trample our loved one's rights. People often push food and liquids on dying patients who no longer wish to eat or drink—or they insist a feeding tube be inserted—either as a misguided expression of their love and concern or out of fear that the person will painfully starve to death.

In fact, according to a 1995 study conducted at Rochester General Hospital in Rochester, New York, starving and dehydration *ease* suffering as the body shuts down, whereas forcing food or liquid may actually *intensify* the terminally ill person's discomfort. "Dehydration is one of the body's ways of protecting the patient," explains hospice nurse Mary Ann Reeks. Ellen Wilson, also a hospice nurse, adds, "If care partners give just as much fluid as the patient can take orally, that's usually enough. If an IV is put in, that's when we see a lot of pulmonary congestion, swelling, and vomiting."

Similarly with food: "It's a matter of listening to what the patient's body is telling you," says Nurse Wilson. "If she's able to eat, terrific; if not, then you must accept that." Force-feeding or artificial feeding can exacerbate nausea and vomiting as well as disrupt the bowels, leading to gas, distention, and cramps. "This is a highly emotional issue, one we talk to families about on a regular basis. Food and water are associated with living, and for families to accept that somebody's not eating means coming to terms with the fact that the person is dying."

When Do You Call EMS?

When someone is dying at home, it's hard to resist the impulse to summon emergency medical services. There are only two situations where it is appropriate: when patients have a treatable problem that is causing needless suffering or when symptoms escalate beyond the capability of the caregiver to manage at home.

Dying people suffer falls, broken bones, cuts, burns, and bruises. They need X rays, casts, stitches, and dressings just as anyone would under the same circumstances. Other times, patients may need more care than you can adequately provide at home. While many folks slip away quietly and comfortably surrounded by loved ones, others are fully conscious and suffering intensely until the end. They may experience terrible difficulty breathing, violent seizures, hemorrhages, fevers, or pain that can't be controlled by the family caregivers. Sometimes it's wiser to head for the hospital or an in-patient hospice unit even when a patient has said he prefers to die at home.

Helping a Loved One Die

When death is imminent, there are several things we can do to ease a loved one's passing. Having ensured that extraordinary medical interventions will not be employed and having resolved not to pester our patient to take food,

water, or medicine, our priority now is to keep him comfortable. For most people that means administering adequate doses of medications to control pain, nausea, vomiting, shortness of breath, fevers, seizures, and severe anxiety.

Terminal sedation is the official term used to describe the highly common practice of loading patients with generous doses of narcotics, barbiturates, antiemetics, tranquilizers, and whatever other drugs are needed to minimize suffering. The tradeoff is that the dying person sleeps longer and more deeply. When awake, he is likely to be drowsy and sluggish. The heavy dosages also hasten death to the degree that patients' respirations become shallower; their heart rate and blood pressure drop; they cease to eat or drink; and they no longer move around or cough enough to clear their lungs.

Some sick people take their own lives, but those who do are usually acting out of deep depression and intolerable physical pain. While the public debates rage on about the morality and legality of physician-assisted suicide or "self-delivery," it is critical that caregivers never lose sight of their preeminent task: to prevent needless suffering. *Most patients will never be driven to consider suicide if their depression and pain are adequately medicated.*

But I've also known honorable, courageous individuals who, after long battles with disease and deterioration, said their farewells to their family, retired to the bedroom, and overdosed on sleeping pills they had been hoarding for exactly this purpose. Rather than endure further indignity, they put a stop to it at the moment of their choosing.

Other patients take heart knowing they can check out at any time. George Kingsley seriously considered ending his life when he tested positive for advanced AIDS. He was convinced that he would die soon and horribly.

George ultimately died of his disease —not by his own hand and more than a year later. What kept him going through the worst nights was the abiding knowledge that he *could* end it all if his decline became too much to bear. Once he realized that he had the option of controlling his destiny, the terror largely dissipated. During that time, George found renewed purpose in life, wrapping up prized projects at work, tending to unfinished business with his family, and becoming a lead plaintiff in a landmark U.S. Supreme Court case considering the legality of physician-assisted suicide.

Organizations such as the Hemlock Society and books like *Final Exit* by Derek Humphry, founder of this right-to-die society, not only provide instructions on how one goes about it, they have long advocated for the legal right of patients to determine the time and circumstances of their own deaths. As frightening as self-inflicted death is to contemplate, explicit instructions *are* necessary. Most laymen don't know how to kill themselves dependably. Some people overdose on the wrong combination of drugs, vomit, and aspirate while they're unconscious; they wake up in the hospital attached to a respirator. For patients and families alike, there is nothing more horrifying than a botched suicide. ► *See Appendix B: "Assisted Suicide," page 504.*

* *Although prosecutions are extremely rare, and convictions rarer still, it is against the law in all fifty states for a loved one to administer a potentially lethal dose of medication to a patient with the intent of causing his or her death. As of 1998, Oregon is the only state that allows physicians to prescribe lethal doses of drugs to terminally ill men and women who have executed a written request to die.*

Tough Decisions: Withholding or Withdrawing Treatment

What is "quality of life"? Obviously we each have our own definition. What may seem unacceptable when we're healthy is likely to change when death is no longer an abstract concept but is looming on the horizon. In a 1996 study of seriously ill patients at a North Carolina hospital, six in ten surveyed said that when death approached, they would want medical intervention even if it extended their lives by a mere week. Clearly, not all patients are ready to go.

Most Americans say that being kept alive on a respirator in an irreversible coma does not constitute an acceptable quality of life for them. Instructing your doctor not to resuscitate you when you're dying is one thing; asking loved ones and the medical team to disconnect you from life-sustaining equipment or discontinue medications is something else altogether. These are the toughest decisions any of us will ever make.

When confronted with such harsh choices, many families forget what the patient would want and make decisions based on guilt or misinformation. I've heard doctors and distraught relatives alike contemplate stopping the tube feedings or discontinuing the antibiotics or turning off the respirators. "But we'll be killing him!" they say. At moments like these it's important to remind yourself—and others—that the *disease* is killing your loved one. Our job is to protect him from any suffering or indignity that he would not endure if given a choice.

–10–

Journey's End

Through the fall, my father continued to live alone in the house on Rabbit Creek. In phone conversations he'd tell me and my brothers, "Don't come now. I'm doing good. Wait till I need you." But right after Thanksgiving, Aunt Kitty called to say, "Your daddy's sicker than he's letting on," an assessment confirmed by Dad's wife Mary and next-door neighbor Darlene Twilley.

It was time.

Dave canceled his last week of work and moved in with Bob two weeks after Thanksgiving. John arrived a few days later and stayed through Christmas. When John first walked in the door, Dave warned him that Dad had deteriorated rapidly in just the time that he'd been there. Upon catching sight of Bob lying in bed, John remembers thinking, *My God! Pop looks just like Granddaddy Mac the day before he died.*

Fully aware that this was the last time he'd see Pop alive, John reported back to Army duty on New Year's Day. A few days later I got the call from Dave: "Come now; he's dying." We'd been on the phone every day, and I had been anticipating this cue to join him. I delegated my next month's work once again to generous colleagues at Broadway Cares and flew to Mobile the first week of January.

The week leading up to Bob's death was a blur of mundane nursing and housekeeping chores. By now my father was extremely weak; the cancer had left him emaciated and unable to eat or drink anything substantial in weeks. In spite of almost constant pain and nausea, Dad remained conscious and clear-headed up until the day before he died. His immediate circle of family and friends called or visited daily, often twice a day. He talked on the phone with our brothers Bob and John.

And despite the dire circumstances, Pop, Dave, and I never felt closer.

306

Making the Most of Your Time Together

In spite of the sadness and a loved one's physical suffering, beautiful times can flourish—often when you least expect them. "There can be some very loving times, some very gentle and meaningful times," reflects Betty Lindstrom, who nursed her husband, Clarence, through five years of debilitating Parkinson's disease. "Oh, yes. They made it all worthwhile."

Diane Young, whose father died of complications from Alzheimer's disease: My father was from Ohio; my mom was from New Orleans. They met during World War II when he was stationed in Biloxi, Mississippi. We always said that Daddy was from up north, so he had this sort of cold demeanor. He was a wonderful father and had a wonderful personality. But he didn't like kissing and hugging.

But when my dad was sick, you could kiss him, hold his hand, rub him —things that when he was well would have made him pull away or tense up. My sister and I talk about how nice that was.

Alvin Novick and his longtime lover Bill Sabella continued to enjoy a relatively normal life together up until three months before Bill died of AIDS in July 1992. "That April," he remembers, "we vacationed in Miami Beach even though our principal baggage was for his medications—sixty different oral medications alone!—and IV drugs, an IV pole, needles, and whatnot. I had only a little overnight bag for our clothes. But we had a wonderful time."

Shortly after they returned home to Connecticut, though, the complications of AIDS began to rain down. "Billy had always been very upbeat, brave, and resilient. Then he became resigned." Yet one sun-drenched Saturday morning that July, the two shared one of their happiest days together. "He'd had a nightmare of a night, with perpetual pain. But when he woke up Saturday morning, he didn't ask for any medication. As far as I know, he was pain-free. He actually joined me for breakfast and ate, and was a transformed person. He looked luminous!"

Alvin laughs softly. "It sounds like a bad movie, but it was real life. He called one of his aunts and talked to her for a while, and was so warm and loving with her. Then he said, 'I want to walk in the garden.' We had quite an extensive garden, and Bill loved to work in it. He hadn't had the strength to walk in the garden for weeks.

"I asked him, 'How are you going to do that?'

"But we walked in the garden and sat down at all his favorite places, though it took us two and a half hours to go a few hundred feet. It was like you would want life to be. I guess it was like what you would want *death* to be. I was holding him, and we were together, sharing things that were important to us."

Making Your Peace

As we've observed more than once, people die much the way they lived. Not everybody experiences a deathbed epiphany or comes to some cosmic resolution. Tearful confessions are not always met with open-armed absolution. Illness and death take place in the context of thirty, forty, fifty, or more years of hard-knocks living and imperfect relationships.

The popular notion of "closure" is highly overrated. And while the final hours of life can be a profound shared experience, these fleeting moments rarely allow for profound differences to be completely smoothed over.

It still pains me to say it out loud, but as children my brothers and I were badly abused for years, both physically and emotionally, by our mother. Many years after her death, long after I was a grown man with plenty of life experience and good therapy under my belt, I still bitterly resented my father's unerring knack for disappearing every time Mother lost control and came after one of us kids. Bob and I spoke and visited regularly throughout the intervening years, but we rarely discussed anything more substantial than the weather or fishing. We were not at all close as father and son until I helped him care for his second wife, Lynn, when she was dying.

By the last year of his life, I had begun to feel mean-spirited and cold-hearted for having enforced our estrangement all those years. To Bob's credit, when I was caring for him following his heart surgery, he was very sincere in owning up to the fact that, in his words, "I wasn't the best father." He told me outright that he was ashamed of having let us down repeatedly when we were children, even though at the time he thought that his intervening would have made matters far worse.

In order to avoid walking on eggshells around each other, we both had to 'fess up. "I'm sorry if I haven't been a good son," I told him early on. "But I promise to stay by your side as long as you need me now." I assured him that the past would not stand in the way of his getting whatever care and protection he required from me, and he believed me.

It's somewhat sad to think that it took a major illness to forge this rapprochement, but we came clean with each other. Bob couldn't make up for history, and I probably could never forgive him anyway. But by speaking honestly and directly, we were both better able to treat each other with loving respect and trust during his remaining months.

Keeping expectations in check is crucial, however. When someone you love is dying, it's your last chance to speak up. You'll sleep better after the person is gone if you say what's on your mind while she is alive. To this day I am haunted by all the things, good and bad, I wish I'd told my mother before she died suddenly. On the other hand, it is naive to think that anything we say will change other people. Speak your peace because you need to, not because you think it will suddenly resolve conflicts or improve relationships that years of living have failed to alter.

Ways That Loved Ones Face Death

"Most people that I have been with are sure that they're going to a better life," says hospital chaplain Christine Swift. "I haven't met too many people who thought they were just going to stop existing."

The day before Dennis Rivera died, a priest had just given the thirty-five-year-old cancer patient his last rites when Johnetta Romanowski, his fiancée, walked into the room. Dennis seemed at peace, she says, and unafraid. "He said, 'I'm ready for whatever happens. I've forgiven everybody. I hold no anger. When God wants me, I'll go.'" In between gasps for breath, he talked to Johnetta about her plans. She was just twenty-six.

"What are you going to do after I die?" he asked.

"I don't know," she answered, wiping away the tears.

Johnetta recalls: "He said to me, 'You're young. You'll meet somebody else and fall in love. But I'll always be with you.' He winked. 'I'll just turn my back when you're having sex.'"

It's not unusual for loved ones to feel hurt or abandoned when the dying person has accepted his fate and is ready to go. "I couldn't match my own aspirations with Bill's," reflects Alvin Novick. "He began to welcome death, but I didn't welcome his death at all!

"It was on a Thursday morning that he said he'd had enough. I had been afraid of hearing that. On a cerebral level, of course I understood it. But at the emotional level, I still wanted him here, whatever his condition was. I became extraordinarily anxious, as if I were jumping out of my skin."

Another pattern sometimes seen is patients or loved ones—or both—growing distant as illness worsens and death approaches. During the years that Gerri Clarke assisted her husband, Paul, with home kidney dialysis, she admits that at times, "I could feel myself pulling away emotionally. I guess you do that so that you won't miss them as much should they die."

Rick and Mary Vitro's son was just three months old when his father was diagnosed with AIDS. Much to Mary's frustration, Rick subconsciously distanced himself emotionally from Doug at times. "He didn't want to fall in love with this kid and let this baby fall in love with him because he was going to die."

Whether folks are resigned to their fate or struggling desperately until the bitter end, the caregiver's preeminent task remains to make them as comfortable as possible while they die in their own, highly individual way. After we've said our own piece and given them every opportunity to say theirs, all we can do is offer the quiet comfort of our dependable and continued presence.

Where People Die

Audree Siden knew the ropes when it came to nursing a dying loved one. Her fiancé, Dr. Edmund Slakter, a New York psychiatrist who works with bereaved parents, puts it this way: "More than any of my professional training, I learned how to care for the old and the dying at the University of Audree."

The fifty-seven-year-old woman had cared for her dying husband and her dying mother at home. She'd also looked after two of her closest friends when they were dying of cancer. She had seen the many faces of death as well as the pros and cons of dying at home versus in a hospital, nursing home, or hospice.

Audree had always been an outspoken proponent for the right of sick people to die wherever they wished, and she was an enthusiastic advocate for dying at home whenever it could be managed. Yet when she herself was dying of advanced bladder cancer in 1996, she checked herself into the hospice unit at Calvary Hospital in the Bronx. It seemed an ironic choice, but as Audree said from her deathbed, "I just feel safer here," adding with a laugh, "I never taught my own sons how to put someone on the bedpan!"

There was more to it than that. Audree's decision to die in an inpatient hospice unit was also very much in character for this lifelong caregiver. She was making things easier for her beloved Edmund, her devoted sons, and their wives. Although Audree had never regretted caring for her husband and her mother at home, she was painfully aware of the toll those trying experiences had taken on her three sons when they were growing up. Edmund could easily have afforded whatever home care she required, but Audree chose to spare her family and herself the burdens and indignities of day-to-day nursing tasks. She freed them to spend their time talking, reminiscing, laughing, crying, or simply sitting quietly together until the moment she died on January 10, 1997. She knew exactly what she was doing.

For a number of reasons, a caregiver may not be able to nurse a terminally ill patient at home. Perhaps she isn't physically able to handle the demands, or she can't adequately keep the patient comfortable, or she can't find or afford home care. Or the demands of young children living in the house make home care impractical.

In no way is having to transfer a patient to the hospital, for any reason, a failure on the part of the caregiver. As we've stressed throughout this book, the only failure is when you do not have a plan of action. Whatever you can't or won't do yourself, arrange for it to be done, and done well. ◄ See "Making

Other Arrangements: Home Care, Hospice Care, and Nursing Home Care," page 238.

Creating a Comfortable Space for the Dying

Dying of meningitis in a Paris hotel, Oscar Wilde was reputed to have said, "Either that wallpaper goes, or I do." The physical and aesthetic environment around a deathbed fundamentally affects the comfort and intimacy of the moment for patients and families alike.

If a patient's symptoms are well controlled and the situation at home permits, there's a lot to recommend dying at home. There's far more privacy for everyone. Most nursing care is provided by loved ones instead of strangers. Lighting, noise levels, and foot traffic can be controlled. Families are not relegated to impersonal waiting rooms or commutes back and forth to an out-of-the-way institution.

At home you have a full kitchen, extra beds, private phone, and private bathrooms. Caregivers and patients alike can come and go as they please at all hours without having to worry about their appearance or whether they're in anybody's way. These may not seem significant, but they truly are when you're up and down all night on a death watch that can last for days or weeks.

It doesn't have to be all that different in the hospital or nursing home. Once medical priorities have shifted from treatment to keeping the patient comfortable, we can close the door. Some people splurge on a private room the last few nights. If you work with the nursing supervisor, visitor-control rules can be bent, allowing for more than two visitors at a time and more flexible hours. The hospital or nursing home room can be made less impersonal by adding family photos, a favorite blanket or pillow, and a few potted plants. ◀ See "Personalizing the Hospital Room," page 58.

Other Ways to Create a Comforting Environment for the Dying

Consider the senses. What does the patient see, smell, and hear? Is she hot or cold? What textures does she feel against her skin? Instead of staring at a blank wall, perhaps your loved one would prefer a window view. Are harsh lights glaring in his face, or is the room so dark it seems like a tomb? Is the room cozy or downright stuffy? Does the aroma of food cooking in the kitchen remind us fondly of hearth and home, or violently nauseate the dying person? Maybe the squeals of kids playing in the yard or the TV droning are reassuring sounds of life, or maybe they're intrusive distractions. Is background music or the voices of loved ones in the next room soothing or grating?

Control the flow of visitors. Caregivers often become gatekeepers. We have to help the sick person see whomever he wants, whether that means scheduling visitors and helping the patient dress or sit up. Other times we're forced to explain to distraught friends and family that the dying person prefers to be alone. ("This is not a good time. We're having a rough day. Could you call again tomorrow?") Sometimes we have to enforce time limits on guests who overstay their welcome or patients who tend to overextend themselves— all the while being careful not to seem as if we're holding others at arm's length or isolating the patient.

Don't intrude on privacy and rest. Dying people need to be needed, too. Ask their advice and opinions, and engage them in conversation as long as they exhibit any interest at all. But if they prefer silence and sleep, simply sit there quietly. ◀ See "Learning to Listen," page 197.

Make sure the dying person is never alone. The fear of abandonment is the second most commonly reported source of anxiety among the dying. (The first? The fear that they will die in unrelieved pain.) While many loved ones feel duty-bound to remain at the bedside in the hours leading up to death, other folks make themselves scarce. By avoiding witnessing death firsthand, they are placing their own comfort ahead of the patient's.

If being present is just too much to bear or simply impossible logistically, schedule others to sit with your loved one, particularly if he is conscious. After a loved one dies, the only comfort an absent caregiver will have is knowing that she made sure that person did not feel abandoned in the end. ◄ *See "Some Common Fears and Our Responses," page 198.*

Waiting Room Marathons and Death Watches

It is a beautiful and gratifying experience to stand at the deathbed and assure someone whose life is ending that he can depend on us, that his life is precious, and that life will go on for those he loves. That's why we shouldn't wait until death is imminent to alert family and friends. It's more helpful to let them know "This might be the last time you can see Mom conscious," rather than "Come quick; she's going to die any minute." It's not always easy to know when someone will die, which is why it's so important to spend quality time with the person while he is still alert. Being present at the moment of death pales in comparison to the chance to tell a dying person good-bye and I love you.

This is also no time or place for nosy neighbors or hysterical relatives. As caregivers we need people by our side who can support us, not folks who divert attention from the patient. Likewise, family conflicts should be put on hold. The death watch is all about making the patient feel comfortable and loved, not us.

If a loved one's death comes unexpectedly, we're shocked. If it comes slowly, we're exhausted. Some of the things you'll need to think through before the final moments:

Who must I officially notify? Post the doctor's or the hospice nurse's name and office and beeper numbers in a conspicuous place. Write down the name and number of your contact at the funeral home.

Make a list of family and friends to be contacted when the person dies. Also give some thought to *who* should do the calling. You may be surprised— or even taken aback—at some of the names that show up on your loved one's call list. Keeping a list also helps avoid regrettable oversights or the hassle of chasing down names and numbers when you're at the end of your rope.

Make a list of agencies and service providers to notify. No need to pay an extra day's rent on medical equipment such as hospital beds or waste a trip for the home-care workers. If the sick person has been receiving community services such as home-delivered meals, transportation, or counseling, give the agency a call. In addition, cancel any upcoming appointments with doctors, diagnostic centers, dialysis units, and the like, so as not to inconvenience other ill people.

Two days before Bob died, we could tell the end was very near. The hospice nurse concurred. Pop slept longer and longer, waking rarely and only long enough to use the urinal or wet his mouth with a sip of water. Besides the Compazine for nausea, we were administering morphine suppositories every three or four hours. Even in his sleep he would moan or contort his face in pain, and we'd give him the next dose whether or not it was "time." The fevers came and went. We'd give him Tylenol suppositories, bathe him with cool, wet towels, and change the sheets. By the next afternoon, a Thursday, Bob had stopped waking up and urinating alto-gether. His breathing grew slow, shallow, irregular.

Kitty, Dave, and I didn't sleep that last night. We took turns sitting with Bob until dawn.

"I'm right here, Pop."

"It's okay to let go now."

"I love you."

—11—

Aftermath

Bob McFarlane died a little after two o'clock in the afternoon on Friday, January 14, 1994.

The nurse's aide and I had just finished giving Pop a shave and a bath in the hospital bed. He was unconscious, as he had been for the past twenty-four hours. We rubbed lotion on his face, back, arms, hands, legs, and feet; powdered his privates; remade the bed with fresh, crisp sheets; fluffed the pillows; and expertly rolled him back into position. I remember thinking at the time how proud I was that Dave and I had never once let Dad's skin start to break down. He didn't even have dandruff.

I was headed to the bathroom to empty the washbowls when Dave and Kitty called me back to Bob's side.

He wasn't breathing, but the tough old cuss had fooled us this way many times throughout the wee hours, going as long as ninety seconds without taking a breath, then abruptly starting again. Dave, Kitty, the now wide-eyed nurse's aide, and I stared at Bob for sev-

eral more minutes as Uncle Howard, Uncle Billy, and Dad's friend David Reeves gathered one by one at the foot of the bed, each of them obviously shaken.

Kitty sat holding Bob's cold, blue hand, praying and weeping softly. The next breath never came. Finally my brother said evenly, "That's it. He's gone."

Dave reflects, "It was as if Poppa was just waiting to get all nice and clean before he went."

We called the hospice nurse; she was there inside twenty minutes. She placed a stethoscope to Bob's chest, looked up at Dave and me, and just nodded. Dr. Wiley Justice arrived moments later, dressed in a scrub suit. He was surprised that Mr. Mac had died "so soon," not realizing that Bob's apparent vitality during their recent visit was a Herculean performance that had in fact left Dad prostrate.

Before leaving, both Dr. Justice and the nurse remarked that they had rarely seen a family mobilize so effectively around a dying person, a comforting compliment from a couple of real pros—and exactly what I most needed to hear right then.

Before the quiet and efficient men from the funeral home arrived to hoist Bob's body down the spindly stairs of the stilt house, I witnessed a most remarkable scene: Darlene and Ron Twilley, unsophisticated in the ways of death but wise beyond their years, carried their very young children into Bob's room. Alexandra was three years old at the time; Austin, one.

As Darlene recalls, "When the boys called me, I went over by myself first. I knew I would be really emotional, and I didn't want my kids to see me really crying. Ronnie brought them a few minutes later.

"Austin thought that maybe 'Poppa Mac' was asleep, but we explained to Alexandra that he was really hurting while he was living, and now that he was peaceful, he was up in heaven playing with all those little children up there who had died."

After Bob's body was removed, Kitty and Billy, Howard, and David Reeves each in turn headed home, heartbroken. Watching them drive away, I remember three feelings most vividly: profound relief for Bob, David, and for myself; aching sympathy for Aunt Kitty, who still had her husband's final decline to contend with; and a deep sense of pride in Dad's care team—exactly the kind of stand-up folks I want at my side when my time comes.

The Moment of Death

Alvin Novick: Bill always said that he would die at home, and he did. It was peaceful and uneventful.

Many of us have formed images of death in our minds based on TV and movies. The dying person's cheeks grow rosier, the camera focus softens, and violins swell in the background; the person mumbles something pithy or noble, then suddenly slumps, as if sleeping.

Even if you've witnessed death first-hand, you may still harbor a distorted notion of what to expect, since death can wear a variety of disguises. If you've ever seen someone die while gasping for breath or writhing in pain, you might choose *not* to nurse a loved one at home even though his case is not at all like the previous one. On the other hand, if you've seen only peaceful, silent deaths, you may be thrown for a loop when your current patient furiously lashes out while dying.

Depending on the underlying condition, some dying people have endured so much pain that the progressively higher doses of medicine required for relief eventually render them comatose. If the patient has discussed this with his doctor and medical proxy, he's virtually guaranteed a peaceful death. As my dad said a few days before he died, "Son, can you take the edge off this hurtin'? And if you can't, could you knock me out completely?" But if the medical team is unskilled at elegant symptom management or the patient has refused terminal sedation, some people remain conscious while suffering terribly up to the very end. Whatever the case, the caregiver's job is to know what to do.

In reality, most people die following hours, if not days, of unconsciousness resulting from the cumulative effects of advanced disease, malnutrition, and dehydration. It's a slow fade; death comes so incrementally that you barely notice the actual moment. Their breathing and heartbeat slow profoundly; their pupils dilate and become unresponsive to light; their skin takes on an ever-darkening blue tinge, especially the lips and nailbeds; their bowels and bladders relax totally. They simply slip away bit by bit before our eyes, over a matter of minutes or hours. Others die abruptly—for example, immediately following a massive heart attack, cardiac arrhythmia, or stroke. Most never know what hit them.

Patients with neurological problems or raging fevers may have multiple seizures, even violent ones, a frightening experience for a caregiver who wasn't prepared for this. A few patients "bleed out," losing massive amounts of blood due to a ruptured vessel or clotting disorder. A fatal hemorrhage is awful to look at, but, blessedly, most are sudden and brief.

Eileen Mitzman: *Marni was just getting weaker and weaker, to where she could hardly get out of bed. Over the Fourth of July weekend she developed a fever, and we took her to the hospital.*

The floor was very busy and very short-staffed. I was trying to get a doctor in for about twenty-four hours because Marni was in terrible pain, but nobody came. I was screaming at the desk that I was going to call 911.

When the doctor finally came, he lifted her up, and she just started to gush blood from her nose, ears, and mouth and went into a coma. The next evening the doctor took her off life support.

Probably the worst way to die, and certainly the hardest to witness, is a conscious patient struggling desperately to breathe. Whether it's a result of end-stage emphysema or pulmonary congestion so dense it threatens to drown the person, slow suffocation is a nightmare. Remember that oxygen and many drugs are available to ease breathing or at least reduce the most severe feeling of air hunger. There are tranquilizers and sedatives to ease the panic. There are narcotics like morphine to escape the terror completely.

* *This is one of the rare instances where you might seriously consider placing an imminently terminal patient on a respirator. While the mechanically assisted breathing will almost certainly protract the moment of death, a conscious patient won't have to struggle so hard to breathe.*

Knowing what to expect and approximately when is essential to the caregiv-

er's survival long after the person has died. You can be haunted by terrible visions if you witness a miserable death unprepared; you can beat yourself up for years for not being at a loved one's side when she died.

Mary Vitro says, "I got to the hospital at 9:10, and they told me Rick had died at 9:00. I walked into the room, and he had this horrible expression on his face." It has haunted her ever since. "I felt like, *Oh, my God, I should have been there.*"

Looking back on her own experience, Mary's sister Johnetta Romanowski alternately feels satisfaction from having been at Dennis's side and despondency that she witnessed his death. "I'm glad I was there, I really am," she reflects. "But in a way I wish I wasn't because the flashbacks of the scene are so bad."

Nola Miller: *Walter was so uncomfortable; he was swishing his head back and forth. I asked, "Do you want me to take your oxygen off?"*

"Yes, please, take it off."

So I took off the nasal cannula. I was standing on the right side of the bed, and the gal who helped me take care of Walter stood on the left.

And then . . . he died. I thought, My God, you mean that's all there was to it?"

Whatever the original cause, ultimately we all die the same way. As the brain is deprived of sufficient oxygen, it begins to shut down like an office tower at night, floor by floor, silently and unspectacularly. For the caregiver, the true challenges arise during the moments or hours leading up to death. Knowing what to expect and what to do when things go wrong are the only ways to prepare yourself.

Days or weeks before your loved one's death, ask the doctor—or, better yet, a hospice nurse—to describe specifically when and how death will most likely come. Discuss all the possible scenarios in graphic detail so you're not caught off guard and so you know ex-

actly what to do to ease the person's suffering. Together with the medical team, formulate a backup plan and know whom to call or where to go if things get out of hand.

Phone Calls and Final Arrangements

Whether stunned by the news or simply overwhelmed with relief after a long ordeal, a caregiver's responsibilities do not end when a loved one dies. Before you're able to relax or crawl into your shell, there are still immediate details that must be seen to.

Inform immediate family members and close friends of the deceased. The first calls Dave and I made were to our brothers John and Bobby, who started making their way back home. Then we went down our list of other people to contact.

Funeral arrangements. Before you leave the hospital or nursing home, make sure you or the admitting office has called the mortuary to pick up the remains. If you haven't made prior arrangements, you will have to sign an authorization for the hospital to release the body. ◄ *See "Prearranging the Funeral," page 289.*

Write an obituary. The newspaper will most likely print exactly what you give it, so make sure the obit department gets everything right the first time. (Another good reason to do this in advance.) You'll regret omitting or misidentifying survivors, and you'll have a big mess on your hands if the local paper incorrectly lists the time and location of the funeral or memorial service. Also consider specifying in the obituary a charity to receive memorial donations. Many families prefer tributes more lasting than flowers.

Dave and I put a lot of thought into Bob's obituary. We wanted it to cele-

brate his life, not merely inform people of his death. The opening sentence, which deliberately mentioned his penchant for storytelling and his love of fishing, brought smiles to the faces of everyone who read it.

Order several copies of the death certificate. They're faster and easier to get while the original is being filed, and you'll need multiple copies when you make claims to Social Security and insurance companies, probate the will, and settle financial affairs.

Go to the bank. You'll need to withdraw or transfer enough money to live on until the will is probated or until the bank releases joint holdings to survivors or trustees.

The Funeral

Dave and I found the days leading up to Bob's funeral were less about the rituals of grieving and remembering, and more of a sustained performance to do Dad's memory justice.

What with the phone ringing off the hook, hundreds of mourners pouring through the funeral home, and the constant traffic through Bob's house, Dave and I enjoyed precious little privacy after that first night. Legions of relatives, kindhearted neighbors, and ladies from the church arrived bearing an array of food, flowers, and condolences —along with that very southern expectation of our *undivided attention.*

For me, dealing with most of the visitors proved more of a trial than nursing my dying father had been, a common experience for primary caregivers. What respite we found came only in stolen moments late at night with Kitty or our very closest friends and family. Nice as most people were, I couldn't wait for it all to be over and for everyone to go away.

Dave had completed Bob's funeral arrangements a week before he died, and we scheduled the burial for Monday, three days after his death. There were dozens of people to call with the news, then two days of receiving visitors before the burial.

As any good host knows, greeting hundreds of people you haven't seen in years is an Olympian exercise in planning, discipline, and utterly deliberate poise. My personal theory is that wakes and funerals were invented to keep folks so distracted that they can't fall apart. No matter how upset you are, there are two things you'll later regret not thinking of if you don't tend to them before the funeral:

1. *Keep flawless records of gifts, visitors, and callers.* Place spiral notebooks by the phone and in the kitchen. Write down the callers' names, the date and time of their call, and their phone number (even if they think you have it). Instruct anyone else at the house to do the same. When someone stops by with food, flowers, gifts, or an offer of help, write it down, along with the person's name, address, and phone number. In addition:

- Make sure the mortuary collects the cards from each bouquet before taking the flowers to the cemetery or giving them away.
- Keep all the condolence cards and letters (and the envelopes they came in—you'll need the return addresses!) in one place.
- Label dishes and pans with the name of the owner so you can return them later.
- Keep a guest registry at the funeral parlor in plain sight and encourage everyone present to sign it. Your life will be made far easier when you get around to thanking all the nice people after the funeral.

2. *Carefully choose those who will eulogize your loved one.* You have only one chance to get this right. *Even the most experienced public speakers should write down their remarks.* If you or someone else is apt to be too emotional to speak eloquently, consider asking someone to read for you. Speakers will never do Dad's memory justice or bring any comfort to the assembled mourners if they go off on tangents, get tongue-tied, or simply sob uncontrollably. Don't forget to brief the minister, too.

As if planning a wedding, baptism, or bar mitzvah, consider asking someone to audiotape or videotape the eulogies. It may bring you peace to hear the well-chosen words later when you're less upset. You can also send a copy to any bereaved loved ones who were unable to attend.

The funeral came off without a hitch only because we had thought of everything in advance. Dave had even draped Bob's casket with pine boughs and Spanish moss instead of flowers, crowning the motif with a couple of bamboo fishing poles. He placed a favorite pipe in Pop's folded hands and stuffed a pack of chewing tobacco in his suit pocket. Those small touches moved many people to tears and prompted many others to recount their fondest memories of Dad.

After the burial, we fed scores of friends and family at Bob's house, then once again found ourselves alone. And there was still more to be done.

Final Details

Dave, his busiest professional season now on hiatus, agreed to stay on to distribute to family members or sell off the contents of Bob's house, garage, workshop, and boathouse, now the property of the Twilleys. There were also Dad's insurance and banking affairs to settle.

By the time my brother had wrapped up Bob's estate, Aunt Kitty was hospitalized for bladder surgery at the same time a series of devastating strokes left Uncle Billy totally incapacitated. Dave ended up staying in Mobile another six weeks after Bob died, until Kitty was well and Billy was buried. It was an impressive achievement of endurance and compassion.

Personal possessions must be sorted

INSIDE INFORMATION

Many financial advisers recommend waiting at least six or eight months before selling the family home or other major holdings. Not only do you want to avoid acting on impulse while you're upset and vulnerable, but there are serious tax consequences to consider carefully as well as the vagaries of the local real estate market to master.

---

and given away or sold, a tedious and heartbreaking task to many. In addition, a quick review of the Personal Legal Inventory in chapter 9 gives you an idea of just how much important paperwork follows a loved one's death.

Bills and taxes must be paid; Social Security, pension, and life insurance survivor's benefits applied for; the will submitted for probate; titles to real estate and automobiles transferred; bank accounts turned over to trustees or heirs—and virtually all of these transactions will require certified death certificates as well as a copy of the will or your appointment as executor.

Grieving and Getting On with Life

There are as many different ways to grieve as there are people, and there is enough published advice on the subject to fill hundreds of excellent books. Survivors may experience a wide spectrum of intense emotions and intrusive thoughts, or not. Either way, they find their identity fundamentally changed, no longer the parent or lover or provider or caretaker they once were. There are some predictable pitfalls, however, for which the recently bereaved must remain alert:

Folks sometimes underestimate the gravity of their loss until months or years later. They seem to be coping well, only to find themselves overwhelmed with sadness on an anniversary or a holiday. On those occasions, surround yourself with understanding friends and family instead of trying to maintain a stiff upper lip.

Others fail to recognize the symptoms of clinical depression. This is a medical condition that disables and kills if left untreated. A shocking percentage of elderly Americans die within a year of their spouse. One can't help but wonder if they simply gave up hope or lost the will to live. Recently bereaved people should evaluate themselves regularly for depression during the year following a loved one's death and alert the medical team if symptoms persist for more than a couple of weeks. ◄ *See "Common Signs of Depression," page 192.*

Some people act rashly or make decisions they later regret. Try to resist the temptation to quit your job, sell the house, move in with family, or move away until you've experienced the full range of emotions that come with profound loss. Instead, consider taking a leave of absence, visiting with family or friends, or going on a long vacation.

There are those who crawl into a hole, a natural instinct when feeling vulnerable. While privacy is also important to healing, don't try to grieve alone. Visit the bookstore and read everything you can on grief, loss, and recovery. You'll find surprising sources of practical advice and inspiration. Talk to a pastor or mental health professional who is experienced in bereavement counseling.

For more information or referrals call:

☎ Widowed Persons Service, American Association of Retired Persons, 601 E Street, N.W., Washington, DC 20049; 202-434-2277.

☎ The THEOS Foundation, 1301 Clark Building, 717 Liberty Avenue, Pittsburgh, PA 15222; 412-471-7779.

☎ American Psychiatric Association, 1400 K Street, N.W., Washington, DC 20005; 202-682-6000.

☎ American Psychological Association, 750 First Street, N.E., Washington, DC 20002-4242; 202-336-5500.

☎ National Association of Social Workers, 750 First Street, N.E., Washington, DC 20002-4241; 800-638-8799.

Most important of all, reach out to others and learn from those who have been down the road before you. The everyday angels introduced throughout this book provide just a sample of the wisdom and insight to be gained from those who have survived this journey.

Aunt Kitty: I had never spent a night by myself in forty-one years. The kids started trying to come over and stay with me, and I said, "I've got to do it. I've got to prove to myself I can." So I did. I just came right back in this house and—I won't lie—prayed all night long because I was scared out of my wits! But after the first night, I was fine.

Alvin Novick: I find survivor's guilt very hard to interpret in myself and in others because I think that living on borrowed time has been an element of my entire life.

When I was nineteen years old, I was a prisoner of war in Germany during World War II. Most of the soldiers I was captured with didn't survive, and most of the soldiers who stayed behind as active infantrymen didn't survive, either.

The HIV epidemic has repeated this pattern for me in almost exactly the same way because I'm HIV negative.

Most of the people that I knew and cared about in 1978, 1980—not just Bill—are dead. Almost all. Maybe all.

It has gotten easier, but it hasn't gotten good.

Eileen Mitzman: When you lose your parents, you lose your history; when you lose a child, you lose your future. I lost my father—a wonderful, wonderful man—when he was sixty-one years old, and it was devastating. But compared to the loss of my child? It's not even in the same ballpark.

Naomi Black: Our family has become very close since our daughter died. The first year, it was kind of like we couldn't do anything without the whole bunch of us being there, to prove that we were all still here except for Nancy.

Debbie Bryant: It has taken me a long time to mourn for my mother because I had suppressed so much of it. It took me ten years before I returned to her grave, which was very hard for me to do. When I finally went, it wasn't as hard as I thought it was going to be. I'm surprised at how many times I've been back since then.

"No Regrets"

Whatever the future holds, the enormous sense of satisfaction from having cared well for your loved one will stand you in good stead the rest of your life. "After Walt died," says his wife, Nola Miller, "I could say right away, 'No regrets.' I felt very complete about it. This was probably the most magnificent experience I could ever have. Not just being there when he died but that whole last year of caring for him. The sharing. The loving. All of it. It was a gift."

Two days after Bob's funeral, I said good-bye to Dave and got on a plane headed for Nashville. Trying to focus on Broadway Cares's star-studded concert at the Grand Ole Opry felt alien and surreal after what I'd just been through, but I needed to get back to work, to life.

As I relaxed into my seat for takeoff, I was overcome with a bittersweet feeling of deep satisfaction. I was intensely proud of my father's courage and dignity, and my family's manifest compassion.

You done good, kids, I thought, and fell asleep without a knot in my stomach for the first time in nearly a year.

PART TWO

The Everyday Angel's Cram Course in Adult Medicine

—12—

Caring for Someone with Cancer

Johnetta Romanowski and her fiancé, Dennis, were looking forward to welcoming in the new year in their new apartment in the Bronx, New York, when the shortness of breath and coughing fits that had bothered Dennis for months began to worsen. Johnetta convinced him to see a doctor. Because lung cancer is extremely rare in people Dennis's age, thirty-four, both she and his physician initially suspected pneumonia or possibly tuberculosis.

Dennis went into the hospital Christmas night 1990 and was diagnosed with advanced lung cancer a week later —on my twenty-sixth birthday. The symptoms had started in the fall. We had a hill near our apartment, and every time he'd walk up it, he'd get winded.

Every morning he'd wake up coughing and choking. Then he began spitting up blood. Dennis drove a taxi. One day while driving across a bridge he threw up so much blood, he

thought he was going to die right there. I told him, "The only Christmas present I want is for you to go to the hospital."

The doctor who gave us the diagnosis seemed as stunned as we were. He said, "It shocks me to see this because you're so young." At first the doctors thought they could surgically remove the cancer. But when they opened Dennis's chest, they discovered the tumor had wrapped itself around a major artery. At that point the plan switched to chemotherapy and radiation therapy, in the hope of shrinking the tumor enough to eventually be able to operate.

By the summer, though, it was clear he wasn't responding to the drugs. That's when the doctor began talking about "keeping Dennis comfortable" instead of a possible cure. He died in the hospital in October.

Advances in treatment have enabled medicine to prolong the survival time for many forms of cancer. But with peo-

323

ple living longer in general, both the incidence (1.4 million cases in 1997) and the overall number of deaths (560,000) continue to climb so that by the year 2000 cancer is expected to overtake heart disease as America's number one killer.

The term *cancer* actually encompasses more than 115 diseases, each a separate entity. Anyone caring for a person with cancer needs to remember that, because inevitably friends and acquaintances will inundate you with accounts of cancer patients they've known—how this one beat the odds and survived, how that one died within months of diagnosis.

Though well meaning, the folks sharing these stories may not know enough to provide critical details such as the type of cancer, the point at which it was detected, the patient's prior health, how aggressive it was, when it took place, and so forth. Each of these factors is going to sway the ultimate outcome to some extent.

We're not implying that you summarily dismiss other people's cancer experiences. But when talk turns to treatment and survival, it's important to listen critically and not be overly encouraged or discouraged by what you hear. An individual is not a statistic. This is true of all diseases, naturally, but perhaps none more so than cancer.

What Is Cancer?

No matter where cancer takes hold in the body, it begins with a single errant cell. Normally the billions of cells in our bodies divide to form identical new ones when old cells wear out, in a tightly controlled process. But roughly once every one million replications the daughter cell departs with a mutation in its genetic material. Why this happens is not fully understood, though it is probably traceable to a genetically acquired sensitivity to *carcinogens*, cancer-causing culprits known to initiate cell damage. Examples include to-

bacco smoke, the sun's ultraviolet rays, and asbestos fibers.

This event alone does not cause cancer. It takes other carcinogens—or co-carcinogens, cancer promoters that cannot trigger the disease by themselves—to convert the defective cell into a cancer cell. Alcohol, for instance, can activate the cancer process in the esophagus, liver, and oral cavity.

Cancer cells proliferate uncontrollably, crowding out normal cells until eventually they form a mass of excess tissue called a *tumor*. A *benign* tumor is noncancerous and rarely life threatening; once removed it usually does not come back. A *malignant* tumor, however, is cancer. Unless arrested, it may grow large enough to impair the function of major organs, rob them of essential nutrients, or burrow through to adjacent organs. Or it may shed cells that the circulatory system whisks to distant parts of the body where they latch onto tissue and spawn new tumors. Whichever route it takes, a cancer that spreads is said to have *metastasized*.

Patients and caregivers alike often find this confusing. Cancers are named for the original, or *primary*, malignancy. (Growths elsewhere are called *secondary* tumors.) For instance, a patient whose ovarian cancer has spread to the liver has *metastatic* ovarian cancer of the liver, not liver cancer. And the cancerous cells in the liver are ovarian cancer cells.

Symptoms of Cancer

An important point to remember is that early-stage cancer rarely brings pain. In fact, the symptoms associated with cancer often suggest far less serious conditions. Blood in the stool: Is it symptomatic of colorectal cancer or hemorrhoids? Nevertheless, any of the following should be brought to a doctor's attention immediately:

- Persistent changes in bowel or bladder habits

- A sore that does not heal
- Unusual bleeding or discharge
- Thickening or a lump in the breast or another part of the body
- Frequent indigestion
- Difficulty swallowing
- Change in a wart or mole
- Chronic cough or hoarseness
- Persistent, unexplained fatigue or flulike symptoms

How Cancer Is Diagnosed

Depending on the suspected cancer site, the doctor will examine the patient, take a thorough medical history, and order one or more of the following types of tests:

- Imaging (X ray, mammogram, CT scan, ultrasound, radionuclide scan, MRI scan)
- Endoscopic exam in which a thin, flexible, lighted viewing instrument (an endoscope) is inserted through the nose, mouth, urethra, or anus. The name of each test is derived from the organ being inspected. An examination of the entire colon is called a colonoscopy. An examination of the larynx is a laryngoscopy. And so on.
- Laboratory tests of the blood, urine, or other body fluids
- Biopsy

Imaging, endoscopy, and laboratory tests can disclose the presence of an abnormality, but confirming a verdict of cancer requires a *biopsy:* harvesting a small tissue sample with a needle, scalpel, or other specialized tool for examination under a microscope. This is done by a *pathologist* who is trained to identify disease according to its cell type. Sometimes exploratory surgery is necessary for obtaining the biopsy specimen.

What Is Staging?

Once cancer has been verified, additional tests may be carried out to determine its progression, or *stage.* Is the tumor limited to the primary organ? Has it infiltrated the lymphatic system,

the network of vessels that transport lymph fluid throughout the body, helping to combat infection? *Oncologists*—doctors specializing in treating cancer—express staging on a scale of 0 to IV, with stage 0 (also referred to as *carcinoma in situ,* meaning confined to the original site, or noninvasive) indicating the least degree of involvement, and stage IV, the most. It is simply a common language to help physicians plan appropriate treatment. These classifications vary from cancer to cancer so that two tumors with the same stage may have radically different prognoses.

In principle, the earlier cancer is detected and treated, the greater the odds of achieving a *remission.* Dr. LaMar McGinnis, medical director of the cancer center at DeKalb Medical Center in Atlanta, defines remission as "an interval in the growth of the cancer." A person in remission exhibits no signs or symptoms, and tests reveal no evidence of cancer even though malignant cells may still lurk in the body. Each year that the disease remains dormant, the outlook for long-term survival brightens, with five years from the time of diagnosis often used as a landmark for gauging the success of treatment. But does that mean the patient is cured?

"It is difficult with most cancers to use the word *cure,*" emphasizes Dr. McGinnis. "The significance of the survival time varies tremendously. With colon cancer, survival beyond three years is considered very encouraging, whereas both breast cancer and melanoma may recur as many as twenty or thirty years later. That is why cancer patients are followed for life in tumor registries."

Caregivers and patients need to interpret survival rates cautiously. The fact that only 25 percent of women with stage III ovarian cancer live five years doesn't mean your stepmother won't be one of them. On the other hand, the grim prognosis reflects the severity of her disease.

A cancer that comes out of remission may surface in the original site or in another part of the body. Generally, but not always, recurrent cancers are more aggressive and more difficult to tame.

How Cancer Is Treated

Surgery, radiation therapy, and chemotherapy constitute the main forms of cancer treatment. The goal may be therapeutic (to attempt a cure) or *palliative*—that is, to make patients more comfortable by alleviating symptoms caused by the tumor. For instance, men whose prostate cancer encroaches on the urinary tract, making it difficult for them to urinate, may receive radiation to shrink the malignancy.

Increasingly, says Dr. McGinnis, "we use what we term *adjuvant* therapy. Instead of relying on surgery, having the cancer spread, and only then using chemotherapy, we may use surgery, radiation, and chemotherapy concurrently." Today chemotherapy sometimes precedes surgery, to whittle a tumor to a more operable size. That would be called *neoadjuvant* therapy. Or the cancer-destroying drugs may be given after the operation to pick off any stray cells still roaming the body. In esophageal cancer, oncologists are experimenting with giving both radiation therapy and chemotherapy during surgery. On the following pages we describe each of these measures as well as less frequently used therapies: hormonal therapy, biological therapy, and bone marrow transplantation. ◄ *See "What Are Clinical Trials?" page 229.*

Surgery

Six in ten cancer survivors owe their lives to surgery, which remains the primary treatment for many types of cancer. The surgeon tries to remove the tumor as well as a *margin* of surrounding normal tissue to reduce the chances of leaving behind any malignant cells. The fear that operating on a cancer patient scatters or hastens the disease is myth. (But try convincing some folks otherwise. My aunt Kitty fervently believes that my father's heart surgery stirred up his lymphoma.)

Obviously, the side effects of surgery can vary greatly depending on the tumor site, the type of operation, the patient's age, health, and condition, and so forth. Chapter 3 discusses at length what caregivers need to know about tending postoperative patients.

Radiation Therapy and Its Side Effects

Radiation therapy aims high-energy rays directly at cancerous cells with the intent of damaging or destroying them so they cannot mature and divide. It is the preferred therapy for Hodgkin's disease, laryngeal cancer, and oropharyn-

---

INSIDE INFORMATION

When bathing a loved one undergoing radiation, be careful not to wash off the "bull's-eye." Ask a member of the radiation department for a few rolls of adhesive tape, and place the tape gently over the marks. Should they begin to fade, alert the radiation therapist. The only time to reapply them yourself is if you think they will vanish before the next appointment, and then be sure to tell the therapist. The ink can rub off on clothing, by the way, so until treatment ends, patients might want to wear older garments or those made of fabrics that are less likely to stain and easily washable. Some medical centers permanently tattoo tiny dots on the spot to be irradiated, making such precautions unnecessary.

geal cancer, and is incorporated into the treatment of many other cancers.

The rays all home in on rapidly dividing cells, whether cancerous or not, so that normal cells invariably get in the line of fire. To spare healthy tissue as much as possible, patients initially undergo what's called a *simulation*. Here they lie under an imaging X-ray machine for half an hour to two hours while a *radiation therapist* maps out the precise area to be radiated, marking the skin with ink or dye.

External radiation is typically administered on an outpatient basis five days a week over six or seven weeks or, if used for palliative purposes, two to three weeks. Because normal cells recover faster than cancer cells, the weekend respite gives them an opportunity to heal while the bloodstream carries off the dead cancer cells to be excreted naturally.

Still, anticipate side effects. There's no telling which adverse reactions the person we are caring for will experience, if any. Everybody—and every body—is different. As you can see from the information in the sidebar, the radiation site, referred to as the *port* or *field*, greatly influences the temporary side effects that may arise.

The following are more general side effects liable to crop up whatever the treatment area:

Skin Inflammation

The skin is the organ most likely to incur injury from the powerful rays. Usually people experience nothing more serious than dryness, redness, and tenderness, comparable to a sunburn. These effects typically subside soon after therapy ends, although some folks find that the treated patch retains its "tan."

More severe reactions can inflict lasting damage on the skin, hair follicles, and sweat glands, which is why it's important to inspect the skin daily. Alert the radiation therapist if the skin ap-

---

Potential Side Effects of Radiation Therapy

To the Head and Neck
Mouth redness and irritation, dry mouth, difficulty swallowing, changes in taste or no sense of taste, nausea, earaches, swollen or droopy skin under the chin, changes in skin texture, stiff jaw, hair loss

To the Chest
Difficult or painful swallowing, persistent cough, fever, shortness of breath

To the Breast
Lump in the throat, dry cough, stiff shoulder, soreness and swelling in the breast from a buildup of fluid, reddened or deeply tanned skin

To the Stomach and Abdomen
Upset stomach, nausea, vomiting, diarrhea

To the Pelvis
Upset stomach, nausea, diarrhea, bladder irritation resulting in uncomfortable or frequent urination

General
Deficiencies of white blood cells (leukopenia) and/or platelets (thrombocytopenia)

◄ *See chapter 3 to learn which medications or medical procedures are generally ordered to control these symptoms, as well as caregivers' skills for prevention and management.*

---

pears bright red or purple, or if you notice scaling, peeling, blisters, or what is called "weeping," where the skin becomes wet and sore.

How It Is Managed. The radiation-therapy department at New York's Memorial Sloan-Kettering Cancer Center typically treats redness, irritation, and itching with an ointment called Aquaphor. Should the skin show signs of breaking down, the patient wears a sterile dressing over the wound and may be advised to forgo therapy for several days to allow for healing.

Skin exposed to radiation demands tender, loving care. Throughout treatment and for several weeks afterward, patients and caregivers should observe the following do's and don'ts:

- Check with the doctor before using any lotions, soaps, deodorants, medicines, perfumes, cosmetics, talcum powder, or depilatories. Besides possibly irritating the skin and undermining healing, such products can actually interfere with the treatments themselves.
- Wear loose, soft, unstarched clothing —preferably made of cotton—over the affected skin.
- Wash skin gently *using lukewarm water only* and pat dry. Never rub, scrub, or scratch.
- Whenever possible, substitute paper tape for cloth tape, taking care to apply it outside the irradiated area.
- If shaving is necessary, consult the doctor or nurse, who will probably advise using an electric razor.
- Avoid applying extreme heat or cold (hot-water bottles, ice packs) to the area.
- Before venturing into the sun, protect treated skin with light clothing. The doctor may also recommend using a PABA (para-aminobenzoic acid) sunscreen or a sunblock with a sun protection factor (SPF) of at least 15.

◀ See "Skin Care," page 116.

Fatigue

Several weeks into treatment you can expect a loved one undergoing radiation to start feeling tired and weak. For one thing, the body has to expend tremendous energy healing itself. Stress, too, contributes to the fatigue, which often lingers four to six weeks following the final session.

How It Is Managed. No magic bullet here. The best we can do is encourage loved ones to rest as much as possible during these few weeks. Now is an opportune time to recruit other family members and friends to pitch in with daily chores, errands, and driving the person to and from medical appointments.

Appetite Loss

People receiving radiation have plenty of reasons not to feel like eating. Irradiation to the head and neck can alter one's sense of taste and make swallowing painful, while treatment to the stomach and abdomen frequently leaves patients queasy and unable to keep food down.

How It Is Managed. An adequate diet is essential for helping damaged tissue repair itself. To circumvent these and other obstacles to a healthy appetite, you'll need to rely on the tricks in chapter 3 for making food more palatable and easier to swallow. ◀ *See "Tips for Stimulating Appetite," page 159.*

Aside from occasional dizzy spells, Dennis Rivera tolerated radiation to the chest extremely well. "On days when he was scheduled for therapy," says Johnetta Romanowski, "he'd drive his taxi to the hospital, have treatment, then get in the cab and go right to work." The procedure itself is as painless as being X-rayed.

When things are running smoothly, a typical appointment takes fifteen to thirty minutes, including setup time. But prepare yourself and your loved one for delays. Equipment breaks down, other patients arrive late, and emergencies crop up. Any one of these can create a daylong backup. Of the time in the treatment room, a mere one to five minutes is actually spent sitting or lying under the imposing apparatus, which rotates to treat from different angles.

A new technique called *hyperfractionated radiation* therapy divides the daily radiation dose into several smaller amounts that are administered several times a day, every four to six hours. It is typically performed on an outpatient basis, with patients returning home between treatments. While the constant round-trips make this method more disruptive to patients' and caregivers' schedules, certain tumors appear to respond more favorably to the hyperfractionated doses.

What Is Internal Radiation Therapy?

As its name implies, *internal radiation* entails implanting a tiny sealed container of radioactive material directly into cancerous tissue, or as close to it as possible, under local or general anesthesia. This allows for a greater total dosage over a shorter period of time than external therapy, and the concentrated dosage exposes fewer normal cells to the harmful effects of radiation. Afterward the radioactive material can be removed, something usually done without an anesthetic at the bedside, or it can be left permanently in the body where it rapidly decays. Radiation oncologists often lean toward internal radiation for treating cancers of the prostate, cervix, uterus, breast, thyroid, head, and neck, sometimes in conjunction with external radiation.

Contrary to popular misconception, patients undergoing external radiation do not emit radioactivity. People with low-dose implants actually can, however, and must be hospitalized for the one to seven days of treatment. Remind other visitors to sit at least six feet from the bed and to stay no longer than thirty minutes. You might also let friends and relatives know that some medical facilities won't allow women of childbearing age or children under eighteen to visit

implant patients; they should call the nurse's desk on the floor in advance to inquire about hospital policy.

Chemotherapy and Its Side Effects

Surgery and radiation therapy are *local* treatments. Chemotherapy, which literally means chemical treatment, fights cancer *systemically* throughout the body by way of the bloodstream. It is considered the primary treatment for leukemia, lymphoma, and multiple myeloma, and an adjuvant therapy for many other cancers. In a recent development, oncologists are testing drug therapy's effectiveness as a preventive measure against secondary cancers.

Although more than a quarter of a million *antineoplastic* agents have been tested for their cancer-inhibiting properties, only sixty or so have been approved as safe enough for patients. How do they work? Basically, explains Dr. McGinnis, "the medications block the cancer cell's ability to mature or reproduce through a variety of ways." That is why oncologists may prescribe *combination chemotherapy* incorporating drugs from one or more families of antineoplastics.

Most of the agents used are too toxic to be ingested orally or are not readily absorbed that way, and so they must be delivered to the bloodstream intravenously. Because repeated needle stickings can cause veins to deteriorate, and the caustic drugs can irritate the blood vessels, a flexible plastic tube may be surgically implanted in a large vein in the upper chest or elsewhere in the body. The medication is then injected directly into this catheter, sparing patients the pain and anxiety of having members of the medical team poke around for a healthy vein. ◄ *See "Central Venous Catheters," page 150; "The Situation: Venipunctures," page 64.*

Several factors will determine how frequently your loved one receives

Potential Side Effects of Chemotherapy

Gastrointestinal Distress
Nausea, vomiting, appetite loss, diarrhea, pain and cramping, constipation

Mouth, Gums, and Throat Problems
Dry mouth, sores in the mouth and throat

Nerve and Muscle Problems
Tingling, burning, weakness, or numbness in the hands and/or feet; loss of balance; clumsiness; difficulty walking; muscle soreness, tiredness, weakness; difficulty picking up objects; jaw pain; hearing loss; stomach pain; neuralgia; and deep nerve pain

Skin and Nail Problems
Redness, itching, peeling, dryness, acne, brittle and cracked nails, darkened skin along the veins used for injecting or infusing chemotherapy, tissue damage from IV drugs leaking out of a vein

Hair and Scalp Problems
Partial or total hair loss anywhere on the body, tender scalp

Kidney and Bladder Problems
Pain or burning during urination, frequent urination, reddish or bloody urine, fever, chills

Fluid Retention
Swelling or puffiness in the hands, feet, or abdomen; labored breathing upon exertion

Sexual and Reproductive Problems
Women: irregular menstruation, unusual bleeding, or none at all during treatment; temporary or permanent infertility; menopauselike symptoms such as hot flashes and vaginal itching, burning, or dryness.

Men: temporary or permanent infertility

Blood Disorders
Deficiencies of red blood cells (anemia), white blood cells (leukopenia), and/or platelets (thrombocytopenia)

◄ *See chapter 3, to learn which medications or medical procedures are generally ordered to control these conditions, as well as caregivers' skills for prevention and management.*

---

treatment: the drug or drugs to be used, the severity of disease, and the oncologist's preference. The two most common schedules call for administering chemotherapy five days in a row every four weeks or on a weekly basis. If combination therapy has been prescribed, the medications may be alternated rather than administered all at the same visit. As for the duration of treatment, that can range from three months to three years. The drugs are dispensed in three cycles—*induction, consolidation,* and *maintenance*—with intervals of rest in between to allow the body to recover and build healthy new cells.

Like radiation therapy, chemotherapy intercepts dividing cells without differentiating between malignant ones and normal ones. "The major effect is on cancer cells, since they undergo the most rapid division," says Dr. McGinnis. But the cells that make up hair follicles, white blood cells, and the lining of the digestive tract *also* reproduce at an accelerated pace—the equivalent of waving a red flag in front of a bull. "That's what leads to some of the more typical side effects," he explains, "such as hair loss, infection, nausea, and vomiting."

Virtually any chemotherapy medication can bring on the latter. Debbie Bryant, a caregiver from Alabama, remembers that her terminally ill mother grew so sick and nauseous, "she eventually discontinued the drugs." In the nearly twenty years since Maida Bryant had colon cancer, dosages have been refined, reducing many unwanted symptoms. Plus, we now have more effective medications on hand for relieving nausea and vomiting.

Johnetta Romanowski: Dennis would get so sick from chemotherapy that for the first four months of treatments he had to be hospitalized each time and knocked out on Benadryl and Ativan so he could sleep through the entire twelve hours.

One day his sister-in-law happened to be watching TV and overheard something about a new drug called Zofran, which numbs the part of the brain that tells the body it's going to be sick. It was being given to chemo patients on a trial basis. She told me about it, and the next time we saw Dennis's doctor I asked him if we could try it. Once Dennis started taking the Zofran, he was able to receive the same chemo regimen as an outpatient without getting sick and without needing the Benadryl and Ativan, so he was up and alert. It made a huge difference.

Nothing could counteract some of the more bizarre side effects Dennis experienced, such as the ringing in his ears and the numbness in his feet. As with radiation, everybody responds differently. The person you are caring for may develop only a few of these complications, most of which disappear upon the completion of treatment or soon after. Still, acquaint yourself with the possible hazards beforehand so you'll be able to anticipate your loved one's needs and report any unusual or serious reactions to the oncologist, who can then modify the dosage or change medications accordingly.

Blood Disorders

One of the most potentially dangerous side effects of chemotherapy is its tendency to suppress the bone marrow's production of red blood cells, white blood cells, and blood platelets.

Red cells *(erythrocytes)* transport oxygen throughout the body. When chemotherapy reduces the ranks of these vital couriers, patients become *anemic* and are susceptible to fatigue, dizziness, chills, and shortness of breath.

Five types of **white cells** *(leukocytes)* team up to disarm potentially harmful assailants in the circulation. At insufficient levels, a person is said to be *immunocompromised*, with little resistance to infections of the lungs, urinary tract, mouth, skin, rectum, reproductive tract—you name it. Symptoms include fever, sweating, chills, diarrhea, redness or swelling, severe cough or sore throat, burning upon urination, vaginal itching, and unusual vaginal discharge.

Platelets *(thrombocytes)* prevent uncontrollable bleeding by converging on wounds and releasing substances that form a jellylike plug, or *clot*, over the broken blood vessel. At the same time they instruct the vessel walls to constrict. Those whose platelet output dwindles are prone to bleed and bruise easily, even from minor injuries. Be on the alert for unexplained black-and-blue or purplish marks, nosebleeds, and bleeding gums, as well as bloody urine, black or bloody stools, and red spots beneath the skin.

✚ *Any of the above-mentioned symptoms warrants a phone call to the doctor.*

Radiation therapy, too, can diminish platelet and white-cell counts, especially when a large area of the body is being treated. But generally, anemia, leukopenia, and thrombocytopenia present more of a worry for people on chemo. Bear in mind that many forms of cancer require both therapies, sometimes concurrently.

How They Are Managed. The day of each treatment, blood is drawn and the three components measured. This is called a *complete blood count (CBC)*. If the level of platelets or white cells is low, therapy may be postponed until it returns to a safe range. That might take one day, two days, or two weeks. Those of us accompanying loved ones to appointments should be prepared for the

---

TIME SAVER

When a person undergoing chemotherapy lives a distance from the medical facility, ask the oncologist to arrange for a local laboratory or doctor's office to perform the CBC a day or two before treatments. In this way you can avoid the inconvenience and stress of making a long trip only to learn that your loved one's counts are down, forcing a delay of chemo. Then you must either drive all the way home or check into a motel indefinitely.

---

possibility of turning right around to go home. In situations where the sick person isn't able to drive, we may find ourselves arranging for transportation several days in a row—however long it takes the blood count to rebound.

Should the level of red cells or platelets drop dangerously low, they will be added intravenously. ◄ *See "Arranging Blood Donations," page 45.*

Drug therapy is also used. A biologic agent called *filgrastim* (brand name: Neupogen) stimulates the bone marrow to turn out more neutrophils, the most abundant type of white blood cell. *Epoetin alfa* (Epogen, Procrit), also given intravenously, steps up red cell production in a similar fashion.

Special Care: When a Loved One on Chemotherapy Develops Anemia. Until she's feeling better, encourage her to sleep longer than usual at night, nap during the day whenever possible, and scale back on activities.

Shortchanged of oxygen, people with anemia may grow dizzy if they stand up too quickly from a sitting or prone position. Remind loved ones to rise to their feet slowly.

See to it that her diet includes foods rich in iron, which promotes red cell production. Excellent sources include lean meat, oysters, egg yolks, kidney beans, spinach, kale, raisins, carrots, apricots, whole wheat bread, and that perennial favorite, liver.

Special Care: When a Loved One on Chemotherapy Develops Immunosuppression. A person who is immunocompromised can reduce his risk of infection by observing such basic daily habits as washing his hands frequently; taking care to avoid cuts, scrapes, and cracks in the skin; and keeping away from people with colds, measles, the flu, and other communicable diseases. ◄ *See "Safeguarding Patients Against Infection," page 105.*

Special Care: When a Loved One on Chemotherapy Develops Clotting Problems. Check with the doctor before administering any medication. Aspirin, aspirin-free pain relievers, and steroids, for example, all have anticoagulant properties and interfere with clotting. Also ask if the person should abstain from alcohol. It, too, has been known to impair coagulation.

Take extreme care not to inflame or tear the skin or the fragile mucous membranes of the mouth, nose, rectum,

---

INSIDE INFORMATION

Some divisions of the American Cancer Society provide free transportation to and from treatment. In the event that no volunteer drivers are available, the organization reimburses patients for the cost of public transportation.

☎ If you have questions, call 800-227-2345.

---

and gastrointestinal tract, which in these patients could induce excessive bleeding. Therefore:

- Do not take temperature rectally.
- Make sure the person cleans his teeth using a soft-bristle toothbrush, never dental floss or toothpicks.
- Remind him to blow his nose gently and not to use his fingers.
- Keep nasal passages and lips moist with a lubricant such as K-Y Jelly or petroleum jelly.
- Follow chapter 3's dietary measures for avoiding constipation, and refrain from serving peanuts, popcorn, and other coarse foods that are difficult to digest and apt to irritate the digestive tract.
- If your loved one is up and about—cooking, ironing, gardening, and so forth—encourage him to protect his skin against burns and injuries with oven mitts or heavy gloves.

Hair Loss (Alopecia)

We don't want to downplay the psychological trauma experienced by people who see their hair fall out gradually or in clumps, a common side effect of chemotherapy and also of cranial radiation. What could be a more conspicuous reminder of the life-threatening disease lurking within? It's enough of a struggle for the seriously ill to hold on to their self-identity without suddenly feeling less attractive as well.

Not all chemotherapeutic agents cause hair loss. When it does occur, typically after several rounds of treatment, the strands may grow thinner or fall out altogether. One aspect of alopecia from systemic cancer treatment that patients find most upsetting at first is that it can affect hair anywhere on the body, including the eyebrows, underarms, and pubic area. But once cancer patients overcome their initial shock, anger, and depression, most come to view hair loss as a reasonable price to pay for a chance at prolonging their lives and possibly attaining a cure. To be frank, a bout of unrelenting diarrhea or another of chemotherapy's nastier side effects usually puts alopecia in perspective. Gradually patients begin to accept the face in the mirror as their own. If anything, hair loss may be more disturbing to other people until they, too, grow used to the sight.

When chemotherapy radically changes someone's appearance, consider gently forewarning any first-time visitors you think may have a hard time masking their shock or discomfort. Their obvious reaction will only reinforce any self-consciousness the sick person may be feeling. On the other hand, don't draw undue attention to what ultimately should be a minor matter.

✻ *Patients may be heartened to know that hair lost to chemotherapy usually returns once treatment is over, sometimes sooner.*

How It Is Managed. It's often suggested that chemo patients switch to a shorter hairstyle to make their hair appear fuller and thicker. Throughout treatment, it's best for them to use soft brushes, wide-tooth combs, conditioner (to avoid tangles), mild shampoos, and, when blow-drying, a low-heat setting. They should not put their hair up in brush-style rollers or hot curlers, or have their hair dyed or permed.

Some folks are perfectly comfortable going out in public au naturel. Men and women who prefer to cover their heads can choose turbans, scarves, bandanas,

---

The American Cancer Society sponsors Look Good, Feel Better, a one-day course in how to effectively use wigs, makeup, and other accessories while undergoing chemotherapy or radiation.

☎ To learn when the program is coming to a hospital near your loved one, call the ACS at 800-227-2345.

or hats, while a baseball cap twisted backward not only serves its intended purpose but these days puts you at the forefront of popular style. The other option, for either sex, is a wig or a hairpiece.

If the oncologist has said to anticipate alopecia and your loved one thinks she might like to try a wig, take her shopping now. We know plenty of patients who began wearing their wigs from the outset of treatment. With a close match in color and style, they were able to make the transition undetectably once their natural hair did indeed start to fall out.

Other Forms of Cancer Treatment

Hormonal Therapy

Normally, the chemical messengers known as hormones foster good health; they travel through the bloodstream to regulate everything from metabolism to tissue regeneration to personality traits to sexual characteristics. But the female sex hormone estrogen and the male sex hormone testosterone can also stimulate cancer cell growth in the breasts and prostate, respectively.

"Hormonal therapy attempts to block the effects of these hormones," says Dr. McGinnis, "either with drugs or by surgically removing the organ that produces each one." Ironically, one strategy for treating prostate cancer is to administer oral estrogen, which prevents the testicles from manufacturing testosterone. Injecting a synthetic

agonist called *luteinizing hormone-releasing hormone,* or LHRH, produces a comparable effect. As Dr. McGinnis noted, other times the testicles have to be removed in an operation called an *orchiectomy.* Likewise, breast cancer therapy may involve antiestrogen drugs —these days most likely tamoxifen—or taking out both ovaries *(oophorectomy),* the main site of estrogen production.

Biological Therapy

Many cancer researchers look to biological therapy (also referred to as *immunotherapy*) as the cancer treatment of the future. The principle behind it is to harness natural or synthetic substances that enhance the immune system's response to disease.

The first biologic, a family of naturally secreted proteins called *interferon,* was discovered in 1957. Others have emerged since, among them *interleukin-2, colony-stimulating factors,* and *monoclonal antibodies.* The latter, scientifically tailored proteins, can be likened to biological smart bombs that target and affix themselves to malignant cells. Combining them with chemotherapeutic agents makes it possible to deliver the medications directly to the tumor.

According to Dr. McGinnis, progress in this area has been frustratingly slow. "We expected much more from biological therapy earlier," he says. "It is still primarily an adjuvant treatment for advanced cancer" and an investigational therapy at that.

Bone Marrow Transplantation

Bone marrow transplantation (BMT), once strictly experimental, is now considered a standard therapeutic option for certain forms of leukemia and lymphoma. Patient studies are under way to evaluate its effectiveness against other cancers as well.

All hollow bones contain marrow, a network of vessels and fibers that serves as the body's factory for blood components. In leukemia, malignant cells inundate the marrow and disrupt its production of red cells, white cells, and platelets. Aggressive chemotherapy or radiation can exert a similar effect by destroying the soft, spongy material. A BMT replaces the impaired marrow with healthy tissue. For malignancies other than leukemia, the procedure doesn't treat cancer as such; it enables patients to be bombarded with unusually heavy doses and thus stand a better chance of seeing their cancer eradicated. In the process, the existing marrow is all but wiped out, at which point new marrow is infused into the bloodstream—much like a blood transfusion. For people with leukemia, doctors intentionally expunge the diseased marrow along with the tumorous cells, then perform the transplant.

An *autologous* BMT harvests the patient's own marrow during a period of remission when it appears to be disease free. In an *allogeneic* graft, the material comes from a genetically compatible donor, either a close relative—usually a brother or sister—or an unrelated volunteer. Success hinges on how closely the donor's and recipient's marrows match in terms of sharing at least four of six proteins called *human leukocyte antigens* (at least five of six if the donor is not a family member). A simple blood test determines each person's marrow design, or *type*.

Only 30 to 40 percent of patients will have an HLA-compatible parent or sibling. Identical twins possess all six HLA antigens in common, but since they represent a small fraction of all births, such

☎ The National Marrow Donor Program's office of patient advocacy can assist you in selecting a transplant center and can answer questions you may have about your loved one's case. Call 800-526-7809.

syngeneic transplants are extremely rare. The odds of finding a suitable donor outside one's family are slimmer still: between one in ten thousand and one in twenty thousand, according to the federally funded National Marrow Donor Program, which regularly fields calls from transplant centers looking to pair a candidate with one of the nearly 3 million anonymous donors in its computerized international registry. When a match is made, the NMDP arranges for additional testing for the donor and transporting the marrow.

Once an allogeneic donor is identified and consents to the procedure, the patient enters the hospital for seven to ten days of megadoses of chemotherapy and possibly full-body radiation therapy. This preconditioning phase brings him to the brink of death; without the transplant, he will not survive.

Marrow collection, performed under general or local anesthesia, is surprisingly simple. The physician inserts needles into the hip bone until he has extracted one to two pints of liquid marrow. That may sound like a lot, but the fluid removed actually contains no more than 5 percent of the donor's marrow, which replenishes itself within a matter of weeks.

To ensure that an autologous transplant patient's marrow doesn't harbor any undetected cancer cells, the sample may be specially treated, or *purged*. It can then be frozen for up to three years. Allogeneic transplants are carried out as soon as possible. While donors typically go home the next day, recipients spend two to four weeks receiving antibiotic therapy in protective isolation, for that is the amount of time it generally takes new marrow to manufacture enough normal white cells to repel infection.

Of course, as with any organ transplant, whatever remains of the original immune system may reject the graft. Or the reverse may occur. Half of all allogeneic patients suffer *graft-versus-host disease (GVHD)*, a potentially deadly affliction wherein the transplanted marrow mistakes the host's body for a foreign invader and attacks the liver, the skin, or the gastrointestinal tract, or sometimes all three at once. The higher the number of corresponding HLA antigens, the lower the risk of graft-versus-host disease.

How It Is Managed. Until the threat of GVHD subsides—several years in some instances—patients are routinely put on *immunosuppressant agents* such as cyclosporine (brand name: Sandimmune). Their goal is to suppress the activity of the most hostile of the white cells, the so-called T lymphocytes. Should your loved one develop graft-versus-host disease, the physician will likely increase the dosage of the immunosuppressant.

Because of the potential dangers from GVHD, infection, graft rejection and other complications, a marrow recipient can expect to remain hospitalized another month or two. The total recuperation period? That's difficult to say. For some folks a full year passes before they feel physically and psychologically recovered.

A relatively small percentage of cancer patients are able to undergo bone marrow transplantation. Besides the health risks involved and the difficulty of finding a donor, the procedure usually costs in excess of $200,000. Most health insurers cover bone marrow transplantation only for certain diseases. What's more, patients and their families can expect to incur thousands of dollars in nonreimbursable expenses such as transportation to a transplant center and lodging. ▶ *See Appendix B:* *"Bone Marrow Transplantation," page 505.*

Potential Complications of Advanced Cancer

The ways in which cancer can bring about death are as varied as the number of malignant diseases themselves. "A tumor may expand to such an extent that it interferes with the function of one or more organs, causing them to fail," explains Dr. McGinnis. Cancerous tissue eventually consumed such a large portion of Dennis Rivera's right lung that "he had just 10 percent breathing capacity left," says Johnetta Romanowski. Toward the end of his life, her fiancé repeatedly gasped for air, despite the aid of an oxygen tank.

"Also," says Dr. McGinnis, "the rapidly growing cancer cells have a generally debilitating effect on the entire body, sapping nutrients and strength necessary for life. That is why wasting often occurs." Debbie Bryant watched her fifty-three-year-old mother wither from 125 pounds to 75 pounds, her constitutional reserve and resistance to infection depleted. "By the time Mom died, she was so small that I could pick her up myself."

Recommended Reading

The following are available free from the National Cancer Institute (800-422-6237). In Oahu, Hawaii, call 524-1234; call collect from other Hawaiian islands.

- "What You Need to Know About Cancer"
- The "What You Need to Know About . . ." series of booklets on each of two dozen forms of cancer
- "Chemotherapy and You: A Guide to Self-Help During Treatment"
- "Radiation Therapy and You: A Guide to Self-Help During Treatment"

The following are available free from the Leukemia Society of America (800-955-4572).

- "Acute Lymphocytic Leukemia"
- "Acute Myelogenous Leukemia"
- "Acute Myelogenous Leukemia"
- "Chronic Myelogenous Leukemia"
- "Multiple Myeloma (MM)"
- "Hodgkin's Disease and the Non-Hodgkin's Lymphomas"

The following are available free from the American Brain Tumor Association (800-886-2282).

- "A Primer of Brain Tumors"
- "About Metastatic Tumors to the Brain and Spine"
- "Coping with a Brain Tumor, Part I: From Diagnosis to Treatment"
- "Coping with a Brain Tumor, Part II: During and After Treatment"

–13–

Caring for Someone with Cardiovascular Disease

Audree Siden, who nursed her Russian-born mother in her East Side apartment in Manhattan for nine months, recalls:

My mother had suffered from congestive heart failure for a number of years but managed it quite comfortably with medications that reduced the fluid buildup in her lungs. Even at eighty-eight she was active, living by herself in upper Manhattan, traveling, taking the bus downtown to Bloomingdale's and Carnegie Hall.

Late one night in June 1992 she called and said, "I'm not doing well." Now, Mae was not the kind of woman to complain, so those words were a call to immediate action. Edmund, my fiancé, is a doctor. He could tell from her voice that the fluid was high up in her chest, and he summoned an ambulance. By the time we got to her home, the paramedics were there. My mother had to be hospitalized.

She grew frailer and weaker, then she became depressed over being in the hospital. Mae's essence had always been her spirit, so I promised that she would never see the inside of a hospital again. I brought her to my home.

My mother worried that her staying with me would curtail my life and my activities, but my partner and I were able to run our belt-manufacturing business from the kitchen table. Mom was a great craftsperson herself; she loved to see the colors and the beadwork and the designs we were creating. Later, when she could no longer get out of bed, I would bring the belts to her and ask, "Which one do you like?" If she didn't have the strength to talk, she would point.

All of this was taking place during the preparations for my oldest son's December marriage. I was caught between the generations very clearly. Mom came to the wedding, looking glamorous. Then she let go. She told me,

"That's it, I've had enough. I wish to finish my life now." About two and a half weeks before she died, in March, she said her last words: "What would I have ever done without you?"

The heart represents many things—love, courage, happiness—but above all it is a symbol of life. Few sounds are as comforting as its steady, pulsating rhythm. In the course of an average lifetime, a heart beats more than 2.7 billion times.

No larger than a fist, this muscular pump consists of four chambers: an upper pair, the left *atrium* and the right atrium, and below them the left and right *ventricles*. What we refer to as a heartbeat is actually the sound of the organ filling, then its chambers contracting, in a tightly coordinated sequence that propels the blood from one section to another through flaplike portals known as valves. The blood follows a sort of figure-eight pattern as it pulses into the right side of the heart and out to the lungs—where carbon dioxide is cast off and fresh oxygen absorbed—and then into the left side of the heart and out to the arterial system.

The heart belongs to the *circulatory system*. *Arteries*, wide elastic tubes buried deep within the body, carry oxygenated blood from the heart. In order to nourish all tissues, they feed smaller *arterioles*, which branch off into vast beds of microscopic *capillaries*. It is here, through the membranous capillary walls, that the blood and tissues exchange products. Tissue cells load up on fresh oxygen, nutrients, and other essential substances while relinquishing waste materials and carbon dioxide.

On its return trip to the heart, the deoxygenated blood travels the venous system, with detours made through the liver and the kidneys for filtering out impurities. The network of veins mirrors the arterial system but in reverse: Capillaries open into larger *venules*, which converge into still wider *veins*. Every minute all five quarts of blood complete a circuit from the heart, out to the body, and back to the pump.

Causes of Cardiovascular Disease

Each year more than 700,000 Americans lose their lives to cardiovascular diseases such as congestive heart failure, heart attack, and arrhythmias. We use the term *cardiovascular disease* rather than "heart disease" because, as cardiologist Dr. Gerald Fletcher of Atlanta's Emory University Hospital points out, "all three of these are usually related to coronary artery disease." (*Cardio* pertains to the heart; *vascular*, to blood vessels.)

Coronary artery disease falls under the broader category of *atherosclerosis*, which when translated from the Greek vividly describes its effect on medium- and large-size arteries. *Athero* means fatty, gruel-like; *sclerosis*, hard. Over time, fats, cholesterol, and other matter in the blood build up on arterial walls like sludge clogging a pipe. *Plaque* accumulation may also cause the walls to harden and thicken, further narrowing the passageway through which blood can flow—or closing it off completely. Doctors refer to any degree of blockage as an *occlusion*.

All muscles need regular deliveries of oxygen and nutrients, none more so than the heart muscle itself. Two large vessels, the left and right coronary arteries, snake down either side of the heart. Each supplies smaller branches that spread out like tributaries across the surface of the muscular cardiac wall, or *myocardium*.

In coronary artery disease, one or both arteries becomes obstructed or constricted, depriving the heart muscle of blood. This condition, *myocardial ischemia*, may produce chest pains known as *angina pectoris*—or, if the heart is completely starved of oxygen, it may induce a heart attack. An occluded coronary artery also serves as a popular haunt for blood clots *(thrombi)*, which can plug up the vessel *(coronary thrombosis)* and trigger a heart attack.

Heredity predisposes some men and women to cardiovascular disease, but to a large extent it is preventable. Smoking, high blood pressure, and high blood cholesterol—*each* on its own—doubles a person's risk, while obesity and physical inactivity play supporting roles.

Types of Cardiovascular Disease

Heart Attack (Infarction)

Myocardial infarction, the medical term for a heart attack, refers to the irreversible cell death *(necrosis)* that a portion of heart muscle sustains when denied oxygen by obstructed or constricted coronary arteries. Infarctions erupt most often in the left ventricle, the chamber that bears the heaviest workload. The longer or more severe the restriction of blood flow to the heart, the greater the damage.

Heart attacks strike 1.5 million men and women annually, killing 500,000 and disabling countless more. Survival depends on the extent of necrosis, which causes scar tissue to form over the now useless muscle area. If the blood deficiency is corrected quickly enough, the heart grows healthy tissue and can regain some of its lost function. A so-called massive heart attack, says Dr. Fletcher, damages "approximately 40 percent of the heart's muscle mass."

Symptoms of a Heart Attack

Myocardial infarction frequently announces its imminent arrival with several classic warning signals. The most common is an intermittent or persistent sensation of pressure, tightness, or pain that begins in the chest but may radiate to the shoulders, neck, and arms.

Women often exhibit different symptoms. They may feel a recurrent pressure or tingling *anywhere above the waist* when exerting themselves or experiencing intense emotions.

Dr. Fletcher, also a professor of cardiology at Emory University School of Medicine, notes, "I have a lot of heart attack patients who perceive the discomfort of heart pain as shortness of breath." While *dyspnea* can in fact be a sign of heart attack, it typically accompanies chest pain, along with nausea and vomiting, sweating and light-headedness or fainting.

All caregivers should acquaint themselves with these harbingers, whether caring for a cardiovascular disease patient or not, because a heart attack can ambush anyone fitting the high-risk profile described earlier, such as the 50 million people with elevated blood pressure and diabetics, half of whom die prematurely from myocardial infarction.

What to Do if a Loved One Suffers a Heart Attack. Recognizing the warning signs and responding promptly is critical. According to the American Heart Association, fatal heart attacks usually occur within two hours of symptom onset. Yet about 50 percent of all heart attack victims wait at least that long before seeking medical attention.

Expect your loved one to protest going to a hospital. "It's only chest pain," he'll say. "I get it all the time. It'll go away." Don't be dissuaded. Insist he lie down and loosen any constrictive clothing, then call an ambulance or take him yourself to a facility that offers twenty-four-hour emergency cardiac care.

Not all myocardial infarctions produce the indicators mentioned above. In fact, it's possible to have a heart attack without truly realizing it, as Grady McCool discovered. In 1972 the forty-nine-year-old realtor and builder was showing a home to a prospective client when suddenly, says his wife, Allene, "he was so short of breath, he couldn't walk back to the car without stopping.

"Because he had been a smoker, his first thought was emphysema. But a coronary arteriogram and some other tests showed that he'd had a heart attack, although they couldn't pinpoint the time." Grady, one of the first patients in Jackson, Mississippi, to undergo coronary bypass surgery, is retired now and a grandfather of eight. The years since his heart attack have been largely healthy ones, tarnished only by a few scares. Most involved occasional attacks of angina pectoris, a common manifestation of coronary atherosclerosis.

What Is Angina?

The acute chest pain called angina pectoris feels similar to an infarction. As with a heart attack, a reduction in oxygen to the heart stimulates what Dr. Fletcher describes as "a dull ache," not unlike the feeling you get in your thigh when riding a bicycle up a hill. But here the ischemia is fleeting and does not decimate myocardial tissue.

Both physical exertion and emotional stress can set off angina. In fact, some heart patients claim to have known in advance that a certain activity or situation would incite an attack. Grady McCool, who had been a football coach ("and a type A person all the way," says his wife), learned it was best for him to take a tranquilizer before attending sporting events or to avoid them altogether.

The fifteen minutes or less it takes for angina to subside can seem like an eternity to the person experiencing it. Help her to a sitting position; this eases breathing. Above all, maintaining your composure, encouraging her to relax in your most soothing voice, and staying calm can go a long way toward mitigating the severity of an episode. Some angina patients need only to rest until the pain ebbs; others, however, may require oxygen and medication.

How to Administer Nitroglycerine. In most cases, the first line of defense remains *nitroglycerine* tablets, which Dr. Fletcher describes as "an old-fashioned drug but still a very good one. You place it under the tongue and allow it to dissolve." Nitroglycerine, a *coronary vasodilator,* improves blood flow to the myocardium and lowers blood pressure by enlarging the coronary arteries and the veins that return blood to the heart. Should the pain fail to pass after five minutes, administer a second pill, reminding your patient not to swallow. After five more minutes, if the pain persists, try another tablet.

"If it's not relieved properly after the third nitroglycerine," says Dr. Fletcher, "take the patient to an emergency room immediately." *Be careful not to give more than three pills*, for the dilating action can send blood pressure plummeting precipitously—even to the point of bringing about acute circulatory shock, a potentially fatal condition. The same holds true for nitroglycerine mist: Use it a maximum of three times, with a five-minute interval between each spray.

INSIDE INFORMATION

See to it that an angina patient taking nitroglycerine

- keeps it nearby at all times but not in a pocket—the pills are highly sensitive to heat, including body heat. The tiny glass bottle they come in makes an ideal container, or ask your pharmacist for a pill box;
- replaces the cap tightly and opens a new bottle every three months—nitroglycerine is most effective when fresh;
- avoids taking extremely hot showers or standing suddenly—the lowered blood pressure may cause dizziness and fainting, leading to a bad fall.

In addition to relieving acute anginal pain, quick-acting coronary vasodilators may also be used preventively to halt an impending attack; the slower-release types are for long-term treatment. Two other families of drugs, *beta-adrenergic blockers* and *calcium channel blockers*, work somewhat differently against angina. Beta-blockers such as propranolol (brand name: Inderal) moderate the heart's workload, while diltiazem (Cardizem) and other calcium channel blockers are particularly effective for angina brought on by coronary artery spasm.

How a Heart Attack Is Diagnosed

The steps taken depend on whether the patient is stable or in the throes of an acute myocardial infarction. An example of the first situation would be a patient who arrives at the hospital complaining of chest pain from the night before but is not currently experiencing discomfort—what Dr. Fletcher calls "a questionable heart attack." Once the physician has examined the patient and taken a thorough medical history, she will most likely order

- an electrocardiogram (EKG/ECG) to detect abnormal heartbeats, areas of damage, insufficient blood flow, and heart enlargement;
- a blood test to look for elevated levels of several enzymes, evidence of cell death.

The results of these two procedures, reviewed together with the clinical symptoms, are usually sufficient for making a diagnosis. Subsequent testing to confirm the cause and the extent of the heart attack might include

- cardiac catheterization/coronary arteriography;
- echocardiogram;
- radionuclide scan;
- magnetic resonance imaging (MRI) scan.

When all signs point to a heart attack in progress and time is of the essence, the emergency medical technicians first make sure that the victim is breathing and getting sufficient oxygen, then they correct any life-threatening abnormal heartbeats *(arrhythmias)* while conducting a continuous EKG in the ambulance. Upon the person's arrival in the emergency room, doctors immediately take an arteriogram "to find out where the blockage or the spasm is," says Dr. Fletcher. ▶ *See "Arrhythmias," page 344.*

How a Heart Attack Is Treated

Because blood clots touch off a stunningly high proportion of myocardial infarctions—more than nine in ten, by some estimates—the immediate course of action is often intracoronary thrombolysis therapy.

Intracoronary Thrombolysis Therapy. In this revolutionary technique, the medical team catheterizes the troublesome coronary artery and injects a *thrombolytic agent* (streptokinase, urokinase, or tissue plasminogen activator, also referred to as TPA) that breaks up the thrombus and restores blood flow. "Thrombolysis therapy has proved very effective at preventing heart muscle damage," Dr. Fletcher says. The window of opportunity for salvaging dying myocardial tissue is a narrow one, however—four hours or less from the onset of the attack. Plus, the clot-dissolving drugs work best when used within one to three hours of clot formation. Both points underscore the importance of getting heart attack victims to a medical facility at once. In about half of all heart attack deaths, the victims die *before reaching the hospital* because they waited too long to summon help.

To prevent future occurrences of clotting, survivors may receive *anticoagulants* or *antithrombotics*, two groups of medications that interfere with thrombus formation. Warfarin (brand name: Coumadin) and heparin are the two most widely used examples of the former; antithrombotics include a number of aspirin products.

As much as thrombolysis therapy saves lives, it is not a permanent remedy for people with sclerotic or plaque-choked coronary arteries. For them the ensuing weeks are likely to include angioplasty or bypass surgery, a pair of interventions also used to improve blood flow to the heart and reduce the chance of future heart attacks in patients suffering from frequent or disabling angina.

Coronary Angioplasty. Percutaneous transluminal coronary angioplasty (PTCA), the less invasive of the two interventions, uses a tiny balloon to widen the coronary artery's inner cavity, or *lumen*. After the patient has been given a local anesthetic, the physician makes a small slit in the skin above an artery in the groin or chest. Guided by high-speed X-ray "movies" called *fluoroscopy*, he threads a thin plastic tube through the arterial system until it reaches the obstructed coronary artery or arteries.

Next, a balloon-tipped catheter is passed inside the first tube and is advanced to the blockage site. Expanding the balloon compresses the plaque against the vessel wall and dilates the lumen. Then the doctor deflates the balloon and carefully withdraws the tube and the catheter. Whereas bypass surgery requires a hospital stay of up to a week or more, balloon angioplasty patients can usually go home in a day or two.

PTCA has its drawbacks. About 25 percent of the time, the plaque or constriction recurs, typically within six months. At this point the procedure may be repeated, or bypass surgery may be recommended as a more lasting solution.

Coronary Artery Bypass Graft. When clogged coronary arteries restrict blood flow to the myocardium, small collateral vessels—normally microscopic in size—enlarge and open, providing the blood an alternate route to the heart muscle. Not everyone's auxiliary circulation is sufficient to prevent myocardial ischemia, but having adequate collateral circulation may spare a person from a potentially fatal infarction.

The principle behind coronary bypass surgery is much the same: taking a segment of a healthy blood vessel from elsewhere in the body—usually the leg or the chest—and constructing a "detour" around the blockage. If, say, a dam of plaque occupies the middle of a coronary artery, the surgeon grafts one end of the vein above the obstruction and the other end below it, permitting blood to once again flow to the myocardium. During the operation, a *pump oxygenator* takes over the functions of the heart and lungs. The device (also called a heart-lung machine) siphons off the patient's blood, adds oxygen, then pumps it back through the circulatory system.

Multiple grafts may be performed at the same time. Grady McCool underwent quadruple bypass surgery: Three of his major arteries were almost fully plugged up, and a fourth was moderately occluded. "The doctor said he probably wouldn't have lived thirty days without the operation," Allene McCool recalls. At the time, the procedure was still new enough that no one could predict her husband's long-term prognosis. "We were told, 'Live as normally as you possibly can; just know your limitations.' And that's exactly what we've tried to do."

Bypass surgery can vastly improve a heart patient's quality of life, but it is not a cure. Unless survivors monitor those contributing factors within their control (diet, blood pressure, smoking, obesity, and so on), the atherosclerosis is liable to cause more damage. As it is, bypass recipients face an increased risk of recurrence. The grafts sometimes collapse after surgery or, for a number of reasons, don't function properly.

Plus, some doctors contend that the transplanted veins—especially those from the leg—attract plaque faster than natural coronary arteries.

Cardiovascular Rehabilitation. According to the American Heart Association, two in three patients survive a first heart attack. "Most stay in the hospital five to ten days," says Dr. Fletcher, "and are in cardiovascular rehabilitation— oftentimes doing exercises—within four to five weeks." A growing number of medical centers and independent facilities offer formal inpatient and out-patient programs to help survivors and their families adjust to life following a heart attack.

☎ The cardiologist will most likely recommend a local rehab program, but should you need additional help finding one, call the American Association of Cardiovascular and Pulmonary Rehabilitation in Middleton, Wisconsin, for free referrals, 608-831-6989.

An essential component of rehabilitation is to start patients on aerobic conditioning, which has been found to speed recovery. Regular exercise strengthens the heart, improves circulation, and controls weight. However, no cardiac patient should attempt any physical activity without the supervision of a physician, who will tailor an appropriate regimen based on a leisurely *submaximal EKG exercise test*, used to measure a person's cardiovascular capacity during minimal exertion.

A well-structured rehabilitation program also addresses the psychological fallout from a heart attack, either through professional individual counseling or group therapy with other coronary patients. "Depression," says Dr. Fletcher, "is a very common problem," particularly in men and women used to leading busy, fast-paced lives who must now scale back their activity level. "But most heart attack victims do well," he adds, "and can be back to physically active lifestyles in a very short period of time. The problem is keeping them mo-tivated so that they continue to comply with the rehabilitation program, keep their weight off, and so forth." Caregivers can have a huge impact in terms of preventing backsliding just by being a supportive presence in patients' lives.

"It's very important that men and women who have had heart attacks have somebody around to nurture them and make them feel better," says Dr. Fletcher. "Patients who live alone tend to become fearful, lonely, depressed, and in general do very poorly."

But Is It Covered? Medicare pays for cardiac rehabilitation following an acute myocardial infarction as long as a physician deems it necessary.

Arrhythmias

The thought that electricity controls the heart is a sobering reminder of just how fragile life can be. But each beat indeed begins with an electrical impulse generated by the *sinoatrial (SA) node*, a knot of specialized cells located at the top of the right atrium. The signal radiates across to the left atrium and down the right atrium to a mass of conducting tissues called the *atrioventricular (AV) node*, which transmits it along special "power lines" to the ventricles below. In the fraction of a second it takes the impulse to traverse the heart, the atrial muscles contract, then the ventricle muscles, pumping blood through the chambers and out to the rest of the body.

Normally the SA node discharges sixty to one hundred times per minute. When physical exertion or emotional stress places additional demands on the heart, this natural pacemaker picks up the tempo. Everyone's heart pounds or flutters from time to time. (How many love songs contain the lyric "My heart skipped a beat"?) Conversely, cardiac contractions slow down during sleep. Although these meet the definition of arrhythmia—a disturbance in heart rhythm—fleeting *palpitations* or dizzy sensations are usually no cause for alarm.

But a sustained arrhythmia may seriously diminish the heart's pumping capacity, whether the irregularity is excessively slow or fast. During *bradycardias* (which literally means "slow heart"), contractions may slacken to such a degree that the heart and brain are deprived of oxygen and may even cease functioning. *Tachycardias*, a racing heart, may also reduce the pumping action by preventing the heart chambers from filling properly with blood.

Of the two, tachycardias are more dangerous, particularly those that originate in the ventricles. The abnormally rapid heartbeat associated with *ventricular tachycardia* may progress to *fibrillation*, where the muscles contract so chaotically that the pump just quivers frantically, depriving the body—and, in the process, itself—of oxygen. Ventricular fibrillation is the number one cause of abrupt heart stoppage, or *cardiac arrest*.

"These are the hearts we say are 'too good to die,' " says Dr. Fletcher. "At autopsy they may appear totally normal, with no heart muscle damage at all." Denying even a tiny area of cardiac conduction tissue its customary meal of oxygen can provoke a fatal arrhythmia. "Frequently," he adds, "the initial problem is bradycardia, which compromises the blood supply to the heart, then degenerates into tachycardia." Combined, the dozen or so subcategories of this disorder account for more than 3.8 million new cases and 44,000 deaths annually.

Causes and Symptoms of Arrhythmias

Imbalances in the blood of *electrolytes*, electrically charged particles that facilitate ignition and conduction in the heart cells, may stimulate an arrhythmic attack. The same is true of nicotine, cocaine, or other recreational drugs and prescribed cardiac medications, including antiarrhythmic drugs. No factor, however, looms larger than underlying cardiovascular disease. The scarring and abnormal tissue formations linked to atherosclerosis, hypertension, and others can impede the electrical signals that set contractions in motion. This condition, *heart block*, often generates bradycardia. In some tachycardias, the impulses lock into perpetual orbit around the inert tissue and never reach their destination.

Whenever a blockage interferes with normal conduction, or the SA node malfunctions, cells elsewhere in the atria and ventricles automatically emit signals in an effort to maintain the cardiac rhythm. Sometimes, though, these subsidiary pacemakers fire too rapidly, touching off tachycardias. If the transmission stems from the lower chambers, the result is ventricular tachycardia; uncontrolled electrical activity arising from the upper chambers produces the wildly irregular heartbeat of *atrial fibrillation*. Similar deviations in conduction bring on other forms of arrhythmia.

The symptoms of bradycardias are fatigue, light-headedness, confusion, and loss of consciousness.

The symptoms of tachycardias are shortness of breath, palpitations, sometimes chest pain, light-headedness, and loss of consciousness in especially severe cases.

How Arrhythmias Are Diagnosed

As with a heart attack, a patient's condition largely determines which tests are performed. Someone in the grip of ventricular tachycardia or fibrillation would be hooked up to an EKG machine to chart electrical impulses through the conduction system. Severe arrhythmias like this, says Dr. Fletcher, are treated at once with electrical and chemical *cardioversion*, *cardiopulmonary resuscitation (CPR)*, and a broad array of drugs, with an eye toward stabilizing the heart function and maintaining blood flow to the brain and heart. "But if it's a lower grade arrhythmia, where it's not necessarily life-threatening at that point, we usually bring the person into the hospital for further testing."

Because an electrocardiogram can document arrhythmias only while they are in progress, the cardiologist may send a stable patient home wearing a portable monitor in the hope of catching a rhythm disturbance in the act. A *Holter* monitor records electrocardiograph signals continuously for twenty-four hours; an *event monitor* allows for days or even weeks of monitoring via telephone. When the patient feels the arrhythmia coming on, she dials the monitoring station or activates the device's memory herself.

Another technique is literally to provoke an episode. People whose arrhythmias seem to come on after physical activity may be asked to pedal a stationary bike or walk on a treadmill, in what's called an *exercise EKG* or *stress test*.

A more reliable method of "turning on" arrhythmias, *electrophysiologic studies (EPS)*, requires local anesthesia. With fluoroscopic X rays showing the way, electrode catheters are inserted into a leg vein or artery, inched toward the heart, and positioned in the right atrium and ventricle. By electrically stimulating the heart, a physician can induce dormant bradycardia or tachycardia, then stop it. EPS far surpasses electrocardiography when it comes to pinpointing the source of an arrhythmia. And, adds Dr. Fletcher, the ability to ignite and defuse an attack "enables us to test the effectiveness of the drugs used to treat arrhythmias."

How Arrhythmias Are Treated

In an emergency situation—a life-threatening ventricular tachycardia, for instance—the medical team moves quickly to stabilize the frenetic, ineffective heartbeat with intravenous drugs and possibly cardioversion, while maintaining respiration and blood flow to the brain and heart.

Drug Therapy. To immediately restore an orderly heart rhythm, physicians administer medications that act on pacemaker, or conductive, tissue. Oral and intravenous *antiarrhythmic* agents—a broad category that encompasses beta-blockers, calcium channel blockers, and other types of drugs—slow down the pace at which tachycardiac impulses are discharged or relayed. When bradycardia is the culprit, beta-blockers speed up the rate of ignition or improve transmission.

Long-term drug therapy, one means of treating tachycardia, is recommended cautiously because of antiarrhythmics' unusually harsh potential side effects. (Drug therapy for bradycardia is strictly a temporary measure.) Paradoxically, these medications may *increase* the frequency of other arrhythmias or spur new ones that are even more severe than those being treated.

Cardioversion. To quickly decelerate an uncoordinated or futile heartbeat and return control of cardiac rhythm to the SA node, an electric shock is applied to the chest wall with metal paddles connected to a generator. Another method delivers the current directly to the myocardium through electrodes during heart surgery.

Patients with a history of chronic arrhythmias may be candidates for permanent cardioversion, or *cardioverter defibrillator implantation*. As the name suggests, it involves inserting a device about the size of a cigarette lighter beneath the skin on the left side of the abdomen. Electrode leads extend to the heart. Anytime the pulse generator detects ventricular tachycardia or fibrillation, it automatically administers an electric shock, disrupting the arrhythmia.

Artificial Pacemaker. An artificial pacemaker, used to correct chronic bradycardias, can be thought of as the implantable defibrillator's counterpart. It, too, consists of a pulse generator (about the diameter of a silver dollar) and thin wire leads that are anchored to the heart muscle. The unit emits a brief electrical signal to keep the heart beating within the normal range. This implant goes under the skin below the collarbone or ribs, where it can remain for several years before a replacement is necessary.

Ablative Techniques. *Ablation* means to remove from the body, and until recently the only way to take out or destroy the cardiac tissue responsible for tachycardia was surgically. A newer, increasingly popular approach, *transcatheter therapy*, involves inserting an electrode catheter through a vein and into the heart—as if conducting an electrophysiologic study—and eradicating the specific tissue creating the errant impulse with *electrocautery*. The technique cures a number of patients and eliminates the need for continuing antiarrhythmic medication.

Congestive Heart Failure

The term *congestive heart failure* is something of a misnomer. It implies an abrupt, total loss of function, much like a cardiac arrest, when in fact the heart's pumping ability degenerates gradually, often over a period of years. The disease typically affects the left ventricle first, then ultimately the right.

In *left-sided heart failure*, the damaged or overworked heart keeps pumping but less efficiently than before. "It cannot eject the proper amount of blood to meet the needs of the rest of the body," explains Dr. Fletcher, "causing blood and fluid to back up into the lungs." This is called *pulmonary edema*.

The opposite problem, poor cardiac input, characterizes *right-sided heart failure*. Here the heart fails to adequately fill with blood because its muscles have lost their elasticity. The blood builds up in the body's veins, particularly those in the legs, ankles, and feet. Over time, the excess fluid *(hypervolemia)* seeps out of the blood vessels and collects in different tissue spaces, causing swelling *(edema)*. A destructive cycle may develop where the kidneys—denied their usual supply of oxygen—don't skim waste products from the blood thoroughly. The body then retains sodium and water that normally would have been disposed of in urine, which serves to increase the fluid volume.

Diminished cardiac function is a natural consequence of aging, but many of the 400,000 cases of heart failure diagnosed each year are attributable to underlying cardiovascular disease. The most common cause is uncontrolled hypertension, which multiplies a person's risk twentyfold. "Heart failure also frequently occurs as a complication of a heart attack," points out Dr. Fletcher. "Usually, the more severe the attack, the more likely you are to have heart failure." Still other conditions can set the stage for heart failure:

- Arrhythmias
- *Rheumatic heart disease*, which damages heart valves
- *Cardiomyopathy*, a disease of the heart muscle
- Congenital heart defects
- Impaired circulation in the lungs resulting from *chronic obstructive pulmonary disease, pulmonary fibrosis*, or a blood clot *(pulmonary embolism)* may bring on a type of right-ventricular failure known as *cor pulmonale* ▶ *See "Caring for Someone with COPD: Cor Pulmonale," page 389.*

For a while the weakened pump manages to compensate—masking the problem and delaying symptoms—by making several adjustments. The chambers enlarge, enabling them to accept a greater quantity of blood and thus dispatch more to the body; the myocardium thickens so that the heart expels blood more forcefully; and the heart rate increases to improve the circulation.

But eventually these adaptive mechanisms can no longer offset the encroaching deterioration, and symptoms begin to emerge. Severe heart impairment often interferes with even simple physical activity so that patients may no longer be able to care for themselves. About two in three heart failure patients die within five years of the diagnosis. According to the National Heart, Lung and Blood Institute, the condition snatches 39,000 lives annually and contributes to the deaths of another 225,000 with ailments such as cancer and emphysema.

Symptoms of heart failure include shortness of breath; fatigue; persistent wet cough; anxiety; blood-flecked sputum; raspy, shallow breathing, wheezing, or gurgling; rapid pulse; inability to sleep; and profuse perspiration *(diaphoresis)*.

The symptoms of associated fluid retention and edema are swollen feet, ankles, legs, wrists, hands, and, sometimes, abdomen, and abrupt weight gain (approximately two to four pounds within four days).

Pulmonary Edema and Pleural Effusion

Most respiratory problems associated with advanced heart failure reflect pulmonary edema. The excess fluid pools in the lung, turning the empty, elastic sac into a wet sponge. Now incoming air must wade through this soggy tissue in order to reach the capillaries and oxygenate the blood. This forces the already overburdened heart to work that much harder to dispatch blood to undernourished muscles and tissues. The added strain further decimates its pumping capacity, and the lack of oxygen causes patients to tire easily. Around and around it goes in a downward spiral.

When air moves through liquid in the lungs, it produces an abnormal noise called a *rale* (pronounced *rahl*). There are approximately a dozen different kinds, each named for its distinctive sound: bubbling rale, dry rale, gurgling rale, and so on. "Gurgling" is the word Audree Siden uses to describe her mother's voice the night Mae Weisenberg called to complain of not feeling well, although rales aren't always audible without a stethoscope. She recalls, "It sounded as if Mom was literally under water, drowning in her own fluid." In a sense that's exactly what was happening.

Fluid can also leak into the airtight narrow compartment between the two layers of the *pleural membrane* that encases each lung. This is called *pleural effusion.* As the space fills with liquid, pressure builds. Unless the overload is corrected, the organ may collapse *(pneumothorax)* like a punctured tire.

How They Are Managed. Pulmonary edema and pleural effusion are typically remedied by way of intravenous diuretic drugs. ▶ *See "How Heart Failure Is Treated," page 350.*

Difficulty Breathing (Dyspnea)

Labored breathing is the most common indication of heart failure. In the disease's early stages, this happens strictly during physical activity. However, as the heart weakens and the lungs grow more congested, patients may feel short of breath even when at rest.

People with severe pulmonary edema often find it difficult to catch their breath while lying down, which, needless to say, makes sleep hard to come by. They may bolt upright in the middle of the night, gasping for air. Such attacks are often accompanied by wheezing and coughing that brings forth sputum flecked with blood.

How It Is Managed.

- Positioning. Folks unable to breathe freely except when sitting up are said to have *orthopnea.* It's best for them to sleep in a semivertical position, either in a raised hospital bed or reclining chair, or propped up by two or more pillows in bed. During the day, try to see to it that they spend some time sitting in a chair.
- Oxygen Therapy. Because heart failure is almost always degenerative, dyspnea can be expected to crop up most of the time in patients with pulmonary edema. Some spells may be so acute that the patient requires supplemental oxygen until the underlying problem is resolved.

✳ *Anytime loved ones complain of shortness of breath, don't hesitate to take them to the hospital emergency room.*

Patients able to breathe partially are given oxygen through a mask. But when a person's respiration is impaired to the point where too little oxygen is reaching the blood, the hospital staff may put her on a *mechanical respirator.* This forces air into the lungs by way of an *endotracheal tube* inserted into a nostril or the mouth and passed down into the windpipe.

"These episodes are usually short-lived," says Janice Fleischman-Eaton, cardiology outpatient coordinator at Stony Brook University Hospital and Medical Center in Stony Brook, New York. "Once the diuretics take off the excess fluid, patients tend to feel better relatively quickly." Should dyspnea become a recurrent problem, the physician may prescribe continuous home oxygen therapy, with the oxygen delivered through a nasal cannula. ◀ *See "Administering Supplemental Oxygen," page 175; "Insomnia and Other Sleep Disorders," page 172.*

How Heart Failure Is Diagnosed

The symptoms of heart failure are often so unmistakable, says Dr. Fletcher, that it's not unusual for a cardiologist to commence treatment on the basis of a medical history and physical examination alone. (An electrocardiogram is obtained routinely in heart patients.) If more information is needed to reach a diagnosis, the doctor may order

- an echocardiogram to visualize heart size, shape, and movement, and to calculate the amount of blood pumped during contractions;
- a chest X ray to ascertain the heart's size and shape, to detect the presence of congestion in the lungs, and to rule out other conditions that can overload the heart and cause it to fail. Though rare, two examples include

acute anemia and an overactive thyroid gland *(thyroxicosis)*.

How Heart Failure Is Treated

Heart failure brought on by cardiac overload is curable either by remedying the primary illness (like the pair mentioned above) or by surgically correcting an anatomical flaw such as a defective heart valve. But the villain behind most instances of heart failure—damaged heart muscle—can be only partly rehabilitated. Therefore, extending survival time and minimizing symptoms become the goals of therapy.

Success lies partly with the patient, who from now on must adopt heart-healthy habits. That means no smoking, little or no alcohol, losing excess weight, eating a low-fat, low-salt diet, and exercising at the duration and intensity recommended by the doctor. For most folks this requires a radical change in lifestyle. To what extent a caregiver should try to enforce these measures depends on the patient's prognosis. In the case of someone reasonably expected to weather the medical crisis, by all means encourage, remind, tease, beg, cajole, nag, bribe—do whatever it takes. But when a person is undeniably approaching the end of her life—a realization that often arrives with startling clarity, by the way, even if you've never been though this before—a caregiver's focus shifts from making her well to keeping her comfortable.

Drug Therapy. In treating congestive heart failure, the cardiologist's immediate aims are to strengthen the pump's contractions, ease its workload, and counteract fluid retention in the lungs and elsewhere in the body. Physicians rely on a different type of medication to tackle each job: *digitalis glycosides* such as digoxin (brand names: Lanoxin, Lanoxicaps), *Angiotensin Converting Enzyme (ACE) inhibitors* (captopril/Capoten), and *thiazide diuretics* (hydrochlorothiazide/Hydrodiuril).

In addition, a person with pulmonary edema may be given the analgesic narcotic morphine to ease his anxiety and make it easier to breathe, and a drug called aminophylline that dilates the bronchial tubes and increases the heart's output.

Surgery. When all other methods fail to control the symptoms of congestive heart failure, a *heart transplant* may be the lone remaining option for selected patients. The frequency of these operations has risen dramatically—from 57 in 1980, to 721 in 1985, to approximately 2,000 annually since 1990—but at present they benefit only a small percentage of coronary patients. While awaiting a suitable donor, a search that can take months or years, some candidates improve sufficiently through other therapies to take themselves off the transplant list. One temporary measure is the *left ventricular assist device*, a mechanical pump that can be surgically implanted in the chest. The LVAD attaches to the heart and assumes practically all blood-pumping activity. In 1995 the Food and Drug Administration (FDA) approved its use for longer-term therapy to benefit patients who are considered poor transplant candidates.

A few medical centers offer an experimental operation called *cardioplasty* in which the surgeon detaches a back muscle, wraps it around the heart, then stitches the muscle to the heart. An implanted electric device stimulates the muscle, which contracts, squeezing the heart so that it pumps blood to the body.

Potential Complications of Advanced Cardiovascular Disease

The major forms of heart disease intertwine so that one may arise as a deadly complication of another—perhaps a fatal arrhythmia initiated by heart failure that developed in the wake of a heart attack. Heart patients also have twice the risk of suffering a cerebrovascular stroke; for those with high blood pressure, the odds climb higher still.

There is also *cardiac death/sudden cardiac death*. A healthy-looking sixty-year-old man is playing a round of golf when he suddenly clutches his chest and crumples to the ground. Minutes later he is dead of cardiac arrest, in which the heart abruptly stops beating effectively. Nearly half of those struck down by cardiovascular disease ultimately die in this manner.

What makes sudden cardiac death particularly devastating for family and friends is that it often comes without warning. The person may not have appeared ill or even been diagnosed with heart disease, although an underlying cardiovascular disorder is almost always found in SCD victims. "Cardiac arrest can reflect heart failure or shock from a heart attack," says Dr. Fletcher. "But it is primarily related to a disturbance of cardiac rhythm"—usually ventricular tachycardia, proceeding to ventricular fibrillation.

How It Is Managed. There's an added tragic dimension to this: If treated within minutes, some cardiac arrests can be reversed. In our fictional example, an emergency rescue team arriving on the scene would have applied electric defibrillator paddles to the duffer's chest to jolt his heart back to a normal rhythm while keeping death at bay through cardiopulmonary resuscitation. ◄ *See "Cardiopulmonary Resuscitation (CPR)," page 181.*

In contrast to the sudden loss of life from cardiac arrest, people with congestive failure often fade out like the embers of a fire, in what can be considered a relatively peaceful death. Mae Weisenberg slipped into a semicoma before dying quietly in bed two weeks later.

Audree Siden: *My mother was perfectly comfortable during those last few weeks. Her breathing was shallow but never labored, with no gasping of any sort and no struggling for air.*

When she started to become somewhat comatose from not eating, and too weak to speak, her eyes would open from time to time, and she would pick up my hand and kiss it and hold it. I kept music on for her all the time.

Every time I went in her room, I wondered, "Will this be the moment?" On the morning of March 19, 1993, my mother didn't look any different from the four times I'd been in during the night. Her eyes were closed. But when I took her pulse, there was none. My fiancé was here, and he confirmed that, absolutely, she had died.

I remember how very, very quiet it was.

Recommended Reading

The following is available free from the American Heart Association (800-242-8721):

- "Heart and Stroke Facts"

The following are available free from the National Heart, Lung and Blood Institute Information Center (301-251-1222):

- "Facts About Angina"
- "Facts About Arrhythmias/Rhythm Disorders"
- "Facts About Coronary Heart Disease"
- "Facts About Heart Failure"
- "Facts About Heart and Heart/Lung Transplants"

—14—

Caring for Someone with Cerebrovascular Stroke or Traumatic Brain Injury

The **Reverend** Harry Cole was in his church office preparing the next morning's Easter Sunday sermon when the telephone rang. It was Thomas, the oldest of his three stepchildren, calling from Baltimore's Maryland General Hospital.

"Something's wrong with Mom!" he blurted, obviously distraught. Jackie Cole had been rushed by ambulance to the emergency room after complaining of a violent headache, followed swiftly by dizziness, difficulty speaking, and numbness in one arm—all distinct signs of a cerebrovascular stroke. Reverend Cole, a Presbyterian minister, sped to the hospital. There he learned his forty-year-old wife had suffered a pair of massive brain hemorrhages and was in a deep coma. The doctor in ER painted a bleak picture, saying that patients with such severe bleeding in the brain usually die within forty-eight hours. All we can do, he told the anguished minister, is wait.

Jackie's stroke changed our life forever. One day I was part of a fairly normal family, and within the blink of an eye, everything just turned around.

At first I was intensely angry. I went home that night and pounded the bed while I prayed, asking why this had happened. When I woke the next morning, I realized it was Easter, which is the day Jesus "woke up." But Jackie didn't wake up. It seemed an ironic injustice.

The first week, I basically lived at the hospital, as did everyone else, because at that point we weren't sure whether Jackie would live or die. But as things began to level out, a routine developed where I would spend time at the hospital in the morning, go to my office, come back in the afternoon, go home, then return to the hospital in the evening. There wasn't much I could do. Jackie was in a deep coma and didn't respond to anything.

Seeing her lying there was surreal

352

in many ways. From the first minute, I never fully believed what was happening.

Roslyn Travers (a pseudonym), forty-three, has worked in medicine her entire adult life. In 1983, the year her younger brother, Duane, was critically injured in a car accident that left him permanently brain-damaged, she was a respiratory therapist. Perhaps because of her medical background, much of Duane's care has fallen to Roslyn, now director of respiratory therapy at a southern hospital.

My brother was in a coma for three days. During the first twenty-four hours, they weren't sure if he was going to live or not. He quit breathing at one point, and they had to intubate him. But once that was done, Duane started breathing on his own again, and so he didn't have to go on a ventilator.

The following Thursday morning is when he first responded to us. He squeezed our hands. At first I was so happy; I felt as if God had answered my prayers. But as Duane began to come out of the coma, he didn't recognize us, didn't know us, didn't know anything.

It took me a good while to accept Duane's condition. It just broke my heart, because you grow up with somebody, you love them, and then all of a sudden, overnight, they're entirely different. And I'd feel so guilty, because sometimes I'd think, Lord, maybe he just should have died.

Cerebrovascular stroke and traumatic brain injury mainly occur at opposite ends of the age spectrum. Stroke, the foremost disabler and third-ranking cause of death in the United States, usually menaces the elderly; its frequency doubles with every decade after age fifty-five. TBI, which you may hear referred to as a *head injury*, is the number one killer of people ages one to forty-five. Both inflict damage on the brain. But whereas traumatic brain injury stems from an external source—most often the whiplike motion of a person's head striking a windshield in a car accident—a stroke, also called a *cerebral vascular accident (CVA)*, is triggered by an internal event.

What Happens in a Stroke?

Fully one-quarter of the blood pumped from the heart is routed to the brain by way of four major arteries and their branches: the two *carotid* (pronounced kah-rot'id) vessels in the front of the neck and a pair of *vertebral* arteries in back. A network of cerebral and cerebellar arteries carries blood within the brain. Should any of these rupture or develop a blockage, cutting off circulation to an area of the brain, a stroke occurs. More than 150,000 men and women lose their lives to this disease each year.

Ischemic Stroke

Of the 500,000 strokes that occur annually, approximately four in five are *ischemic*, prompted by an obstructed or constricted cerebral artery. Just as impeded blood flow to the heart muscle (myocardial ischemia) induces a myocardial infarction, or heart attack, in a *cerebral infarction*, brain cells deprived of oxygen and nutrients wither and die within minutes unless there is sufficient *collateral circulation* to reroute the stalled blood to the brain. Appropriately, the National Stroke Association refers to a stroke as a "brain attack."

Because the cerebrovascular and cardiovascular networks both belong to the circulatory system, stroke and heart attack share most of the same risk factors. At the top of the list: high blood pressure, associated with as many as nine in ten strokes, and the degenerative arterial disease *atherosclerosis*.

The latter is the chief cause of *cerebral thrombosis*, by far the most common form of stroke. As Dr. Fletcher McDowell, executive director of the Burke Rehabilitation Hospital in White Plains, New York, explains, "Atherosclerosis does its dirty work by scarring the inner lining of the vessels in the neck or in the brain." Over time, fatty deposits such as cholesterol infiltrate the damaged *lumen* and adhere to the arterial wall, which hardens and narrows. The site around the jaw where the carotid arteries divide happens to be an especially attractive hangout for *plaque*.

As plaque continues to build up, like barnacles on a ship's hull, the obstructed opening becomes a potential snag for the formation of a blood clot, or *thrombus*. This further barricades the passageway or stops circulation altogether. Cerebral thrombosis tends to occur early in the morning or at night when a person's blood pressure is naturally low.

Atherosclerotic arteries also make convenient traps for a *cerebral embolism*, the instigator of roughly one in ten strokes. Embolisms are blood clots that detach from the inner lining of a blood vessel (usually in the heart), get swept through the circulatory system like a piece of debris in a flood, and block, or *occlude*, an artery—in this case, a cerebral artery. (*Embolus*, incidentally, means *plug* in Greek.)

About 15 percent of cerebral embolisms can be traced to a type of cardiac arrhythmia called *atrial fibrillation* (AF). The connection is as follows: In atrial fibrillation, the heart's upper left chamber, the left *atrium*, contracts frantically—up to four times as fast as a normal rhythm—and out of synch with the rest of the heart. Instead of the blood's being pumped efficiently through the heart and out to the body, too much stagnates in the atrium. "This," explains Dr. McDowell, "considerably increases the chances of a clot forming there and breaking off."

Untreated AF magnifies a person's chances of suffering a stroke fourfold to sixfold. Physicians steady the irregular heartbeat with electrical stimulation *(cardioversion)* or drug therapy and may also put the patient on an *anticoagulant* such as warfarin (brand name: Coumadin) to foil clot formation.
◄ *See "Caring for Someone with Cardiovascular Disease: Arrhythmias," page 344.*

In Brief: High Blood Pressure and Stroke

Blood pressure is expressed in two numbers, such as 140/90. The first represents *systolic* pressure—that is, the force that blood exerts against the arterial walls as the heart is pumping. The second number denotes the pressure during the *diastole* phase of the cardiac cycle when the heart is "at rest," filling between contractions. A person whose blood pressure *consistently* measures 140/90 or higher is said to be hypertensive. As many as 50 million Americans have chronically high blood pressure, or hypertension. The means by which this disease initiates stroke are as numerous as its causes, which include family history, age, being overweight, smoking, excessive drinking, inadequate exercise, and diabetes.

High blood pressure lays the foundation for a cerebral thrombosis by causing arterial walls to thicken and deteriorate; it elevates the odds of a cerebral hemorrhage from a burst vessel by weakening the walls and causes blood clots to tear from arterial walls, possibly resulting in a cerebral embolism. In addition, it hastens several forms of heart disease that increase the danger of a stroke. ◄ *See "How to Measure Blood Pressure," page 140.*

Symptoms of an Ischemic Stroke

Knowing the symptoms of a stroke, be it ischemic or hemorrhagic, can spell the difference between life and death or between full recovery and lifelong disability. As with a heart attack, swift medical intervention is crucial, for a stroke not only irreparably destroys the brain cells it robs of oxygen but also imperils tissue outside the original area of infarction. In what is called *secondary injury*, the dying cells activate an electrochemical chain reaction that envelops neighboring cells. The longer the deprived area of the brain must wait for blood to bring it oxygen and carry away waste products from the deteriorating cells, the more serious and widespread the damage.

Because a cerebral vascular accident can crop up as a complication of other diseases, among them heart disease and diabetes, all caregivers should familiarize themselves with the signs of stroke. "The most common phenomenon," says Dr. McDowell, "is numbness, weakness, or paralysis on one side of the body," typically in the face, arm, or leg. Other symptoms include

- sudden blurred or diminished vision in one or both eyes;
- difficulty speaking or grasping simple statements;
- dizziness and loss of balance or coordination, particularly in combination with other symptoms;
- unusual confusion, disorientation, or loss of conciousness.

Transcient Ischemic Attack

About one in ten strokes is telegraphed by a transient ischemic attack days, weeks, or months beforehand. This so-called little stroke, explains Dr. McDowell, "is a temporary disturbance in cerebral circulation severe enough to produce symptoms in areas of the brain that stop functioning due to the decreased blood flow."

The signs, similar to those of a permanent stroke, "come on abruptly, then disappear, usually after ten to fifteen minutes. This happens because some-

times the body's natural system of dissolving blood clots activates quickly and restores normal blood flow."

Though TIA leaves behind little permanent damage, it is a significant event and often the prelude to an impending cerebral vascular accident. Nearly 40 percent of people who have experienced at least one transient ischemic attack subsequently suffer a stroke—one in five within a month; one in two within a year. Should the person you're caring for complain of fleeting stroke-like symptoms or should you observe them yourself, contact a physician immediately.

A diagnosis of TIA typically raises suspicions of carotid artery disease, which, if the occlusion is severe enough and surgically accessible (that is, in the neck), warrants *carotid endarterectomy*. This operation to strip the arteries of plaque is described on page 358.

Patients who are not suitable surgical candidates are treated with drugs that impede clotting: anticoagulants and/or *platelet inhibitors*. Platelets are the component of the blood that scurry to injury sites to stanch bleeding and seal wounds. Inhibiting agents, explains Dr. McDowell, "prevent the accumulation of platelet debris inside an artery, which may further block circulation." As a preventive measure, TIA patients usually receive aspirin or ticlopidine (Ticlid).

Hemorrhagic Stroke

Hemorrhages, the type of stroke that incapacitated Jackie Cole, are far less common than ischemic infarctions but far more deadly. Here a defective artery in the brain bursts, spilling blood into the tissue *(intracerebral hemorrhage)* or into the surrounding subarachnoid space *(subarachnoid hemorrhage)*, which is filled with cerebrospinal fluid to absorb shock.

Hemorrhages inflict double damage. Not only do cells asphyxiate from the derailed oxygen supply, but the pool of escaped blood compresses adjacent tissue and interferes with brain function. Half of all cerebral hemorrhage patients die from this increased pressure. However, those who survive often recover more completely than do victims of ischemic strokes. Once the pressure brought on by a hemorrhage gradually subsides, tissue may return to its previous state, whereas cells fatally starved of oxygen cannot regenerate.

What triggers a hemorrhage? One cause is chronic high blood pressure, which wears down arterial walls until eventually one springs a leak. Another frequent perpetrator is an *aneurysm*, a tiny blood-filled sac that balloons from a weak spot in a vessel, particularly one outside the brain in the subarachnoid space. ("Aneurysm" comes from the Greek word for a "widening.")

"Nobody's quite sure why aneurysms form and burst," says Dr. McDowell. "They may be congenital defects, and as time goes by the wall weakens and bulges, then weakens and bulges some more. Finally it becomes too weak and bursts open."

The source of Jackie Cole's stroke remained a mystery for three months, until enough of the excess blood in her brain receded into the arteries to allow for a clear X-ray view of the original site. A CT scan revealed that a rare *arteriovenous malformation (AVM)*, present since birth, had ruptured. Most people who have one of these internal time bombs can go their entire lives without even knowing it, but in this case the tangled mass of abnormal blood vessels made its presence known dramatically.

Symptoms of a Brain Hemorrhage

A hemorrhagic stroke may produce the same symptoms as an ischemic stroke, but it comes on without warning. Its most telltale sign: a sudden, excruciating headache, sometimes accompanied by nausea, vomiting, and loss of consciousness.

Traumatic Brain Injury

A driver slamming headfirst into the windshield. A woman slipping on the ice and striking the back of her head against the sidewalk. A boxer taking a jolting right hook to the jaw. The impact from each of these external forces can cause a cerebral hemorrhage, not to mention substantial brain damage.

More than 2 million traumatic brain injuries occur annually, most of them categorized as mild or moderate. We're going to focus on severe head trauma, which affects 150,000 people each year. Dr. Jam Ghajar, a neurosurgeon at Manhattan's New York Hospital and chief of neurosurgery at Jamaica Hospital/Cornell Trauma Center in Jamaica, New York, defines a severe head injury patient as "someone who comes into the hospital in a coma," unconscious and unresponsive.

Traumatic brain injury snatches 75,000 to 100,000 lives, usually at the time of the accident or within two hours of hospitalization. Of those who survive the precarious hours, days, or weeks in the hospital intensive care unit, 70,000 to 90,000 will be permanently disabled and require various degrees of ongoing attention. Another 2,000 will exist in a prolonged coma, or *persistent vegetative state*. Like any patient bedridden for an extended length of time, they are susceptible to a host of potentially terminal complications. Although PVS patients are cared for in inpatient settings, where their needs are tended to by the nursing staff, caregivers have a vital role to play. With the comatose person unable to communicate, it's up to us to keep close tabs on the caliber of medical care.

What Happens in a Closed Head Injury

Sadly, the car crash that damaged Duane Travers's brain and nearly cost him his life is an all too common occurrence. According to the Brain Injury Association, automobile accidents are responsible for half of all traumatic brain injuries. Falls (21 percent), assaults and violence (12 percent), and sporting and recreation accidents (10 percent) comprise the other major causes.

To illustrate what happens in a *closed head injury,* the most common type of traumatic brain injury, let's use the example of a man driving down a street—minus a seat belt—at forty miles per hour. Suddenly the car in front of him brakes sharply. The sound of squealing rubber gives way to a deafening crash as the driver plows into the other vehicle. The momentum hurls him forward into the windshield.

"This is called an *acceleration/deceleration injury.*" says Dr. Ghajar, who likens the brain to a Jell-O mold inside a rigid container. In the collision, it rocks back and forth on its stem and ricochets off the interior of the skull, which is not only hard but has bony ridges. Between the blow to the head and the impact from the brain striking the cranium, nine in ten victims of a severe head injury suffer one or more brain bruises called *contusions.* What's more, the force of the crash can tear vessels in the head, causing blood to seep into the brain itself *(intracerebral hematoma)* or between the brain and the skull *(subdural hematoma).* As with a hemorrhagic stroke, the mass of displaced blood exacerbates brain damage by exerting pressure on the tissue.

Contusions and hematomas are *focal lesions*—that is, injuries confined to a specific part of the brain. *Diffuse lesions* involve several areas, the cells of which have been temporarily or permanently distorted by all the jarring and jostling. The most serious type of dispersed impairment, *severe diffuse axonal injuries,* is distinguished by damage to both the brain stem and brain axons. The stalklike stem serves as the hub for regulating such vital functions as heartbeat, breathing, and swallowing, while axons are neurofibers that assist chemical transmissions

from the brain to the rest of the body. Even a mild diffuse axonal injury causes unconsciousness; patients with the harshest form are likely to remain deeply comatose for some time. A number will die. Those who emerge from their vegetative states usually exhibit significant deficits in intelligence, sensation, and movement.

The second category of traumatic brain injury, an *open head injury,* refers to direct brain damage from, say, a bullet or a knife that pierces the scalp and skull and enters the brain. Naturally the magnitude of the damage depends on the size, force, and path of the penetrating object, which can shred soft tissue and nerve fibers as well as send bone fragments tearing into the brain like shrapnel.

Diagnosis and Treatment of Stroke and Traumatic Brain Injury

Because brain trauma patients are frequently rushed to the emergency room from the scene of an accident, they generally come under the care of a trauma team composed of surgeons, nurses, and various medical specialists. "Many times," explains Dr. Ghajar, "these patients not only have a head injury but also associative injuries such as bone fractures, abdominal injuries, and so on. Once they are stabilized, or if they have only a head injury, a CT scan is taken to make sure they don't have a large hemorrhage that requires immediate neurosurgery."

A CT scan is also the preferred diagnostic tool for patients suspected of having suffered a stroke. According to Dr. McDowell, its detailed three-dimensional images can confirm a cerebral hemorrhage "with 95 to 97 percent accuracy. If we see no evidence of bleeding in the brain, the assumption is that the patient has had a thrombotic or embolic occlusion of a vessel." A bedside examination also provides clues as to whether the stroke is ischemic or hemorrhagic.

Other measures for diagnosing stroke include

- magnetic resonance imaging—to establish early on whether or not the brain has been deprived of blood flow and to what extent. In this respect, an MRI is superior to a CT scan. However, says Dr. McDowell, computed tomography remains the preferred method of determining the type of stroke because "MRI does not distinguish hemorrhage very well";
- Doppler ultrasound—to detect blockages of the carotid arteries by pressing a pencil-like probe to the neck or eyelids and listening to the blood flow.

Medical interventions to treat a cerebral vascular accident or traumatic brain injury must be implemented right away, because the window of opportunity for minimizing damage shuts quickly. Following the onset of an ichemic stroke, says Dr. McDowell, doctors have a mere four hours, "and maybe even less time than that," in which to return sufficient blood flow to an area of the brain and halt permanent cell destruction. This is done through surgery, drug therapy, or both. Carotid endarterectomy and aneurysm surgery pertain only to stroke patients. *Craniotomy*, a term that describes any operation on the cranium, is used to treat both blood clots and bleeding inside the skull.

Craniotomy

Two weeks after his car accident, Duane Travers underwent surgery to remove from his right frontal lobe a hematoma that had turned up on a subsequent brain scan.

After making an incision in the scalp, the surgeon opens a small hole or larger flap in the skull in order to expunge the blood mass. Here, too, time is of the essence. A National Institute on Neurological Disorders and Stroke study found that the survival rate for patients operated on within two hours of sustaining a head wound was more than 70 percent, as compared to 5 percent when more than six hours elapsed between injury and surgery. Craniotomy, which calls for general anesthesia, is also used to eliminate blood clots from cerebral arteries following thrombotic or embolic strokes.

Carotid Endarterectomy

In carotid endarterectomy, a vascular surgeon opens a clogged carotid artery at the site of the blockage, strips it of plaque, then closes the newly unobstructed vessel. This approach, introduced in 1954, has been shown to benefit stroke survivors and symptomatic patients with *severe* arterial narrowing (severe defined as 70 percent or more). In a pivotal 1994 study, however, carotid endarterectomy was found to halve the risk of stroke in patients with significant blockages but no outward signs of cerebrovascular disease. During the operation, performed on patients under general or local anesthesia, the surgeon installs a flexible shunt that detours blood around the fatty deposit and preserves the flow to the brain.

Aneurysm Surgery

For someone who survives a subarachnoid hemorrhage, "the chances of a recurrence are quite high," says Dr. McDowell. "The way we prevent another aneurysm from bursting is to surgically cut off the blood flow into it. There have been hundreds of different ways of doing this." One involves injecting acrylic cement into the tiny sac. The most prevalent method is to place a titanium clip around the aneurysm's necklike opening, damming it shut. This microscopic surgery requires general anesthesia. The skull is opened and the brain drawn back, or *retracted*, so that the surgeon can gain access to the aneurysm. If a burst arteriovenous malformation caused the stroke, the knot of blood vessels is surgically removed (excised).

Drug Therapy

In the wake of an ischemic stroke, anticoagulant drugs such as heparin or Coumadin are often administered to prevent the blood clot from enlarging. A revolutionary drug called tissue plasminogen activator, or TPA (brand name: Activase), actually halts a stroke in progress by dissolving blood clots and reinstating the cerebral blood flow. A major 1995 study published in the *New England Journal of Medicine* found that patients given TPA intravenously within three hours were at least 30 percent more likely to avoid permanent disability than those not given the enzyme drug.

Neurologists are extremely excited about an experimental group of drugs, *neuroprotective agents* such as antioxidants and glutamate inhibitors, which safeguard neighboring cells from the devastating chemical chain reaction we described earlier. Like tissue plasminogen activator, these drugs must be administered soon after a stroke to be effective.

Since hemorrhagic stroke patients frequently have elevated blood pressure, they may receive antihypertensive medications to bring it down to normal—but no lower than that. "What we don't want to do," Dr. McDowell explains, "is bring the pressure down so low that other, intact areas of the brain are deprived of blood flow and die."

Potential Acute Complications and How They Are Managed

Physicians refer to the initial damage from a stroke or traumatic brain injury as the *first injury.* "This can be quite minor in a lot of people," notes Dr. Ghajar. But the patient is by no means out of danger. The next few weeks are charged with tension as the medical team watches closely for indications of secondary injuries, the aftershocks following the earthquake. Nearly four in ten stroke victims die within thirty days. For those who survive this critical period, the outlook for long-term survival brightens significantly.

The gravest delayed reaction, swelling of the brain, typically manifests two to three days after a severe stroke—closer to the time of a traumatic brain injury. Although you may hear this complication described as *cerebral edema*, the term actually applies specifically to an overaccumulation of fluid in the brain. Another suspected cause is an increase in cerebral blood flow, which forces the vessels—and, in turn, the brain—to enlarge. Generally, the greater the original damage to the brain, the greater the swelling and potential for further harm.

Constricted by the skull, the brain has little room for expansion before the *intracranial pressure (ICP)* builds up precariously. "If the pressure gets too high," Dr. Ghajar explains, "not enough blood reaches the brain, causing a massive stroke." In addition, severe swelling can compress important structures at the base of the brain and interfere with respiration, blood pressure control, and other vital functions. "During the patient's first week in the hospital," he says, "our major job is to minimize swelling," a task aided immensely by the use of *intracranial pressure monitoring.*

What is intracranial pressure monitoring? Here's another opportunity for everyday angels to earn their wings and perhaps save a life. Stroke or TBI patients may have dangerously high levels of intracranial pressure from swelling well before symptoms appear. Neurologists can continuously track this, though, by drilling a small *burr hole* in the skull and fitting it with a tiny sensor.

Although a bit of a stretch, think of it as a dipstick for measuring the pressure of the cerebrospinal fluid that fills the four pockets of the brain known as *ventricles*.

Should the pressure rise above normal, steps can be taken to control the swelling early on and avert additional brain damage. For instance, says Dr. Ghajar, "Whenever the brain pressure gets too high, we insert a catheter [through the burr hole and directly into a ventricle] and siphon out the fluid." The problem is, according to a study conducted by the Brain Trauma Foundation and coauthored by Dr. Ghajar, only one in three trauma centers routinely monitors intracranial pressure.

It's safe to say that most caregivers probably wouldn't be aware of the importance of measuring intracranial pressure—at least not until they'd had time to read up on stroke or brain trauma, as you're doing. Ideally, for the patient's sake, a friend or family member asks the attending neurosurgeon within the first twenty-four hours whether or not ICP monitoring is under way.

If the reply is no, ask for an explanation. Now, there are circumstances that might not warrant monitoring, at least in the hospital's view. For example, since arriving in the emergency room, the patient may have shown steady improvement. Or perhaps, to be blunt, the trauma team does not expect the person to survive the next forty-eight hours but isn't saying this to the family. The decision might boil down to dollars and cents: Does the patient meet the hospital's criteria for justifying the expenditure?

Chapter 1, "The Hospital and the Medical Team: Who's Who and What's What," discusses when it is appropriate to register a complaint about the quality of medical care and to whom, going up the ladder of command if necessary. This is not one of those times. Aside from stating your case, realistically there's not much you can do to insist

that doctors institute ICP monitoring. The purpose of asking is to at least eliminate the possibility of an oversight or lapse in communication, which in the bustle of ICU can happen. Another reason for raising the issue is that you'll probably receive a more honest assessment of the patient's condition.

A second question to ask: Is *hyperventilation* being used? This controversial technique for decreasing intracranial pressure accelerates the speed of a mechanical ventilator so that the patient breathes rapidly and shallowly. While this indeed lowers pressure inside the skull by causing the cranial blood vessels to contract, it also diminishes the deliveries of blood and oxygen to undamaged areas of the brain. The same Brain Trauma Foundation study cited above found that while 95 percent of the trauma centers surveyed practiced hyperventilation, more than one in four did so in a manner that was potentially dangerous, leaving their patients' brains virtually depleted of precious oxygen.

One in ten people with a severe head injury sinks into a persistent vegetative state; the percentage among stroke patients is smaller. Like anyone who is bedridden and/or unconscious for a long period of time, they make inviting targets for pneumonia ("the most common cause of death in these patients," says Dr. Ghajar) and other complications that may endure as a chronic or permanent condition: urinary incontinence; bedsores; infections; indigestion; dependent edema; bone, muscle, and joint pain; chronic constipation; foot drop; fever; venous thrombosis; and phlebitis.

Then you have still more serious hurdles, described below, that may arise as a direct result of the stroke or traumatic brain injury. According to Dr. Ghajar, "If we can minimize the risk of a second injury and keep patients stable, they will have a good outcome. But if we cannot control these things, the prognosis is poor."

Impaired Respiration

Damage to the brain stem, whether from a stroke, injury, or swelling, can depress normal breathing.

How It Is Managed

"Patients who have stopped breathing on their own, or breathe so irregularly that they're not providing their body with enough oxygen, are generally put on artificial ventilation," says Dr. McDowell. The breathing machine attaches to either an endotracheal tube or a tracheostomy tube, although anyone requiring mechanical respiration at home would almost certainly have had a trach implant by the time of his discharge from the hospital. ◄ *See "Mechanical Ventilation," page 175.*

Heart Attack

Earlier in this chapter we looked at the intimate connection between stroke and heart disease, and how both stem from a general deterioration of the arteries. Typically, says Dr. McDowell, atherosclerosis surfaces in the aorta. Next it affects the coronary arteries and then the cranial arteries so that "by the time people suffer a stroke, they usually have compromised cardiac function. In the stress of the stroke, a small percentage have fatal heart attacks."

How It Is Managed

Patients may receive intracoronary thrombolysis therapy, coronary angioplasty, or coronary artery bypass surgery. ◄ *See "Caring for Someone with Cardiovascular Disease: How a Heart Attack Is Treated," page 342.*

Difficulty Swallowing (Dysphagia)

Because the brain stem regulates our swallowing mechanism, a stroke or head injury involving this part of the brain may leave someone unable to chew and swallow properly. Instead of food or liquid traveling down the esophagus and into the stomach, sometimes it inadvertently slips into the trachea and spills into the lungs. As Dr. Ghajar explains, "This causes pneumonitis," an inflammation of the lungs that can progress to what's called *aspiration pneumonia.*

How It Is Managed

To avoid aspiration, patients who are semiconscious or unconscious receive food via a *nasogastric (NG) tube* inserted through the nose and into the stomach. For someone in a prolonged coma, we bypass the upper digestive tract altogether: An artificial opening, or *gastrostomy,* into the stomach permits food and other nutrients to be delivered directly by way of a surgically implanted *"G" tube.* Conscious patients are also candidates for either method, but many need only to be carefully positioned and watched during mealtimes. ◄ See *"Difficulty Swallowing (Dysphasia)," page 165; "Tube Feedings and Total Parenteral Nutrition (TPN)," page 166.*

Pulmonary Embolism

Since the majority of stroke patients are predisposed to developing blood clots, they are prime candidates for a pulmonary embolism: a vagrant clot that breaks off from its original site and plugs up a blood vessel in the lungs. This can cause pulmonary bleeding or infarction, severely damaging the lung as well as precipitating right ventricular heart failure known as *cor pulmonale.* ► See *"Caring for Someone with COPD: Cor Pulmonale," page 389.*

Preventive Management

Prevention is waged on two fronts: deterring clot formation with anticoagulant medications and improving sluggish circulation (a major cause of venous thrombosis) through exercise. Elastic stockings can enhance blood flow in the legs, which is where thrombi often develop. ◀ See "Circulatory Complications," page 178.

Incontinence

During the first twelve months following a stroke, fully half of all survivors find themselves unable to control their bladder and, to a lesser extent, their bowels. Since cerebral vascular accidents mostly afflict the elderly, stroke-induced incontinence sometimes compounds preexisting urinary tract problems. Incontinence is not commonly associated with traumatic brain injury, with the exception of comatose patients.

The bladder, which temporarily stores the urine received from the kidneys, depends on the central nervous system for instructions on when to release its contents to the urethra. If a stroke incapacitates the portion of the brain responsible for transmitting these messages, the bladder never receives the nerve stimulation that prompts its muscular wall to contract and its cylindrical neck to open. The result is *uninhibited neurogenic bladder*, a condition characterized by frequent involuntary urination of little volume.

As you'll read later on in this chapter, stroke survivors (and TBI patients) are often subject to depression. A number of antidepressant medications have what's called an *anticholinergic* effect. Anticholinergics give rise to *urinary retention* by inhibiting the bladder mus-

cle from contracting. The bulb-shaped organ accumulates urine until it distends like a balloon filled to the bursting point. When the two ureter tubes from the kidneys expel more urine into the bladder, the excess is forced out through the urethra. You may hear this referred to as *overflow incontinence*. Also, a cough, a sneeze—anything that places stress on the abdomen—may permit urine to escape *(stress incontinence)*. Retention can lead to urinary tract infection and kidney failure, both potentially fatal conditions.

How It Is Managed

Upon admittance to the hospital, stroke patients are routinely catheterized to prevent urine from collecting in the bladder. An indwelling drain soon becomes a trap for bacteria itself, though, and should be cleaned and irrigated by the nursing staff daily and the drainage system changed regularly.

A long-term strategy for managing stroke-induced incontinence usually begins with *bladder training*. Briefly, the program is designed to help patients learn to control urination or to avoid accidents by voiding frequently at regular intervals.

If these techniques fail, step two is to consider drug therapy. For stroke patients taking antidepressants, changing to a medication with less anticholinergic activity may be all it takes to correct urinary retention. For those with uninhibited neurogenic bladder, the reverse is true: The stronger the anticholinergic, the greater its relaxing effect on the hyperactive bladder.

Between bladder training and drug

INSIDE INFORMATION

If you're caring for a stroke patient who is feeling depressed and anxious *and* suffers from incontinence due to a hyperactive bladder, ask the doctor about prescribing imipramine (brand name: Tofranil) or amitriptyline (Elavil, Endep, and others). These versatile antidepressants boast anticholinergic properties, and they help control anxiety and pain as well.

therapy, by the end of the second year following a cerebral vascular accident, the incidence of urinary incontinence shrinks by more than half. ◄ *See "Incontinence," page 170.*

Potential Long-Term Effects of Stroke and Severe Traumatic Brain Injury

Once a stroke or TBI patient has been stabilized medically, relief can turn to foreboding, as the magnitude of the aftereffects becomes evident. Family members worry what the future will hold, both for them and for their loved one. Will the patient ever be the same? Will *anything* ever be the same?

Roslyn Travers: Eventually Duane got to where he would recognize us and could have more of a conversation, but he was still just so childlike. He'd say things that didn't make sense. I kept asking the doctor, "How long will it be before we know if there's been permanent brain damage?" He said, "Not for a good year, because it takes the brain so long to heal."

It is not unusual for a stroke or severe head injury to assault more than one area of the brain, resulting in various neurological deficits. Whether a person comes away with multiple disabilities, one, or none depends on the location of the brain injury as well as its severity. Each of the brain's three principal structures regulates specific faculties. The *brain stem*, situated at the base of the brain, serves as the command center for breathing, heartbeat, blood pressure, and other essential functions, while the *cerebellum*, nestled under the cerebrum at the rear of the skull, oversees balance, walking, and talking.

The *cerebrum*, the largest part of the brain, is divided into two hemispheres, with the left half governing the right side of the body, and the right half orchestrating the left. Thus, an injury to the right brain frequently causes paralysis or weakness of the left side, and vice versa. Other deficits are affiliated with damage to a particular side or can be narrowed down further still to one of the brain's four sections: the *frontal lobe* at the forehead, the *temporal lobe* at the temple, the *parietal lobe* at the side, and the *occipital lobe* at the back of the skull.

Throughout this chapter we've emphasized the similarities between stroke and traumatic brain injury. One important distinction between the two is that stroke generally affects a single part of the brain, yielding a specific deficit, whereas a severe head injury may be both focal and diffuse, sending waves of damage rippling through several areas. Still, victims of stroke and TBI must struggle with many of the same long-term effects. ◄ *See "When a Loved One Suffers from Brain Function Impairment," page 202.*

Paralysis/Weakness

Three in four stroke survivors experience partial paralysis on one side of the body. This is called *hemiparesis; hemiplegia* denotes total paralysis, also on one side. The motor dysfunction might seize the entire hemisphere or confine itself to an arm or leg.

Jackie Cole had *quadriparesis*, partial paralysis of all four limbs. At the time of her discharge from Maryland General Hospital—five months to the day after her stroke—she was still wheelchair-bound, unable to stand or walk. Quadriparesis is associated with widespread damage deep within the brain, either from a severe head wound or a stroke. In Jackie's case, the blood from her ruptured vessel flooded the subarachnoid space. Then it infiltrated the ventricles that tunnel down into the brain.

As you can see from the chart, other

Potential Impairments from Stroke and Severe Traumatic Brain Injury, According to Location of Injury

Left Cerebral Damage	Right Cerebral Damage
Physical Deficits	
• Right side paralysis • Right side vision loss • Right side sensation loss • Right side neglect	• Left side paralysis • Left side vision loss • Left side sensation loss • Left side neglect
Cognitive Deficits	
• Aphasia • Impaired memory, reasoning, logical thinking	• Problems with perception and with judging spatial relationships • Impaired short-term memory
Psychological, Social, Behaviorial, and Emotional Deficits	
• Inappropriate emotional responses	• Inappropriate emotional responses • Impulsivity

Cerebellar Injury

Physical Deficits

• Poor balance and coordination • dizziness

Psychological, Social, Behavioral, and Emotional Deficits

• Inappropriate emotional responses

Brain Stem Injury

Physical Deficits

• Slurred speech • Difficulty swallowing
• Impaired breathing • Unstable blood pressure
• Impaired vision and hearing
• Full or partial paralysis on one or both sides of the body

Psychological, Social, Behavioral, and Emotional Deficits

• Inappropriate emotional responses

neurological deficits can further hamper mobility, setting the stage for a potentially serious fall. For a caregiver, this may require having to assist the person with walking and with performing everyday tasks such as bathing, eating, or dressing—an enormous responsibility. ◄ See "Turning, Maneuvering, and Lifting," page 132; "Bathing," page 112; "Safety Measures for Around the Home," page 76; and "Tips for Preventing Falls," page 134.

Contracture

Paralysis predisposes patients to contracture, in which muscle tissue shrinks (atrophies) and loses its ability to stretch. Within twenty-four hours of Jackie Cole's stroke, her hands began to curl up like claws. The toes, feet, ankles, knees, arms, and shoulders, too, can angle inward, causing painful cramping. If joints stay contorted for too long, patients may end up permanently disabled. The threat of contracture is twice as great for the brain injured, whose joints may not only stiffen but turn bonelike, or *ossify*.

Preventive Management

Contracture and atrophy are often preventable through what are called *passive range-of-motion exercises*, in which a nurse, nurse's aide, physical therapist, or physical therapy aide carefully rotates, flexes, and extends the immobilized person's joints. The likelihood of forestalling contracture from setting in improves if the bedside therapy begins shortly after a stroke or TBI victim's admission to the hospital, regardless of whether or not he is conscious. As patient advocate, it's up to us to see to it that this is being done. Once the immediate crisis subsides, ask the nurse or therapist to teach you how to perform these exercises, which are described in chapter 3. ◀ *See "How to Perform Passive Range-of-Motion Exercises," page 136.*

Hemispheric Neglect

Damage to the right brain, particularly from stroke, can bring about a curious phenomenon called *left side neglect*, in which the afflicted person fails to acknowledge objects, people—anything —on her left side. If asked to draw a clock, for example, she may crowd all the numbers on the right side and leave the left half blank. Or she may eat only the food on the right half of a plate, ignoring the rest unless somebody turns the dish around. Not surprisingly, the inability to perceive half their world can leave these patients accident prone and dependent on others.

How It Is Managed

When someone has left side neglect, help him to compensate by placing objects on his identifiable side. Hang all clothes on the right side of the closet, put all socks on the right side of the dresser drawer, and so on. Your first step, though, should be to rearrange the person's bedroom so that all furniture is on the same side as the door; otherwise, he may not be able to find his way out of the room.

Anytime you notice an instance of neglect, gently bring it to the person's attention. The National Stroke Association suggests posting simple written messages around the house, such as a note taped to the right side of the bathroom mirror reminding someone with left side neglect to turn his or her head while shaving or putting on makeup.

Persistent Headaches

In most cases, the chronic headaches brought on by severe head trauma can be relieved sufficiently through extrastrength Tylenol, says Dr. Ghajar. "What you don't want to do," he cautions, "is give any medication that will make the patient sleepy or impair his neurological status, such as narcotics."

Speech/Language Loss (Aphasia)

Aphasia robs one in five stroke survivors of their ability to communicate. Although "aphasia" is derived from the Greek word *aphatos*, meaning "not speak," this cognitive disorder can also jumble the faculties necessary for listening, reading, or writing—and at a number of levels. For example, people with speech-related aphasia may have any of the following problems:

- Producing the proper sounds (*apraxia*)
- Using the appropriate words (*dysnomia*)

- Putting the words in the correct order
- Interpreting conversational cues, such as knowing when to let other people speak

Likewise, where listening is concerned, aphasics may find it difficult to

- listen attentively;
- understand the meaning of a sentence even though they hear and understand the individual words;
- recall the information they recently heard;
- grasp innuendo, sarcasm, jokes, or wordplays.

Victims of severe brain trauma do not experience aphasia per se, but their deficits in the areas of learning, comprehension, and formulating language may result in comparable communication impairments. According to Dr. Nathan Zasler, director of the Brain Injury Rehabilitation Program at Sheltering Arms Hospital in Richmond, Virginia, severe TBI often causes *dysarthria*, which he describes as "injury to the neurofibers that control the muscles around the mouth or the tongue." Dysarthrics formulate their thoughts normally but have trouble enunciating them. Depending on the degree of paralysis, speech can range from slurred to unintelligible. The effect is not unlike trying to talk after being given a shot of Novocain.

How It Is Managed

◄See "When a Loved One Has Impaired Communication Skills," page 208. ► See "Speech-Language Therapy," page 368.

Changes in Behavior and Personality

When talking about her brother, more than once Roslyn Travers laments, "He's just not the same." As distressing as it can be to witness the physical toll from stroke or severe brain injury, the most painful consequences are often those that alter a loved one's intellect, memory, or personality—elements that we identify as the essence of their being. Jackie Cole, for instance, lost her history. The usual pattern is for brain damage to wipe out sections of recent memory, says Dr. McDowell, "whereas long-term memory can remain intact." Yet Jackie's recollection of the past was so riddled with holes, her husband had to recount their years together to her. Fortunately, her personality survived.

It goes without saying that each patient's case is unique. But in general, the cognitive deficits from stroke typically affect perception and communication, while those from severe head trauma tend to manifest as learning impairments. However, cognitive changes seem to be less common in people with TBI than personality changes, which, while harder to quantify, can be every bit as disabling.

One common characteristic of both stroke and TBI is apathy. Men and women who once burned with intensity may now seem indifferent toward life, their emotions blunted. Other patients have difficulty controlling their emotions, a general effect referred to as *emotional lability*. They may erupt in laughter, tears, or anger at the most inappropriate moments. These outbursts then end as abruptly and inexplicably as they began. Duane Travers exhibited the loss of inhibition, self-control, and social skills frequently seen in people who have sustained a frontal lobe injury. "This will sound terrible," says his sister, "but that first year, I was embarrassed to go out with him in public."

Depression

More than half of all stroke survivors plunge into depression six months to two years later. TBI patients, too, are prone to depression and such attendant side effects as appetite loss, fatigue, sleep disturbances, and anxiety.

How It Is Managed

In order for depression to be treated effectively, it is imperative that a physician determine its cause, which in survivors of stroke or severe head injury is due partly to the brain's psychophysiological response to the injury *and* partly to the person's psychological reaction to what's happened. "The patients themselves know there's been a change," explains Dr. Ghajar, "and they become very depressed."

Roslyn Travers's voice aches as she recalls driving her brother to an Austin nightclub. "We were riding along, and he said to me, 'I'm not the same anymore, Roslyn, am I?'

"I didn't know how to reply. 'Well, yeah, Duane,' I said. 'You have a little problem walking and stuff, but everything's fine.'

" 'No,' he insisted, 'I'm just not the same.'

"And he has never discussed it since."

Most abilities diminished by stroke or severe head trauma return, either partially or fully, within the first several weeks, as numerous brain cells that were damaged but not destroyed resume activity. In addition, the brain compensates for its losses by reorganizing itself, assigning functions to other, undamaged areas. While this natural healing process is under way, the medical team evaluates patients to see if they can profit from rehabilitative therapy.

Rehabilitation

"It used to be that stroke patients were more or less written off and put in a back room," says Dr. Glen E. Gresham, professor of rehabilitative medicine at the State University of New York at Buffalo. "Then research showed that rehabilitation can help many of them improve greatly and do very well." The National Stroke Association estimates that with appropriate rehabilitative treatment, seven in ten stroke survivors can learn to handle daily activities again and regain their independence. Many brain trauma patients also benefit from rehabilitation, which consists of three main components: *physical therapy*, *occupational therapy*, and *speech-language therapy*.

Physical Therapy. Exercises and training designed to improve problems with walking, balance, and coordination often begin while patients are still confined to the hospital bed. The range-of-motion exercises mentioned earlier as a hedge against potentially crippling muscle contracture make up the first level of physical therapy.

"As soon as the patient has been stabilized medically," explains Dr. Gresham, "the staff should move on to further mobilization: having the person sit up and move around in bed and, eventually, transfer to a wheelchair." In 1995 a panel headed by Dr. Gresham issued the first national guidelines and recommendations for stroke treatment. According to the eighteen health care experts commissioned by the federal Agency for Health Care Policy and Research, early mobilization not only helps avert the common complications of prolonged bed rest, it promotes a quicker return of motor and mental functions.

* *If you feel that the medical team is slow to start physical therapy, raise these points with your loved one's doctor. Be aware, though, that it is best to delay mobilizing a patient if he or she*

- is comatose or nearly comatose;
- recently suffered a hemorrhagic stroke;
- recently suffered a related heart attack;
- has neurological signs or symptoms indicating an expanding stroke. "The classic," says Dr. Gresham, "is a patient who is admitted to the hospital with weakness in the left arm and leg, and the next day has complete paralysis";

- feels faint and experiences a sharp drop in blood pressure upon sitting up or standing, a condition known as *orthostatic hypotension;*
- has a blood clot in the leg. Physical therapy should wait until the thrombus has been disintegrated with medications; otherwise too much movement could jar it loose, resulting in an embolism.

Occupational Therapy. Folks often confuse this with vocational training. The mission of occupational therapy is to reacclimate patients with the basic skills of daily living—eating, cooking, dressing, bathing, writing—and, if necessary, to learn new ways of mastering them, such as doing things one-handed.

Speech-Language Therapy. A *speech-language pathologist* teaches patients to retrieve language skills and educates family members on how to communicate more effectively with a speech- or listening-impaired person. This specialist is also versed in helping patients surmount swallowing difficulties.

Deciding on the Proper Rehab Setting

Inpatient or outpatient? Individual services or a comprehensive program? Matching a patient with an appropriate regimen of rehabilitation "is very, very important," stresses Dr. Gresham, who also serves as director of rehabilitation medicine at Buffalo's Erie County Medical Center. There are several options:

Hospital Inpatient Programs. These are found in rehabilitation units of acute care hospitals or in special rehabilitation hospitals. These comprehensive programs, staffed by the full range of rehab specialists, tend to be the most demanding physically and mentally for patients.

Hospital-Affiliated Nursing Home Programs. Found in or adjacent to the hospital, they are intended primarily for survivors expected to improve enough within two to three weeks that they can continue their therapy in another setting.

Private Nursing Home Programs. These programs are found in freestanding nursing facilities. The level of rehabilitation may be comprehensive or limited. Generally, the programs are less intensive than hospital inpatient programs.

Outpatient Programs. Hospital outpatient departments and freestanding outpatient clinics offer these programs. They provide both multidisciplinary therapy and individual services, though hospital day programs are often more intensive. Patients typically spend several hours at the facility three to five days per week. The advantage is that the patient is able to live at home. The disadvantage is that the patient and family must arrange round-trip transportation.

Home Programs. Physical therapy, occupational therapy, and speech therapy can all be carried out at home, either separately or as part of an all-encompassing program. In-home therapy carries two major advantages: many patients function better in familiar surroundings, and they acquire their new living skills in the same environment where they will be applied.

Someone with only a mild deficit in one area—say, hemiparesis of the left leg—may do just fine receiving physical therapy at an outpatient facility or at home. Patients with a broader range of problems often require inpatient treatment that incorporates the three major therapies and possibly recreational therapy, group activities, psychological counseling, and so on.

Then there are those whose limitations are either so great or so slight that no rehabilitation is recommended. For instance, a person with a severe learning deficit may be better off in a nursing facility or at home. By the same token, someone who incurred minimal damage may not have much to gain. "It's with the middle group," says Dr. Gresham, "that we can see a great amount of improvement." The key, he says, is to select therapy that matches the patient's goals, interests, and abilities. Although the hospital staff will suggest specific programs, ultimately the final determination is up to the patient. Bear in mind, however, that in the wake of a stroke or severe head injury, a survivor may have difficulty processing information or expressing her wishes.

Discuss the matter of rehabilitation with your loved one. What does he hope to achieve? To walk again, at least with the aid of a cane or a walker? This is a reachable goal for most survivors. To drive a car? Possibly, but not everyone will be able to attain the level of independence desired.

Convey the patient's ambitions to the hospital staff. Do they seem realistic? Setting impractical goals may doom the person to failure. But if they are too low, he may not receive all the services he truly needs. And if the goals don't correspond to his interests, he may grow bored and pursue therapy halfheartedly. In order to be effective, therapy requires patients' total commitment and a lot of hard work.

Answering the questions in Table 14, devised by the Agency for Health Care Policy and Research panel, should help point you and your loved one in the right direction. Its treatment recommendations take into account such factors as the patient's medical condition, ability to learn and level of physical endurance, the nature and severity of functional handicaps, and the support available at home. Encourage the person to share your findings with his doctor, or do so together.

According to Dr. Gresham, the same criteria cannot be applied exactly to people with severe head injuries. One major difference in recoveries from stroke and TBI, he points out, is that "traumatic brain injury patients are usually rehabilitated physically much more quickly than they are cognitively and socially." Still, enough parallels exist to make this a worthwhile exercise for TBI patients, their caregivers, and their doctor.

If rehab is recommended, "the patient should be transferred to a rehabilitation facility as soon as medically stable," says Dr. Gresham. That doesn't leave much time for asking questions and researching what's available. As such, many families are forced to make this important decision virtually in the dark. "I get many calls from very sophisticated people," reflects Dr. Gresham, "and they have no idea whether or not they're doing the right thing."

Whenever possible, visit the facilities under consideration. Since survivors of stroke or traumatic brain injury are liable to be physically disabled at this point, write down your impressions and report back to them. Then, together, weigh the following points:

Choosing a Rehabilitation Program

- Does the program provide the services your loved one needs?
- Does it match his abilities, or is it too demanding or not demanding enough?
- When visiting a prospective facility, ask if it actively involves patients and family members in rehabilitation decisions and if caregivers are encouraged to participate in some rehabilitation sessions and practice with the patient.
- Don't underestimate the importance of location. Is the facility close enough that family members can visit easily?
- If this is an outpatient program, is transportation provided?

TABLE 14
Which Rehabilitation Setting Is Best for Your Loved One?

After each answer, follow the arrow, which will direct you either to another question or to the recommended form of therapy.

1. Is your loved one medically stable or moderately stable?
   ❑ No ▶ Recommendation: Delay your decision on rehabilitation until the patient is fully stabilized. Until then, recuperation should continue at home or in a nursing facility.
   ❑ Yes ▼

2. Does your loved one have a functional disability? This encompasses bowel or bladder control, cognition, emotional health, pain management, swallowing, language dysfunction, and problems carrying out the activities of daily living.
   ❑ No ▶ Recommendation: No rehabilitation is necessary.
   ❑ Yes ▼

3. Does your loved one have more than one functional disability?
   ❑ No ▶ Recommendation: individual rehabilitation services performed at home or on an outpatient basis.
   ❑ Yes ▼

4. Is your loved one able to learn and expected to make functional gains?
   ❑ No ▶ Recommendation: *custodial care* at home or in a long-term-care facility. Custodial care, which entails helping patients with the activities of daily living, can often be rendered by people who have no professional training, such as family members.
   ❑ Yes ▼

5. Does your loved one have the endurance to sit for one hour and participate actively in rehabilitation?
   ❑ No ▶ Recommendation: rehabilitation in a setting such as a nursing facility or a home program with low-intensity services.
   ❑ Yes ▼

6. How much assistance does your loved one need with mobility or with activities of daily living?
   ❑ Independent ▶ Go to question 8.
   ❑ Needs moderate, maximal, or total assistance ▶ Go to question 10.
   ❑ Needs supervision or minimal assistance ▼

7. Is adequate support available at home?
   ❑ No ▶ Recommendation: a brief inpatient program in a nursing facility or an intermediate care facility.
   ❑ Yes ▶ Recommendation: a home rehabilitation program or an outpatient program. A brief inpatient program in a nursing facility may be called for if the person has multiple, complex deficits.

8. Can your loved one manage more complex tasks such as fixing meals, housekeeping, using the telephone, driving, shopping, and writing checks?
   ❏ No ▶ Go to question 9.
   ❏ Yes ▶ Recommendation: a home rehabilitation program or outpatient rehabilitation service as needed.

9. Is adequate home support available?
   ❏ No ▶ Recommendation: rehabilitation services in a nursing facility or another supervised-living setting.
   ❏ Yes ▶ Recommendation: home or outpatient rehabilitation services as needed.

10. Can your loved one tolerate intense rehabilitation of three or more hours per day?
    ❏ No ▶ Recommendation: rehabilitation in a setting such as a nursing facility or a home program with low-intensity services.
    ❏ Yes ▼

11. Does your loved one need medical care or monitoring 24 hours a day?
    ❏ No ▶ Recommendation: rehabilitation in a setting with intense services and adequate medical coverage, such as an inpatient rehabilitation hospital, a nursing facility, or a home program.
    ❏ Yes ▶ Recommendation: an inpatient rehabilitation hospital or a nursing facility with intensive rehabilitation program capabilities and adequate acute medical care coverage.

• Is the program accredited and state licensed? To find out the latter, call your state department of health; its number is listed in the "State Government Offices" section of the phone book. As for verifying accreditation, contact the two organizations that accredit rehabilitation facilities:

☎ Commission on Accreditation of Rehabilitation Facilities
4891 East Grant Road
Tucson, AZ 85712
520-325-1044

☎ Joint Commission on Accreditation of Healthcare Organizations
One Renaissance Boulevard
Oakbrook Terrace, IL 60181
630-792-5000

• Ask around about the facility's reputation for quality. What has the patient's physician heard about this program? Ask if you can be put in touch with patients who have undergone rehabilitation there, as well as their caregivers.
• If you plan on hiring an individual practitioner or if you want to check the credentials of the staff at a rehabilitation center, confirm that the person is licensed by inquiring at your state's licensing board for each profession: physical therapy, occupational therapy, speech-language pathology, and so forth. Practitioners may be licensed by the same board, separately, or, in some states, not at all, and are typically overseen by the department of health or education.

☎ To obtain the phone number, your best bet is to dial directory assistance for your state's capital and ask for the specific licensing board. Knowing the practitioner's license number is helpful, but a search can be conducted based only on his or her last name. Be wary of anyone who refuses to give you his license number (which, incidentally, is public information).

☎ The American Speech-Language-Hearing Association Information Resource Center (10801 Rockville Pike, Rockville, MD 20852-3279, 800-638-8255) certifies over 65,000 speech-language pathologists nationwide and can refer you to members in your area.

- Not to be overlooked: To what extent, in actual dollars and cents, does Medicare, Medicaid, or private insurance cover the costs of the program? The hospital social worker can help you find out.

How You Can Help During Rehabilitation

Rehabilitation can be a time of conflicting emotions for patients and their caregivers, with elation resulting from today's progress possibly giving way to discouragement by tomorrow's setback. Our role during this period demands the balancing skills of a high-wire act as we try to impart a sense of optimism yet remain realistic; encourage the person but not load on pressure; accept obstacles in the road to recovery but not give up prematurely. Here are several ways to help loved ones benefit from rehabilitation as much as possible:

- Encourage the person to take part in decisions relating to his therapy.
- Participate in the education programs offered to family members on how to be of help.
- Attend several rehab sessions to see what's involved.
- Help the person practice the skills learned in physical therapy and occupational therapy. This should continue unfailingly even after rehab ends.
- Work with the person at discovering new ways to do things and to solve problems brought on by her impairments.
- Resist the understandable urge to do everything for the survivor of a stroke or brain injury. Determine which tasks she can perform herself, and then *let her do them!*

But Is It Covered?

Nearly three in four stroke patients are age sixty-five or older and therefore most likely will have health insurance under the federal Medicare program. Victims of traumatic brain injury, who tend to be substantially younger, usually rely on private health insurance or, if they qualify, Medicaid, the state-administered federal plan that provides coverage to low-income individuals and families.

Although Medicaid benefits vary from state to state, it generally covers some portion of rehabilitation therapy expenses, as do many private policies. Medicare is uniform throughout the country.

☎ Since benefits may change from year to year, order "The Medicare Handbook." This informative booklet, revised annually, is available free from the Health Care Financing Administration's Medicare Hotline (800-638-6833) and from the Social Security Administration (800-772-1213). ◄ See "How to Get the Most out of Health Insurance," page 280; "Medicare," page 278; and "Medicaid," page 279.

Whoever the carrier is, it will undoubtedly insist on documentation from the physician saying not only that the patient would benefit from rehabilitation but also from a particular form of therapy. Another reason we suggest you refer to Table 14, "Which Rehabilitation Setting Is Best for Your Loved

One?," is that the recommendations developed by the Agency for Health Care Policy and Research panel conform closely to the policies of Medicare, Medicaid, and most private insurers.

Insurance benefits for rehabilitation generally end once progress levels off, a point that may arrive after weeks, months, or longer. Dr. McDowell, also a member of the AHCPR panel, says bluntly, "The person who has had a stroke is not going to be the same as before, either physically or intellectually. Generally, if people recover much function, they do so in the first three months. After that, any changes that occur are minor. Their caregivers should understand that and not spend huge amounts of time, effort, and money trying to obtain that last ounce of function through endless therapy."

Recovery from severe head trauma tends to take longer. In fact, three months isn't even ample time for a long-term prognosis—something that, understandably, often frustrates family members. "You really have to wait six months to truly be able to say how the patient will turn out," says Dr. Ghajar. "A person could be in a vegetative state for up to six months and still make a good recovery." By the time a year has passed, however, the ramifications of the accident are apparent, and, for better or worse, "the person is considered 90 percent of where he's going to end up."

Roslyn Travers calls her brother's improvement after thirteen months in an Austin, Texas, residential program "remarkable."

"Once Duane came back home he was a lot better," she recalls, "and he continued to improve for the next two or three years. Then he seemed to peak, and ever since he's been about the same. Now it takes people a little while to know something's wrong with him. He still has the limp and the weak arm, and his short-term memory is really bad, but he'll carry on a big conversation with you." Although Duane lives in his own apartment, "he can't pay bills, and he has to have close supervision. He still stays with me a good bit on weekends."

Jackie Cole's recovery was excruciatingly slow but more complete. After awakening from her coma in mid-May, she spent two months in the rehab unit at Maryland General Hospital, then was transferred to Baltimore's Montebello Rehabilitation Hospital. She lived there three months before finally returning home to her family in time for an especially joyous Thanksgiving.

Today, the only visible remnant of her stroke is a slight stiffness when walking. The main lasting handicap, says her husband, "is a significant loss of short-term memory, which is fairly permanent." The Reverend Cole wrote about Jackie's and his ordeal in a book (his third) entitled *One in a Million*. "This was not a total fairy tale," he reflects. "I suppose in some ways we're still working out the story."

Jackie is among the 35 percent of stroke survivors who recuperate almost completely or with minor impairments. Forty percent incur moderate to severe deficits and require special care, and 10 percent must be placed in long-term care. In a National Institute of Neurological Disorders and Stroke study of traumatic brain injury survivors, half exhibited what researchers termed a "good" recovery after three months or more. Thirty-five percent were left moderately disabled; 10 percent, severely disabled; and 5 percent remained in a persistent vegetative state.

Potential Life-Threatening Complications

"Most people who survive a stroke generally die of heart disease," says Dr. McDowell, pointing to the underlying atherosclerosis that often precipitates both diseases. "A person's chances of living five years after a stroke without developing serious heart disease are

Examples of Antihypertensive Medications

Type	Generic Name	Brand Name
Thiazide diuretics	hydrochlorothiazide	Esidrix
Beta-blockers	acebutolol	Sectral
Vasodilators	minoxidil	Loniten
ACE inhibitors	enalapril	Vasotec
Calcium channel blockers	nifedipine	Procardia

not very great. And if they already have heart disease, their chances of its becoming more serious are extremely high." Another potentially serious complication is a second stroke, which happens to 14 percent of survivors within a year, and to 25 to 42 percent within five years.

For most stroke patients, those forbidding statistics should be enough to motivate them into giving up harmful habits that contribute to high blood pressure, which, as we know, figures prominently both in stroke and in cardiovascular disease. That means abstaining from tobacco and most alcohol, exercising, taking off those extra pounds, and adhering to a low-salt, low-fat, low-cholesterol diet.

What about reducing emotional stress, which many folks associate with hypertension? To be sure, learning to modulate our reactions to life's daily pressures can enhance mental health, and for that reason alone we would recommend investigating any of the stress-reduction techniques explained in chapter 3. (That goes for caregivers, too.) But you may be surprised to learn that the only link found thus far between stress and stroke is that it may send a person reaching for a smoke, a drink, or a container of ice cream. In fact, although we know how to control high blood pressure, in nine of ten cases its causes go unidentified.

In addition to recommending changes in diet, physical activity, and so forth, your loved one's physician may prescribe antihypertensive medications from one or more drug categories: *thiazide diuretics, beta-blockers, vasodilators, angiotensin converting enzyme (ACE) inhibitors,* or *calcium channel blockers.*

Because survivors of severe head trauma may have sustained other injuries in the accident, they can acquire an assortment of health problems over the years. One complication that appears to be directly related to the brain injury itself bears enormous ramifications both for the patient and the caregiver: a higher-than-average incidence of Alzheimer's disease, the irreversible degenerative condition that slowly brings on senile dementia, leaving its victims completely dependent.

Roslyn Travers is already preparing for the inevitability of one day having to care for her brother full-time again. Duane has been diagnosed with hepatitis C, a puzzling form of liver disease that can lead to cirrhosis or cancer. The faulty memory and fleeting concentration caused by brain damage had relegated him to menial work, mostly raking leaves and doing odd jobs for his father. Duane is so fatigued from the hepatitis, however, that he cannot do that anymore.

"My mother, who lives in the same apartment complex as Duane, is his guardian," she says. "But Mama's seventy-six; she's not going to be around. And my father's seventy. Somebody will have to look after my brother and be his guardian.

"Even before we found out about the hepatitis, my husband and I were planning to build a garage or a room in back, because we knew that one day Duane would have to go somewhere. Then lo and behold, the next thing we knew, my husband's eighty-four-year-old mother began going downhill and couldn't be left on her own anymore. So we're now in the process of building a little guest house in the back for her.

"And eventually," she says in a voice full of acceptance but brimming with sadness, "Duane will be living there."

Recommended Reading

The following is available free from the Agency for Health Care Policy and Research Information Clearinghouse (800-358-9295):

- "Recovering After a Stroke/Patient and Family Guide"

The following is available free from the American Heart Association (800-242-8721):

- "Heart and Stroke Facts"

The following are available free from the National Institute of Neurological Disorders and Stroke (800-352-9424):
- "Head Injury: Hope Through Research"
- "Stroke: Hope Through Research"

The following are available free from the National Stroke Association (800-787-6537):
- "Stroke Treatment & Recovery"
- "Home Exercises for Stroke Survivors"
- "Understanding Speech and Language Problems After Stroke"
- "Living at Home After a Stroke"

–15–

Caring for Someone with Chronic Obstructive Pulmonary Disease

(Emphysema and Chronic Bronchitis)

When **Nola J. Miller** of Centerville, Utah, met her future husband, Walter, she was a forty-two-year-old divorcée with six children; he was a forty-eight-year-old bachelor and avid gardener who worked for the Union Pacific Railroad. "A very unusual man" is how she affectionately describes her late husband, adding, "I adored him." The couple wed a year later, in 1976.

Walter Miller had been a heavy smoker since his teens. "This man smoked more than you could ever imagine," says Nola. "I tried my very best to encourage him to quit. I never nagged him or told him he couldn't smoke in the house—although I did say, 'You're going to have to scrub the yellow walls.' He'd tried quitting over the years, but he was so addicted to those cigarettes, he just wasn't able to handle it." Increasingly, Walter began to experience the shortness of breath and crushing fatigue symptomatic of chronic obstructive pulmonary disease.

We both were aware of the symptoms, but he would not go to a doctor because every time he went, they would tell him he'd have to quit those damn cigarettes. The year before he was finally diagnosed, in 1984, he lived in constant fear of not being able to smoke. It was as if he thought each cigarette would be his last.

Walter had been ill with a cold for about three weeks but still refused to go to a doctor. My husband loved his yard and his garden. Though it was November, we hadn't had any snow, so he went outside to mow the lawn. I was inside doing housework. After a while, I couldn't find him. I started calling around the house and discovered him in bed. He had a warmup suit on and was under all the covers, yet he was shivering.

I said, "Do you think you're ready to see a doctor now?" That evening he finally agreed to go to the emergency room at Holy Cross Hospital in Salt Lake City. It turned out that Walter had *emphysema* and *pneumonia in both lungs.* The staff asked him, "How did you get in the hospital?"

He said, "I walked in." (I had led him to the door.)

They replied, "You could not have!" Walter had so little oxygen in his blood and in his body, they didn't know how he'd managed to walk in there. That's how critical his condition was.

He immediately went on two liters of oxygen per minute twenty-four hours a day and was hospitalized for five days. The day he was to be discharged, I received a phone call at work. "We need someone to be at your house so we can bring the oxygen."

"The what?" I knew nothing about this. The oxygen company delivered the tank, so that when I picked Walter up at the hospital and brought him home, he already had his oxygen here.

And for the next eight years, until he died, that was our life.

Have you ever physically exerted yourself to the point that you were left gasping for breath and feeling as though you could barely move another muscle? If so, then you have some idea of what it can be like to suffer from advanced-stage chronic obstructive pulmonary disease, or COPD. Now imagine feeling that exhausted and desperate for oxygen merely from raising an arm to comb your hair. For some patients with this progressive, incurable disease, the second leading cause of hospitalization in the United States, physical activity becomes a distant memory as they edge ever closer to death.

The term *COPD* embraces a handful of diseases that obstruct air flow to the lungs, but it pertains primarily to *emphysema* and *chronic bronchitis*, which afflict an estimated 2 million and 12.5 million Americans, respectively. Although each may arise independently of the other, "patients typically have both," says Dr. Norman H. Edelman, chief of pulmonary medicine at Robert Wood Johnson University Hospital in New Brunswick, New Jersey.

All told, COPD places fourth on the list of fatal ailments, accounting for over 100,000 deaths annually. Asthma, a condition marked by recurrent episodes of labored breathing due to inflammation of the air passages, is generally *not* classified as a chronic obstructive pulmonary disease.

Chronic Obstructive Pulmonary Disease and the Lungs

To appreciate how COPD brings on such devastation, it helps to have a basic understanding of the lungs, two elastic sacs comprised of spongy tissue and intertwining networks of blood vessels and airways. The lungs lie on either side of the heart and occupy most of the chest cavity, encaged by the ribs. They are the principal organs of the *respiratory system*, which delivers life-sustaining oxygen to the blood and discards carbon dioxide, a waste product of the body's cells.

Oxygen makes up one-fifth of the air we breathe. Each breath's tour through the respiratory tract begins in the nose or the mouth, where it is warmed and moistened. Next it flows down through the throat *(pharynx)*, the voice box *(larynx)*, and the windpipe *(trachea)*. The trachea forks into two tubes, the *mainstem bronchi*, with the left bronchus routing air to the left lung, and the right bronchus leading to the right lung.

The lungs inflate to accommodate the inrushing air, an action prompted by the *diaphragm.* Wedged snugly beneath both lungs, this large dome-shaped muscle compresses and flattens every time we inhale, enabling the organs to expand.

The bronchial tract resembles a pair of inverted trees: Each main stem of the bronchus divides into two secondary bronchi, which fan out into more than one million *bronchioles.* These feed clusters of tiny round air sacs called *al-*

veoli (a single one is an *alveolus*); over 300 million in all.

Likewise, the blood vessels in the lung become progressively smaller as they branch out from the large *pulmonary trunk* exiting the heart to the *pulmonary arteries*, to the *pulmonary arterioles*, and finally to microscopic *pulmonary capillaries* enmeshed in the membranous wall of each alveolus. All these conduits relay *venous* blood —"used" blood, you could call it, since it has been depleted of oxygen and is suffused with carbon dioxide—that the veins have recirculated to the heart.

Time for the crucial exchange of gases: Oxygen from the alveoli filters into the capillaries, while carbon dioxide from the capillaries permeates the alveoli. *Pulmonary venules* and *veins* then return the reoxygenated blood to the heart for distribution to the entire body via the arterial system.

With the transaction completed, the abdominal muscles initiate the mechanical sequence of *expiration:* By contracting, they nudge the diaphragm back into position against the lungs. The pressure expels the carbon dioxide–laden air from the alveoli (picture air escaping from millions of tiny balloons), which backs up through the ever-enlarging passageways and out the nostrils.

Normally this entire process—from the moment air enters the respiratory system to the moment it exits—repeats about every four seconds.

Everyone's ability to move air in and out of the lungs diminishes slightly with age. But people with chronic obstructive pulmonary disease lose a profound degree of respiratory function. To what extent this impacts on their daily activities, says Dr. Edelman, "varies according to who they are and what they do, and a number of other factors." A person with only 30 percent *total lung capacity* (one of many test measurements used to quantify respiratory function) may be able to lead a relatively normal life, whereas another COPD patient with 60 percent lung capacity may be completely incapacitated.

As Dr. Edelman noted earlier, emphysema and chronic bronchitis conspire together most of the time. Although the two diseases affect the airways of the lungs similarly, they carry out their destruction in different ways.

Emphysema breaks down the elastic alveoli walls to leave behind large, useless pockets called *bullae*. Since the air sac tissue is what surrounds and buttresses the bronchioles, with its deterioration the corridors narrow and collapse, trapping the "stale" outgoing air in the lungs during exhalation.

Airway constriction is also a hallmark of chronic bronchitis. In addition, the inner lining *(mucosa)* of the air passages secretes excess lubricating *mucus*, which plugs the already slender openings and further interferes with the air's commute to and from the lungs.

Combined, emphysema and chronic bronchitis throw the gas exchange between the air sacs and blood vessels dangerously out of balance. Two things happen: After a while, the overburdened respiratory muscles can no longer propel enough air to the surviving alveoli, a condition known as *hypoventilation*. What's more, COPD destroys not only air sacs but the capillaries serving them, so that some alveoli possess an ample volume of air but too few operative blood vessels for carrying out an effective swap of gases. Or vice versa. Either way, this shortchanges the bloodstream of oxygen and causes carbon dioxide to build up.

What Causes Chronic Obstructive Pulmonary Disease?

That's an easy one: Smoking is responsible for more than eight in ten COPD-related deaths. The smoke is believed to hike the level of *elastase*, an enzyme that breaks down the chief component (*elastin*) of the lungs' connective tissue and consequently gives rise to chronic obstructive pulmonary disease.

However, a small percentage of people develop COPD due to a hereditary deficiency of a protein in the blood, *alpha-1-antitrypsin (AAT)*. AAT, produced by the liver, protects elastin from the ruinous effects of elastase. Approximately seventy thousand Americans have this genetic shortage, which can hasten the onset of COPD—normally a disease of old age and middle age—particularly if they smoke.

Early Symptoms and Diagnosis

Because chronic bronchitis often precedes emphysema, COPD first emerges as a mild, nagging "smoker's cough" that yields clear phlegm, usually upon awakening. If this becomes a morning ritual for six out of twelve months or for at least three months a year for two consecutive years, the bronchitis is considered chronic.

Another early sign of COPD is feeling winded and fatigued after even minimal exertion. Unfortunately, sufferers often ignore these symptoms. "There's frequently a lot of denial," Dr. Edelman observes. "People don't appreciate how short of breath they are. They'll say, 'Oh, I'm just out of shape' or 'I'm getting older.'" By the time manifestations first appear, the insidious disease has already ravaged lung tissue along with some measure of pulmonary function. Both losses are generally irreversible. However, if COPD is detected at this stage, before it has run rampant, the effects are largely manageable.

COPD can't be diagnosed on symptoms alone, but complaints of coughing, labored breathing, and weakness point strongly in that direction, especially if the patient has a history of smoking. The following procedures provide a definitive answer: a physical exam, chest X rays, a series of breathing tests known as pulmonary function tests, and blood-gas analysis—repeated blood tests to assess the concentrations of oxygen and carbon dioxide in the arterial blood, as well as its *pH*, the balance between acids and alkali (substances capable of neutralizing acids). Too much of one or the other can be fatal.

People with severe COPD typically have low oxygen and high carbon dioxide levels, and a low pH, meaning more acid than alkali. All indicate an inadequate blood gas exchange in the lungs.

Symptoms and Complications of Advanced COPD

As in Walter Miller's case, it often takes pneumonia or some other emergency before people with symptoms of COPD finally seek medical attention. By then, however, the disease is usually too far along to be diverted from its fatal course.

The goal of treatment, then, becomes symptom control, to make people more comfortable and to prolong their lives. Airway obstruction is partially correctable with smoking cessation and rehab; at first you can expect to see some improvement in your loved one's lung function. But over the next four or five years, COPD becomes increasingly debilitating. According to the National Heart, Lung and Blood Institute, part of the National Institutes of Health, the median survival time for COPD patients who have lost two-thirds of their normal lung function when diagnosed is ten years.

Shortness of Breath (Dyspnea)

Air hunger, or *dyspnea*, during physical activity is a fact of life for most people with early-stage COPD. "When the disease becomes more severe," says Dr. Edelman, "they may become dramatically, remarkably short of breath" following even modest exertion. Nola Miller recalls the dashes to the emergency room on those occasions when "Walter simply couldn't catch his breath. I would either call an ambulance or get him into the car and make the drive myself," she says. "He'd be admitted to the hospital, given medication and special breathing treatments we didn't have at home, and then released after five or six hours."

How It Is Managed

No Smoking. "The most important step is to give up cigarettes," says Dr. Edelman. "It's important for people to know that it's never too late." Although stopping smoking cannot undo existing lung damage, it does decelerate the disease process. If a smoker with COPD quits before his condition turns serious, he eventually will see his rate of lung deterioration return to that of a nonsmoker.

Walter gave up smoking the night he was diagnosed, much to Nola's astonishment, for as abysmal as he felt on the car ride to Salt Lake City, he nevertheless fished out a cigarette from his pocket and lit up. At 2:00 A.M., when his exhausted wife was putting on her coat to leave the hospital, she asked if there was anything she could get him.

"I would like a Coke and a cigarette," he said.

Nola recalls, "He was sitting there with oxygen on at the time." She replied coolly, "I will be glad to get you the Coke, and you can talk to the nurses about the cigarette." He never had another one.

Not to sound pessimistic, but the majority of COPD patients have smoked most of their lives. For them to give up tobacco permanently is extraordinarily rare. The psychological and physical cravings for nicotine are usually so overpowering that not even the prospect of death—and a rather agonizing

one at that—is incentive enough. Diane Young, a caregiver from New Orleans, tells of how her emphysemic mother continued to smoke until just days before she died.

"We had to have people with her to move the oxygen tank out of the room so that she could have a cigarette," she says. Oxygen and open flame, of course, make for a dangerously combustible combination. With that in mind, if a terminally ill patient receiving oxygen therapy insists on smoking, it's more sensible to assist them than risk having them sneak a cigarette, nod out, and set the bed ablaze or possibly cause an explosion.

Enrollment in a formal smoking-cessation program may be of value for someone in the early stages of COPD, although the recidivism rate far outnumbers the success stories. But if it's understood that death is inevitable, let's not try to enforce what amounts to a profound transformation in behavior—as I saw my father do with my stepmother when she was dying of emphysema and lung cancer. Relaxing on the back porch at night with a smoke and reminiscing was one of her few remaining pleasures. While Dad tried to keep Lynn from her cigarettes at all costs, I would slip her the whole pack.

Pulmonary Rehabilitation. Some COPD patients benefit from a pulmonary rehabilitation program where they learn ways to breathe more effectively. For instance, a person with advanced disease often has a flat, weak diaphragm, the muscle that works the lungs like a bellows. *Abdominal breathing,* also called *controlled deep breathing,* is a method for employing the diaphragm to its maximum capability instead of relying solely on the chest muscles.

Ask a respiratory therapist or nurse to demonstrate this and other breathing exercises so that you can help your loved one practice until it becomes second nature, as well as coach her through spells of respiratory distress.

> ☎ **For free referrals to a pulmonary rehab program:**
>
> call the American Association of Cardiovascular and Pulmonary Rehabilitation in Middleton, Wisconsin, at 608-831-6989.

Understandably, it's a terrifying sensation to feel as though you cannot draw a breath. "When Walt couldn't breathe," recalls Nola, "absolute fear would set in, which only exacerbated the problem." Calming the person down using light massage and relaxation exercises will enable him to focus on recapturing a breathing rhythm.

Pulmonary rehab also incorporates general exercise training. Its purpose, explains Dr. Edelman, is "to condition the rest of the body to utilize oxygen more efficiently, thereby placing less of a demand on the lungs," and to strengthen the diaphragm and abdominal muscles. Whether or not our loved one belongs in rehabilitation is a matter to take up with the doctor. If the person is beyond the point of making progress, the experience can prove deeply upsetting, as it did for Walter Miller. The June before he died, he entered a pulmonary program conducted at Holy Cross Hospital.

"He failed it miserably," says Nola. "He was in such pain, and the staff kept insisting that he do more than he was capable of. To stay in the program, Walt had to pass certain evaluations, but he couldn't do it, so they transferred him to a nursing home." ◄ See "Difficulty Breathing (Dyspnea)," page 174.

Drug Therapy. *Bronchodilators*, a family of drugs that open constricted air passages by relaxing the smooth muscles, are generally the preferred medication for facilitating breathing. Examples include isoproterenol (brand name: Isuprel), metaproterenol (Alupent), and theophylline (Marax). A sec-

ond choice may be dexamethasone (Decadron) and other *corticosteroids*, synthetic hormones that reduce airway inflammation.

Bronchodilators can be taken orally, rectally, or by intravenous injection. They also come in an inhalable solution that is poured into a *nebulizer*, a machine that dispenses the medication as a fine mist to be inhaled through a mouthpiece. In-home breathing treatments, lasting five to fifteen minutes, become part of a COPD sufferer's daily routine. The following recommendations from the American Lung Association can help make therapy pass more easily for patients:

- Ideally, keep all equipment set up in one place permanently. If your loved one takes treatment during the daytime, you might want to try a spot near the kitchen or bathroom, since the equipment needs to be cleaned afterward. If breathing therapy is called for at night, consider the bedroom.
- Here's the perfect arrangement: a small table with a drawer or a flat-top desk placed in front of a window (one with a view, thank you). When treatment is over, be sure not to leave any medications sitting in the sun.
- Place an egg timer, kitchen timer, or alarm clock nearby so the person can time his treatments.
- If medication must be measured using an eye dropper, squeeze out any air bubbles first.
- Tubes, mouthpieces, and medicine cups can be stored in one or two plastic storage boxes—approximately 6 by 8 by 2½ inches—with locking tops. You can keep them inside a small drawer and out of sight.
- Thoroughly clean and sterilize all equipment as directed. There are several methods for this, so don't worry if someone else with COPD or their caregiver does this differently from you. Just make sure you store them dry so as not to introduce germs into the lungs.

- If your patient likes to listen to the radio or watch TV during treatments, use an earpiece because the equipment can be noisy. To muffle the machine's motor or compressor, set it atop a rubber typewriter pad or some folded fabric.
- If there is not enough mist, check all the hose couplings, which may have worked loose. A simple hand-tightening should solve the problem. Two other troubleshooting suggestions: Detach and wash the hose to clean out a possible clog or increase the machine's flow rate to push more gas through.
- When disassembling the equipment for cleaning following therapy, you may have difficulty tugging the plastic hose off. This is usually easier to do while the nebulizer is running.
- Some machines have a small air filter that must be changed periodically. Request extras from the supplier.
- Most home medical equipment can be purchased, which in the long run may prove cheaper than renting. However, you would then have to pay for repairs should something malfunction or break. Ask the supplier for prices and compare.

The complications that *corticosteroids* can stir up are worth mentioning. In their inhalable form, these medications "tend to produce relatively few side effects," says Dr. Edelman. Patients spray the medicine into their mouth using a handheld device called a *metered-dose inhaler*. But the roster of side effects from oral steroids when taken for weeks or months "is very long and very serious." Among them are mood swings, indigestion, ulcers, and bone fractures. "Patients will tumble out of bed or slip on the floor and break a bone," says Dr. Edelman, who advises, "Homes should be adapted very carefully to minimize the opportunities for falls."

Walter Miller went on the anti-inflammatory agent prednisone. "He suffered a fractured back from it," says Nola. For the last seven months of his life, "his back fractured every four or five weeks." To allay the pain, doctors prescribed morphine, one of the most potent *narcotic analgesics*. It is not uncommon for COPD patients to require *tranquilizers* as well to ease anxiety. Walter was given alprazolam (brand name: Xanax), a controlled substance. Since you may find yourself doling out medicine at home, it's important to bear in mind that these categories of drugs depress breathing, and dosages must be heeded precisely.

For the 1 to 3 percent of COPD patients with the alpha-1-antitrypsin deficiency, treatment includes *AAT replacement therapy*, in which the missing protein is delivered to the bloodstream through an intravenous drip once a week for life. The disruption to patients' lives is one drawback of replacement therapy; its exorbitant cost is another. ◄ *See "Tips for Preventing Falls," page 134.*

Oxygen Therapy. COPD patients with inadequate concentrations of oxygen in the blood *(hypoxemia)* may need to go on supplemental oxygen, for if not remedied, hypoxemia can progress to *hypoxia*—a state where the body's cells receive such meager rations of oxygen that they begin to die. Pulmonologists typically recommend continuous oxygen therapy—yes, twenty-four hours a day—for anyone whose blood oxygen levels are low while resting, sleeping, or during mild exertion. COPD patients expected to remain on supplemental oxygen indefinitely are usually administered low concentrations of oxygen at a flow rate of one to four liters per minute.

"Putting a patient with low blood oxygen levels on continuous oxygen will extend his life," asserts Dr. Edelman. "There's no question." The added time needn't lack quality, either. During the first seven years that Walter Miller was on oxygen therapy, he and his wife continued to lead an enviably active lifestyle.

INSIDE INFORMATION

The National Heart, Lung and Blood Institute discourages COPD patients from taking "combination" drugs that blend more than one bronchodilator plus a sedative and sometimes an *expectorant* (to loosen and expel mucus secretions from the air passages). There are many over-the-counter brands available, including Primatene tablets, Quadrinal tablets, and Marax syrup.

While these combo platters sound wonderfully versatile—and, indeed, are useful in treating other respiratory conditions—they don't always achieve a safe balance between the dose of the methylxanthine bronchodilator and the other ingredients, resulting in unwanted side effects. What's more, the sympathomimetic contained in such compounds, ephedrine, is less effective than other bronchodilators and can generate nervousness and agitation, hence the need for the counteraction of the sedative. The expectorant component, too, may not work satisfactorily for all patients and may also cause side effects.

Nola Miller: When Walt went on the oxygen, there was an immediate change. His skin no longer seemed gray; he looked beautiful, healthy. We would put an oxygen tank in the back of the car and travel. He really kept going and continued to be very self-sufficient.

I encouraged that, though there were times when I would overchallenge him. Once we were on our way to a wedding reception, and I was walking way too fast. He stopped me and asked, "What are you trying to do to me!"

At first Walter wore a *nasal cannula.* It's a simple device: a two-pronged soft plastic nosepiece that fits into the nostrils and attaches to a flexible tube connected to the oxygen tank. An elastic strap or a plastic tube over the ears or under the chin holds it in place. The steady stream of pure oxygen tends to dry out the nose, mouth, and throat, which can be very bothersome for patients and make them vulnerable to infection.

After three years, Walter's pulmonologist recommended exchanging the cannula for a *tracheostomy,* which according to Dr. Edelman is fast becoming the preferred route for delivering oxygen to people with chronic obstructive pulmonary disease. Here a surgeon creates an opening through the neck and into the windpipe, then implants a permanent tube. Now the unit can be connected directly to the "trach." The oxygen passes through a humidifier first, greatly reducing problems with dry throat.

A note of caution: At home and in the hospital it's very important to administer the exact level of oxygen prescribed by the physician. This is true for all patients but particularly those with COPD. Very often your instinct is to give as much as possible because the person is so obviously deprived, with a bluish cast to his skin (a condition known as *cyanosis*). But too much oxygen can actually depress breathing further. The body has grown so used to working with little oxygen that the inflow of supplemental oxygen fools the brain's respiratory center into thinking the person has enough. In response, it slows down breathing or possibly stops it altogether. ◄ See "Dry Mouth," page 161; "Sore Mouth or Throat," page 161; and "Administering Supplemental Oxygen," page 175.

Mechanical Ventilation. When patients cannot breathe adequately on their own, a mechanical *ventilator,* or *respirator,* must do part or all of the work for them. The machine, which attaches to the tracheostomy tube, drives air into the lungs, forcing both them and the chest to expand. "Until recently," says Dr. Edelman, "this could be done only in hospitals. More and more, though, we're putting patients on ventilators at home. But it requires an extraordinary home environment with devoted caregiving to make it work." ◄ See "Mechanical Ventilation," page 175.

Chronic Coughing

The nagging cough that heralds early COPD rarely worsens over time, unlike most other symptoms of the disease. Nonetheless, patients may be subject to violent hacking that prevents them from catching their breath and leaves them feeling sore—and frightened—afterward. In the midst of one of these convulsive coughing fits, people sometimes lose control of their bladder or bowels.

How It Is Managed

We *want* COPD patients to cough, nice and deeply, to rid the respiratory tract of mucus. But if incessant coughing is causing pain and interfering with sleep, a physician will likely prescribe a cough suppressant, also known as an *antitussive*. Those containing narcotics (codeine, dilaudid, and hydrocodone are just a few) depress breathing somewhat and must be used with caution. As for how to handle *stress incontinence*, a sanitary pad or adult diaper worn inside undergarments is often all that's necessary to prevent a potentially embarrassing accident and keep your loved one dry should one occur. ◄ See "Incontinence," page 170; "Chronic Coughing," page 178.

Difficulty Expelling Secretions

As the disease advances, the sputum from the lungs turns thick and gummy, making it extremely difficult for patients to clear their respiratory tracts. Compounding the problem is the fact that people with COPD frequently cough ineffectually. The effort merely exhausts them, and so over time they may resist even trying to cough up phlegm.

How It Is Managed

Suctioning. If necessary, you can suction secretions from the airways using a device called an *aspirator.* Ask the doctor to prescribe one and show you how to use it safely. ◄ See "Using a Suction Device to Clear the Airway," page 177.

Inhalation Therapy. Patients inhale bland aerosols, usually consisting of saline solution or bicarbonate of soda, which dilute and loosen sputum. Bronchodilating drugs may be added.

Drug Therapy. Expectorant medications have a similar effect on airway secretions, making them easier to bring up and expel.

Hydration. See to it that your loved one drinks plenty of fluids daily, whether it's water, bouillon, or fruit juices. This not only liquefies mucus but it restores the fluid loss commonly seen in COPD patients due to their increased respiratory rate, mouth breathing, and frequent expectoration. Placing a vaporizer or humidifier in the person's room is another good way to help loosen secretions. The moist air can make it harder to breathe, however, in which case the machine should be turned down or off until the dyspnea passes.

Postural Bronchial Drainage, Chest Percussion, and Controlled Coughing. Chapter 3 describes all three techniques for raising phlegm.

Appetite Loss

"Emphysema," says Dr. Edelman, "is one of the most wasting diseases we know. Appetite loss can be a major problem for these patients, and they usually lose a lot of weight." Toward the end of Walter Miller's life, his daily diet consisted only of Jell-O and, at most, one can of Ensure, a liquid nutritional supplement.

One cause of this is purely anatomical. "In COPD the lungs remain partially inflated and constantly press down on the stomach," Dr. Edelman explains, "which leaves little room for food." Conversely, a full belly compresses the lungs, interfering with breathing. To this add the persistent shortness of breath, coughing, fatigue, and disagreeable taste in the mouth from medications, dehydration, and spitting up mucus, and you can see why a person with chronic obstructive pulmonary disease might eventually lose interest in food and become malnourished.

How It Is Managed

Once the body depletes its reserves of glycogen and fat, it begins to break down muscle tissue for fuel. That is why the National Heart, Lung and Blood Institute recommends COPD patients eat a diet high in protein, which builds and repairs muscle. Good sources include meats, poultry, fish, dairy products, eggs, and beans.

What if the person you're caring for doesn't want scrambled eggs, doesn't want a piece of grilled chicken, doesn't want fish, but craves linguine with clam sauce? Fix him a plate. Ultimately, the day's menu becomes whatever appeals to him. And remember: Never pressure sick people to eat if they say they're not hungry.

With COPD patients it's best to serve six smaller meals rather than the customary three so as not to overload the stomach. In order to process a large meal, the digestive system has to divert oxygen-carrying blood from other areas of the body to the stomach. Since these folks may have too little circulating oxygen to begin with, the less time and energy digestion takes, the better. ◀ *See "Tricks for Stimulating Appetite," page 159.*

Insomnia

Most people with severe COPD can only daydream of enjoying a night of uninterrupted slumber. They awaken frequently—short of breath, perhaps seized by a smothering sensation—and must sit up and cough, sometimes for several minutes. It's not unusual for them to have to sleep in a semi-sitting position, either propped up by pillows or in a raised hospital bed or reclining chair.

"For the last eleven months, Walter was never able to lie down again because he couldn't breathe," says Nola Miller, who describes her husband's sleep as "very erratic." A second obstacle to restful sleep is the disruptive effect that too little oxygen and too much carbon dioxide in the blood has on the central nervous system, particularly the brain.

How It Is Managed

Your loved one's doctor may order a sleeping aid or sedative. As with antidepressants and tranquilizers, these medications depress breathing and should be dosed with great care. ◀ *See "Insomnia and Other Sleep Disorders," page 172.*

Depression

Certainly any terminal illness is capable of plunging a patient into despair. But people with advanced COPD are especially prone to depression because the disease so drastically alters their way of life *for years.* Imagine the frustration of having to go about your day "in slow motion," as Nola puts it, while carting around a portable oxygen tank—a painfully conspicuous reminder of a life fated to be cut short.

"Around 1987, Walter started getting quite depressed about the fact that he was on oxygen," says Nola. "He also had to deal with the fact that he'd worked so hard to get himself into this position, having smoked for forty-seven years. His own sense of guilt was far worse than anything I could have said." It should go without saying that now is no time for I-told-you-so's; it is time for infinite compassion.

How It Is Managed

Antidepressant medication is used. Psychotherapy, counseling, or a support group conducted by a professional therapist may also prove worthwhile. ◄ *See "Depression," page 191.*

Other Potential Complications

The debilitating effects of end-stage COPD eventually confine most patients to bed. During the last few months of Walter Miller's life, he could manage only the two halting steps necessary to transfer from his wheelchair to his electric recliner, then back again. At this point a caregiver must watch for the many medical problems that threaten all immobilized patients. ◄ *See chapter 3, "The Everyday Angel's Cram Course in Essential Nursing Skills," page 101.*

How COPD Is Treated

A COPD patient's only hope for long-term survival is a *lung transplantation.* Unfortunately, "the numbers of lung donors is so small," says Dr. Alfred Munzer, "the procedure is not widely performed" and is not a realistic option for the vast majority of cases, most of whom are too sick to survive the surgery. In 1994 the number of lung transplants performed was 688, up from just 2 in 1985.

Bullectomy, the surgical removal of large bullae (the empty, enlarged lung compartments), offers relief for one type of emphysema called *bullous emphysema.* But can it be considered a cure? "There has always been a lot of controversy over how effective bullectomy is," says Dr. Munzer, codirector of pulmonary medicine at the Washington Adventists Hospital in Takoma Park, Maryland, and former president of the American Lung Association. "Certainly it can help people who have a very large bulla that is compressing normal lung tissue."

A variation on bullectomy, *lung volume reduction surgery,* has shown promise for its ability to excise not just large bullae but smaller diseased sections of the lung as well, improving the efficiency of the lungs. Realistically, the best outcome most people with COPD can expect is to see their lives extended and symptoms kept at bay temporarily. If your patient wants to investigate having this specialized operation, be sure you consult a thoracic surgeon who has at least several dozen lung volume reduction surgeries under his belt, because in inexperienced hands, the procedure carries a high mortality rate.

Potential Life-Threatening Complications

Walter Miller's condition declined sharply beginning in late 1991. By this time he had been diagnosed with a malignant tumor in his prostate. On Christmas Day he complained of not being able to breathe and asked his wife to drive him to the hospital. A pulmonary function test showed no lung capacity whatsoever. Between the advancing lung disease and cancer, "for the next six months he lived in and out of the hospital," says Nola Miller.

In June she was informed that her husband could die "any day" and asked if she wanted him to remain hospitalized. "I said, 'No. I want him to die at home in bed with me.'" Walter went home to live out the remainder of his life, which, it would turn out, surpassed all expectations.

"My husband couldn't walk to the bedroom anymore," Nola recalls, "so we fixed a place in the kitchen for his recliner. Since I still worked during the day, I'd hired an aide. During the day, she'd take Walt outside on the deck, which he loved, and let him sit in the sun with the birds fluttering around. It was beautiful. And he had all his animals. This one little dog slept by him every night."

As with many bedridden patients, Walter's skin became increasingly delicate. "On November 16, a Monday, the community service nurse called me at work," Nola remembers. "She said, 'We need to have an electric hospital bed delivered. Your husband's bedsores are getting much worse, and I can't turn him because he is always sitting.' I made arrangements to have a bed delivered the next day.

"It was a brand-new one. They took it out of the cardboard casing and put it together. Walt looked at that bed and started to cry. He said, 'No! No!' I am convinced he knew that if he got in that bed, he would die.

"The aide and I lifted him into the bed. He just sat there and pointed to his wheelchair and said, 'That! That!' I'll never forget it as long as I live," she says, crying. "He wanted to be back in his wheelchair."

Pulmonary Infection

Because their lungs serve as traps for bacteria, people with chronic obstructive pulmonary disease are susceptible to severe respiratory infections. "The biggest problem," says Dr. Edelman, "is *infectious pneumonia*," a deadly disease that inflames the lungs. When respiratory function is dangerously compromised, as in COPD, virtually any pulmonary infection can mushroom into a life-threatening crisis. That's why

we pluck used tissues from the garbage pail and examine the patient's sputum daily. Any of the following early traces of respiratory infection should be brought to a physician's attention immediately:

- a change in color from clear to yellow or green
- a thicker consistency
- an unusual odor
- the patient's complaining of a foul taste in the mouth
- fever

How It Is Managed

Antibiotics are administered.

Respiratory Acidosis

Carbon dioxide circulates through the bloodstream in the form of carbonic acid. The body rids itself of this and other acids two ways: through the air expelled by the lungs and through the urine excreted by the kidneys. *Respiratory acidosis* refers to the overaccumulation of carbon dioxide in the blood of people with poor pulmonary function. By retaining a type of salt known as bicarbonate, the kidneys can compensate and preserve a reasonably even *acid-base balance*. But should even a minor respiratory infection develop, further impairing the beleaguered lungs' ability to discard carbon dioxide, the kidneys may no longer be able to pick up the slack. If not corrected, acute respiratory acidosis can trigger cardiac arrest or respiratory failure.

The blood-gas analysis referred to earlier as a diagnostic measure is repeated at regular intervals to monitor COPD patients' oxygen–carbon dioxide levels. "At first it was every month, then every three months," says Nola Miller. To that add the blood studies that must be performed whenever the patient is taken to an emergency room complaining of respiratory distress, to gauge the diffusion of oxygen and carbon dioxide in the lungs. "We were always so wor-

---

INSIDE INFORMATION

To prevent bleeding from an arterial needle "stick," pressure should be applied to the puncture site for 5 minutes; up to 10 minutes if the blood was taken from the larger, more accessible *femoral* artery in the groin. But blood-gas analyses are often carried out in emergency situations, when the medical team is anxious to learn the results, so it's not unusual for the technician to finish drawing the blood, place it on ice, and then rush off to the lab. Should blood leak out, the patient will wind up with a painful bruise, or *hematoma*, around the site. Repeated stickings also cause scar tissue to build up; then another artery has to be stabbed.

Therefore, anytime you're with a patient and a member of the hospital staff comes to draw blood gases, see to it that she compresses the puncture site for the full 5 minutes. Or better yet, do it yourself. Just press your thumb on the spot and hold it there gently but firmly, all the while looking at a clock or watch. Don't go by what *feels* like 5 minutes; you'd be amazed how slowly time passes when you're doing this. Sometimes a technician will place gauze and tape over the wound as a substitute measure. Not good enough. Get out your trusty thumb. It's a simple but important maneuver, one that can spare patients needless pain later on.

---

ried each time," says Nola, "wondering, *How is he doing?*"

People with COPD come to dread blood-gas analysis for another reason: They hurt. Ordinarily, the sample is drawn from the *radial* artery in the wrist. Whereas many large veins run near the surface of the skin, big arteries lie deeper in the tissue, making for a more elusive target. When I was training to be a respiratory therapy technician, we students had to practice performing blood-gas analysis by sticking needles into one another's arteries. I'll say one thing: You get *real* good *real* fast. But even experts often strike or pass close to the bundles of nerves that surround the radial artery.

Imagine how excruciating this can be for someone who is short of breath, anxious, and restless. A patient in respiratory distress may have blood taken every fifteen to thirty minutes until the supplementary oxygen and intravenous injections of bicarbonate bring his Pa_{CO2} (partial pressure of carbon dioxide in the arterial blood) and Pa_{O2} (partial pressure of oxygen in the arterial blood) under control.

How It Is Managed

Ventilation is improved either by natural means or with the assistance of a mechanical respirator, to return blood levels of oxygen and carbon dioxide to the safety zone.

Secondary Polycythemia

In response to the shortage of oxygen in the blood, the body steps up production of the red blood cells that tote oxygen throughout the bloodstream. This is beneficial, to a point. *Polycythemia*, the overabundance of red blood cells, ultimately inflames matters. The blood thickens, impeding its flow and curtailing the supply to vital tissues. Among these is the brain, thus accounting for symptoms such as impaired mental ability, irritability, headache, dizziness, and fainting.

Secondary polycythemia produces two readily identifiable signs: *clubbing* of the fingertips and toes, and cyanosis. The viscosity of the blood also invites clots to form, always a dangerous development.

How It Is Managed

Oxygen therapy is used.

Respiratory Failure/ Ventilatory Failure

A pulmonary infection, a plug of mucus in an airway, or added strain on the lungs can send COPD patients into respiratory or ventilatory failure. Put simply, the lungs and heart are no longer able to satisfy the body's demand for oxygen, not even while at rest, and the cells asphyxiate.

You may hear the two terms used interchangeably. Although respiratory failure and ventilatory failure may occur in tandem, and the effects of each are largely the same, they stem from two separate, albeit related, malfunctions. *Respiratory failure* refers to a poor exchange of oxygen and carbon dioxide within the lungs. In *ventilatory failure* the problem is one of faulty lung mechanics, which prevents the organs from expanding and deflating properly. This can develop as a direct complication of COPD (a blocked air passage, for instance) or as the cumulative result of years of respiratory deterioration. I've seen the disease leave patients so generally weakened that the effort to breathe simply was too exhausting for them.

The warning signs of respiratory and ventilatory failure aren't readily distinguishable from the familiar symptoms of late-stage COPD or heart disease: dyspnea, wheezing, apprehension, and worsening cyanosis, with the nail beds and lips turning a darker blue. But as the condition progresses, neurological symptoms begin to emerge due to the lack of oxygen to the brain. Patients become drowsy and mentally confused, and may slip into a coma.

Nola Miller kept working throughout her husband's illness, taking time off as needed. As much as she wanted to lie next to him at night, the couple agreed that she should continue to sleep in the bedroom, so that she could get a decent night's rest. One evening as Nola was saying good night, Walter asked plaintively, "When you go to bed, where do you go?"

"That broke my heart," she recalls. "He no longer remembered what the rest of the house looked like. So I drew him a floor plan."

How It Is Managed

For respiratory failure, oxygen therapy is used and possibly mechanical ventilation. For ventilatory failure, mechanical ventilation is used and possibly oxygen therapy.

Cor Pulmonale

As damage to the small blood vessels of the lungs mounts, "the right chamber of the heart has to work harder to pump the blood through the remaining healthy vessels," explains Dr. Edelman. In order to carry out its increased workload, the chamber, or *ventricle*, enlarges and thickens. This is *cor pulmonale*, a serious cardiac condition that can end in right-side heart failure. "You have to remember that most of these people smoke," Dr. Edelman points out. "So more often than not, in addition to their lung disease, they also have intrinsic heart disease."

Symptoms mirror those of congestive heart failure brought on by other causes: profuse perspiration *(diaphoresis)*, labored breathing, palpitations, and chest pain. Eventually the liver and kidneys lag behind on filtering the blood of toxins and waste products, and disposing of them via the urinary tract. In what is called *edema*, the excess fluid saturates body tissues. "Patients typically get lots of swelling in their feet and legs," says Dr. Edelman, "and sometimes higher up in the body."

How It Is Managed

Oxygen Therapy and Bronchodilating Drugs. These remedy the lack of blood oxygen and relieve dyspnea.

Diuretics diminish fluid retention and bring down the swelling.

Digoxin, a member of the *digitalis* family of chemical agents that act upon heart muscle, intensifies the force of the heartbeat. It is prescribed cautiously in COPD patients, particularly those with low blood oxygen levels, as the drug may provoke abnormal cardiac rhythms known as *arrhythmias*. ◄ See "Caring for Someone with Cardiovascular Disease: How Heart Failure Is Treated," page 350.

Nola Miller had been terrified that her husband would choke to death and there would be nothing she could do to help him. Late on the afternoon of November 19, 1992, Walter Miller, sixty-five, died quietly, his wife at his side just as they had wished.

Recommended Reading

The following is available free from the American Lung Association (800-586-4872):

• "Around the Clock with COPD"

The following is available free from the National Heart, Lung and Blood Institute Information Center (301-251-1222):

• "Chronic Obstructive Pulmonary Disease"

-16-

Caring for Someone
with Diabetes

Suzanne Hardy, fifty-three, of Pomona, California, is the mother of four grown daughters. Her second youngest, twenty-eight-year-old Kristin, has been diabetic since the age of two. "From the time she was little," says Suzanne, "I taught her that it was her disease, and she's always tried to take good care of herself. When Kristin was eight, she started giving herself insulin injections. We never made a big deal out of it. It was just part of her routine, and she wasn't treated differently from anybody else."

"Outgoing" and "vivacious" are the words Suzanne uses to describe her daughter, who at twenty-one was just beginning to savor life on her own. Kristin had an apartment and worked as a manager at a supermarket. That's when the truce she appeared to have forged with her diabetes shattered, abruptly ending her independence. "Anything that can happen to a diabetic has happened to her," sighs Suzanne, Kristin's full-time caregiver ever since. "It's been one thing after another."

First it was discovered that the young woman had symptoms of diabetic retinopathy, an eye disease common to diabetics and a major cause of blindness. After a half-dozen laser surgeries, the Hardys were assured that the retinopathy had been apprehended early enough to preserve Kristin's sight. "But it seems as if anytime we're told something isn't going to happen, that's exactly what happens," Suzanne says matter-of-factly.

One day Kristin woke up and couldn't see out of one eye at all; the retina had torn. That entailed a long operation. A few days after she came home from the hospital, she woke up and couldn't see out of the other eye.

Kristin had already developed a complication called gastroparesis, where the stomach doesn't empty properly. She has nausea and vomiting,

391

and is fed through two tubes. She also has a catheter in her chest because she frequently needs IV hydration and medication. For the first couple of years—until they put these tubes in her so I could take care of her at home —I'd say she spent two to three weeks out of every month in the hospital.

My daughter is also quite hypertensive, so that has to be dealt with, too. In addition to monitoring Kristin's blood glucose level every four hours, I have to check her blood pressure and other vital signs around the clock. It doesn't give me much free time. If she's having a good day, I'll go out for an hour or so, but if she's sick or in a lot of pain, or if her blood sugar is too low or too high, then I can't leave.

We've had some real scares. A couple of years ago, when she had one complication right after another, Kristin became so weak, we didn't know if she was going to make it or not.

Diabetes, the fifth most deadly of all diseases, tends to get taken for granted —except, that is, by anyone diagnosed with it. Most folks, it's probably fair to say, fail to appreciate diabetes's potential dangers, regarding it as a disruptive nuisance, perhaps, but largely manageable.

To be sure, the majority of diabetics do learn to live with the illness, so that the dietary restrictions, exercise regimen, blood tests, and, for many, self-administered insulin injections become part of their daily routine. But there is nothing at all routine about diabetes, which casts an ominous shadow over the rest of one's life. Even if carefully controlled, this incurable disease can damage blood vessels and nerves, predisposing its victims to serious long-term complications such as kidney disease, coronary artery disease, and stroke.

According to Dr. Kathleen Wishner, an endocrinologist from Pasadena, California, and past president of the American Diabetes Association, diabetes accounts for far more deaths than the approximately 60,000 recorded by the Centers for Disease Control and Prevention. "We estimate that 178,000 people lose their lives annually to diabetes," she says. "And even that figure is probably too low, because somebody may die of coronary artery disease secondary to diabetes, yet the cause of death will usually be listed as coronary artery disease."

What Is Diabetes?

Diabetes interferes with *metabolism*, the fundamental process by which the body harnesses food for energy and growth. When we eat, the digestive system converts food into chemicals. Sugars and starches *(carbohydrates)* get broken down into *glucose*, a simple sugar and the body's principal source of fuel.

After being absorbed in the stomach, glucose enters the general circulation to be taken up by cells throughout the body. Normally, in response to this influx of "blood sugar," beta cells scattered across the surface of the pancreas secrete *insulin*, the hormone that regulates glucose metabolism. Besides signaling tissue cells to burn blood sugar for energy, insulin directs the liver and the muscles to store excess glucose as *glycogen*. The body can then draw upon these reserves as needed.

Diabetes assumes one of two forms. Approximately one in twenty diabetics has type I disease, the kind afflicting Kristin Hardy. Ordinarily, the body's immune system defends against infection by attacking germs, bacteria, and other foreign invaders. But in type I diabetes, it mistakenly annihilates the beta cells, shutting down insulin production. Therefore, people with this type of diabetes, also referred to as *insulin-dependent diabetes*, must receive daily injections of the hormone. Type I diabetes usually develops around puberty; accordingly, it used to be called juvenile diabetes.

The other 95 percent of diabetics

have type II, formerly known as adult-onset diabetes because it typically arises after age forty and is seen primarily in men and women fifty-five or older. Unlike type I, type II is not an autoimmune disorder but a condition of *insulin resistance:* Although the pancreas secretes insulin, the body's cells do not react to it. Consequently, they aren't able to import glucose from the blood for energy.

Type II disease also goes by the name *non-insulin-dependent diabetes*, which is misleading. For a time it can often be kept in check with diet, exercise, and oral agents that stimulate the pancreas to release insulin. But eventually the drugs no longer compensate for the body's lack of response to the hormone, so that nearly four in ten people with adult-onset diabetes end up on injectable insulin.

Both forms of the disease bring about the same net effects: an unhealthy accumulation of unused glucose in the blood and a body deprived of its customary energy supply and forced to burn its own muscle and fat instead, with potentially devastating results.

Diabetes specialists have yet to pinpoint its causes, but a propensity for the disease appears to be genetically programmed. Someone with a diabetic parent or sibling has a 5 to 15 percent chance of developing it. The risk spirals in proportion to the number of relatives touched by the disease, the severity of their disease, and where they nest on the family tree. Three of Kristin Hardy's paternal uncles were diabetic.

A second factor for type II diabetes is obesity. Four in five people with non-insulin-dependent diabetes are overweight. Most overweight people's bodies do not assimilate glucose adequately; the ability dwindles in relation to how heavy they are. Fortunately for these folks, the pancreas usually manages to step up sufficient production of the hormone to keep their blood sugar reasonably normal. Given the correlation between obesity and insulin insensitivity, weight control becomes an essential component of diabetes management.

Symptoms of Diabetes

The symptoms are as follows:

- Frequent urination
- Ravenous appetite
- Rapid weight loss
- Irritability
- Weakness and fatigue
- Nausea or vomiting
- Tingling or numbness in the feet or hands
- Insatiable thirst
- Frequent infections
- Sores that heal slowly
- Bladder infections
- Drowsiness
- Blurred vision
- Itching

The symptoms tend to emerge suddenly and harshly. But a person can harbor non-insulin-dependent diabetes for years without noticeable symptoms; in fact, half of the 16 million diabetics in the United States don't even realize they have it and thus are not under proper medical care.

Regardless of whether diabetes comes on abruptly or gradually, its earliest symptoms are usually the same. When blood sugar rises to where the kidneys can no longer reabsorb glucose, it spills into the urine. Sugar is an *osmotic* agent, meaning that it pulls water along with it as it travels through the urinary tract and out the body. This explains the incessant urination and unquenchable thirst characteristic of diabetes. The constant intake and outflow of fluid plays a game of tug-of-war with the body's cells, which alternately expand and contract, leading to symptoms such as blurred vision.

How Diabetes Is Diagnosed

Each year, 500,000 to 700,000 people are diagnosed as diabetic. Frequently an acute event brings them to the doctor, or the disease is picked up during a routine checkup. "If you were to appear in a doctor's office complaining of extreme thirst and frequent urination," says Dr. Wishner, "the first thing that might be done is to test the urine for sugar, which normally would not be present." A positive result, while inconclusive, suggests diabetes and indicates the need for more definitive studies:

Two abnormal test results using any of the following three tests *on two separate days* confirm diabetes:

1. The preferred test is a *fasting blood glucose test*, which is performed after the person has fasted for eight hours. Abnormal result: greater than 126 milligrams per deciliter (mg/dL).
2. A *random blood glucose test* can be given at any time and requires no fasting. Abnormal result: greater than 200 milligrams per deciliter.
3. For an *oral glucose tolerance test*, patients drink an extremely sweet glucose solution, to gauge their body's reaction over the next several hours. This test requires ten hours of fasting beforehand. Abnormal result: greater than 200 milligrams per deciliter.

Once a diagnosis has been established, blood is tested for levels of electrolytes and ketones as well as substances called blood urea nitrogen (BUN) and creatinine, to assess kidney function. Urine, too, is examined for traces of protein or albumin, early indicators of kidney disease.

How Diabetes Is Treated

Caring for an ailing person with diabetes usually involves having to manage the disease against the backdrop of one of the serious long-term complications spelled out earlier or an unrelated illness such as cancer, Parkinson's, or Alzheimer's. When a loved one is too fragile to look after himself, it falls to us to maintain the delicate balance between proper eating habits and administering diabetes medication—quite possibly while contending with the effects of the concurrent sickness as well. Without a doubt it's an awesome, complicated responsibility, especially if you've seldom or never had to do this before.

Each day brings the continuing challenge of keeping the blood sugar pendulum from swinging beyond the parameters of safety. Straying too far in either direction can bring on *hyperglycemia* (an elevated concentration of glucose in the blood) or *hypoglycemia* (not enough). *Blood glucose monitoring*, a daily home test described below, yields this crucial feedback from which endocrinologists tailor an individualized treatment plan.

Generally, we want to keep the blood sugar level between 70 and 120 milligrams per deciliter of blood. A diabetic advised to maintain stricter control might be given a narrower range: perhaps 80 to 110 before meals, and no higher than 120 to 140 two hours after eating. Someone else, however, might be able to tolerate an upper boundary of 160 without suffering hyperglycemic symptoms.

Be forewarned: At times you may feel like a contestant in a greased watermelon race. Just when you think you have your loved one's blood glucose level under control, it slips out of your grasp for one reason or another: A cold, emotional stress, or a change in activity level can alter the body's ability to burn glucose. You're aiming at a constantly moving target, so don't get overly discouraged should you miss from time to time.

Because diabetes has no cure, the long-range goal of treatment is to prevent the associated life-threatening and debilitating consequences. A ten-year government-funded study completed in 1993 found that stringent control significantly reduced the rates of kidney, nerve, and eye complications in people with type I diabetes. "We assume the same holds true for type II disease," says Dr. Wishner.

Obviously we're not as concerned that elderly or terminal patients might develop kidney disease down the line.

However, unless our loved one is on the threshold of death, we still try to contain blood sugar levels for the sake of safety and comfort. Hypoglycemia and hyperglycemia, besides being potentially fatal, make patients extremely ill.

"Your control might be a little looser," advises Christine Beebe, director of the diabetes centers at the St. James Hospital and Health Centers in Chicago Heights, Illinois. "So instead of trying to get an average level of, say, 130, maybe we let them hover between 150 and 200 more frequently than we would someone who is thirty years old and healthy otherwise."

Blood Glucose Monitoring

Everyone's blood sugar level fluctuates throughout the day. But with diabetes, the body loses its ability to automatically regulate the amount of glucose in the blood whenever it rises too high or falls too low.

This simple blood test, performed several times a day, reveals patterns in the body's reactions to certain foods, insulin, oral medications, exercise, and so on. Based on the information, your loved one's physician can then fine-tune drug dosages, mealtimes, and food choices in an effort to balance carbohydrate intake and insulin in the body. While the doctor sets the broad parameters on a day-to-day or hour-to-hour basis, patients or care partners make the necessary adjustments themselves; with experience, most come to feel very much at ease doing so.

Until only recently, diabetics measured blood sugar at home by dipping a tablet or chemically treated paper strip in their urine. A change in color indicates the presence of glucose, which tells you the kidneys are having to skim excess sugar from the blood. Monitoring the blood itself affords a far more accurate reading and stands as the preferred testing method. Most diabetics can test themselves, but if you're caring for someone who is very ill, this task may fall to you. Dr. Wishner says that in her experience "most people get over the initial fear of sticking somebody's finger for blood. When we have patients who are homebound, everybody participates in blood glucose monitoring. Even someone who says, 'I could never do that,' soon comes to understand that if he doesn't, the patient will feel worse."

How often do you perform the test? That depends. If your loved one has type I disease, perhaps two to four times daily. People with non-insulin-dependent diabetes may be able to get away with fewer than that. Remember, the purpose of blood glucose monitoring is to problem-solve. The repeated fingersticks sting like the devil, especially if you're old and sick, because your pain tolerance and patience are shredded. So we do this as sparingly as possible. Once we're comfortable with the person's blood sugar levels before and after meals, two tests a day should be sufficient for stable, well-regulated patients.

"Alternate your times," advises Christine Beebe, "so that at the end of the week the doctor can see a couple of blood sugars before breakfast, a couple before lunch, and a couple before dinner. You'll have a daily profile without having to stick the person four to seven times."

How to Test Blood for Glucose.

1. Gather together cotton balls, a pen, a logbook or record sheet, a clock or watch, and your implements for sampling blood and measuring blood glucose:

- A *lancet*, a tiny needle that resembles a pushpin; or a spring-loaded automatic device. One popular brand, the Penlet, is about the same size and shape as a fountain pen.
- A *reagent strip* coated with a substance that makes it change color according to the amount of sugar in the blood. The testing strips can also be read in conjunction with a small electronic *glucose meter*, which displays the result as a digital readout.

INSIDE INFORMATION

The earlobes make excellent locations for obtaining blood; they are highly vascular but not as sensitive as the fingertips. Another point to consider: When people's fingers are pricked again and again, household tasks such as slicing a lemon or washing dishes in detergent can make them feel as if they're on fire.

---

2. Choose any fingertip for drawing blood; for subsequent stickings, use different fingers.

3. Wash your hands with an antibacterial soap and dry them thoroughly. Or wipe rubbing alcohol on the puncture site and let it evaporate.

4. With the person's hand resting against a table or other hard surface, softly squeeze the fingertip between your thumb and forefinger.

- *When using a lancet,* twist off the plastic cap, exposing the pinlike needle. Grasp the blunt end with two fingers of one hand and jab the fingertip or earlobe.

- *When using a mechanical device,* insert a new lancet, place the instrument against the fingertip, and press the button. In an instant the needle pierces the skin.

5. Gently "milk" the finger until a sizable drop forms.

- *When using a reagent strip,* before you begin, remove one strip from the vial, making sure to replace the cap tightly. Hold the strip up to the fingertip and let the blood thoroughly cover the treated square. Don't rub or spread it around. If the sample smears, get another strip.

  Wait one full minute while holding the strip perfectly flat, then lightly wipe off the blood with the cotton ball. Wait another minute. (Note: Times vary somewhat from brand to brand.) Printed on the vial are two columns of colored blocks, each representing a specific level of blood glucose. Compare your strip to the column marked "two minutes."

Which block does it most closely resemble? That is the person's blood-sugar level. If none matches exactly, average the two numbers together. For instance, should the color fall between the blocks labeled 180 mg/dL and 240 mg/dL, your loved one's concentration of blood glucose is roughly 210 mg/dL. Anytime a reading exceeds 240 mg/dL, wait a minute, then hold the strip against the "three minutes" column.

- *When using an electronic meter:* "These machines are so simple to use," says Suzanne Hardy, who has had to test her daughter's blood sugar ever since Kristin lost her eyesight. "You just turn on the power, insert the test strip, place a drop of blood on it, and wait about a minute for the number to appear." Many hospitals and physicians recommend the One Touch II blood glucose meter, which stores the most recent 250 results, including time and date. Still newer devices just now reaching the market will make fingersticks a thing of the past. The patient merely places his finger on the machine and gets his reading.

6. Enter the level in a logbook or record sheet, along with the time of day you performed the test. If your loved one's blood sugar is elevated, jot down anything you believe might have caused this, such as an extra helping of carbohydrates or a fever.

Share this information with the doctor during the patient's quarterly visits, at which a highly sensitive *glycohemoglobin test* is conducted to measure the average blood sugar level over the past thirty to sixty days. When blood glucose drifts into hyperglycemia territory, excess glucose sticks to the hemoglobin molecules that endow blood with its red color and remains there until the blood cells die. It's a valuable test because patients often have a habit of downplaying (subconsciously and otherwise) the number of occasions when their blood sugar spiraled out of control. Like archaeological artifacts, the glycohemoglobins rarely lie, alerting the physician that either treatment or the patient's adherence to treatment could stand improvement.

The Diabetic Diet

Good nutrition benefits all patients, of course, but for the person with diabetes it is a crucial part of treatment. And if he has non-insulin-dependent diabetes, eating the proper foods in the proper amounts is his best protection against precarious peaks or valleys in blood glucose. While overseeing a diabetic's diet is a considerable responsibility, bear in mind that a registered dietitian will have devised the basic eating program. If you're going to be fixing the meals, arrange a consultation with the dietitian, who can explain the specific guidelines for your patient as well as the rudiments of managing diabetes dietetically. Even if you've never so much as glanced at a food nutrition label before, grasping these principles really isn't all that difficult. Essentially, we're concerned with carbohydrates, fats, and protein—the three nutrients in food that furnish energy—and their impact on the diabetic's blood glucose, body weight, and cardiovascular health. Mind you, there is no single "diabetic diet." The exact proportions of carbohydrates, fats, and protein allowed by your loved one's dietitian will hinge on how efficiently the person's body metabolizes each of these substances. But your basic blueprint looks like this:

Finding a Registered Dietitian

Upon a diagnosis of diabetes, the endocrinologist will refer your patient to a dietitian; in fact, most endocrinology practices have one on staff at least part-time.

☎ The American Diabetes Association (800-DIABETES) and the American Dietetic Association (800-366-1655) can also provide you with names of certified professionals in your area.

- Carbohydrates: 50 to 60 percent of a person's total daily calories
- Fats: less than 30 percent
- Protein: 10 to 20 percent

The dietitian will have calculated how many calories your loved one needs per day based on age, weight, and activity level. A *calorie* is the unit used to express food's fuel value. Consume more calories than your body can burn, and the balance is stored as fat.

Let's suppose the dietitian has recommended your patient consume 2,000 calories per day. Of that total:

- 1,000 to 1,200 calories (50 to 60 percent of 2,000) should come from carbohydrates.

  * *Since 1 gram of carbohydrate yields 4 calories, that's 250 to 300 grams.*

- Fewer than 600 calories (30 percent of 2,000) should come from fats.

  * *Since 1 gram of fat yields 9 calories, that's 67 grams.*

- 200 to 400 calories (10 to 20 percent of 2,000) should come from protein.

  * *Since 1 gram of protein yields 4 calories, that's 50 to 80 grams.*

Protein. "There has been a revolution in the way we look at the diabetes diet," says Christine Beebe. Years ago the emphasis was on protein, which comes from meat, poultry, fish, dairy products, eggs, peas, and dried beans. In order to keep blood sugar normalized, "we felt we had to give protein at every meal and snack."

It turns out that protein has relatively little effect on blood glucose unless a diabetic eats large quantities in one sitting. Devouring a seven-ounce steak at dinner, for instance, is apt to send blood sugar into the stratosphere. Stick to serving smaller portions—three or four ounces—and you won't have to concern yourself with protein. According to Beebe, "Very seldom do people eat more than the daily maximum allotment" of 10 to 20 percent. Another advantage of moderate protein intake is that it may delay the progression of diabetic kidney disease.

Fats. Fats have an indirect bearing on blood glucose in that a fat-heavy diet can contribute to obesity. Excessive body weight, you'll recall, is associated with insulin insensitivity, which hampers cells from using glucose properly and leads to a buildup of sugar in the blood. Obesity also abets chronically high blood pressure, or *hypertension*, a major cause of cardiovascular disease, cerebrovascular stroke, and kidney disease. When a person is extremely ill, however, we banish all thoughts about weight control and set our sights strictly on balancing blood sugar.

More important than the quantity of fat is the type. *Saturated* fat—from animal meat, butter, lard, shortening, and palm and coconut oils—raises the level of *cholesterol*, a fatlike substance, in the blood. People with high blood cholesterol are more likely to develop *atherosclerosis*, in which fatty deposits called *plaque* clog the arteries feeding the heart and brain. If the blockage obstructs blood from reaching these organs, a heart attack or stroke occurs. ◄ *See chapter 13, "Caring for Someone with Cardiovascular Disease"; chapter 14, "Caring for Someone with Cerebro-*

vascular Stroke or Traumatic Brain Injury."

Diabetes predisposes patients to atherosclerosis, although the exact link between the two is not known. Consequently, we want to restrict saturated fat to 10 percent. Instead, serve products containing *polyunsaturated* or *monounsaturated* fat, both of which are found in nuts and vegetable oils and can help lower blood cholesterol. Polyunsaturated fat is found in corn, sunflower, safflower, and soybean oils. Monounsaturated fat is found in canola, olive, and peanut oils.

Carbohydrates. Carbohydrate-laden foods make up at least half a diabetic's diet and are the ones we focus on most. In fact, we suggest forgetting about fats and protein initially, until you've gotten the hang of maintaining normal blood glucose levels by parceling out carbs appropriately throughout the day.

"Then you can do more fine-tuning," suggests Christine Beebe. "For instance, maybe we see the person's blood cholesterol is still elevated, so we further restrict fats." The Centers for Disease Control recommends that daily cholesterol consumption not exceed 300 milligrams. "You have to take it in steps."

Why the accent on carbohydrates? Because the body converts sugars and starches to glucose. In the past, dietitians honed in primarily on sugar, which was considered to be to high blood glucose what pepper is to sneezing. But the body makes no distinction between the two. As Beebe explains, "The old theory was that sugar changed into glucose molecules more rapidly than starch and therefore would give you a very high blood sugar response, whereas bread, rice, and potatoes wouldn't. We now know it's the total quantity of carbohydrate that makes a difference, regardless of where it comes from."

Formulating the Diet

In developing an individualized meal plan, dietitians usually start by evaluating the patient's current eating habits. "Most older people are pretty well set in their ways as to what foods they like," says Beebe. "So we spread those out over the course of the day based on how to get the best blood sugar responses." Blood glucose testing will indicate whether carbohydrates need to be added or deducted, and when. "If someone is eating 90 grams of carbs at lunch and we consistently see high blood sugars two hours later," Beebe explains, "I might suggest pulling a few grams from lunch and putting them elsewhere."

For diabetics who do not need supplementary insulin, eating about the same quantity of food around the same time each day helps stabilize their blood sugar level. Once you've hit upon the volume of carbs your loved one can tolerate at each meal and snack without trespassing into hyperglycemia, stay within that carbohydrate budget.

Insulin-dependent patients have more flexibility because they can adjust the dosage of insulin to counterbalance a carb-heavy meal. On the other hand, mealtimes must conform to their insulin schedule to ensure that their bodies have enough insulin to handle the influx of glucose.

Based on our 2,000 calorie diet, let's look at where those carbohydrates might fall. Most people are least tolerant of starches and sugars in the morning, when the body produces various hormones that antagonize, or work against, insulin. Of the three main meals, breakfast will likely feature the fewest carbs. Out of our 250 total grams for the day, 60 might be allocated for breakfast, 75 for lunch, and 90 for dinner, with the remaining 25 going toward a snack or two.

Counting Carbohydrates: Gauging Grams or Using the Exchange Lists. How do you know the nutritional

contents of the foods you're serving? One way is to consult one of the many nutrition guides—available in almost any bookstore—that list the amounts of carbohydrates, fats, and so on found in a wide range of packaged and unpackaged foods, and then tally up the totals.

Or you can refer to "Exchange Lists for Meal Planning," a booklet published jointly by the American Diabetes Association and the American Dietetic Association. It is available from either organization for $1.50. The exchange lists group together foods with nearly identical values of carbs, fats, protein, and calories *per serving* (more about this in a moment), so you can trade any item for another without having to get out a calculator.

There's the Fat Group, the Meat and Meat Substitute Group, and the Carbohydrate Group, which is subdivided into "starch," "fruit," "milk," "other carbohydrates," and "vegetables." You're not going to see significant swings in blood sugar from veggies. Besides the fact that they're low in carbs, most folks don't eat them in large volumes anyway, so serve them freely.

To illustrate how to use the exchange lists, let's prepare a dinner of chicken, rice, vegetable, bread, and beverage. Remember, the dietitian has given us 90 grams of carbs to "spend" as well as approximately 35 grams of protein, 25 grams of fat, and 700 calories. While you don't have to worry about slightly overshooting your protein target, with carbohydrates we want to come within roughly 3 grams of a bull's-eye.

What if Dad wants pasta instead of rice? Not a problem. You'll find both on the starch list, along with nearly six dozen other foods that contain 15 grams of carbohydrate, 3 grams of protein, 0 to 1 gram of fat, and 80 calories. However, the portion sizes vary: One-third cup of rice has the same nutrients as one-half cup of pasta. Since we can afford 30 grams of carbohydrate from grains at this evening's meal, Dad can enjoy a full cup of pasta as opposed to

TABLE 16.1

Food	Carbohydrates (grams)	Protein (grams)	Fat (grams)	Calories
Lean white-meat chicken with skin (4 ounces)	0	28	12	220
Rice (²/₃ cup)	30	6	0–2	160
Whole wheat bread (1 slice)	15	3	0–1	80
Steamed broccoli (1 cup)	10	4	0	50
Apple juice (1 cup)	30	0	0	120
Totals	85	41	15	630

two-thirds of a cup of rice, or double the "starch exchange" listed.

Substitutions are by no means limited to the same food group, which opens up countless variations in meal planning. Dad may announce that there's nothing he'd like more than ice cream for dessert. According to the "other carbohydrates" list, half a cup contains 15 grams of carbohydrate and therefore can be exchanged for any starch. So either forgo the slice of bread or serve half as much pasta, and you're still within dinner's total allowance of 90 carbs.

"You can work in whatever a person wants," Christine Beebe emphasizes. "What really irritates many people in my profession is someone telling a seriously ill elderly patient, 'You can't have ice cream! You have diabetes!' If the primary goal is to keep people nourished, you give them whatever they want, especially elderly patients. It's not that difficult," she says of managing a diabetic patient's eating habits, "as long as you don't make it complicated."

Constant Carbohydrates: Foods for Sick Days. A patient with diabetes needs to follow her regular diet and meal timetable even on days when she doesn't feel well. But what if someone is so sick that the mere thought of eating makes her queasy, or she throws up the little food she does eat? Then we switch to soft foods and liquids high in the carbohydrates necessary for

avoiding treacherously low blood sugar. Each item below contains 15 grams.

- Fruit juice: ⅓ to ½ cup
- Fruit-flavored drinks: ½ cup
- Nondiet soda: ½ cup
- Regular Jell-O: ½ cup
- Popsicle: ½ twin
- Sherbet: ¼ cup
- Hot cereal: ½ cup, cooked
- Milk: 1 cup
- Thin soups (vegetable, chicken noodle): ½ cup
- Thick soups (cream of mushroom, tomato): ½ cup
- Vanilla ice cream: ½ cup
- Sugar-free pudding: ½ cup
- Regular pudding: ¼ cup
- Macaroni, rice, noodles, mashed potatoes: ½ cup, cooked

Not only are these easier to keep down than solids, but they convert to glucose more rapidly. Soft or liquid carbs are also ideal for anyone who has difficulty swallowing.

Provided that your loved one can ingest something solid, try crackers or toast, which boast ample carbs but little fat. Like liquids, low-fat foods don't sit in the stomach, leaving patients feeling uncomfortably full. You can get 15 grams of carb from one slice of toast, three graham crackers, or six salted crackers.

A general guideline for aiding digestion and perking up the appetite is to offer patients smaller, more frequent meals instead of the customary three. While this applies to diabetics, it does complicate matters somewhat. You'll have to rely on blood glucose readings to guide you in adjusting insulin dosages as well as in selecting the *type* of insulin (short-acting, rapid-acting, intermediate-acting, long-acting) best suited to the modified eating pattern. "If you're serving six small meals a day," Christine Beebe suggests, "it's sometimes best to go with a combination: intermediate-acting, to cover the between-meal periods, *and* short-acting." Raise this matter with your patient's endocrinologist or diabetes counselor.

Exercise

The enduring rewards of daily physical activity parallel those gained from a high-carbohydrate, low-fat diet: regulation of weight, blood pressure, and blood cholesterol. Since muscles burn more fuel when put to work, exercise also delivers an immediate benefit by lowering blood sugar. At the same time, the body disperses extra glucose and fats to its cells for energy, so engaging in rigorous activity before insulin or oral medications have had time to take effect causes blood sugar to rise. Conversely, physical exertion on an empty stomach sends the level plummeting. Just as diabetics must eat according to a schedule, they need to plan strenuous activity around meals and medication.

By "exercise," obviously we don't mean that older people or the seriously ill should huff and puff along with Cindy Crawford or Jake. Twenty-minute walks several times a week are ideal. But even patients confined to bed or a wheelchair can be shown simple movements that will help keep blood sugar in check. Whatever the regimen, it should always be established by the physician.

Oral Agents

Three in four people with adult-onset diabetes start out on oral *hypoglycemic agents* such as chlorpropamide (brand name: Diabinese) and tolbutamide (Orinase), which cue the pancreas to secrete more insulin. Rarely is this a permanent solution: Six in seven diabetics receiving diabetes pills no longer respond to the medication within ten years and have to be placed on insulin.

Insulin

Until the discovery of insulin in 1921, people with diabetes had but weeks or months to live. Three-quarters of a century later, injecting it under the fat in the skin, or *subcutaneously*, remains the only method of delivering insulin to the bloodstream, although experts predict that in the not too distant future, insulin will be available both in pill form and as a nasal spray.

There are approximately thirty brands of commercially prepared insulin, derived from beef or pork pancreas, or genetically engineered to duplicate the structure of human insulin. As you can see from Table 16.2, the four main groups of insulin vary drastically in terms of the time each takes to begin working (onset), reach its maximum effect (peak), and fade from the circulation (duration). The reason for the wide variances in time is that diabetics absorb and utilize insulin in their own way —for that matter, a patient may respond differently to the same dosage at different times.

TABLE 16.2
Types of Insulin

Type	Onset	Peak	Duration
Short-acting (regular)	30 minutes	2 to 4 hours	4 to 8 hours
Rapid-acting (Humalog)	1 hour	3 hours	6 hours
Intermediate-acting (NPH and Lente)	4 to 6 hours	4 to 14 hours	14 to 24 hours
Long-acting (Ultralente)	6 to 14 hours	14 to 24 hours	20 to 36 hours

Our objective is to synchronize the injection with digestion so that the insulin enters the bloodstream around the same time as glucose from broken-down food. Pinpointing the correct moment comes through experience and the results of repeated blood glucose testing.

Conventional therapy calls for two injections a day, typically one before breakfast and one prior to dinner. But the growing trend, particularly for type I disease, is to administer three or four shots of short-acting insulin with the aim of keeping the blood sugar level as close to the desired range as possible. While disruptive—you have to test blood glucose four or more times a day and adjust dosages, food intake, and activity levels on the basis of the results—intensive therapy affords more freedom when it comes to eating and exercise. "Because the insulin doesn't last all day," explains Christine Beebe, "patients don't have to eat or exercise at a specific time."

An alternative to repeated injections is an *insulin infusion pump*, a battery-operated device that looks like a pocket calculator and can be clipped to a belt loop. The pump delivers a continuous low rate *(basal rate)* of regular insulin by way of a plastic tube attached to a needle inserted beneath the skin in the abdomen and taped in place. Patients or caregivers can manually dispense extra boosts of insulin *(bolus doses)* prior to eating. The pump is not without drawbacks: It is uncomfortable to wear during sleep and cannot be taken into the shower or bath.

Whether given via pump or syringe, intensive insulin therapy is highly involved and hikes the risk of severe hypoglycemic reactions. For a seriously ill elderly person, most diabetes specialists would probably feel that the disadvantages outweigh the benefits and recommend the standard morning and evening shots, often a *mixed-dose* regimen that combines fast-acting insulin with one of the longer-lasting types. To spare patients twice the number of injections, we administer these together.

NPH and regular insulins come pre-mixed in 70/30 or 50/50 ratios. While convenient, obviously you cannot modify one amount without affecting the other. Type I diabetics are often on what's called a sliding scale, their dosages contingent on their blood sugar level. Kristin Hardy's dosages fluctuate so frequently, says her mother, "it's very confusing even to nurses who have worked around diabetics." If premixed solutions aren't practical, we mix the insulins ourselves, either ahead of time or just prior to injection. Consistency is important, so stay with whichever procedure the doctor recommends.

How to Mix Insulins in a Syringe.

1. Wash your hands with antibacterial soap.

2. Start with the long-acting insulin. Use an alcohol swab to clean the vial's rubber stopper.

3. Following the calibrations on the syringe's clear barrel, pull back the plunger to the prescribed number of in-

sulin *units*. Insulin is a potent drug, and so measurements must be painstakingly precise. Most insulin manufactured in the United States is U-100 concentration, meaning it consists of 100 units of insulin per milliliter (mL) or cubic centimeter (cc) of solution.

4. With the needle inserted in the top of the bottle—but not making contact with the solution itself—inject air by pushing down on the plunger.

5. Pull out the syringe.

6. Repeat steps 2, 3, and 4 with the bottle of regular insulin. *Then leave the needle in the vial.*

7. Invert both the vial and the syringe and withdraw the prescribed units of regular insulin.

8. Once again, clean the top of the longer-acting insulin bottle.

9. Turn the vial and syringe upside down and extract the number of units needed to complete the *total* dosage. Example: If the syringe contains 20 units of regular insulin and you need 10 units of longer-acting insulin, draw the plunger back to 30 units.

10. Remove the needle and lay it down so that it does not touch anything.

Tips on Injecting Insulin. Needles are so sharp nowadays that insulin shots rarely hurt. As a matter of fact, patients often find the fingersticks for blood glucose testing far more irritating. An insulin injection is like administering any other fluid subcutaneously, a technique we describe in chapter 3, "The Everyday Angel's Cram Course in Essential Nursing Skills." There are, however, some points unique to giving insulin that you should know:

◆ *Match insulin strength with syringe size.* If you're injecting U-100 insulin, make sure the calibrations correspond accordingly.

◆ *Don't inject cold insulin.* Insulin manufacturers advise refrigerating insulin, but cold insulin can make shots more painful. Warm up the vial by gently rolling it between your palms be-

fore filling the syringe. Or keep your current bottle at room temperature. If you purchase more than one vial at a time, store these in the fridge until you're ready to use them.

◆ *Extreme temperatures ruin insulin.* The American Diabetes Association warns never to store insulin at temperatures below 36 degrees or above 86 degrees; likewise, don't put the bottle in the freezer or in direct sunlight.

◆ *Examine the vial before using.* Regular insulin should appear perfectly clear; intermediate insulins, cloudy. Should you notice floating pieces, clumps, or crystals in the bottle, return it to your pharmacy. Similarly, check the expiration date: After having been open for more than thirty days, insulin may lose its potency.

◆ *Rotate injection sites.* Vary the spots on the body where you give injections. For one thing, this prevents the formation of unsightly lumps or small "dents" in the skin *(lipodystrophy)*; though harmless, these interfere with the action of insulin. Here are some of your most accessible targets: the outer area of the upper arms; just above and below the waist, but not within a two-inch circumference of the navel; the upper buttocks, just behind the hip bone; and the front of the thigh, midway to the outer side, four inches below the top of the thigh to four inches above the knee.

For optimum results, once you've settled on a general area for each shot—perhaps the stomach for the morning injection and an arm for the evening injection—stay within that region. This will help ensure consistency in the timing and action of the insulin.

◆ *Never administer a different type of insulin* unless prescribed by your loved one's doctor.

◀ *See "Injections," page 146.*

> **Diabetes and Infection:**
> **A Vicious Cycle**
>
> Poorly controlled diabetes lowers the body's natural resistance against infection, which in turn exacerbates diabetes.

Acute Complications of Diabetes

Even with impeccable management, Dr. Wishner points out, "patients find their blood sugar frequently rises above normal." A cold or infection is apt to set off hyperglycemia because the body responds to fever by accelerating metabolism and discharging its stockpiles of glucose into the bloodstream. By the same token, anger, fear, or any intense emotion that unleashes *adrenaline* may exert a similar effect, as the potent hormone induces the liver to distribute glucose for added energy. "If Kristin just gets nervous," Suzanne Hardy says, "it can make her blood sugar go up."

At levels above 180, a person may experience symptoms such as those below, as well as the persistent thirst and urination diabetics know so well.

- Fatigue
- Blurred vision
- Nausea or vomiting
- Appetite loss
- Abdominal pain
- Dehydration
- Rapid breathing
- Dizziness
- Confusion, disorientation
- A feeling of panic
- Loss of consciousness
- Bed-wetting at night

Whereas hypoglycemia steals up suddenly, hyperglycemia often emerges over a period of hours or days so that a person may become depleted of fluid and life-sustaining electrically charged particles in the blood *(electrolytes)* from urinating so frequently. Losing electrolytes such as magnesium and potassium triggers a number of serious bodily disturbances, among them diminished reflexes, convulsions, and irregular heartbeats known as *cardiac arrhythmias.*

How It Is Managed

Administering oral hypoglycemics or a dose of fast-acting insulin will usually lower blood sugar to an acceptable level, preempting a major crisis. Never assume that a diabetic doesn't need his medication just because he's not eating. Naturally, with the patient ingesting fewer carbohydrates, you cut down the amount of insulin accordingly. Christine Beebe explains: "If the person normally eats 75 grams of carbs at lunch and takes six units of insulin to cover that, and now there's no way he can keep down more than 45 grams, you might reduce the dosage to four units. Otherwise he's going to get low blood sugar from too much insulin."

Call the Doctor or Go to the Emergency Room When:

- the blood glucose remains at 240 or higher;
- the person can't keep food or liquids down after more than 6 hours. The physician may recommend taking her to a hospital emergency room, where fluid and electrolytes will be restored intravenously;
- the person loses 5 pounds or more;
- the person's temperature exceeds 101 degrees Fahrenheit;
- the person has severe diarrhea;
- the person has difficulty catching her breath or seems disoriented, lethargic, or inordinately drowsy.

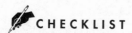

CHECKLIST

When a Person with Diabetes Is Ill

❑ Test blood sugar every 4 hours or before each meal.

❑ Hydrate! Hydrate! Hydrate! Preventing dehydration is a prime concern with any patient but particularly someone with elevated blood sugar. During bouts of hyperglycemia and illness, see to it that your loved one drinks at least half a cup to three-quarters of a cup of water, decaffeinated herbal tea, or sugar-free soda every 30 to 60 minutes.

❑ If your loved one is ambulatory, weigh him once a day.

❑ Take his temperature every morning and evening.

❑ Every 4 to 6 hours, monitor for signs of labored breathing, excessive drowsiness, or fuzzy-headedness.

❑ Write down all the above information for the person's physician.

Diabetic Ketoacidosis/ Hyperglycemic Hyperosmolar Nonketotic Coma

Hyperglycemia can culminate in either of these critical coma-inducing conditions. "Ketoacidosis," Dr. Wishner explains, "occurs almost exclusively in type I diabetes when insulin is not available to assist in utilizing sugar for energy and the body must burn fat instead." Fat metabolism in the liver yields three by-products called *ketone bodies*, two of which are acids. The liver cannot break down the ketones, so it circulates them to other tissues, which convert the bodies to a usable form of fuel.

One of insulin's vital tasks is to limit ketone production. In its absence, the liver churns them out indiscriminately, flooding the bloodstream with toxic quantities. The ensuing upsurge in acid disrupts the crucial balance between acidity and alkalinity of body fluids. Unless the chemical equilibrium is restored by administering insulin and fluids, headache and weakness may give way to stupor, unconsciousness, coma, and ultimately death.

"Ketoacidosis is particularly life-threatening because oftentimes its symptoms are confused with the flu," Dr. Wishner points out, "delaying the diagnosis of a diabetic condition." One way to detect ketoacidosis is to sniff the person's breath, which will often have a sweet, fruity smell. "Tutti-frutti breath," doctors and nurses call this. Were it not for the fact that Kristin Hardy's father had three diabetic brothers and instantly recognized the aroma, the two-year-old's diabetes might have gone undiscovered until it was too late.

"We almost lost her then," Suzanne remembers. "Kristin's blood sugar was so high it was completely off the charts, and she was in a coma. The doctors thought she had mumps or encephalitis. When her daddy leaned over the crib to kiss her, he could smell the ketones on her breath. He grabbed the pediatrician and asked if he had checked for diabetes, which, despite the family history, he had not. Needless to say, my husband was *very* upset."

Hyperglycemic hyperosmolar nonketotic coma (HHNK), another metabolic disorder capable of rendering patients comatose, sends blood glucose soaring to levels of 600, 800, and beyond, but without producing ketoacidosis. Two potential symptoms mirror those of a stroke: paralysis on one side of the body *(hemiplegia)* and impairments of communication and comprehension, known collectively as *aphasia*. Hallucinations, seizures, and sensory deficits such as partial blindness number among its other effects.

When an elderly person has adult-onset diabetes, it's important to be aware of these signs. HHNK, fatal in ap-

---

INSIDE INFORMATION

Testing your loved one's urine for excess ketones *(ketonuria)* can alert you to impending ketoacidosis before severe symptoms appear. According to the Centers for Disease Control and Prevention, whenever someone with diabetes becomes acutely ill from hyperglycemia or has a blood glucose reading of 240 or more, run the test every 4 hours or each time he urinates.

It's simple to do. Ketostix, available in most pharmacies, are chemically impregnated pads mounted on polystyrene sticks. Either catch the sample in a cup and dip in a stick or hold it directly in the stream of urine. Wait 40 seconds, then compare it against the accompanying color chart. A change from beige to 1 of 5 positive color blocks tells you the ketone level, from a trace amount (5 mg/dL) to a large amount (160 mg/dL). Share any positive result with the doctor promptly.

---

proximately half of all cases (as compared to fewer than one in twenty for ketoacidosis), accosts mostly non-insulin-dependent diabetics sixty and older. While the high mortality rate is due in part to the advanced average age of those who develop the disorder, many times its symptoms go unheeded.

How It Is Managed

Both diabetic ketoacidosis and hyperglycemic hyperosmolar nonketotic coma should be considered critical situations. Emergency room treatment consists of insulin therapy, to bring down blood glucose, and replacing lost fluids and minerals intravenously.

Our experience with balancing blood sugar and restoring fluids for this particular person will dictate whether or not we try to intervene or proceed straight to the hospital. A seasoned care partner has probably been here before and has some sense of whether or not she's getting a handle on the situation. But anyone new to this shouldn't hesitate to contact the doctor. And if he isn't available *immediately*, dial 911 or bring your loved one to the nearest ER. Although ketoacidosis builds up slowly, patients can barrel downhill too quickly to try winging it.

Hypoglycemia

While diabetes is by definition a condition of elevated blood sugar, the opposite problem can crop up. You may hear hypoglycemia referred to as an *insulin reaction.* Indeed, administering too high a dosage in relation to the amount of food consumed can push blood sugar below 60, the line dividing hypoglycemia and a normal blood glucose level. But then, so can missing a meal, eating later than scheduled, or unplanned demanding exercise. Early signs of abnormally low blood sugar—headache, trembling, drowsiness, heavy sweating, heart palpitations, hunger pangs, nausea, a tingling sensation, vision impairment—sound frightening but are actually easily reversed with prompt and proper care.

How It Is Managed

Diabetics often feel a hypoglycemic attack coming on. *If your loved one is conscious and able to swallow,* immediately give her one of the fast-acting sugars listed below, followed by a complex carbohydrate like a piece of bread.

- ½ cup of fruit juice or *non-diet* soda
- 3 teaspoons of sugar, honey, or grape jam
- 5 Lifesavers mints, 6 jellybeans, or 10 gumdrops

Each equals roughly 10 to 15 grams of sugar. In fifteen minutes, measure the blood glucose again. Have the person eat another 10 to 15 grams of sugar every quarter hour until her level returns to at least 70. Keep these items on hand at all times; in fact, it's a good idea to get into the habit of stocking up whenever you go grocery shopping so you're never caught short. At drastically low levels, your patient may need oral glucose, which comes in tablet, gelatin capsule, and liquid forms. If the person is not housebound, be sure she carries some with her wherever she goes.

A situation where the patient cannot swallow calls for injecting 1 milligram of *glucagon*, a hormone that prompts the liver to release stored glucose. This can be done subcutaneously or directly into a muscle (*intramuscularly*) anywhere on the body. Since he may be too disoriented to wield a hypodermic needle himself, you may have to assume this responsibility.

Or try a packet of glucose gel, the kind that comes in first-aid kits. You see long-distance runners pop them in their mouths routinely during marathons to ward off nausea. Simply squeeze the gel onto a finger and rub it under the person's tongue or between their cheek and gum, where it will be absorbed into the body.

Diabetics can tolerate hypoglycemia briefly without adverse effects, but should the blood sugar level linger below 60 for too long, depriving brain cells of glucose, a host of serious symptoms may arise: difficulty awakening, confusion, combative behavior, hallucinations, and convulsions. Eventually the person lapses into a deep coma and can die.

"This can happen very quickly," notes Suzanne Hardy, "and you have to act very quickly." In the past, she has given her daughter intravenous injections of sterile 50 percent glucose, a measure usually reserved for severe cases. However, Kristin, with her array of medical problems, has a permanent catheter implanted in a large vein in her chest. Suzanne inserts the needle into the opening of the plastic tube. Unless the person you're caring for has a similar port, a physician or nurse will be administering glucose and all other intravenous medications.

Call the Doctor or Go to the Emergency Room When:

- symptoms don't improve noticeably *after the first snack;*
- you've had to inject glucagon, since blood glucose levels can drop abruptly again thirty minutes to two hours later;
- your loved one experiences a series of attacks over several days or two or more within twenty-four hours. The physician needs to determine what's causing the hypoglycemia; lowering the dosage of insulin or diabetes pills sometimes solves the problem.

As with dangerously high blood glucose, a caregiver who has dealt with hypoglycemic attacks before can roll with it a bit, tweaking the patient with sugar and watching for symptoms to relent. When you've never faced this before, you can give your loved one something with sugar and take her straight to the emergency room.

Kristin's condition is "brittle," meaning that some days her glucose level swerves wildly from one extreme to the other. "I have seen her with a 30 blood sugar in the morning," says Suzanne, "where she's needed intravenous glucose, and then watched it go as high as 800 by nighttime."

Long-Term Complications of Diabetes

Other serious complications may beset a diabetic as a result of associated injuries to nerves and blood vessels. Doctors divide diabetes-related vascular disorders into two categories. *Microvascular disease*, a factor in serious ailments of the kidneys, eyes, and nerves, causes the body's small blood vessels to thicken, weaken, and ultimately leak, slowing circulation. *Macrovascular disease*, which affects veins and arteries, can culminate in heart attack, stroke, and impaired blood flow to the lower limbs. Although endocrinologists don't fully understand why these complications frequently accompany diabetes, "all theories," says Dr. Wishner, "point to the effects of high blood sugar."

Then we have the manifold health problems attributable to *diabetic neuropathy*, or nerve disease, of the *peripheral* nerves in the extremities and the *autonomic* nerves that govern mostly internal organs of the cardiovascular, gastrointestinal, and urogenital systems.

Peripheral Neuropathy

Diabetic neuropathy of the legs, feet, and fingertips seldom brings about intense pain; rather, patients usually describe a tingling feeling. More common still is the reverse: numbness that comes on furtively.

How It Is Managed

With conscientious blood glucose management, foot and leg pain usually subsides on its own. However, three categories of medication are available: capsaicin (brand name: Zostrix), a topical analgesic cream; anticonvulsants; and tricyclic antidepressants. Antidepressants? Yes, because people with neuropathies may become depressed. It's unclear whether this is a direct effect of the neuropathy or a psychological response to the discomfort, but treatment focuses on relieving both the pain and the depression. ◄ *See "Fundamentals of Pain Management," page 154.*

Foot Ulcers

When peripheral neuropathy and peripheral vascular disease operate in tandem, a diabetic can find himself with a gaping foot ulcer. What typically happens is, a seemingly innocuous sore or blister goes unnoticed due to the lack of sensation in the lower limbs. This, coupled with the deficient blood flow to the area, allows the wound to fester. Should gangrene or other severe infections set in, the patient faces the prospect of amputation. Diabetics account for half of the 100,000 nontraumatic amputations performed each year.

Dr. Wishner recalls one case of diabetic foot ulcers that, she says, "remains burned in my memory." A patient came in for a routine checkup. "When we looked at his foot, we found a huge ulcer on the bottom of it. We took an X ray and saw that he had a *sewing needle* embedded in his foot. Who knows how long it had been there, yet he couldn't feel it."

Preventive Management

Tending to an ailing person with diabetes calls for devoting special attention to the feet. Inspect them each day for blisters, cracks, cuts, or scratches, remembering to check soles, heels, and between the toes. If your loved one is able to do this herself, give her an unbreakable hand mirror.

Other steps to proper foot care:

Wash the feet each day in warm water (90 to 95 degrees), but don't let them soak, which can dry out the skin and create a breeding ground for infection. Afterward, dry thoroughly, once again taking care not to overlook the toes, for moisture invites germs.

If the skin is dry, gently massage in a thin coat of moisturizer or lanolin-based foot cream. ◄ *See "Skin Care," page 116.*

We don't want a ragged toenail to inadvertently break the skin. The best time to trim toenails is after bathing and drying the feet, when the nails are softer. Cut straight across, following its contour, then smooth the corners with an emery board. If the person has thick, brittle toenails, leave the job to a doctor, nurse, or podiatrist. The same holds true for removing corns and calluses. Let a podiatrist or nurse show you how to manage them properly with a pumice stone, emery board, or callus file. Don't use over-the-counter corn plasters or liquid corn or callus removers.

To keep the person's feet warm at night, slip on a pair of socks made of cotton, which help keep feet dry. Folks plagued by numbness should *never* be tucked in with a hot-water bottle or heating pad: They may wake up with a nasty burn and not even realize it.

Remind your loved one not to cross her legs; doing so can further compress nerves and blood vessels. Poor circulation in the lower extremities predisposes a person to *dependent edema*, characterized by fluid retention and swelling, and to clotting. As a precaution, encourage him to get into the habit of elevating his feet whenever seated or lying down.

Anyone with insensitive feet should have them examined by a physician at least four times a year. For convenience sake, perhaps this can be done at the same time as the quarterly glycohemoglobin tests.

Most important of all: Insist your patient wear shoes *and* socks whenever he's out of bed. "After twenty years, I still have to remind Kristin at least once a day to put something on her feet," says Suzanne Hardy. "She'll say, 'Oh, Mom, I'm just getting up to go to the bathroom.' But that's all it takes for her to step on something."

Before shoes are put on, feel inside for pebbles and other foreign objects, nail points, torn linings—anything that could conceivably injure the feet. When buying a new pair, make sure the person feels comfortable in them; too snug or too loose a fit can raise blisters. Also, let your loved one break in new shoes by wearing them around the house a few hours at a time for several days.

Drug therapy may be used to improve circulation to the legs and feet, thereby promoting faster healing. The doctor may prescribe a blood-thinning medica-

tion, Trental, known generically as pentoxifylline.

How It Is Managed

Should a foot ulcer develop, therapy consists of *antibiotic medications*, to stem infection, and seeing to it that the patient keeps his weight off the wound until it mends. Sometimes total bed rest may be necessary.

Foot ulcers can be mighty stubborn, often coming back in the same spot. Your loved one's physician may recommend a pair of extra-deep shoes designed to redistribute weight. In one study of patients who had suffered foot ulcers, only one in five who wore special shoes experienced a recurrence, as compared to four in five who resumed wearing their street shoes. Medicare helps pay for one pair of therapeutic shoes and orthotic inserts per year for anyone with severe diabetic foot disease. If other treatment methods fail, the physician may consider vascular surgery to improve circulation to the damaged area.

Gastroparesis

Peristalsis is the continuous wavelike action of digestive-tract muscles as they push food from the stomach to the small intestine and beyond while at the same time churning, liquefying, and mixing it with digestive juices. In gastroparesis, a form of autonomic neuropathy, damage to the nerves that spontaneously set the contractions in motion prevents them from transmitting impulses properly. Food lingers in the stomach, giving rise to symptoms such as nausea and vomiting, bloating, abdominal pain, persistent fullness, and a lack of appetite. The delayed digestion can also create problems when trying to time insulin injections following meals.

Gastroparesis may occur sporadically, coming on during episodes of elevated blood glucose and then subsiding once the level is brought under control.

For people who go for long periods of time with high blood sugar, the condition often turns chronic, as in Kristin Hardy's case.

"She gets hungry and wants to eat," says her mother, "then ten minutes later she'll say, 'I wish I hadn't done that,' and end up throwing up. If she throws up twice in one day, she knows that she can't have anything by mouth other than ice chips for the rest of the day." When the symptoms are especially severe, Suzanne bypasses the stomach and feeds her daughter liquids through a "J" tube permanently implanted in the *jejunum*, the middle portion of the small intestine. According to Dr. Wishner, few diabetics require tube feedings.

How It Is Managed

Two drugs, metoclopramide (brand name: Reglan) and cisapride (Propulsid), have been found to strengthen peristalsis and relieve nausea, though their effectiveness wanes over time. During bouts of gastroparesis, serve your patient several small meals throughout the day and stay away from high-fat foods. "We've tried everything," Suzanne sighs. "It just doesn't work. Kristin is nauseous most of the time and is never entirely pain free despite fairly regular pain medication." ◀ *See "Managing Pain," page 152; "Indigestion and Nausea," page 162; and "Tube Feedings and Total Parenteral Nutrition (TPN)," page 166.*

Constipation

As with gastroparesis, if diabetic neuropathy dulls the nerves that activate peristalsis in the colon, a patient's bowels grow sluggish. "It's a constant problem," says Suzanne. "We always have to be careful not to let Kristin get too backed up."

How It Is Managed

Neuropathy-related constipation can be difficult to treat. Our chief concern is correcting high blood sugar. Patients may also benefit from drinking plenty of liquids, eating a high-fiber diet, and taking natural fiber preparations such as Metamucil. ◀ *See "Constipation and Gas," page 167.*

Diabetic Diarrhea

According to Dr. Wishner, so-called diabetic diarrhea "occurs frequently at night" and can last anywhere from a matter of hours to several weeks.

How It Is Managed

Antidiarrheal medications (loperamide, diphenoxylate, and atropine are three examples) or antibiotics such as tetracycline or metronidazole are used. Other approaches include serving high-fiber foods and encouraging the person to move her bowels regularly. ◀ *See "Diarrhea," page 169.*

Incontinence

If the nerves that control the rectum and the bladder sustain damage, patients may not be able to sense when it's time to defecate or urinate. People with *diabetic bladder dysfunction* also have difficulty emptying their bladders completely. This renders them susceptible to recurrent urinary tract infections, which consequently may hasten the progression of renal disease or exacerbate existing kidney problems.

How It Is Managed

Bowel and bladder training programs and biofeedback techniques are used. ◀ *See "Incontinence," page 170; "Urinary-Tract Infections," page 172.*

Diabetic Retinopathy

Diabetes is the leading cause of blindness in the United States. In the course of their lifetime, seven in ten people with insulin-dependent disease will develop *proliferative diabetic retinopa-*

thy, the principal threat to a diabetic's eyesight.

Initially, tiny blood vessels in the light-sensing *retina* at the rear of the eye become swollen and leak fluid. At this stage, referred to as *background retinopathy*, vision may blur. Most of the time the disease halts there. But in its proliferative form, knots of new vessels branch out. They may rupture and bleed into the transparent gel that fills the center of the eye. What's more, scar tissue can build up near the retina, shifting the lining out of position.

Preventive Management

Even if your loved one hasn't complained of problems seeing, make sure that he has his eyes examined annually by an *ophthalmologist* (not an optometrist). Timely *photocoagulation* can reduce a patient's risk of vision loss by more than half. The surgical procedure entails using a laser beam to seal off bleeding blood vessels and burn away *(cauterize)* new growths.

How It Is Managed

In instances where retinopathy is too advanced for laser surgery, an operation called *vitrectomy* may be able to partially restore sight. Here the eye surgeon extracts the blood-clouded gel (the *vitreous body*, hence the procedure's name) and replaces it with clear fluid.

Potential Life-Threatening Complications

For people with insulin-dependent diabetes, diabetic renal disease looms as the major threat to life. After twenty years, nearly four in ten require *dialysis* or kidney transplantation in order to survive. "Kristin has the beginnings of kidney problems," her mother says grimly. "We know it's just a matter of time." Given the fact that renal failure accelerates the onset of retinopathy,

neuropathy, and other diabetes-associated complications, diabetics are often put on dialysis sooner than other patients with dwindling kidney function.

Someone with adult-onset disease has more to fear from heart attack and stroke, which combined kill eighty thousand diabetics every year. Fifty percent of all diabetics die prematurely of heart attacks; those who recover survive half as long, on average, as nondiabetic heart attack victims.

Preventive Management

Kidney disease, heart attack, and stroke share one common risk factor: hypertension. For a diabetic expected to overcome a critical condition, controlling high blood pressure becomes crucial. A class of antihypertensive agents, *angiotensin converting enzyme (ACE) inhibitors*, appears to prevent or delay kidney failure in people with diabetes. Apart from medication, the primary strategy for lowering blood pressure calls for a diet low in fat, salt, and cholesterol; exercise; and giving up harmful habits such as smoking.

At each of the quarterly glycohemoglobin tests, your loved one's physician should measure blood pressure. In addition, a person with diabetes should receive the following evaluations at least once a year:

- Blood creatinine test to assess kidney function
- Urinalysis, looking for evidence of protein or albumin, an early indicator of diabetic renal disease
- Blood cholesterol test
- Electrocardiogram (EKG) to monitor heart function

◄ See chapter 13, "Caring for Someone with Cardiovascular Disease"; chapter 14, "Caring for Someone with Cerebrovascular Stroke or Traumatic Brain Injury." ► See chapter 19, "Caring for Someone with Kidney Disease."

Suzanne Hardy: For me the hardest part is having to accept that this is the way things are, and there's nothing I can do about it. The disease is more powerful than I am. All I can do is try to make Kristin comfortable.

I feel it's my duty to care for her. When you bring a child into this world, you do so with the knowledge that that child is your responsibility. And I know that the law says that once they reach eighteen that's no longer so, but I think you have a moral responsibility. Plus, Kristin's such a neat person, I can't imagine not doing it or turning her over to the state.

She would die if she had to go into some nursing home. And it wouldn't take very long.

Recommended Reading

The following are available free from the National Diabetes Information Clearinghouse (301-654-3327):

- "The Diabetes Dictionary"
- "Insulin-Dependent Diabetes"
- "Non-Insulin-Dependent Diabetes"

The following is available for $1.50 from the American Diabetes Association (800-342-2383) and the American Dietetic Association (800-366-1655):

- "Exchange Lists for Meal Planning."

–17–

Caring for Someone with AIDS/HIV

(Acquired Immunodeficiency Syndrome/
Human Immunodeficiency Virus)

Dr. **Alvin Novick,** seventy-two, a professor of biology at Yale University in New Haven, Connecticut, and his companion, Bill Sabella, had been together for more than ten years when Bill was diagnosed with AIDS in 1989. Bill, then in his mid-forties, retired from his job with the Yale–New Haven Medical Center AIDS care program. For the next two and a half years, says Alvin, "we pretty much enjoyed life together." He continues,

Until July 1992, Bill was doing pretty well. He'd gained weight rather than lost weight and looked good. He was totally independent in the sense of making all his own decisions and self-administering his oral and IV medications, which took about eight hours a day. Sixty different oral medications!

Then he started to become partly confused and forgetful. Bill also developed a severe inflammation of the optic nerve, which depleted his vision. That was very discouraging to him. He felt

he could no longer manage things by himself, so I took over his care more and more.

Among the population as a whole, the mortality rate from AIDS appears to have plateaued, at least for now. For the first time since the epidemic began in 1981, the first half of 1996 saw a 13 percent drop in the number of AIDS-related deaths from the same period the year before. However, deaths rose 3 percent among women, who now account for one in five cases. Approximately 40 percent of female patients contract the HIV retrovirus that causes AIDS through heterosexual contact, proof that it does not discriminate on the basis of sexual orientation.

Early on in the epidemic, AIDS was widely perceived as preying almost exclusively on gay men and intravenous drug users—hence the government's slow initial response (some would say indifference) to the escalating health crisis. Meanwhile, to most folks outside

413

the gay community, the horror of AIDS remained largely abstract.

Eileen Mitzman, one of the founders of Mothers' Voices, an AIDS education and advocacy organization, laughs as she recalls her reaction upon learning her twenty-four-year-old daughter Marni had AIDS. It was 1989, and Eileen was sitting at the bedside of her dying mother in a Florida hospital when her husband called from New York with the shocking news.

"I said, 'Neil, don't be ridiculous,'" says Eileen, sixty-three. "'*Girls* don't get AIDS.'" According to Eileen,

Marni was a free spirit, exciting, exceptionally beautiful. She lived with us the last six months of her life.

She'd been infected by a boy from our neighborhood in Bayside, New York. Later on she told us that he had been involved in IV drugs. When Marni's doctors suspected she had AIDS, naturally they asked if she had ever slept with an IV drug user. By then she and her boyfriend were no longer seeing each other. She called him and told him. He went for the test, and he was HIV positive. They had been very much in love and resumed the relationship. Also, after Marni was infected, she thought, Who else am I going to see? But then when he started to get sick and not feel well, and she started to get sick and not feel well, they split up for good, about six months before Marni died, over the Fourth of July weekend in 1991.

The boy came to her funeral, and we never heard from him again. I have no idea what happened to him.

In the spring of 1981, I was working as an administrator for a Madison Avenue hospital-management firm, hiring and scheduling the physicians for the emergency room and house staff at more than a dozen New York City hospitals. Throughout my social circle I became known as "the hospital guy"; inevitably, whenever anyone had a question relating to health care, they'd come to me for advice.

One day an acquaintance called, deeply distressed. His lover was deathly ill with three extraordinarily rare infections, diseases you *might* see only in a transplant patient taking immunosuppressant drugs to prevent organ rejection or in a cancer patient whose immune system had been ravaged by chemotherapy or radiation therapy. This thirty-five-year-old man was neither.

It was probably the fifth such call I'd received over the past year from gay men or their lovers, all describing equally bizarre constellations of symptoms that bewildered their doctors. While five cases hardly constituted an epidemic, clearly *something* was going on. Yet I couldn't find a single medical professional who was even aware of this phenomenon.

Out of frustration I contacted Arthur Bell, an openly gay gossip columnist at *The Village Voice*. "You're about the tenth person who's called me," he said. "You ought to talk to Larry Kramer; he's obsessed about this." Kramer, a novelist, playwright, and movie producer, was renowned in the gay community. "By the way," Bell mentioned, "the newspaper just ran an item about some gay cancer."

The article, tucked away in the July 3, 1981, edition of *The New York Times*, described a mystifying outbreak of a virulent, seldom-seen skin cancer, Kaposi's sarcoma, among forty-one young gay men in New York City and San Francisco. Many of them had also developed serious viral infections such as cytomegalovirus (CMV) and herpes simplex. This came on the heels of a June report from the federal Centers for Disease Control noting five cases of the rare pneumocystis pneumonia in Los Angeles. Here, too, the victims were young, gay, and male. What's more, all had CMV and candidiasis, a fungal infection. Today, any one of these conditions denotes acquired immunodeficiency syndrome, or AIDS, which was still a year away from receiving a name.

As subsequent accounts of Kaposi's sarcoma, pneumocystis pneumonia, and other lethal afflictions surfaced over the following months, a group of us formed an organization: Gay Men's Health Crisis. GMHC's first major project was to publish a comprehensive booklet titled "Questions and Answers About AIDS." One answer that would remain elusive for another couple of years was the cause of the disease.

The booklet contained a hot line number—my personal answering service. At most, I figured, we'd hear from a handful of people. Instead, more than one hundred calls came each night, from every region of the country. Over the course of the next decade, what began as an obscure disease snowballed into the leading killer of Americans ages twenty-five to forty-four. Through 1994, AIDS had infected more than 440,000 men, women, and children, claiming some 270,000 lives. While the rate of new infections has leveled off, it shouldn't lull anyone into presuming the storm has passed. For one thing, no cure exists. This, coupled with continued unsafe sexual practices among many heterosexuals and homosexuals alike and the upsurge in needle drug use, has prompted grim predictions of continued waves of new infections.

What Is AIDS? What Is HIV?

Acquired immunodeficiency syndrome and human immunodeficiency virus are inextricably linked, for it is HIV, discovered in 1984, that sets the stage for AIDS. The *retrovirus* disables the body's *immune system*, our natural defense against disease, leaving its victims vulnerable to an array of deadly cancers and opportunistic infections. "People

don't die from the virus itself," explains Dr. Howard Grossman of St. Luke's–Roosevelt Hospital in New York City, "but from the associated illnesses." Half of his private patients are HIV-positive.

HIV attacks the immune system's most valuable and versatile component: a specialized group of white blood cell called *T-lymphocyte helpers*. Lymphocytes, in addition to eradicating harmful invaders, or *antigens*, govern the entire immune process. The T helper cells (also known as *T4* or *CD4* cells) activate other T cells and signal *B-lymphocytes* to manufacture *antibodies*. These molecules adhere to specific antigens, marking them for the *natural-killer T cells* that come along to finish off the intruder.

HIV is transmitted primarily through unprotected sexual intercourse with someone who harbors the retrovirus or by way of blood on an infected needle. Upon entering the body, HIV infiltrates the CD4 cells, transforming them into tiny virus mills that disperse copies throughout the bloodstream and the lymphatic vessels. For the first few weeks the virus mass-produces itself unopposed, until the body launches an immune response.

Although HIV can take as long as eight, ten, twelve, or more years to progress to AIDS, it assails the immune system from the moment of entry. But once the body mounts its vigorous counterattack, the combatants hammer away at each other like a pair of evenly matched prizefighters.

Ultimately, however, the tenacious retrovirus prevails. Little by little it kills off CD4 cells. As the number of T-helper cells dwindles, not only does the body become increasingly defenseless against the proliferating HIV particles but it is unable to identify and destroy cancer cells and opportunistic microorganisms. These bacteria, fungi, viruses, and protozoa, which ordinarily reside harmlessly in the body, can turn deadly in someone profoundly immunocompromised. A person is diagnosed as having AIDS if he develops any of the illnesses listed in the chart below *or* if his CD4 count drops below 200 per cubic millimeter of blood. A normal level is approximately 1,000. Like most people with AIDS, Bill Sabella exhibited several AIDS-defining conditions.

"He had zero T4 cells for at least two years," says Alvin Novick. At the time of diagnosis, Bill was suffering from candidiasis of the esophagus, one of the most common manifestations of AIDS. Over the next three years he developed cytomegalovirus retinitis, a viral infection of the retina that can cause blindness, and the bacterial infection mycobacterium avium complex (MAC).

Keep in mind that many of these conditions are exceptionally rare. Although any can be fatal in a person with immunosuppression, some AIDS illnesses that posed a grave threat to life only a few years ago are now highly treatable, PCP being the prime example. "In the early days of the AIDS epidemic," says Dr. Grossman, "pneumocystis pneumonia is what killed most people. It's still the leading AIDS-indicator disease, but today people rarely die from it." Caring for someone with AIDS therefore often involves nursing him through multiple critical episodes, with periods of relative health in between. Once Marni Mitzman survived her initial bout of PCP, she felt generally good for the next two years. "When she went for her monthly checkups," her mother recalled, "the doctor would say, 'If I didn't know why she was here, I wouldn't know why she was here.' "

AIDS Illnesses from Most Common to Least Common

1. Pneumocystis carinii pneumonia
2. HIV wasting syndrome
3. Esophageal candidiasis
4. Tuberculosis
5. Kaposi's sarcoma
6. Mycobacterium avium complex or M. kansasii
7. Recurrent pneumonia
8. Encephalopathy
9. Herpes simplex
10. Cytomegalovirus
11. Toxoplasmosis
12. Cryptococcosis
13. Cytomegalovirus retinitis
14. Cryptosporidiosis
15. Candidiasis of bronchi, trachea, or lungs
16. Immunoblastic lymphoma
17. Other mycobacterium
18. Progressive multifocal leukoencephalopathy
19. Histoplasmosis
20. Primary central nervous system lymphoma
21. Burkitt's lymphoma
22. Invasive cervical cancer
23. Coccidioidomycosis
24. Salmonella
25. Isosporiasis

The Illnesses of AIDS

The conditions profiled below rank among the most prevalent and serious of AIDS's many identities.

Pneumocystis Carinii Pneumonia

Roughly one in five HIV-infected men and women develop PCP at some point. As with Marni, its cough, chest pain, fever, and shortness of breath are often how AIDS makes its presence known. Because in 1989 the young woman did not fit the then existing stereotype of someone with AIDS, her pulmonary doctor initially suspected lupus, an autoimmune disease, as the cause. It was only after she saw an infectious diseases specialist that Marni was diagnosed with PCP and, consequently, AIDS.

AIDS ILLNESSES

Opportunistic Infections

Bacterial Infections

- Tuberculosis in the lungs or any other site
- Mycobacterium avium complex or M. kansasii that has spread outside the lungs or throughout the body
- Other mycobacterial diseases that have spread outside the lungs or throughout the body

Fungal Infections

- Candidiasis (thrush) of the mouth, esophagus, or vagina
- Candidiasis of the bronchi, windpipe, or lungs
- Cryptococcosis that has spread outside the lungs or throughout the body
- Histoplasmosis that has spread outside the lungs or throughout the body
- Coccidioidomycosis that has spread outside the lungs or throughout the body

Protozoal Infections

- Pneumocystis carinii pneumonia (PCP)
- Toxoplasmosis of the brain
- Chronic intestinal cryptosporidiosis lasting longer than one month
- Chronic intestinal isosporiasis lasting longer than one month

Viral Infections

- Herpes simplex characterized by chronic ulcers persisting longer than one month; or bronchitis, pneumonitis, or esophagitis
- Cytomegalovirus disease of organs other than the liver, spleen, or lymph nodes
- Cytomegalovirus retinitis causing loss of vision

Miscellaneous Infections

- Two or more episodes of viral, fungal, or protozoal pneumonia within one year
- Recurrent salmonella septicemia

Cancers

- Kaposi's sarcoma (KS)
- Immunoblastic lymphoma
- Primary CNS (central nervous system) lymphoma
- Burkitt's lymphoma
- Invasive cervical cancer

Others

- HIV-related encephalopathy, a term encompassing any degenerative disease of the brain; also known as HIV dementia
- Progressive multifocal leukoencephalopathy, a particularly aggressive disease that affects the white matter of the brain
- HIV wasting syndrome

How It Is Managed

Without question the greatest boon to prolonging survival for people with AIDS thus far has been the introduction of *trimethoprim-sulfamethoxazole* (brand names: Bactrim and Septra), a synthetic antibacterial medication. Both TMP-SMX and another drug, *pentamidine* (Pentam), typically clear the infection inside three weeks' time. "Within three days of treatment," Eileen Mitzman recalls, "Marni's PCP was gone."

Tuberculosis

Until the discovery of antibiotics in the 1940s sent tuberculosis the way of the five-cent plain, it inspired fear on an even greater scale than AIDS does today. Consumption, as this once incurable bacterial infection was called, killed more Americans than any other disease. How ironic, then, that tuberculosis owes its recent resurgence partly to HIV's weakening of the immune system sufficiently for the bacteria to gain a foothold and inflame the lungs, producing chronic coughing and coughing up of blood, chest pain, fever, night sweats, fatigue, swollen lymph glands, and weight loss. TB can also spread to the bones, brain, and kidneys.

What distinguishes tuberculosis from the other AIDS opportunistic infections is that it is communicable. Even people with healthy immune systems can catch TB from inhaling a contagious patient's airborne germs, which, incidentally, can hover in the air indefinitely. Therefore, until a physician declares the infection under control, we need to wear a mask whenever coming into close contact with a TB patient. As an additional precaution, caregivers should undergo a simple skin test (known as the *Mantoux method* or *PPD*) to screen for evidence of TB exposure. While a positive result may indicate only the presence of the bacterium and not an active infection, you can expect to be placed on antibiotics temporarily.

How It Is Managed

Antibiotics and antituberculosis agents are used.

Mycobacterium Avium Intracellulare Complex

A close cousin of tuberculosis, this bacterial infection is caused by mycobacterium avium and mycobacterium intracellulare, a pair of bacteria so much alike that they are referred to jointly as mycobacterium avium intracellulare complex. Whereas TB can occur anywhere across the CD4 cell spectrum, MAC typically develops in people with levels below 100, bringing on chronic fever, night sweats, weakness, severe anemia (a deficiency of red blood cells), and marked weight loss.

How It Is Managed

This infection is treated with an antibiotic in combination with either an oral chemotherapeutic agent (ethambutol; brand name: Myambutol), an antileprosy agent (clofazimine; brand name: Lamprene), an antimicrobial agent (ciprofloxacin; brand name: Cipro IV), or an antimycobacterial agent (rifabutin; brand name: Mycobutin).

Cryptosporidiosis

Until 1980 or so, cryptosporidiosis had never been reported in humans. But 1994 brought nearly one thousand cases of the protozoal infection, which can cause chronic diarrhea. It is not uncommon for patients to have more than a dozen explosive, watery stools a day for *months* on end, leaving them dangerously malnourished, dehydrated, and depleted of essential minerals.

How It Is Managed

To date no medication has proved effective for treating cryptosporidiosis;

drugs are prescribed to manage diarrhea and other gastrointestinal symptoms, along with aggressive replacement of fluids, electrolytes, and nutrients. ◄ *See "Diarrhea," page 169.*

Toxoplasmosis

Most of us have unknowingly been infected with toxoplasmosis, a protozoal infection, but our immune systems disarm the tiny organisms before they do any harm. In people with depressed immunity, however, toxoplasmosis can inflame the brain; its symptoms include intense headaches that respond poorly to pain medication, fever, visual changes, seizures, paralysis on one side of the body *(hemiplegia)*, confusion, lethargy, and delusions.

How It Is Managed

The infection is treated with an antiparasitic, pyrimethamine (brand name: Daraprim), and one or more antibiotics.

HIV Encephalopathy (HIV Dementia)

As many as four in five people with AIDS experience complications involving the central nervous system. Cryptococcosis, a fungal infection, often causes meningitis, an inflammation of the membranes encasing the brain, while two cancers, Kaposi's sarcoma and CNS lymphoma, sometimes spawn brain tumors. Any of these, along with toxoplasmosis, can lead to the mental disorder *dementia*, characterized by altered intellect and personality.

HIV dementia also stems directly from the retrovirus's effect on the brain. In contrast to the abrupt personality changes that generally signal an adverse drug reaction or the rapid progression of an AIDS illness, Dr. Grossman points out, "HIV dementia creeps up slowly."

How It Is Managed

No specific therapy exists other than antiviral medications prescribed to slow or halt HIV from replicating itself and antibiotics for other underlying infections. ◄ *See "When a Loved One Suffers from Brain Function Impairment," page 202.*

Kaposi's Sarcoma

KS, the fifth most common manifestation of AIDS, can be described as an opportunistic cancer. Until the emergence of AIDS, it was exceptionally rare, confined mainly to elderly men and organ transplant recipients. Highly treatable, this "classic" form of Kaposi's is often little more than a cosmetic nuisance, producing one or more benign *(noncancerous)* skin tumors that usually remain localized.

But in a person whose natural defenses are down, the malignant cancer that develops in blood vessel walls comes on so suddenly and with such severity that it is designated *epidemic* Kaposi's sarcoma to distinguish it from its comparatively mild relation. Here innumerable blue, brown, or purple lesions riddle the skin. "Highly aggressive Kaposi's can block blood flow, causing swelling known as edema," says Dr. Grossman. "We see this mostly in the legs." Eventually, KS almost always infiltrates internal organs such as the lymph glands and the gastrointestinal tract. Patients who succumb to the cancer itself and not to a concurrent opportunistic infection, as is typically the case, usually die from Kaposi's sarcoma of the lungs.

How It Is Managed

Lesions that are relatively small in size and in number can often be eradicated surgically or melted away with radiation therapy. Chemotherapy, for fighting cancer throughout the body, must be used cautiously, since anticancer agents suppress immunity and could conceivably throw the door wide open to potentially lethal infections.

HIV Wasting Syndrome

A number of HIV-related illnesses cause wasting, a term that describes all too vividly the shocking physical deterioration frequently seen with end-stage AIDS and cancer. The person appears emaciated, listless, consumed by illness —just wasting away.

When wasting occurs in the absence of an underlying infection or cancer, patients are said to have HIV wasting syndrome, defined as "a loss of at least 10 percent of body weight within approximately one month," according to Dr. Grossman. Other symptoms include fever, diarrhea, and weakness, each lasting more than thirty days.

HIV wasting is what claimed Marni Mitzman's life. "About six months before Marni died," says her mother, "she started to lose weight. Gradually she got weaker and weaker, to where she could hardly get out of bed."

How It Is Managed

Diet and Nutrition. Just a few added pounds of body weight can give patients the edge they need to overcome opportunistic infections, so one of a caregiver's most crucial tasks is to see to it that a loved one with AIDS who is still able to fight for life stays well nourished.

This is no small challenge. If you scan Table 16.1, "Common Symptoms of AIDS Illnesses," you'll see that most of these conditions give rise to gastrointestinal distress of some kind. "Marni was able to eat only yogurt and certain soft foods," says her mother. "The rest she would throw up." In addition, many of the medications prescribed to control HIV and manage infection can make patients nauseous and rob them of their appetite.

Expect to confer closely with the physician and the hospital dietitian on ways to prevent malnourishment and weight loss, preferably before they spin out of control. Ideally, we try to get the person to obtain his recommended intake of nutrients and vitamins through the diet. But sometimes it is necessary to rely on supplements. The high-protein drinks favored by body builders come in handy when a loved one experiences difficulty swallowing solid food, perhaps due to an inflamed esophagus, a symptom of candidiasis as well as cytomegalovirus. Appetite stimulants (including marijuana) are also part of a caregiver's arsenal when malnutrition presents a serious threat to life.

In some cases, you may find yourself administering liquid nutrients *intravenously* via a central catheter surgically implanted in a major vein in the chest, either because your loved one cannot ingest solid food or on account of *malabsorption*, another contributor to wasting. In this condition, the intestinal tract sustains such damage—from a variety of causes—that it no longer adequately absorbs nutrients from the partly digested food sent its way by the stomach. Instead of being utilized for energy, building and repairing body tissues, and so on, excessive amounts pass out of the body in the stool.

Exercise. Physical activity prescribed by the doctor joins healthy eating as part of the strategy to prevent wasting. The goal is to build lean muscle mass to maintain weight and mobility. Even stretching exercises can benefit people with HIV, not only physically but in terms of helping to alleviate stress, a known tax on the immune system. ◀ See *"Types of Infection and How to Prevent Transmission," page 106; "Tricks for Stimulating Appetite," page 159; and "Tube Feedings and Total Parenteral Nutrition (TPN)," page 166.*

How HIV Is Diagnosed

Understandably, the decision whether or not to undergo screening for the HIV retrovirus can be an agonizing one. Who wants to chance learning he has an incurable, life-threatening infection? The nagging suspicion that they may have been exposed is often enough to compel some men and women to seek testing, though they may not show any signs of disease whatsoever. Other times it takes an alarming symptom before someone goes for testing.

Two frequent harbingers of compromised immunity are oral candidiasis, which produces patchy white plaques on the mouth and tongue, and herpes zoster, the painful blisters better known as shingles. While neither falls under the heading of AIDS, doctors often see a precipitous drop in CD4 cell levels soon after either infection.

The blood tests routinely used to diagnose HIV, *enzyme-linked immunosorbent assay (ELISA)* and the *Western blot*, don't actually detect the retrovirus but rather the antibodies that the immune system manufactures after sighting it. ELISA, quick and inexpensive, is performed first, with a negative finding considered definitive. Given ELISA's high sensitivity, should the result come back positive, the more specific Western blot is conducted for confirmation. "If the Western blot is positive," says Dr. Grossman, "there almost isn't any question that the person has HIV." Combined, the two laboratory procedures (home-testing kits are also available) are more than 99 percent reliable.

However, the retrovirus can elude both techniques during its first three to six weeks in the body because the immune system may not yet have deployed a sufficient number of antibodies to register on the test. For this reason it's recommended that HIV testing be repeated three months later. (Antibody testing and CD4 counts are now joined by routine measurements of *viral load*, the actual concentration of viral particles in the blood.)

A negative result is bound to induce a tremendous sigh of relief. But even if the physician delivers devastating news, it's usually best for patients to know their HIV status; for one thing, so that they don't unwittingly infect someone else, and, for another, so that treatment—limited though it may be—can begin promptly.

How HIV/AIDS Is Treated

Tragically, the optimism of the late 1980s that a cure or vaccine for HIV and AIDS was around the corner has yielded to discouragement, frustration, and anguish over the harsh realization that, for the foreseeable future, many more people will die from this terrible disease. HIV is a cunning infection, mutating to resist the full effects of the drugs leveled at it thus far.

Until something more effective comes along, doctors currently adopt a two-prong treatment strategy: contain the retrovirus with antiviral agents and, where applicable, use medications *prophylactically* to stave off opportunistic infection. The ultimate goal, of course, is to keep HIV-positive patients healthy indefinitely. I know folks who were diagnosed with the retrovirus well over a decade ago. Through timely treatment, observing a healthy lifestyle, and, possibly, fate, good fortune, divine providence—call it what you will—their CD4 levels remain above the critical zone, and they have either recovered from life-threatening AIDS-related illnesses or managed to sidestep them altogether. Even people with counts below 200 can remain stable for years.

Antiviral Therapy

As of 1997, the Food and Drug Administration (FDA) had approved five *nucleoside analog* antiviral agents: ZDV, or zidovudine (brand name: Retrovir); ddI (didanosine; Videx); ddC (zalcitabine; Hivid); d4T (stavudine; Zerit); and 3TC (lamivudine; Epivir). Although none eradicates the retrovirus, according to Dr. Grossman, "all have been shown to slow the progression of

---

INSIDE INFORMATION

Unless your loved one's physician has a busy AIDS practice, don't expect to be routinely offered combination antiviral therapy. The average internist or general practitioner may not be well versed in the benefits of multidrug treatment and will likely start HIV-positive patients on ZDV only. Another factor here is that, by and large, medical insurers do not reimburse for combination therapy. Therefore, patients or their care partners should take it upon themselves to inquire about trying this promising strategy.

---

the disease" by inhibiting it from replicating.

ZDV, introduced in 1985 as AZT, was once the first line of defense; today it is frequently combined with other nucleoside analogs, as well as a new family of anti-HIV drugs known as *protease inhibitors:* saquinavir (Invirase, Fortovase), crixivan (Indinavir), ritonavir (Norvir), and nelfinavir (Viracept). Patients on combination therapy are prescribed anywhere from two to four medications, though most take three— for example, ZDV, 3TC, and one of the protease inhibitors; or ZDV, ddI, and a drug called nevirapine (Viramune), which belongs to yet another category. Studies show that these so-called AIDS cocktails decelerate the disease's progression significantly. In the near future we can expect *monotherapy*—relying on a single drug—to become synonymous with malpractice.

The conventional wisdom used to be to commence therapy as soon as a person traversed from HIV to full-blown AIDS, and to refrain from prescribing these medications as long as the CD4 count exceeded 500, the border separating normal from low ranges. This strategy has come under fire, the rationale being that it makes more sense to start treatment earlier—in other words, to bring down the viral load *before* the T cells are wiped out.

Controversy also rages over the question of when is the optimal time for patients whose CD4 levels hover between 200 and 500. Proponents of early intervention contend this approach reduces hospitalizations for AIDS-related illnesses. The counterargument is that the antivirals are toxic and can make patients sick. Serious side effects include anemia; bone-marrow suppression leading to a drop in white blood cells *(granulocytopenia);* nerve damage; and *pancreatitis*, a potentially deadly inflammation of the pancreas.

A 1995 British study found that while early treatment did indeed defer the onset of AIDS illnesses, in the end it did not ward off death, a conclusion that corroborated an earlier European study. Since AIDS treatment remains an uncharted region, with no definitive guidelines, the decision of when to initiate antiviral therapy belongs to the patient—or should. In my experience, most doctors will accede to the patient's wishes.

AIDS Treatment and Prevention

Since 1987, survival time has increased from twenty-four months to forty months for people with CD4 cell counts under 200, and from fourteen months to nineteen months for people with one or more AIDS conditions, a development many attribute to earlier detection and improved therapies for HIV-related illnesses but especially to preventive treatments.

While many AIDS illnesses continue to thwart a cure (cryptosporidiosis, Kaposi's sarcoma, and HIV lymphomas spring to mind), physicians do wield formidable ammunition against several, most notably acyclovir (brand name: Zovirax), for treating herpes; fluconazole (Diflucan), for candidiasis; and ganciclovir (Cytovene), for cytomegalovirus. Still, whenever possible, it's far preferable to avoid active infection in the first place. Each bout of PCP, for instance, injures the lungs, and the drugs used in treatment inflict further harm on the entire body. Even patients who go on prophylactic therapy once they've recovered from the pneumonia have a 10 to 20 percent chance of a recurrence within twelve months. What's more, it is believed that a single outbreak of PCP inflates a person's odds of developing another opportunistic infection.

The central factor in the extended survival rates cited above has been the evolution of PCP prophylaxis—the oral medications trimethoprim-sulfamethoxazole and Dapsone, and aerosol pentamidine (brand name: NebuPent). TMP/SMX, favored by many doctors, bears a dividend in that it may also ward off toxoplasmosis and bacterial infections. Meeting any of the following conditions qualifies a person for immediate preventive therapy:

- a CD4 count below 200
- a prior episode of PCP pneumonia or any AIDS condition
- a CD4 count under 250 *plus* night sweats, weight loss, or the disease *hairy leukoplakia*, which produces thick white patches inside the mouth.

Two other potentially fatal AIDS conditions warrant prophylactic strategies. To safeguard against mycobacterium avium intracellulare complex, an oral medication called rifabutin (brand name: Mycobutin) is often prescribed for people with CD4 counts under 200. Effective preventive treatment also exists for MAC's microbiological kin, tuberculosis, in the form of an antibiotic, isoniazid (INH). The federal Agency for Health Care and Policy Research rec-

ommends that any HIV-infected person who tests positive for TB but does not have the active disease receive isoniazid prophylactically for a full year.

Clinical Trials and HIV/AIDS

A number of promising drugs are available to patients only through clinical trials, studies conducted to test a new treatment's effectiveness and safety. Because the available therapies for HIV and most manifestations of AIDS are of relatively limited value, having access to experimental treatments before they've been fully tested should constitute standard care.

This points up the importance of seeing to it that a loved one be treated by an AIDS specialist, someone who's attuned to developments in research. "With this disease," Dr. Grossman emphasizes, "things change too quickly for a physician to rest on textbook knowledge."

When the government and the medical establishment were slow to mobilize at the outset of the epidemic, many people touched by AIDS took matters into their own hands. Out of necessity, an information underground sprung up: Gay Men's Health Crisis in New York, Project Inform in San Francisco, as well as other, similar organizations. Their newsletters and telephone hot lines keep patients and caregivers abreast of the latest in cutting-edge treatment, open clinical trials, and new applications for existing drugs. Bill Sabella's MAC responded "miraculously," says Alvin Novick, to clarithromycin, a ubiquitous antibiotic that "was still unlicensed at that point" for the treatment of mycobacterium avium intracellulare complex.

Upon a loved one's diagnosis of HIV, we strongly urge you to plug into the network and make use of these invaluable resources. (For more information about each, turn to "AIDS/HIV" in Ap-

☎ If you are seeking an AIDS special-ist, call the 24-hour National HIV/AIDS Hotline (800-342-2437), operated by the Centers for Disease Control and Prevention. It refers callers to specialists in their area.

pendix A.) "Because of the high-tech na-ture of HIV care and the fact that many of the diseases and the drugs we use are poorly understood," says Dr. Grossman, "patients and their caregivers need to have a good sense of what's going on." ◄ *See "What Are Clinical Trials?," page 229.*

Managing Symptoms and Side Effects

A caregiver to a person with AIDS may be called upon to manage a broad spec-trum of symptoms. Table 17.1 lists those commonly associated with specific AIDS illnesses. Among the symptoms typically encountered are fever, night sweats, fatigue, weakness, weight loss, and chronic diarrhea. Many of these may also occur as side effects from the medications used in treatment. Diar-rhea and another frequent consequence of AIDS, peripheral neuropathy, bear special mention; although not unique to AIDS, both are particularly severe in people with this disease.

Chronic Diarrhea

As Mary Vitro can tell you, the violent, unrelenting diarrhea often seen with AIDS-related opportunistic infections presents one of a caregiver's more de-manding challenges. Her husband, Rick, contracted HIV from a transfusion dur-ing surgery in 1984, one year before the government implemented measures for testing the safety of the nation's blood supply. Five years later he came down with shingles, then the flu and night sweats that literally soaked the bed-

sheets. His doctor blamed the mys-terious symptoms on stress. The HIV infection went undetected until Rick was hospitalized for what turned out to be PCP pneumonia, indicative of full-blown AIDS.

"Rick had a couple of bouts of diar-rhea that covered the walls," recalls Mary. "I would say stupid things to him like, 'You really need to try to get to the bathroom.' He would tell me, *'But I can't.'* The first time it happened, I thought to myself, *Uh-uh, I'm not do-ing this."* But she did, nursing Rick throughout his two years of illness.

How It Is Managed. ◄ See *"Diar-rhea," page 169.*

Bedsores (Pressure Ulcers)

Days or weeks of incessant watery bowel movements contribute to wast-ing, which in turn may give rise to another serious problem: bedsores. "To-ward the end," says Mary, "Rick was all bone. In the hospital two weeks before he died, he developed a horrible, pain-ful bedsore right on his tailbone—just this huge gaping *hole* in his body." Peo-ple with AIDS, encumbered by a deteri-orating immune system, "heal very poorly," Dr. Grossman points out. "In many cases it becomes extremely diffi-cult to get bedsores to close up." Be-cause these people's bodies are all but defenseless against infection, tech-niques for preventing pressure ulcers become of utmost importance.

How It Is Managed. ◄ See *"How to Prevent Pressure Ulcers," page 118; "How Pressure Ulcers Are Treated," page 120.*

Peripheral Neuropathy

Three in ten people with advanced AIDS suffer painful nerve damage in the feet, legs, and/or hands, while virtually all late-stage disease produces some de-gree of peripheral neuropathy. "The most common complaint initially," says

Dr. Grossman, "is a tingling sensation." Later symptoms may include a lack of sensation to heat and cold, ulceration, burning, and sharp pain.

A few months before Bill Sabella's death, Alvin Novick recalls, "he developed a very severe nerve inflammation in his face that didn't respond to any treatment. It was excruciatingly painful around the clock, and Bill didn't handle pain particularly well." The nerve damage may stem from the HIV retrovirus itself but also from ddI, ddC, and, to a lesser extent, d4T.

How It Is Managed. Neuropathies believed to have arisen due to drug toxicity generally subside once the medication has been discontinued temporarily or permanently. Unfortunately, no therapies exist for pathologic nerve damage. Physicians can only treat symptoms, and even then, sighs Dr. Grossman, "not always with the greatest relief."

"Frequently," he continues, "we have to employ unusual means to manage them": acupuncture; narcotic analgesics; antidepressants such as amitriptyline (available under several brand names); and mexiletine (Mexitil), a dual antiarrhythmic and local anesthetic. One potential treatment for HIV-associated peripheral neuropathy currently under study in patients is *nerve growth factor (NGF)*, a drug that may be able to help repair damaged nerves. ◄ *See "Managing Pain," page 152.*

Of the thousands of phone calls I answered while manning the Gay Men's Health Crisis hot line, one remains forever engraved in my memory. It came from a man with late-stage AIDS who had just been discharged from a New York hospital. He had no money, no medical insurance, and no place to stay. When I contacted his mother in Virginia, she said in a frightened, resigned voice, "Tell him to come home. I'll take care of him." I arranged to have the man's belongings sent there and purchased a bus ticket for him.

He arrived at his mother's to find a return ticket to New York pinned to the front door, along with a note that read, "I'm sorry, I can't do it," and wound up back at Manhattan's Port Authority bus terminal penniless. After making a few phone calls, I found him a place to stay in the Brooklyn home of an Episcopal priest. The man died there a few nights later.

It's difficult to imagine families turning their backs on dying children, yet it happens. On the other hand, I can offer countless stories of folks who transcended whatever fears they held about AIDS or about what the neighbors might think, or their own intolerance and prejudices, and embraced a terminally ill son, brother, or uncle with love and compassion.

"At the time our daughter was diagnosed," reflects Eileen Mitzman, "many people were not going public with their disease because of the stigma attached. But one of the first things Marni said to us, as soon as she could catch her breath from the pneumonia, was 'You *must* tell your friends—every one of them—because they're the only ones who will be able to help us.' And our friends were fabulous."

To be sure, attitudes toward AIDS have generally grown more enlightened than in the early years of the crisis. Yet this disease remains shrouded in ignorance and bigotry, and is unique in that it is probably the only terminal illness where patients and caregivers cannot necessarily count on support from others.

Mary Vitro, who had moved into a new middle-class development in Clearwater, Florida, one year before her husband's diagnosis, chose to tell only a handful of neighbors. "People didn't know as much about AIDS back then as they do now," she reflects. She was all too aware of the fate of the Rays, a family in nearby Arcadia whose three sons, all hemophiliacs, contracted HIV from tainted blood products. The townspeople by and large shunned the family. Not long after a suspicious fire burned their home to the ground, the Rays, targeted by bomb threats, moved elsewhere.

TABLE 17

Condition	Fever	Night sweats	Fatigue/ weakness	Weight loss	Chronic diarrhea	Abdominal pain/cramps	Nausea/ vomiting	Dizziness	Itchy, rashy skin/ skin lesions
AIDS-related lymphomas	✔	✔	✔	✔					✔
Candidiasis				✔					
Cervical cancer									
Coccidioidomycosis	✔		✔	✔					
Cryptococcosis	✔		✔				✔		✔
Cryptosporidiosis and isosporiasis	✔		✔	✔	✔	✔	✔		
Cytomegalovirus	✔			✔	✔	✔			
Encephalopathy and leukoencephalopathy	✔		✔				✔		
Herpes simplex									
Histoplasmosis	✔	✔		✔	✔		✔		✔
Kaposi's sarcoma	✔	✔		✔	✔				✔
MAC/MAI	✔	✔	✔	✔	✔	✔	✔	✔	
Pneumonia	✔								
Pneumocystic carinii	✔	✔			✔				
Salmonella	✔				✔	✔	✔		
Toxoplasmosis	✔								
Tuberculosis	✔	✔	✔	✔					
Wasting syndrome			✔	✔	✔	✔			

Ricky Ray, the oldest boy, would die of the disease at age fifteen in 1992.

Mary Vitro: *I was so isolated. I had no one I could talk to. Everyone said, "Don't tell your neighbors." The people across the street and maybe one other couple were the only people who knew what I was going through. One friend at work knew, and she was very supportive.*

But there really wasn't a lot of support for me. Most of it came from my in-laws, who moved down to Clearwa-

Common Symptoms of AIDS Illnesses

Chronic coughing	Appetite loss	Difficulty swallowing	Swollen lymph glands	Confusion, delirium, altered mental state	Difficulty breathing	Constipation	Others
			✔				
		✔					White patches on gums, tongue, or lining; vaginal candidiasis causes itching, burning, vaginal discharge
							Abnormal vaginal bleeding
✔							
	✔			✔	✔		Mild headache and intermittent fever from meningitis; bacterial pneumonia
	✔					✔	Dehydration, electrolyte imbalances
		✔					Blurry vision progressing to blindness; pneumonia
		✔		✔			Loss of vision, lack of coordination, headaches, seizures
							Shingles: painful blisters on the rectum, mouth, genitals, face, chest
			✔				Bacterial pneumonia
✔	✔		✔				Anemia, poor blood clotting, enlarged liver and spleen
✔				✔	✔	✔	Chest pain, blood-streaked phlegm, dehydration
✔	✔				✔		
				✔			Seizures, paralysis on one side of the body, and severe headaches from encephalitis; changes in vision
✔			✔				Chest pain, coughing up blood

ter to help us, and my family and friends back in New York. I couldn't have gotten through this without them.

With AIDS I think the hardest thing to handle is the hopelessness of it. Which drug is going to work? How does it work? Nobody knows; they can only guess. In the end, nothing's going to work. I hate to sound so pessimistic, but it's true. It's a terrible, terrible disease. ► To find a support group specifically for people with AIDS and/or their caregivers, see Appendix A: "AIDS/HIV," page 489.

Recommended Reading

The following is available free from the Agency for Health Care Policy and Research Information Clearinghouse (800-358-9295):
- "Understanding HIV"

The following is available free from the American Foundation for AIDS Research (800-392-6327):
- "AIDS/HIV Clinical Trial Handbook"

The following is available free from the AIDS Treatment Data Network (800-734-7104):
- "Treatment Review," a newsletter published eight times a year

The following is available free from the CDC National HIV/AIDS Clearinghouse (800-458-5231):
- "AIDS/HIV Treatment Directory"

The following is available free from Gay Men's Health Crisis Hotline (212-367-1000):
- "Newsletter of Experimental AIDS Therapies," published monthly

The following are available free from Project Inform Treatment National Hotline (800-822-7422):
- "PI Briefing Paper," published three times a year
- "Guide to the Management of Opportunistic Infections"

–18–

Caring for Someone with
Liver Disease

Naomi and Wyman Black of Rochester, Minnesota, raised eight children, four boys and four girls. In 1977 their second oldest daughter, fifteen-year-old Nancy, was diagnosed with chronic hepatitis non-A/non-B, now known as hepatitis C. While this virus can lead to liver failure directly, its more typical pattern is to progress to cirrhosis, the most deadly of all liver ailments.

"At the time," says Naomi, sixty, "the doctors didn't really know what Nancy's long-term prognosis would be, although they did say she probably wouldn't have a long life." Every few years a serious complication would land the young woman in the hospital. Nevertheless, says her mother, "she was determined to live her life normally."

Nancy had very much come to terms with her illness and knew that she could die at any time. But she never dwelled on it. She studied computer science at Mankato State College, was

a straight-A student, and got married. In 1987 my daughter had a liver transplant at the Mayo Clinic here in Rochester. The doctors never said it was a cure, but because she was young and otherwise healthy, they did feel she had a very good chance of leading a much longer life. Two years later she and her husband, Gary, had a son, Jacob, then another son, Patrick, the following year.

The last two years of her life, Nancy's health was really pretty good, although she did have a problem with her spleen. The doctors were concerned and talked about possibly removing it. They didn't want to operate, though, unless it was absolutely necessary. On June 6, 1993, the spleen ruptured, and Nancy hemorrhaged to death. She was thirty-one, four months pregnant with her third child.

Each year some forty thousand people die from chronic liver disease, a category that includes hepatitis, cirrhosis, and other disorders. This chapter fo-

429

cuses primarily on cirrhosis, the liver ailment responsible for the vast majority of those deaths and the seventh leading killer in the United States.

The Liver

The liver lies wedged up against the diaphragm in the upper right portion of the abdomen. Part refinery, part storehouse, it is one of the body's most vital components as well as the largest solid organ. Dr. Bruce Bacon, director of gastroenterology and hepatology at St. Louis University Health Sciences Center in Missouri, enumerates just some of its many functions.

"To begin with, the liver processes all the nutrients, vitamins, and minerals from food into forms the body can use," he explains. "Similarly, it detoxifies and metabolizes drugs, alcohol, and other potentially harmful chemicals in the blood and also stores blood, vitamins, fats, and glycogen." *Glycogen* is the stored form of digested sugar, or *glucose*, our principal source of fuel. Whenever the body's cells need quick energy, the liver reconverts glycogen to glucose and releases it into the bloodstream for distribution. What's more, the dark red gland manufactures an array of important chemicals and substances, including proteins, cholesterol, urea, bile, and digestive enzymes.

Cirrhosis, a degenerative disease, interferes with these life-sustaining functions by irreparably destroying the cells of the liver and leaving behind thick scar tissue. Ordinarily the liver has a remarkable capacity to regenerate itself, but the accumulating scar tissue gradually obstructs blood from delivering essential nutrients to the organ's remaining healthy cells, which subsequently wither and die. Have you ever seen photographs of a normal liver and a severely cirrhotic liver? The contrast is startling. Whereas the normal liver appears smooth, the scarred liver resembles an alligator's scaly coat. The damaged organ also contracts in size.

When it can no longer function adequately, a person is said to have progressive liver failure.

Causes of Cirrhosis

Chronic Alcoholism

The liver routinely neutralizes alcohol's harmful effects on the body as long as its owner drinks in moderation. However, years of excessive consumption (what constitutes "excessive" can vary widely from one person to the next) causes liver tissue to become inflamed, a condition known as *alcoholic hepatitis*. Unless the person stops drinking, the inflammation will advance to *alcoholic cirrhosis*. In the United States, alcoholism is to blame for more than half of all cases of cirrhosis.

Chronic Active Viral Hepatitis

Scientists have identified at least eight types of *viral hepatitis*, a contagious disease that attacks liver cells: viruses A through E, plus several others tentatively accorded their own letter names. Unlike *acute* hepatitis, which typically resolves in a matter of weeks or months without inflicting permanent damage, *chronic* hepatitis can progress to cirrhosis. Only types B, C, and D have been documented to assume the chronic form. Of these, says Dr. Bacon, "hepatitis B and hepatitis D do not commonly cause cirrhosis." However, of the approximately thirty thousand men and women who incur chronic hepatitis C each year, "about 20 to 30 percent go on to develop cirrhosis." The virus, which can also culminate in primary liver cancer, advances extremely slowly. On average, cirrhosis doesn't emerge for ten to twenty years after the initial infection; cancer, for thirty years.

Discovered in 1989, hepatitis C is very much an enigma. While it's confirmed that people can contract the disease through contaminated needles, hemodialysis treatment for kidney failure, and, rarely, blood transfusions, in four in ten cases the source of transmission remains a mystery.

Nancy suffered such serious complications from hepatitis C that a liver transplant offered her the only realistic hope for survival. Transplants are still relatively uncommon, however. Treatment sometimes calls for subcutaneous injections of the *immunological* agent interferon alfa-2b (brand name: Intron-A) three times a week for six months. Patients—and caregivers—are taught to administer the shots.

Interferon, a natural substance produced by the body, stimulates noninfected liver cells to inhibit the hepatitis virus from replicating. Currently the only approved treatment for hepatitis C (and B), it is not without drawbacks. The medication is expensive and frequently produces debilitating side effects. Then there's the question of its effectiveness. Only one in four patients sees her hepatitis C go into remission for an extended period of time. What's more, it is not yet known whether interferon deters the virus from ultimately proceeding to cirrhosis or cancer.

Several other liver diseases can also give rise to adult cirrhosis of the liver:

* *hemochromatosis*, in which excess iron collects in the liver and other organs;
* *Wilson's disease*, characterized by an accumulation of copper;
* *Primary sclerosing cholangitis*, the buildup of bile in the liver, leading to cell damage;
* *Primary biliary cirrhosis*, a chronic ailment that progressively destroys the liver's bile ducts.

Early Symptoms and Diagnosis of Liver Disease

Because hepatitis and cirrhosis both injure liver tissue, they share many of the same symptoms. "The one I hear from patients most often," says Dr. Bacon, "is fatigue and a lack of energy." In its early stages, liver disease may also bring about:

* indigestion, nausea, appetite loss;
* marked weight loss stemming not only from a lack of interest in eating but from the liver's inability to utilize the nutrients in food;
* diarrhea;
* a propensity for bleeding and bruising due to a decline in certain proteins that promote blood clotting. Patients may experience bleeding gums, tarry stools, frequent and heavy nosebleeds, and bloody vomit.

Dr. Bacon stresses that even people with advanced liver disease may not appear terribly ill. "A lot of times," he says, "the people around them don't believe they're very sick, which of course is very frustrating for patients. I've had situations where husbands and wives come in together, and I'll assure the sick person that their complaints of not feeling well are legitimate. They'll turn to the other and say, 'See, I told you so!' "

Nancy's symptoms were so vague and comparatively mild, recalls Naomi, that she and her husband assumed the teenager merely "had a bad cold." The diagnosis escaped her Mayo Clinic physicians at first. "They said she had pneumonia and needed to rest at home. But a few days later Nancy's joints ached so bad, she could hardly get off the couch. So we took her back to the clinic, they did more tests, and that's when they discovered she had hepatitis."

Oftentimes a physician will suspect liver disease based on just the patient's description of symptoms and a physical examination. A liver that feels sore and swollen, for instance, may signal the onset of liver failure. Although the diseased organ eventually shrinks in size, it expands initially to compensate for cells too damaged to carry out their tasks. The doctor's touching (*palpating*) the area is liable to provoke a deep aching sensation or outright pain.

The next step in confirming a diagnosis involves testing the person's blood for specific enzymes emitted by the damaged liver. Your loved one's doctor may additionally order a *biopsy*, in which a needle is used under local anesthesia to harvest a tiny sample of liver tissue.

A diagnostic workup may also include ultrasound imaging or a CT scan and a laparoscopy, which is performed under local or general anesthesia. The physician inspects the liver through a viewing instrument *(laparoscope)* placed inside a small incision in the abdominal wall.

Managing Symptoms of Liver Failure

Since cirrhosis is incurable, the purpose of therapy is to slow its progression and to control the symptoms and complications that are apt to arise as liver function deteriorates.

Jaundice

In jaundice, probably the symptom most commonly associated with liver disease, bile pigments called *bilirubin* collect in the bloodstream, turning the skin, the whites of the eyes, and other tissues a yellowish hue.

Normally the liver absorbs bilirubin from red blood cells and synthesizes it with cholesterol and other substances to form bile, which is then secreted to the intestines to aid in digestion. But when damaged by cirrhosis or chronic hepatitis, the organ can no longer take in its usual quota, and the orange-yellow pigment accumulates in the circulation.

How It Is Managed

Bile products can also seep into the skin, causing intense itching that may prevent patients from getting a good night's sleep. Thus skin care becomes a paramount concern for caregivers. Conscientious hydration and sponge baths using tepid water and a baking soda product can help alleviate discomfort from jaundice, followed by moisturizing the skin with an emollient lotion. ◄ *See "Skin Care," page 116.*

Gallstones

People with cirrhosis are especially prone to *gallstones*, stonelike masses consisting of crystallized cholesterol and/or pigments from bile. The liver stores this fluid in the *gallbladder*, the small pear-shaped organ located just beneath it. Gallstones range from pebble size to golf ball size, yet they can reside in the gallbladder for years without incident.

Sometimes, though, one or more stones enters the *common bile duct*, the thin conduit that delivers bile to the small intestine, and lodges there. The duct and the gallbladder contract and release, contract and release, in an attempt to extricate the stone. These attacks can be excruciatingly painful. In addition, with the duct blocked, bile can back up into the bloodstream, causing jaundice.

How It Is Managed

The following methods are used:

If your loved one has *cholelithiasis* (gallstone formation), but with minimal or no symptoms, the doctor may elect to merely monitor her condition.

Drug Therapy. For those whose symptoms are intolerable, an oral *gallstone dissolution agent* called ursodiol (brand name: Actigall) can sometimes dissolve the stones, sparing them surgery. Treatment takes several months, however, and does not always whittle down stones completely. What's more, as many as half of all patients suffer a recurrence within five years.

Surgery. Over 400,000 *cholecystectomies*, the operation to remove the gallbladder, are performed each year in this country. A relatively simple surgical procedure, it requires a two- to three-day hospital stay and several weeks of recuperation at home.

Edema/Ascites

Albumin, formed in the liver, is a protein that patrols the bloodstream, regulating the natural seepage of water through the membranous walls of the tiny capillaries and into the microscopic spaces between cells throughout the body. Liver disease curtails albumin production; consequently, the fluid may inundate the tissue of the legs and ankles *(dependent edema)* or pool in the abdomen *(ascites)*. Either condition induces noticeable swelling.

Severe ascites can compress the digestive organs, lungs, and blood vessels, interfering with eating, respiration, and circulation. The symptom isn't life-threatening per se but, Dr. Bacon explains, "people can die from accompanying complications. For instance, the ascitic fluid can become infected, and infections of the abdomen can be quite serious. Or patients develop kidney failure in addition to their liver failure. We call this *hepatorenal syndrome*. It's usually seen in people with severe liver disease and a lot of ascites, and, unfortunately, it is very difficult to treat successfully." ► *See chapter 19, "Caring for Someone with Kidney Disease."*

How It Is Managed

The following methods are used:

Drug Therapy. The doctor will prescribe a *diuretic* drug, which increases urination and rids the body of excess fluid. Restricting salt in the diet helps, too, because sodium causes the body to retain water.

Surgery. Extreme cases may require either of two surgical procedures. In *paracentesis*, patients receive an injection of local anesthetic. The physician then withdraws the ascitic fluid into a *trocar*, a sharp-pointed instrument enclosed in a tube. A more permanent solution is to insert a *peritoneal-venous shunt* consisting of two tubes and a one-way valve. The device, also referred to as a *LeVeen shunt*, continuously drains fluid from the abdomen and returns it to the venous system via a large vein.

Until the ascites is brought under control, keep your loved one's head elevated at least 20 inches in bed. Most patients find that this position allows them to breathe more freely. Placing a pillow under the calves is also recommended to prevent edema of the lower extremities. We never want patients to remain in one position, of course, which impedes circulation and invites the formation of bedsores. As often as possible, help the person lie on her side, propping small pillows around the rib cage for support and another between the knees. ◄ *See "Tricks for Stimulating Appetite," page 159; "Difficulty Breathing (Dyspnea)" page 174.*

Life-Threatening Complications of Liver Failure

As the scarred liver closes itself off to the portal vein that delivers blood from the intestines and the spleen for processing, patients fall prey to a number of serious complications. The flow stalls in the short, thick vein and pressure builds and builds *(portal hypertension)*, until the blood actually forces the creation of new branches, bypassing the liver.

Consequently, waste products, acids, toxins, and bacteria accumulate in the body, causing what Dr. Bacon characterizes as "profound metabolic abnormalities." The overall effect is akin to corrosion clogging a car's fuel line:

INSIDE INFORMATION

Progressive liver failure often makes patients highly sensitive to medications. With the diseased organ unable to filter chemicals at its customary rate, the drugs build up in the system and remain active longer than intended, dulling mental function. Consult with the doctor before giving your loved one *any* drug, particularly pain relievers and sedatives. Attempts should be made to prevent constipation, which can contribute to encephalopathy by detaining toxins in the intestinal tract. ◀ See "Constipation and Gas," page 167.

Eventually the engine breaks down. *Metabolic acidosis* (acid overload in the blood and body tissues), imbalances of crucial minerals called electrolytes, heightened susceptibility to infection, hepatic encephalopathy (see below)— any of these conditions can prove fatal, especially for someone already weakened by liver damage.

Hepatic Encephalopathy

A glut of toxins in the circulation due to liver damage can harm the brain. This is called *hepatic encephalopathy*. Its effects range from poor concentration and hand tremors to confusion and personality changes, to coma and death.

Patients with a history of alcohol abuse are additionally subject to neurological disorders arising from a shortage of *thiamine*, or vitamin B₁. Among other functions, it aids production of body chemicals crucial to the nervous system. Alcohol-related encephalopathy's cluster of symptoms—double vision; paralysis of the eye muscles; *nystagmus*, a rapid, involuntary fluctuation of the eyes; an awkward, unsteady gait; disorientation—often comes on abruptly. Sometimes these are accompanied by memory loss, or *amnesia*.

Oral thiamine supplements usually correct disturbances of the eyes immediately. However, the faculties of walking, thinking, and perception return painfully slowly, if at all. As for patients with amnesia brought on by alcohol-associated thiamine deficiency, the out-

look is bleak. Only one in five recovers fully, and nearly as many die during the acute phase. Sadly, a number of these people must spend the rest of their lives confined in a psychiatric institution.

How It Is Managed

The following methods are used:

Drug Therapy. Most likely the doctor will prescribe a strong laxative such as lactulose syrup (brand names include Cephulac), which absorbs toxins and expedites their removal from the intestinal tract.

Low-Protein Diet. Excessive amounts of unmetabolized protein are believed to be partly responsible for hepatic encephalopathy. Your loved one's physician may therefore also suggest restricting dietary protein so that fewer toxins form in the digestive tract.

Variceal Bleeding

Portal hypertension—the backup of blood in the vein leading to the liver— can bring about other serious complications such as an enlarged spleen and ascites: The increased pressure forces fluid to leak through the liver capsule and into the abdominal cavity.

The biggest problem from portal hypertension is internal hemorrhaging. We explained how the blood, blocked from entering the liver, bores new routes around it. Blood vessels in the stomach and the esophagus also become distended. *Varices* refers to offshoot vessels that become engorged with blood, their walls stretched dangerously thin and prone to rupturing. Variceal bleeding constitutes a medical emergency; its seriousness is compounded by the fact that people with liver disease often have concurrent clotting disorders.

Naomi Black: *When Nancy was in college, the veins inside her burst. By the time we got her to the hospital, she'd lost so much blood, they had to give her seven pints. A few years later she had another bad attack and had to have more blood transfusions.*

How It Is Managed

When it comes to bleeding, there are two concerns:

Controlling Bleeding. "If a patient has catastrophic bleeding," says Dr. Bacon, "you need to get him to a hospital right away." Spitting up bright red blood is an obvious indication that someone is hemorrhaging internally. We should also look for a hard, abnormally distended abdomen and signs of shock, including profuse perspiration, a rapid pulse, cold, wet skin, and falling blood pressure.

Two techniques are commonly used to prevent variceal bleeding. In *sclerotherapy*, a flexible viewing instrument called an *endoscope* is inserted through the mouth and down into the esophagus or the stomach. Then the physician collapses the ruptured veins by injecting them with a hardening solution. Sclerotherapy is also used to rid the skin of *spider naevi*, networks of minuscule spiderlike blood vessels frequently seen in cirrhosis patients.

The other method entails passing a special tube through the nostrils and down into the bleeding site. The device contains three shafts: one leading to a balloon in the stomach, one to a balloon in the esophagus, and one for suctioning the contents of the stomach. Inflating the balloons compresses the varices; ice water is sometimes circulated through the stomach tube to further help control hemorrhaging.

Treating Portal Hypertension. Mild portal hypertension may be able to be kept in check with *beta-blockers*, a family of drugs typically used to treat high blood pressure from cardiovascular disease and other causes. Critical cases, however, call for surgery: either a liver transplantation, described later in this chapter, or a *portacaval shunt*. Here the surgeon connects the portal vein to the large *inferior vena cava* vein, which returns blood from the lower part of the body to the heart, thus allowing for excess blood to drain to the general circulation.

How Liver Disease Is Treated

Whereas cirrhosis brought on by chronic viral hepatitis is usually difficult to halt, the person with early-stage alcoholic cirrhosis stands a chance of averting further liver damage and enjoying years of reasonably healthy living—provided he gives up alcohol completely.

Sad to say, for many drinkers that can be an insurmountable hurdle. Patients diagnosed with alcoholic cirrhosis have drunk heavily for at least ten years, on the average, approximately the same amount of time it takes for *alcohol abuse* to become full-fledged *alcoholism*. Although the American Medical Association classified alcoholism as a disease back in 1956, there are still plenty of folks who feel that addiction of any kind indicates a lack of willpower, a deficit of moral character, and so forth. They believe the alcoholic could give up drinking "if he really tried." What they don't understand or accept is that an alcoholic is not only psychologically dependent on drink but almost always is physically addicted, so that abstaining—sometimes even for just one day—produces withdrawal symptoms ranging from mild (tremors of the hands, nausea, and vomiting) to potentially fatal (grand mal seizures, delirium tremens).

If your loved one is still using alcohol at the time of diagnosis and has a history of physical dependence, the doctor will admit him to a hospital or an alcoholism treatment facility for three to ten days of *detoxification*, in which the body rids itself of the toxic effects of alcohol. Fewer than one in ten alcoholics experiences severe withdrawal symptoms. But because these men and women are often in fragile health—dehydrated, malnourished, and suffering from complications of liver disease— they need to be carefully monitored by medical professionals. Many require tranquilizers and sedatives to help relieve anxiety and agitation, and to enable them to sleep.

The next step is to assist patients in staying sober. For an alcoholic, drinking has often been a way of life if not the very center of life. Among the goals of rehabilitation is to help him discover a new pattern for living as well as to get to the heart of the underlying emotional pain that fueled his excessive drinking in the first place.

According to a survey of substance abuse treatment facilities and their clients, approximately one in ten patients enters a residential facility. Over a twenty-eight-day period, typically, these patients undergo a highly structured program of alcoholism education, individual counseling, group therapy, and, as the day of discharge nears, family therapy. Following their release, *maintenance* therapy continues either at an outpatient facility or through regular attendance at peer support groups such as Alcoholics Anonymous. Outpatient care, by far the most popular form of primary treatment for alcoholism, varies widely in intensity. One program may operate eight hours a day, seven days a week; another, three hours a day, several times a week.

The hot lines listed here can direct you to alcohol abuse treatment programs in your area. Other sources for referrals include psychiatrists, therapists, social workers (either in private practice or at the hospital), clergymen, and family members, friends, acquaintances, or coworkers who have been in rehab themselves.

☎ Alcoholics Anonymous, 212-870-3400

☎ Center for Substance Abuse Treatment National Drug and Alcohol Treatment Referral Routing Service, 800-662-4357

☎ 1-800-COCAINE (800-262-2463)

☎ National Clearinghouse for Alcohol and Drug Information, 800-729-6686

☎ National Council on Alcoholism and Drug Dependence Hope Line, 800-622-2255

Studies comparing the effectiveness of the different modes of alcohol rehabilitation have been inconclusive. The truth of the matter is that the failure rate for treatment as a whole is discouragingly high. Half of all people who complete rehab are back to drinking within three months; more than 90 percent relapse over the next four years. Most of those who manage to maintain their sobriety do so through AA or similarly modeled "twelve-step" peer support programs.

If you're caring for someone with liver disease, chances are you've traveled down this dead end before. We're not suggesting you give up hope, only that you have realistic expectations. When a person has spent the better part of a lifetime viewing the world through the bottom of a bottle, it may be that no type of intervention or any amount of love and support will be able to overcome that.

One incentive for sobriety is the fact that liver disease takes any remaining pleasure out of drinking. Liver patients who imbibe become hellishly sick. An oral drug called disulfiram (brand name: Antabuse), taken daily, works according to a similar principle. It pro-

> If you are caring for someone addicted to alcohol, you need help and support, too. Consider joining AA's sister organization, Al-Anon, a national self-help group made up of family members of alcoholics.
>
> ☎ For a referral to the chapter nearest you, call the Al-Anon World Service Office at 800-344-2666.

duces a heightened sensitivity to alcohol so that even a small sip brings on nausea and profuse vomiting, a throbbing headache, sweating, chest pain, blurry vision, and a sensation of impending death. Antabuse should never be prescribed without the patient's full consent and thorough understanding of its effects.

When nothing seems to be working, perhaps it's time to accept that a loved one is going to die of alcohol-related liver disease. On the average, alcoholism shears twelve to fifteen years off a person's life. Sure, you can hurl yourself into the drama of trying to prevent him from drinking. But no matter how admirable your intentions, you must ask yourself this: Is "saving" this person from drinking by sermonizing, condemning, cajoling, and guilt-tripping really going to save a life? It took your loved one years, perhaps a lifetime, to get to where he is today. Only he can change his course now. Accept that and then move on. Invest your energy and emotions in nursing the person right now, and let both him *and yourself* off the hook.

Diet

As caregiver you may inherit the responsibility of overseeing your loved one's diet at home. Unless the person is about to die, sound nutrition is one of the keys to managing cirrhosis, helping injured liver cells to mend and stemming further deterioration. It's also essential because the body of a person with liver dysfunction is operating at a nutritional deficit, deprived of nutrients, vitamins, and minerals.

These patients are often particularly deficient in protein, which the body uses for energy, building and maintaining tissue, and, for that matter, virtually every bodily function. Make sure that roughly 15 percent of your loved one's daily diet consists of protein, the recommended dietary allowance. So if the doctor or dietitian has suggested your mother eat, say, 1,600 calories a day, the diet should include 192 to 240 calories of protein—or 48 to 60 grams, since each gram of protein equals 4 calories. The Nutrition Facts labels on packaged foods specifies the number of grams of protein per serving.

The challenge in feeding people with liver disease, warns Dr. Kyle Brown, "is that most of them are anorexic. It's a problem getting them to eat enough calories of *any* composition." Those still addicted to alcohol tend to have poor eating habits, but even when drinking is not a factor, the effects of cirrhosis—ascites, nausea, and hormonal changes that influence the appetite center of the brain—often curb the desire for food. "The ascites in and of itself can be a big problem," says Dr. Brown, a gastroenterologist at the John Cochran Veterans Administration Medical Center in St. Louis. "Patients have this fullness in their abdomen, so they just don't feel like eating."

We therefore need to maximize protein and calories without loading on too much fat. Try serving protein-rich foods such as meat, poultry, grains, peanut butter, fish, dairy products, nuts and seeds, and peas, lentils, soybeans, and other legumes. Four ounces of medium-fat beef contains 28 grams of protein, 300 calories, and 20 grams of fat. Chicken breast is an especially good source: A skinless 4-ounce portion packs the same amount of protein but only 140 calories and 4 grams of fat. Don't obsess over protein, however. Our main concern is getting patients to eat, period.

INSIDE INFORMATION

If hepatic encephalopathy becomes a recurrent problem, the physician will likely impose a low-protein diet. In Dr. Brown's view, all too often the restriction is administered prematurely and out of habit.

"It's an appropriate thing to do only after you've ruled out the other causes of encephalopathy, of which there are about half a dozen," he contends. "These patients, by virtue of their liver disease, are already malnourished. Anytime you start fooling around with people's diets, telling them what they can't have, it just makes it harder for them to find foods they want to eat." Should your loved one's physician prescribe a low-protein diet, ask him to reconsider his decision, or justify why he feels it is necessary.

"If they're not interested in food or they don't finish their meals," suggests Dr. Brown, "go for a strategy of small well-balanced snacks throughout the day," including one at bedtime. A healthy person can go without eating between dinner and breakfast, for should the body use up the sugar in the bloodstream during the night, the liver converts its reserves of glycogen to glucose and circulates the fuel as needed. "People with liver disease don't have a normal supply of glycogen," explains Dr. Brown. Ten or twelve hours without food leaves them low on glucose, forcing the body to break down muscle tissue for energy instead.

A low-sodium diet (2 grams a day) is all but mandatory for people with liver disease on account of their propensity for developing edema and ascites. Considering that the average American consumes 2.5 to 6 grams of sodium daily, you can see why Dr. Brown refers to this as "a very difficult restriction for people to live with." ◄ *See "Tricks for Stimulating Appetite," page 159.* ► *See Appendix B: "Dietitians," page 506.*

Liver Transplantation

After Nancy survived a third life-threatening episode of variceal bleeding around Christmas 1985, her physicians decided it was time to seriously consider a liver transplantation.

Increasingly, says Dr. Bacon, "we don't let people get that sick nowadays; we intervene with a transplant sooner." Still, the procedure is relatively rare: 3,922 were performed in 1995. The donor organ must come from a person declared brain dead with a functioning liver and a compatible blood type.

Before a patient's name is listed with the United Network for Organ Sharing (UNOS), says Dr. Bacon, "we have to be sure the rest of his or her body is healthy enough to tolerate the transplant." The grueling, complex operation lasts eight to twelve hours and involves attaching several major blood vessels and bile ducts. In addition, notes Esther Benenson, a spokesperson for UNOS, "Most transplant programs require patients to have demonstrated at least six months of sobriety; some more, some less."

UNOS oversees the distribution of donor organs for the U.S. government. In a major policy change, in 1997 the nonprofit organization moved patients with chronic liver diseases from status one—or top priority for a transplant—to status two or three, depending on whether or not they needed to be hospitalized. Status one is reserved for people suffering from acute liver failure, though naturally there is no guarantee that an organ will be available in time. Chronically ill patients may have to wait longer now for a transplant, but 95 percent of all donor livers go to people with chronic hepatitis C and other chronic liver disorders. According to the American Liver Foundation, 72 percent of liver recipients survive at least three years.

Nancy underwent her transplant at the Mayo Clinic in early December 1987, coming home on Christmas Eve. The major hazard facing a transplant patient is that her body will reject the donor organ, which the immune system perceives as a foreign invader. Consequently, patients must spend the rest of their lives on *immunosuppressant agents*, drugs that, through a variety of mechanisms, neutralize the defense network. Nancy learned to give herself daily injections of cyclosporine (brand name: Sandimmune).

One side effect of immunosuppression is an increased vulnerability to infection. "Nancy got strep throat," recalls her mother. "Another time she had shingles, which was very painful." But other than the concern over her daughter's enlarged spleen, "things seemed good." Then

Nancy and her family were at our house the night she died. We had a few neighbors over and played boccie ball, then they went home at a quarter after eleven. Gary called an hour later to say that she had passed out, and he'd taken her to the hospital. At about a quarter after one, the doctors told us she was gone. Had her spleen ruptured in the hospital, they might have been able to save her. It was very sudden.

With Nancy there had been so many times when we didn't think she was going to make it, so when she did die, we weren't prepared for it because she'd been doing so well.

Recommended Reading

The following are available free from the National Digestive Diseases Information Clearinghouse (301-654-3810):

- "Cirrhosis of the Liver"
- "Cirrhosis—Information Packet"
- "Hepatitis C—Information Packet"

—19—

Caring for Someone with Kidney Disease

It was during a college physical in 1965 that doctors discovered one of Paul Clarke's (a pseudonym) kidneys had stopped functioning. The news came as a shock, for Paul, then eighteen, had never exhibited any symptoms suggestive of a renal problem. But then, people can go their entire lives with one healthy kidney, which ably compensates for the loss of its twin.

Over the next fifteen years Paul married and became an attorney. Other than high blood pressure, he felt fine. But a routine examination revealed that his working kidney was showing signs of chronic renal failure. Paul's wife, Gerri, also a lawyer, recalls, "The doctors said it could take anywhere from one year to thirty years before the kidney totally shut down. It turned out to be a little more than a year. Although Paul's kidney failure was slowly getting worse and worse, he was never so symptomatic that it really affected him. But he and his doctor discussed at length initiating dialysis treatment early so that he wouldn't get to the point where he felt truly horrible. Six weeks before our first daughter was born, in 1980, Paul began hemodialysis at home —at first twice a week, then three times a week. For the next thirteen years this was our life."

More than forty thousand men and women die each year of kidney failure, a state where the identical organs have sustained such extensive damage that they can no longer perform their vital functions, such as ridding the body of chemical waste and excess fluid. *Acute* renal failure, which comes on abruptly due to inflammation, infection, physical trauma, or a reaction to a drug or chemical, is often reversible if the underlying cause can be corrected before the kidneys become permanently damaged.

This is not true of *chronic* renal failure. Three stages mark the gradual and permanent deterioration that occurs over a period of years or decades: *de-*

creased *renal reserve*, *renal insufficiency*, and *end-stage renal disease*. This chapter focuses on the more than 260,000 people living with ESRD. The kidneys are remarkably hardy. Even at this point, with 90 percent of their tissue destroyed, the organs keep working, albeit less efficiently. Generally, however, once renal function dips below 5 percent, a patient will die unless he receives regular *dialysis* treatment—a procedure that takes over the inert kidneys' duties for the rest of a person's life—or a *kidney transplant*.

Although ESRD can be classified as a controllable chronic condition, patients and family members live with the knowledge that a potentially serious complication can erupt at any time. The Clarkes, from New York, were vacationing in Arizona when Paul suffered an episode of renal bleeding.

"It was scary," recalls Gerri, forty-eight. "I had two young children sitting in a hotel room and a husband who was critically ill and couldn't move. I had to race him in a car forty-five minutes to the nearest hospital. Fortunately, the staff there handled the emergency extremely well. Then we were able to get him back home."

The Kidneys

In spite of their small size (four inches long, two inches wide, one inch thick) and weight (4 to 6 ounces apiece), the bean-shaped kidneys receive more blood from the heart than any other organ: 540 gallons every day. What enables each kidney to handle such a massive influx of fluid is a complex network of 1 million filtering units called *nephrons*. After blood is delivered to the kidney by way of the renal artery, it travels through smaller arterioles, which diverge into tiny capillaries. These in turn relay the blood to the *glomerulus*, a tuft of capillaries housed in a cuplike receptacle perched at the end of each nephron. Chronic *glomerulonephritis*, the

form of kidney disease that most frequently progresses to renal failure, is an inflammation of the glomeruli.

Glomeruli act as sieves, retaining blood cells and protein. The fluid portion of the blood *(plasma)*, which contains both essential chemicals and waste products, passes through and then continues along a winding course of fine nephron *tubules*. Cells in the tubule walls reabsorb virtually all the plasma and valuable minerals and salts, and return these to the general circulation. The nephrons also bear the crucial task of correcting the blood's concentrations of water, acid, potassium, sodium, phosphate, and other chemicals based on the body's needs; excess amounts proceed through the urinary tract as *urine*, along with the waste. Of the forty-five gallons of fluid the kidneys draw off from the blood each day, only one and a half quarts reach the *renal pelvis*, the funnel-shaped collecting channel in each organ that drains into the *ureter* tube. From there the urine is stored temporarily in the bladder before being eliminated.

Besides filtering the blood and adjusting the body's equilibrium of acids and nonacids *(bases)*, and water and sodium, the kidneys play an essential role in enabling the bones to absorb calcium; help regulate blood pressure; synthesize vitamins that control growth; and stimulate production of red blood cells, which carry oxygen to all living tissues.

Causes of End-Stage Renal Disease

The hormonal disorder *diabetes* and poorly controlled *hypertension* account for more than half of all cases of chronic kidney failure. Both injure the renal blood vessels, which harden and thicken from the years of wear and tear. The kidney tissue, denied its usual supply of blood, dies off until the damaged organs no longer function efficiently.

Diabetes

People with diabetes must balance a specialized diet with oral medications or injections of insulin, the hormone that under normal circumstances enables the body to burn and store glucose, its chief source of fuel. As we explain later in this chapter, dialysis patients follow an even more rigid meal plan; consequently, caring for a diabetic person with end-stage renal disease can be tremendously complicated. A routine day might involve administering dialysis at home or driving your loved one to and from a dialysis center; testing her blood glucose levels and injecting insulin two, three, or more times; *and* overseeing her diet. Because renal failure hastens several complications of diabetes, diabetics often begin dialysis sooner than other folks with waning kidney function. ◄ *See chapter 16, "Caring for Someone with Diabetes."*

Hypertension

You'll recall that one of the kidneys' numerous functions is to regulate the pressure of the blood pulsing against vessel walls throughout the body. If it's too low, the nephrons flood the circulation with *renin*, which induces the walls to constrict slightly. Too high? The nephrons secrete less of the enzyme, and the muscular walls relax. Renin also assists in controlling the amount of salt and water transferred from the blood vessels to the urine, raising the pressure within the tubular compartments.

Chronically high blood pressure, or hypertension, sets in motion a destructive cycle, with the added stress on the renal vessels impairing the kidneys' blood pressure control mechanism . . . which exacerbates the hypertension . . . which further damages the organs— and so on. (Most men and women with diabetes, incidentally, suffer from hypertension either as a direct complication of the disease or because they're well above their recommended weight.)

Hypertension accelerates the process of *atherosclerosis*, which is perhaps one reason that heart attack and stroke rank behind only infection as the leading causes of death among dialysis patients. Diabetics with end-stage renal disease can't afford to neglect their diabetes, and your loved one's doctor will almost certainly advocate steps to control blood pressure: a low-salt, low-fat diet; exercise; shedding excess pounds; cutting down on alcohol; and giving up smoking. Most ESRD patients are routinely prescribed *antihypertensive medications;* those with high levels of cholesterol and other fatty substances *(lipids)* in their blood may receive *hypolipidemic* drugs as well.

Kidney Diseases

Earlier we mentioned chronic glomerulonephritis, the form of kidney disease that beset Paul Clarke and the third most frequent cause of end-stage renal disease. Another serious threat is a hereditary disorder known as *polycystic kidney disease (PCK)*, in which hollow spaces called *cysts* spring up throughout the organ and infringe on the nephrons. Eventually the kidneys swell to three or four times their normal size and cease functioning. While several other renal ailments can force patients onto dialysis—kidney stones, atherosclerosis of the renal artery, chronic inflammations of the tubules *(pyelonephritis, interstitial nephritis)*—these bare less common causes of ESRD.

Analgesic Drugs

A headline-making 1994 study established a link between end-stage renal disease and heavy, prolonged use of two types of nonprescription pain relievers: *acetaminophen*, the ingredient in such popular brands as Excedrin and Tylenol, and *nonsteroidal anti-inflammatory drugs (NSAIDs)*, such as Motrin and Advil. According to the report, taking one or more pills containing acetaminophen per day—or more than one thousand over the course of a lifetime—doubles a person's chances of eventually having to go on dialysis. Similarly, men and women who consume more than five thousand NSAIDs during their lifetime (not as implausible as it may sound: an average of four pills per week for twenty-five years, or three per week for thirty-three years) see their odds of developing ESRD multiply fourfold.

The implication of the study? If a loved one requires habitual relief for chronic pain—say, from arthritis—you should ask the doctor about possibly prescribing another type of analgesic. Aspirin, even in considerable doses, does not harm the kidneys. However, it and other *salicylates* can generate a different set of problems, including stomach ulcers, gastric bleeding, and impaired blood clotting.

Symptoms of Chronic Renal Failure

The kidneys carry out their assignments so efficiently that renal function can decline to 10 percent—and sometimes lower—before symptoms materialize. Usually the first noticeable signs are fatigue and insomnia, puffiness around the eyes and swelling of the extremities, and an assortment of urinary problems, such as frequent urination (*polyuria*), particularly at night (*nocturia*); a burning sensation upon urinating; difficulty passing urine; bloody urine; and urine that appears frothy.

How Kidney Disease Is Diagnosed

When symptoms point to kidney disease, physicians routinely study the blood and urine for evidence of proteins and other substances indicative of diminished renal function. The most significant of these is *creatinine*, a byproduct of an amino acid produced by the muscles and excreted in urine. A high concentration of creatinine in the blood alerts the *nephrologist* (a doctor who specializes in diagnosing and treating diseases of the kidneys) that the organs are not filtering the blood adequately. Given that the normal blood level of creatinine is one, a level of two denotes 50 percent kidney function; a level of four, 25 percent kidney function, and so on. A blood creatinine level of ten or higher usually signifies total renal failure.

To determine the cause of the kidney disease, your loved one's physician may order:

- an *arteriogram*, in which a contrast solution is injected into a blood vessel and tracked on an X-ray screen as a means of detecting a blocked renal artery.
- one or more of the following lab tests to measure the concentration of glucose in the blood: *fasting blood glucose test, random blood glucose test, oral glucose tolerance test.*
- a *percutaneous kidney biopsy*, in which the physician relies on an imaging technique such as a CT scan or ultrasonography to guide him as he inserts a needle through the skin and into the organ and withdraws one or two samples of tissue. "A biopsy is the only way to definitively state the cause of kidney disease," explains Dr. Allan Hull, former president of the National Kidney Foundation. He adds that fewer than one in ten kidney patients undergo this procedure, carried out under local anesthesia.

Still further diagnostic procedures may be necessary in order to assess the impact of chronic renal failure on the rest of the body: a *chest X ray* to evaluate the heart and lungs; an *electrocardiogram (EKG)* to warn of any cardiac disturbances; and *X rays* to reveal calcium deposits in tissues.

Complications of End-Stage Renal Disease and Their Symptoms

Because the kidneys take part in so many biological processes, ESRD affects literally every bodily system. Symptoms and complications vary in severity from bothersome (nausea, headache, muscle cramps) to potentially fatal (congestive heart failure, cardiac arrhythmias, diminished immunity against infection). Most, including the life-threatening manifestations, usually subside once a person's renal function is restored through dialysis or transplantation surgery. Additional measures may be taken to contain a serious problem or emergency.

Uremia

With the diseased kidneys unable to adequately filter waste products and eliminate them from the body, toxic proportions of urea, uric acid, creatinine, and other substances build up in the blood. This condition, *uremia*, can bring about an array of problems: nausea, vomiting, appetite loss, headache, confusion, dizziness, blurry vision, a urinelike odor to the breath, and elevated blood pressure.

How It Is Managed

Dialysis is used. In *uremic pericarditis*, a serious complication, the heart's tough outer membrane (the *pericardium*) becomes inflamed. Patients typically suffer chest pain and find it difficult to catch their breath. If the underlying uremia is not corrected, the heart may eventually lose elasticity, thus impeding its pumping action.

Hyperkalemia

In the same way that malfunctioning kidneys fail to excrete waste products, *potassium* accumulates in the circula-

tion as well. Potassium, one of the body's electrically charged particles, or *electrolytes*, figures prominently in activating the muscles of the respiratory tract, the intestines, and the heart. Accordingly, the symptoms of *hyperkalemia* include weakness; a tingling sensation in the feet, hands, and tongue; twitching, particularly at night; nausea; diarrhea; muscle cramps; and a sluggish, irregular pulse. At extremely high levels, two grave dangers loom: respiratory paralysis and the irregular heartbeat known as arrhythmias, which can trigger cardiac arrest. ◀ *See "Caring for Someone with Cardiovascular Disease: Arrhythmias," page 344.*

How It Is Managed

A *potassium binder* such as sodium polystyrene sulfonate (brand name: Kayexalate), administered orally or as an enema, binds potassium in the colon so that it can be excreted in the stool. Lowering potassium this way takes hours, sometimes days, and therefore severely hyperkalemic patients may need to begin dialysis at once.

✻ *Hyperkalemia is extremely perilous. When a loved one is diagnosed with ESRD, ask the physician about possibly prescribing a potassium binder as a preventive measure.*

Hypervolemia/Edema

Water makes up roughly 50 percent of our blood. In renal failure, the excess water normally disposed of in urine spills back into the blood vessels. The increased fluid volume, or *hypervolemia*, gives rise to hypertension, which, as you know, afflicts many ESRD patients.

The water can seep out of the vessels and into tissues and body cavities, a condition called *edema*. Its telltale sign is swelling, typically of the hands and feet. People with malfunctioning kidneys may also develop *ascites*. Here fluid collects in the abdomen. Enough liquid may fill this space that the person gains weight suddenly; what's more, the pressure from the expanding peritoneal lining can interfere with breathing, eating, and circulation.

Two critical complications of fluid overload are *congestive heart failure* and *pulmonary edema*. The glut of water in the circulation forces the heart to work harder in order to satisfy the body's demands for oxygen-bearing blood. Eventually it lags behind. When this happens, fluid backs up into the lungs and other tissues. Unless the excess fluid is brought under control, the heart failure and pulmonary edema will compound themselves until the cardiac muscle begins to deteriorate. Symptoms of these interrelated conditions—difficulty breathing, particularly while lying down—constitute a medical emergency and warrant a prompt trip to the hospital.

How It Is Managed

The diuretic medications ordinarily prescribed for hypervolemia and edema work only as long as the kidneys are functioning. A loved one with end-stage renal disease, then, would most likely have surplus fluid pulled off by means of dialysis. If there is evidence of congestive heart failure, the doctor may additionally put the person on the drug digitalis, a *cardiac glycoside*, which intensifies the heart's pumping capacity. ◄ *See "Caring for Someone with Cardiovascular Disease: Congestive Heart Failure," page 347.*

Renal Tubular Metabolic Acidosis

Our health and overall well-being hinge on the balance between so many elements, among them the blood's acidity and alkalinity. Kidney failure impedes the nephron tubules from reabsorbing *bicarbonate* (the electrolyte responsible for neutralizing acids) and rechanneling it to the circulation. This allows so-called *keto acids* to dominate the blood. At first patients may feel weak and complain of a headache. As the acid content rises, the symptoms of *metabolic acidosis* can progress to lethargy, unconsciousness, coma, even death.

How It Is Managed

To restore your loved one's crucial acid-base balance, the medical staff will administer intravenous *sodium bicarbonate*, the main ingredient in over-the-counter antacids such as Alka-Seltzer.

Anemia

The kidneys secrete *erythropoietin*, a hormone that stimulates the bone marrow to produce red blood cells, or *erythrocytes*. Yet another effect of renal failure is a drop in erythropoietin production. This predisposes patients to *anemia*, a shortage of red blood cells. Since these cells ferry oxygen throughout the body, anemic men and women tire easily; in severe cases, physical exertion leaves them short of breath, their hearts pounding, and their pulses racing. Recognizable signs of anemia include pallor of the palms of the hands, the fingernails, and the lining of the eyelids.

How It Is Managed

Patients are treated with injections of synthetic erythropoietin (epoetin alfa; brand names: Epogen, Procrit). In severe cases, transfusions of whole blood or packed red cells are administered.

Renal Osteodystrophy

The bones, too, can incur damage from end-stage renal disease. That is because kidney failure diminishes the blood's level of calcium and allows the blood to retain too much phosphorus, which binds with whatever calcium is available to form the hard, dense material of the bones. When calcium supplies are low, the blood must appropriate it from the bones. Over time, *osteoporosis* develops, with the bones turning brittle and porous and subject to spontaneous fractures. The classic form of the disease produces pronounced curvature of the spine, backaches, and respiratory and digestive problems on account of the rib cage pressing against the lungs and stomach.

Renal osteodystrophy encompasses a group of bone diseases associated with ESRD. Besides osteoporosis, there's *osteomalacia* (characterized by soft, weakened bones), *osteosclerosis* (abnormally hard, dense bones), and *osteofibrosa cystica* (deformities caused by cysts and nodules on the bones). End-stage renal disease also predisposes people to *calcification*. Deposits of calcium phosphate amass in the body's soft tissues, causing itching, inflammation of the membrane lining the eyelids and covering the eyeball (*conjunctivitis*, also known as *pink* eye), and a bony protuberance around the joints in the hands.

How It Is Managed

Dialysis alone cannot sufficiently purge the circulation of phosphorus, and so most renal patients take a second binder, calcium acetate (brand name: PhosLo), with food; the phosphorus remains in the intestine and leaves the body in stool. Once renal osteodystrophy has gained a foothold, dialysis cannot stop it, only slow its progression.

Immunosuppression

Likewise, dialysis cannot fully compensate for the progressive wearing down of the body's natural defenses against pneumonia and other potentially fatal infections. Those of us caring for a person with end-stage renal disease must get into the routine of safeguarding against infection: washing our hands with antibacterial soap, turning bedrid-den patients in order to avoid pressure ulcers, and the other precautions outlined in chapter 3. ◄ *See "Safeguarding Patients Against Infection," page 105.*

Dr. Garabed Eknoyan, chief of renal services at Houston's Ben Taub General Hospital and president of the National Kidney Foundation, cautions that although kidney dialysis patients often lead normal lives for many years, "even the best dialysis restores only about 10 to 15 percent of renal function. That is why some symptoms persist." As caregiver to someone with ESRD, you may encounter problems such as these:

Neuropathy

The term *neuropathy* refers to any of a number of nerve disorders. People on dialysis often complain of leg twitching and muscle cramps, particularly at night, which makes it difficult to sleep. Bear in mind that about one in three kidney patients is diabetic and therefore may also have to cope with the more debilitating effects of what's called *diabetic neuropathy*. These include tingling and numbness in the legs, feet, and fingers, as well as gastrointestinal distress and incontinence resulting from damage to the *autonomic* nerves that control the stomach, bladder, intestines, and many other organs.

How It Is Managed

The exact cause of the twitching and cramping isn't known, but a profusion of phosphorus in the blood *(hyperphosphatemia)* might be the culprit. Cutting down on phosphorus-rich foods such as dairy products and taking a phosphorus binder with meals effectively brings down the blood level. Nevertheless, says Dr. Eknoyan, "the neuropathy associated with ESRD never goes away entirely." ◄ *See "Caring for Someone with Diabetes: Peripheral Neuropathy," page 408; "Managing Pain," page 152.* ► *See "The Renal Diet," page 455.*

Dry, Itchy Skin

Uremia typically leaves the skin dry, itchy, and scaly as the hair follicles exude urea crystals that coat the skin like frost. (In fact, the medical name for this condition is *uremic frost.*) Calcium phosphate deposits, too, produce annoying itching, or *pruritus.*

How It Is Managed

Topical and oral *antipruritic* medications are used. Since ESRD patients are prone to infection, we don't want them scratching so furiously they accidentally scrape themselves, so generously moisturizing the skin with an emollient lotion is a must. Baths containing baking soda also help soothe itching. ◄ *See "Skin Care," page 116.*

Dry Mouth, Altered Taste, and Chronic Thirst

A combination of factors produces the parched mouth, disagreeable taste, and incessant thirst characteristic of end-stage renal disease. One reason is that the saliva of uremic patients contains elevated amounts of urea. "The second reason," explains Dr. Eknoyan, "is that many of these people develop metabolic acidosis. To compensate, they breathe more than you or I would, which dries out their mouth." Third, some of the antihypertensive drugs prescribed to a great percentage of kidney disease patients also dry out the mouth.

How It Is Managed

Whereas ordinarily we would encourage our loved one to drink plenty of water, men and women on dialysis are limited to half a quart to one quart of liquid a day—more if they are still able to empty their bladders. (Many no longer can; Paul Clarke went ten years without relieving himself, until after his kidney transplant. Instead, the urine leaves the body through a surgically im-planted tube that attaches to an external drainage bag, usually worn on the leg.) We want to replace any water lost through urination.

Because renal failure predisposes patients to fluid overload, drinking *too* much is liable to leave them short of breath, with elevated blood pressure and edemic swelling. "Paul would feel all bloated and crummy," says his wife, "from carrying around eight to fifteen extra pounds of fluid."

Obviously, then, alleviating thirst and dry mouth requires a little ingenuity on our part. Lori Fedje, renal nutrition coordinator at the Good Samaritan Hospital dialysis unit in Portland, Oregon, recommends giving patients ice cubes and sour candy to suck on. "Ice," she explains, "tends to go further than water, while sourballs stimulate the saliva glands and help mask the thirst." For combating cotton mouth she suggests squeezing some lemon into drinking water. Have your loved one swish it around in his mouth, then spit it out. This not only freshens but can be repeated as often as he likes.

Another suggestion: encourage patients to brush their teeth, gums, and tongue several times a day to temper unpleasant taste or breath odor. ◄ *See "Keeping Patients Hydrated," page 102; "Intravenous (IV) Injections and Infusions," page 149.*

Depression

Imagine having to carve five hours out of your day for outpatient dialysis three times a week or having to excuse yourself for at least half an hour five times each day in order to dialyze yourself. Small wonder, then, that folks with ESRD frequently become mired in despair, particularly at the start of treatment.

"That's a critical time," observes Charlie Thomas, a renal social worker in the transplant department of Good Samaritan Regional Medical Center in Phoenix, Arizona. "Often, as people approach the initiation of dialysis, they feel absolutely lousy and become less and less able to fulfill their social roles, be it as a worker, a parent, a spouse, or a sexual partner." Changes in circulation, hormones, nerve functioning, and vitality due to chronic kidney failure may dim sexual ability and interest for members of either sex. Depression further compounds sexual disinterest and dysfunction.

"All of those," he continues, "can turn into losses. And while dialysis makes patients feel better physically, their social relationships or feelings about themselves don't necessarily return to normal."

How It Is Managed

By federal mandate, kidney dialysis and transplant programs must employ a master's level social worker to counsel patients and families, with sessions typically beginning during the first few weeks of treatment. Dialysis imposes a rigid new structure on daily life and can drastically alter the dynamics within a household; that's why we strongly encourage patients and those close to them to participate in a support group, which the law requires all programs to offer. Increasingly, says Thomas, the pattern is for several centers in one area to conduct groups cooperatively. ◄ *See "Depression," page 191.* ► *See Appendix A: "Kidney Disease," page 498.*

☎ In addition, both the American Association of Kidney Patients (800-749-2257) and the National Kidney Foundation (800-622-9010) sponsor support groups throughout the country. The NKF also runs a patient-to-patient counseling program.

How End-Stage Renal Disease Is Treated

The artificial kidney machine was invented in 1946. However, for years dial-

ysis was used exclusively to sustain patients with acute renal failure until they recovered. It was only in 1960 that nephrologists began offering the treatment to men and women whose kidneys were irreversibly destroyed from chronic disease. Dialysis stands as one of the pivotal medical breakthroughs of the last half-century. Given the shortage of suitable donor kidneys, only about ten thousand renal patients are fortunate enough to benefit from transplantation surgery each year. Were it not for dialysis, the many thousands of others would die.

Dialysis, explains Dr. Hull, takes over for the impaired kidneys, "pulling off the accumulating poisons in the blood and drawing off excess fluid." *Hemodialysis*, usually administered three times a week in a hospital or a dialysis clinic, uses a mechanical kidney to convey blood from the patient's arm, cleanse it, then return it to the body. Each treatment, conducted by a nurse or a trained technician, takes three to five hours.

In *peritoneal dialysis*, the patient's own peritoneal lining serves as the filter. Patients attach a bag of cleansing solution to a catheter surgically implanted in their abdomen and let the *dialysate* fluid slowly fill the peritoneal cavity. Over the next four to six hours they are free to go about their daily routine as waste and surplus water pass through the membranous peritoneum and into the dialysate. Then patients drain the used solution back into the bag and infuse a fresh two-quart bag. They repeat this process three or four times a day.

For some patients, peritoneal dialysis, introduced in 1976, affords greater flexibility than hemodialysis in that patients can perform their own exchanges at home—or in any clean, well-lit room, for that matter—and tailor the treatment cycle to their daily schedule, whereas people on outpatient hemo must report to the dialysis facility at their regularly appointed time. Should they plan to travel, they have to make arrangements with a hospital or clinic near their destination at least a month in advance. Despite these constraints, four in five dialysis patients receive hemo instead of peritoneal. For one thing, the artificial kidney provides superior filtering. Too, many folks prefer being able to enjoy up to four full days free of treatment as opposed to dealing with it every few hours every day.

Barring circumstances where a person's condition or situation at home dictates one type over another, ultimately it's up to each patient to decide which method of dialysis is most compatible with her lifestyle. Most affiliates of the National Kidney Foundation offer newly diagnosed patients a multisession predialysis education program at which a certified instructor describes each treatment in depth. Some patients, though not all, can change their minds and switch from hemo to peritoneal, or vice versa, at any point.

After investigating their options, the Clarkes settled on home hemodialysis. "For us," says Gerri, "it was really the right decision, because Paul worked full-time the entire thirteen years. If he had a meeting, we could adjust our schedules." With his hectic schedule, Paul considered peritoneal dialysis an unsuitable alternative.

But Is It Covered?

People on dialysis face a lifetime of prohibitively expensive treatment: more than $30,000 annually. Since 1972 the federal government's Medicare insurance program has covered the full amount of approved hospital costs and picked up 80 percent of the tab for dialysis and other medical expenses for anyone with permanent renal failure, regardless of their age. (Two-thirds of dialysis patients are under sixty-five, the age of eligibility for Medicare.)

Still, that leaves 20 percent—$6,000 or so a year, hardly a negligible sum for most folks—plus the monthly Medicare premium ($42.50 in 1996) to be paid. There are several avenues for bridging this gap:

Incentive to Self-Dialyze

Medicare pays for home hemodialysis and peritoneal dialysis beginning with the very first treatment. However, as an incentive for patients to learn to dialyze themselves, coverage for unit dialysis doesn't kick in for three months.

Private Insurance. When someone is insured privately prior to a diagnosis of ESRD, Medicare serves as a secondary payer for the first eighteen months of dialysis. After that the roles reverse, with Medicare becoming the primary payer and the private insurer laying out the remaining 20 percent.

Medigap Insurance. This is a supplemental plan to cover the 20 percent balance as well as Medicare deductibles for hospitalization ($736 in 1996) and medical expenses ($100). Senior citizens can take out Medigap insurance individually or through a group policy, such as those offered by the American Association of Retired People, 601 E Street, N.W., Washington, DC 20049; 800-424-3410. Membership in AARP, an organization for men and women over fifty, costs $8 a year.

Medicaid Insurance. Medicaid provides health coverage to those with limited income and resources. As each state administers its own program, benefits vary, but typically Medicaid pays whatever Medicare does not; in instances where someone fails to qualify for Medicare, Medicaid assumes 100 percent of his medical expenses. Unlike Medicare, Medicaid often funds prescription drugs and transportation to and from dialysis appointments. ◄ See *"Medicaid," page 279.*

State Renal Programs. Roughly half of the fifty states sponsor programs to further help finance ESRD treatment, but only after patients have drawn upon all other available resources.

CHAMPUS/CHAMPVA.   CHAMPUS, which stands for the Civilian Health and Medical Program of the Uniformed Services, is a health benefits program for military retirees and their dependents as well as families of deceased servicemen or those on active military duty. CHAMPVA, the Civilian Health and Medical Program of the Department of Veterans Affairs, covers spouses and children of veterans stricken with an illness or permanently disabled while on active military duty. For the first three months of unit dialysis, CHAMPUS pays 80 percent of all allowable costs; CHAMPVA, 75 percent. At that point Medicare insurance takes over. From then until age sixty-five, both programs bear all secondary expenses as long as the patient is enrolled in Medicare Part B.

For more information contact the military health benefits advisor at a local military hospital. Or call:

☎ CHAMPUS, 303-361-1126

☎ CHAMPVA, 800-733-8387

◄ *See "Veterans and Military Dependents," page 280.*

The dialysis unit's social worker will help your loved one apply for Medicaid. She will also be familiar with additional financial assistance that may be available. For instance, some state renal programs help defray the costs of outpatient medications and transportation, as do the National Kidney Foundation and the American Kidney Fund. Both the NKF and the AKF provide *limited* financial aid and services to patients in need.

The American Kidney Fund (800-638-8299) offers

• modest cash grants for special dietary needs and other treatment-related services and expenses;
• emergency relief following a natural disaster to pay for food, clothing,

household items, utility deposits, and other essential relief services;
• 20 percent copayment for dialysis treatment away from home due to a family or medical emergency.

The National Kidney Foundation (800-622-9010) offers

• free Medic Alert jewelry and cards;
• nutritional supplements to dialysis units for distribution to patients and sometimes free food vouchers at area supermarkets, donated by state affiliates.

◄ *See "How to Get the Most out of Health Insurance," page 280; "Prescription Drug Patient-Assistance Programs," page 275.* ► *See Appendix A: "Kidney Disease," page 498.*

What Caregivers Should Know About Hemodialysis

Sometime prior to the first appointment, people with ESRD undergo an operation to fashion an entrance, or *hemoaccess*, in a blood vessel, usually in the forearm. The preferred technique is to join a vein to an artery, creating what's called an *arteriovenous fistula.* This sizable vessel lies just beneath the surface of the skin. During hemodialysis, one needle is inserted in the vein side and another in the artery side. Both needles attach to tubes, which route the blood to the artificial kidney and back to the circulation.

To be a candidate for a fistula, a person must have healthy blood vessels. "Unfortunately," says Dr. Eknoyan, "well over half of patients end up getting an external shunt"—plastic tubing that protrudes slightly from the arm. The minor surgical procedure for constructing either entry usually requires general anesthesia.

Caring for a Fistula or Shunt

As with any artificial opening in the body, we want to keep the site scrupulously clean. It's also essential to inspect the fistula or shunt regularly for *patency*—that is, to make sure a blood clot isn't plugging up the passageway. "This is very important," stresses Dr. Eknoyan, "because the sooner the problem is detected, the easier it is to declot the vascular access." One time a clot formed in Paul Clarke's fistula while he and his family were on vacation. The problem went unrecognized long enough that he had to undergo a second *fistulization.*

All patients are shown how to check for patency. One way is to feel the spot for a pulse or a slight vibration called a *thrill.* Another is to listen with a stethoscope; a soft *whooshing* sound known as a *bruit* (pronounced *broo-ee*) tells you the blood flow is normal. Ask your loved one, the nephrologist, or the nephrology nurse to demonstrate both techniques for you.

People who tend to clot are frequently put on *anticoagulant* medications. If you're caring for someone with a history of clotting, Dr. Eknoyan recommends checking the venous access several times a day.

A Typical Hemodialysis Treatment

At an outpatient unit, patients can expect to spend three to five hours on the artificial kidney; at home, tack on another hour or so for setup and cleanup. One advantage of home hemodialysis, of course, is no travel time.

For a right-handed person, the fistula or shunt is made in the left arm; for a southpaw, the opposite arm. Although one arm must remain immobilized during dialysis, patients are able to read, watch television, or sleep. "I'd put Paul on the machine when he came

home from work around seven o'clock," says Gerri Clarke. "He did paperwork, caught up on his reading, and ate dinner."

Because home hemodialysis requires another person's assistance, the first several weeks of treatment take place at a unit where a nephrology nurse teaches patients and their care partners how to place the needles in the arm, attach the tubing, and operate and maintain the equipment.

What's in a Number?

Plenty. Either of two measurements, URR and KT/V, reveals how efficiently dialysis treatment eliminates waste from the blood. *URR* stands for *urea reduction ratio*, while *KT/V* represents *clearance* (the quantity of blood cleared of toxins), multiplied by the amount of *time* the patient spends on the machine, divided by the *volume* of urea left in the blood.

Once a month, on the average, blood is drawn before and after a session. If our loved one's unit uses URR, we will want to see at least a 65 percent (0.65) reduction in urea; if it uses KT/V, the postdialysis number should read 1.2 or higher. Ask the dialysis nurse or the physician for the number and enter it in a log. Low numbers are a cause for concern and should be discussed with the nephrologist so that steps can be taken to improve the waste removal. Perhaps treatment needs to be extended or more frequent, or maybe the patient must stick more closely to her diet. People undergoing peritoneal dialysis also have their blood evaluated for urea content.

Side Effects of Hemodialysis

Healthy kidneys are continuously skimming toxins and excess fluid from the blood, whereas hemodialysis must accomplish this task in just a few hours. The rapid changes in the body's chemical balance and fluid level may bring about sundry side effects. Some, such as chest and abdominal pain, are fleeting, occurring ten to fifteen minutes into treatment and lasting but a few minutes. Muscle cramping and hypotension, however, often linger several hours after treatment. *Hypotension*, an abrupt drop in blood pressure, leaves patients weak, dizzy, and nauseous.

We can help loved ones reduce the risk of dialysis-related hypotension by seeing that they restrict their fluid intake as recommended by the physician or dietitian. "In essence," explains Dr. Eknoyan, "they reduce the burden on the machine" so that it doesn't have to remove as much fluid. "Patients who are well managed don't get these symptoms."

It's normal to feel wiped out for several hours after a session as the body adjusts. In the Clarkes' opinion, another benefit of home hemodialysis was being able to dialyze at night. "That way," explains Gerri, "Paul could go right to sleep. By the next morning, he'd be feeling better.

"You have a lot more control at home," she asserts. "Ultimately, it gives you more security even though sometimes you feel as if you're left 'stranded' should a serious problem crop up. But the dialysis unit had someone available to provide assistance twenty-four hours a day, as did the company that leased us the machine, so we always had a lot of backup support."

Our Role as the Patient's Advocate

The amount of control you have over the dialysis relates to the caliber of therapy, which for someone dependent on an artificial kidney becomes a matter of survival. An alarming 1995 *New York Times* investigative report on the quality of hemodialysis care in the United States painted an unflattering portrait of an industry that all too often endangers patients' welfare for the sake of profit. One in four Americans on dial-

ysis dies each year—more than twice the number in Japan, France, or Germany.

In focusing on the country's largest dialysis provider—a company that serves more than forty thousand men and women—the series exposed a number of shoddy (albeit legal) practices, including the use of outmoded, poorly maintained machines and replacing doctors and nurses with underskilled, undersupervised technicians.

One critical point of controversy pertains to the industry at large: patients being shortchanged in terms of time hooked up to the machine. Numerous studies have demonstrated a higher survival rate for people who dialyze longer than the standard three hours. In the United States, kidney patients average ten hours of treatment weekly, as compared to twelve hours in Germany and fourteen hours in Japan.

A second serious concern is the widespread policy of recycling the dialyzer and other disposable equipment. The *dialyzer*—the artificial kidney itself—attaches to the hemodialysis machine. Despite the fact that these filters often bear labels stating SINGLE USE ONLY, the vast majority of facilities reuse them, some as many as *fifty* times. Following treatment, the dialyzer is disconnected, cleaned, coded, and placed in storage until the patient's next visit.

The findings of a 1992 study conducted by the National Institutes of Health revealed a higher death rate among people who dialyzed at centers that used equipment more than once. There are documented cases of patients dying of infections from bacteria-laden secondhand filters or being infused with "purified" blood that in fact contained residues of the bleach and formaldehyde used to clean the equipment. Dialyzers, incidentally, cost as little as $8.50 apiece, while the plastic blood lines, which are difficult to clean thoroughly, go for less than $3.

Unlike in Japan, where multiple use is prohibited, there are no U.S. government restrictions on the number of times a unit can reinstall a dialyzer. In fact, Medicaid guidelines prevent patients from paying for a fresh filter out of their own pockets. Patients who object to receiving dialysis with worn equipment are typically told to go elsewhere—but in many communities there *isn't* anywhere else to go. And even if you could locate a single-use unit nearby, would your loved one's coinsurer pay for it? While Medicare allows recipients to undergo dialysis at any of the more than 2,100 approved facilities around the country, a private payer often directs patients to the center of its choice.

When it comes to other issues concerning care, hemodialysis patients *do* have rights and should not hesitate to exercise them. For care partners, it's time to assume your advocate's role. As often as you can, accompany the person to treatment. Look around. Does the dialysis unit appear clean? Did your loved one receive a minimum of three hours on the machine? You have three options for trying to redress any problems.

The Health Care Financing Administration established seventeen regional *End Stage Renal Disease Networks* primarily as a watchdog for monitoring standards of care and safeguarding patients. (See Appendix A: "Kidney Disease," page 498, for the telephone number of the network serving your state.) "All patients may register a complaint with their network without fear of reprisal," explains Geraldine Rasmussen, executive director of the New York ESRD Network. "The network must investigate every complaint and do everything in its power to correct the problem." If a facility is found to have committed a serious safety violation—unsafe water, hazardous equipment, falsifying records—the network has the authority to shut it down.

Before you set off down that route, however, social worker Charlie Thomas suggests trying to work out problems within the unit first. "I advise patients and families to approach somebody on the staff, the person they trust the most

or with whom they have a rapport," he says. "It may be your unit social worker, the head nurse, or your physician.

"If you don't get satisfaction at that level, then you have more formal options, such as filing a grievance with the ESRD Network. The next step would be to contact your local health department." Dialysis units, whether housed in hospitals or freestanding, are subject to safety regulations set by the state or county health department, which certifies all Medicare facilities. You'll find its telephone number in the Government Listings section of the white pages.

"Support groups are a good resource for people who are frustrated with their unit," adds Thomas. "There you can connect with others who are dealing with the same problems."

Quality varies widely not only from company to company but from site to site within the same company. In the uncommon event that your loved one has the freedom to comparison-shop for a dialysis center, call your ESRD Network and inquire if any grievances have been lodged against the center you're considering. The network can't divulge the exact nature of complaints but can tell you whether or not they've been resolved. When touring a facility, ask patients there to describe the caliber of care. Are they satisfied? Below are some suggested questions for the unit's medical director and other staff members:

- What is your annual mortality rate? *(Compare this against the national yearly average: 23.6 percent. In addition, your ESRD Network can give you mortality rate figures for the state or states within its jurisdiction.)*
- What is your average KT/V or urea reduction ratio? *(The Health Care Financing Administration recommends that clinics meet these standards: KT/V of no less than 1.2, and URR of no less than 65 percent.)*
- How long is each dialysis treatment? *(It should last at least three hours.)*

- Do you have physicians on staff full-time? If not, who is on call for emergencies and when, typically, are they called?
- What is your ratio of registered nurses to patients?
- Does the staff include a renal dietitian? *(By federal law all clinics must employ a renal dietitian.)*
- Can patients refuse a reused dialyzer?
- Do you recycle blood lines?
- Is this a for-profit or nonprofit clinic?

More than six in ten dialysis facilities are run for profit. And with tens of thousands of ESRD patients desperately needing expensive treatment year after year, there is a great deal of money to be made—and hence potential for corruption. *The New York Times* uncovered instances where some for-profit clinics funneled Medicare funds into the pockets of doctors, who reciprocated by referring patients there. While we know of no studies demonstrating that nonprofit dialysis centers offer superior care, Charlie Thomas says without hesitation, "I believe you receive better care in a not-for-profit setting." Most folks, though, don't have a choice.

One heartening development for dialysis patients is the gradual shift toward health maintenance organizations. Yes, HMOs. Despite the trepidation expressed both by medical professionals and the public about the quality of so-called managed care programs, HMO dialysis units have a powerful financial incentive to keep patients healthy and out of the hospital. That same *Times* series looked at a Kaiser Permanente dialysis clinic in Los Angeles. There it found state-of-the-art machines, treatments longer than the national average, and a policy of not reusing equipment if the patient so requests. Even though this particular clinic counted an unusually high percentage of diabetics among its clientele, it boasted markedly lower rates of mortality and hospitalization. By the end of the decade, Thomas predicts, "we'll see more and more kidney patients enrolled in HMO-style programs—hopefully with outcomes that resemble Kaiser Permanente's."

What Caregivers Should Know About Peritoneal Dialysis

Continuous Ambulatory Peritoneal Dialysis (CAPD), the type described earlier, takes around forty minutes per exchange—at least ten minutes to attach the empty bag, fifteen minutes or more to drain the used solution, and another ten minutes to infuse the new bag. If possible, you may want to convert one room into the patient's dialysis area where you store equipment and supplies. The dialysate bags alone—at more than thirty per week—take up a good deal of space. Add to that your clamps, special soap, gauze bandages, sundry gadgets, and so forth.

Two less popular methods of peritoneal dialysis require the use of a *cycler* machine, which connects to the catheter. In *Continuous Cycling Peritoneal Dialysis (CCPD)*, the machine automatically fills and drains the solution from the abdomen every hour and a half while the patient sleeps. *Intermittent Peritoneal Dialysis (IPD)*, the oldest form, typically takes place in a hospital three times a week. The treatments last ten to fourteen hours and must be performed by nurses or technicians.

Side Effects of Peritoneal Dialysis

Because the chemical and fluid exchanges occur more slowly, peritoneal dialysis exerts less stress on internal organs. Its sole serious potential complication is *peritonitis*, an inflammation of the peritoneal lining. Malfunctioning or contaminated equipment, a leaking catheter, tainted solution, an infection at the catheter site—any of these can cause peritonitis, which brings on symptoms such as abdominal pain, fever and chills, nausea and vomiting, diarrhea and confusion. Peritonitis can be deadly if not controlled promptly with antibiotics.

Preventive Management

1. Wash your hands with antiseptic soap before each exchange.
2. Change the sterile dressing over the catheter every day.
3. Slip on a surgical mask every time you open the dialysis system.
4. Perform all exchanges in a clean, dry, well-illuminated room (never the bathroom).
5. Do not use a dialysate bag that has droplets of moisture on the outside, an indication of a possible leak and, consequently, contaminated solution.
6. Encourage your loved one to shower instead of taking long, relaxing baths. Showers are less likely to allow bacteria to infiltrate the catheter site.
7. Follow the procedure *exactly* each time.
8. **Alert the physician** if the skin around the catheter becomes red, warm, swollen, or painful, or if the person spikes a temperature for no apparent reason.
9. **Bring your patient to the doctor or hospital immediately** if the drained solution appears cloudy or if you observe any other symptoms of infection, like fevers.

How It Is Managed

It is treated with antibiotics.

The Renal Diet

Few meal plans are as complicated as the renal diet. On one hand, we're trying to see to it that our loved one takes in ample calories and protein. On the other, we're limiting their consumption of potassium, phosphorus, sodium, *and*

liquids. Compounding the challenge for a caregiver charged with cooking for someone on dialysis is the fact that these folks usually aren't all too keen on eating to begin with. Between the food restrictions, the metallic or urinelike taste in the mouth, the bloated feeling from fluid overload, and other assorted digestive problems, who wouldn't lose his desire for food?

"Malnutrition is quite common with these patients," notes dietitian Lori Fedje, a former chair of the National Kidney Foundation Council on Renal Nutrition. Because the renal diet is so demanding, the dietitian at the dialysis unit typically meets with patients and their caregivers once a month "to review their chemistries and eating habits, and make any necessary dietary adjustments. Then we're available as needed throughout the month."

Although the diets for hemodialysis patients and peritoneal dialysis patients vary slightly, the general principles are essentially the same. Just as a diabetic's chief concern is eating a prescribed amount of carbohydrates, men and women with end-stage renal disease focus on protein, which the body harnesses for energy, to build and repair tissues, and other vital functions.

Protein

People on hemodialysis want to restrict their daily protein intake to 1 to 1.2 grams per kilogram of body weight in order to prevent a buildup in the circulation of its waste product urea between treatments. *One kilogram equals 2.2 pounds; one pound equals roughly half a kilogram.* Thus a person weighing 200 pounds (about 90 kilograms) requires 90 to 108 grams of protein per day, with some protein served at every meal—high-quality protein, by which we mean complete protein from animal sources such as eggs, chicken, fish, and meat. Low-quality protein, derived from vegetables, grains, and other plant sources, contains considerable amounts of phosphorus and potassium, two components people with kidney failure want to avoid. Peritoneal patients can eat 1.2 to 1.5 grams of protein per kilogram because the dialysate absconds with precious proteins normally retained in the blood. Using our example of a 200-pounder, that would come to 108 to 135 grams.

Potassium

"The potassium level," says Fedje, "is probably the strictest part of the renal diet, particularly for hemo patients." With peritoneal dialysis, the continuous blood cleansing "enables us to keep relatively stable levels," she explains. As a result, these patients rarely have to contend with potassium restrictions. But people on hemodialysis must limit their consumption to 2 to 3 grams per day. Foods high in potassium include:

Almonds
Avocado
Bananas
Dried fruits, particularly apricots, peaches, raisins, figs, and prunes
Dry lima beans
Milk and nonfat dry milk
Oranges
Peanuts
Pork
Potatoes
Pumpkin and squash seeds
Sardines
Swordfish
Turkey
Wheat germ

Sodium

In Lori Fedje's experience, renal patients tend to be least compliant with the low-sodium part of the renal diet. "Whereas the symptoms of high potassium disguise themselves, the signs of fluid overload are easy to recognize," she explains. "So if they feel short of breath, they know they can simply come in for dialysis," which pulls off the extra water. In addition to promoting fluid retention, exceeding the rec-

ommended 2 to 3 grams of sodium daily (up to 4 grams for peritoneal patients) sends a person's blood pressure rising and leaves him feeling thirsty.

Phosphorus

Phosphorus, present in all foods but especially milk, cheese, fish, poultry, meat, egg yolk, and dried beans and peas, should be limited to approximately 1,000 milligrams or less a day. You can spare yourself the inconvenience of having to count this mineral by simply keeping dairy products to a minimum.

Few ESRD patients derive sufficient calcium from diet alone. The calcium-based drugs prescribed for regulating the blood's level of phosphorus double as a calcium supplement.

Calories

"End-stage renal disease," says Fedje, "is an extremely *catabolic* illness." That is to say, it robs people of energy and causes muscle to break down, a condition often referred to as *wasting*. "They need more calories than normal to build body tissues and maintain weight." Patients on peritoneal dialysis require 25 to 35 calories per kilogram of body weight per day (2,268 to 2,722 calories daily for a two-hundred-pounder), and those on hemodialysis, 30 to 35 kilograms (2,722 to 3,175 calories daily).

The reason the calorie requirement is less for peritoneal dialysis patients is that the dialysate solution contains glucose, and so, Fedje explains, "patients get an infusion of sugar with each exchange." Although many of these folks are susceptible to heart disease and stroke on account of high blood pressure, we are not as intent on trimming fat as we might be with other hypertensive patients "simply because it is so hard to get them to consume enough calories from other sources.

"However," she emphasizes, "we want to be as cardiac health conscious as we can." Avoid saturated fat and in-

---

INSIDE INFORMATION

The Nutrition Facts label on packaged foods makes it easy to calculate an item's calorie, protein, or sodium content, but how do you determine the amounts of potassium and phosphorus, neither of which is listed? Few books on nutrition include either mineral. One that does is *Bowes and Church's Food Values of Portions Commonly Used* by Jean Pennington. You can find it in bookstores or purchase it directly from the publisher, Lippincott-Raven (800-638-3030).

Usually, though, you won't have to tally up individual minerals and nutrients. The dietitian will compile a roster of permissible foods for meal planning. Ask her for one of the handy 28-page booklets on renal nutrition published by the American Dietetic Association (800-366-1655). The series, "A Healthy Food Guide," addresses the unique dietary needs of folks on peritoneal dialysis and hemodialysis (as well as those with concurrent diabetes) and groups foods according to high, medium, and low levels of both potassium and phosphorus. If your dietitian doesn't have the booklets, you can order all six (single copies are not available to the public) from the ADA.

---

stead serve products containing *polyunsaturated* or *monounsaturated* fat. Both come from vegetable oils and some nuts and seeds, and can help reduce cholesterol.

The Renal Diet and Diabetics

What if your loved one is also diabetic, like so many people on dialysis? Dietitian Fedje calls the renal diabetic diet "a *very* restrictive diet." In addition to monitoring protein, potassium, and the other nutrients and minerals, we must see to it that loved ones get carefully balanced portions of starches and sugars, or carbohydrates. If our patient has insulin-dependent diabetes, we have to coordinate meals and snacks with their hormone injections. Intensive? You bet.

"We try to combine the two diets," Fedje explains. "But because end-stage renal disease is extremely life-threatening, the renal diet tends to take precedence. So we focus on the renal aspects while trying to maintain a normal blood sugar as much as possible." ◄ *See "Caring for Someone with Diabetes: The Diabetic Diet," page 397.*

With or without the diabetic restrictions, Fedje observes, "the renal diet is difficult in that it changes the way people are used to eating." For those of us in charge of cooking, "the most important things are to ensure that patients get adequate protein and calories and maintain their nutritional status. If they're not eating, inform the dietitian and doctor so they can try to come up with other ideas that will work for that patient."

One solution: vitamin supplements containing the recommended daily allowance of vitamins B, C, and folic acid. A word of caution, though: Excessive doses of vitamins B and C may cause a salt called oxalate to build up in body tissues until it forms a hard mass. Do not dispense *any* vitamins—not even over-the-counter brands—without first consulting your loved one's doctor. ◄ *See "Tricks for Stimulating Appetite," page 159.*

Kidney Transplantation

After ten years on dialysis, Paul Clarke asked his nephrologist to place his name on the waiting list for a donor kidney. "He'd had enough," says his wife. With his two daughters entering adolescence and an increasingly busy schedule, he found it harder and harder to set aside the five hours for dialysis three nights a week. And at forty-four, Paul saw his physical condition begin to deteriorate. Dialysis provides stability, whereas kidney transplantation surgery, first performed in 1954, offers the prospect of a long-term solution.

Paul's physician had first broached the idea back in 1980 as an alternative to dialysis. "At that time," Gerri recalls, "the success rate was much lower than it is now. I was pregnant with our first child, and we both felt it wasn't worth taking the risk. We looked into it again five or six years later, but the percentages still weren't very good." By 1991 the survival rates had improved sufficiently that the Clarkes decided to go forward. Today, according to the United Network for Organ Sharing (UNOS), 80 percent of kidney grafts are still working after one year; 75 percent after two years; and 69 percent after three years. (*Graft survival* isn't necessarily commensurate with *patient survival*, as is usually true with other organ transplants. Should the graft fail, renal patients can go back on dialysis indefinitely.)

If the donor organ comes from a living relative rather than someone who is deceased, the figures are higher still— 91 percent, 88 percent, and 84 percent, respectively—for success hangs largely on the similarity between the donor's and the recipient's blood and tissue. A kidney from a living relative usually makes for a closer match. Of the 10,643 transplants performed in 1994, 7,639 utilized cadaver kidneys.

Each year more than thirty thousand renal patients await donor kidneys; only one in three receives one, due to the shortage of suitable donors. The procedure takes three to six hours, and patients typically remain hospitalized for approximately two weeks, the peak time for acute kidney rejection. As with any organ graft, the body's immune system may identify the transplanted new-comer as an invader and seek to obliterate it. "Paul had two minor episodes," his wife recalls. "The first one was on day fourteen, while he was still in the hospital; the second occurred four days after he came home."

But Is It Covered?

As you might expect, the cost of kidney transplantation surgery is exorbitant: $100,000 for the first year and $7,400 each year after that, for drugs and followup visits. Fortunately, Medicare, Medicaid, and most private insurers cover the procedure.

Medicare. The principal payer for the majority of transplant patients also shoulders the expenses of obtaining a suitable donor kidney and the full price of the donor's medical care; this remains in effect for three years following a successful transplant. *Should a loved one's transplant fail at any point thereafter, refile as soon as possible to reestablish coverage for regular dialysis or another transplant.*

CHAMPUS/CHAMPVA. Once Medicare coverage terminates, either program takes over as primary payer for eligible transplant recipients.

Life Following Kidney Transplantation Surgery

A kidney transplant returns a patient's (and his family's) life to normal—not entirely normal, mind you, but certainly much more so than before. In order to ease the threat of chronic rejection, recipients must take *immunosuppressive* drugs for as long as their body continues to accept the kidney. (Medicare covers the cost of all immunosuppressants for *one year* from the time patients are discharged from the hospital.)

Prednisone (brand name: Deltasone), a steroid, is frequently used in combination with two immunosuppressants— azathioprine (Imuran) and cyclosporine

(Sandimmune)—in the hope of reducing the considerable side effects of each. Prednisone, for example, may bring on acne, weight gain, and facial swelling, and has been associated with cataracts of the eyes. And like other steroids, it can cause fierce mood swings and make users extremely cranky. Cyclosporine, too, can produce undesirable side effects, among them inflamed gums and high blood pressure. Most serious of all, it may damage the transplanted kidney itself. What's more, inhibiting the immune system lowers a person's defenses against infection.

"Paul is currently on a dozen pills a day, down from thirty," says Gerri Clarke. "There are some side effects, but they're not nearly as bad as the general effects of dialysis."

Although kidney recipients do not have to follow the full-fledged renal diet, many remain hypertensive and therefore must continue to watch their salt intake. Low-cholesterol, low-fat fare may also be recommended because, as Lori Fedje explains, "the immunosuppressive medications can cause them to have high lipid levels and gain tremendous amounts of weight." On the other hand, she stresses, "a patient could be doing just fine and have no problems."

Transplant patients typically return to the doctor once a month for urine and blood creatinine tests to monitor kidney function, a complete blood count, and another blood test to assess electrolyte balance. Every few months the nephrologist additionally analyzes the blood for cholesterol and calcium, and measures the level of protein in the urine.

Despite the inconveniences, life for the Clarke family has improved immeasurably since Paul's kidney transplant operation. According to Gerri, "Paul's being off dialysis has really changed our family in certain ways. Just having the freedom to go out and do things when-ever you want, without having to worry about getting home in time to put him on the machine! There's also less tension in the house. Although you deal with someone's chronic illness as best you can, clearly it adds an element of tension that affects every member of the household—not just him, not just me, but the kids as well, and everybody else. I've seen noticeable changes in terms of family relationships and flexibility. It's been fabulous."

Recommended Reading

The following are available from the American Dietetic Association (800-366-1655):

- "A Healthy Food Guide: Hemodialysis"
- "A Healthy Food Guide: Peritoneal Dialysis"
- "A Healthy Food Guide: Diabetes and Hemodialysis"
- "A Healthy Food Guide: Diabetes and Peritoneal Dialysis"
- "A Healthy Food Guide: Kidney Disease"
- "A Healthy Food Guide: Diabetes and Kidney Disease"

The following is available free from the Health Care Financing Administration (800-638-6833):

- "Medicare: Coverage of Kidney Dialysis and Kidney Transplant Services"

The following is available free from the National Institute of Diabetes and Digestive and Kidney Diseases (301-654-4415):

- "End-Stage Renal Disease: Choosing a Treatment That's Right for You"

The following is available free from the National Kidney Foundation (800-622-9010):

- "Coping Effectively: A Guide for Patients and Their Families"

—20—

Caring for Someone with a
Progressive Neurological Disease

(Alzheimer's Disease, Parkinson's Disease, and

Amyotrophic Lateral Sclerosis)

No sooner had Diane Young's elderly father-in-law died in a nursing home in 1978 than her own father began to exhibit the exact same symptoms: forgetfulness, confusion, and disorientation. "It was unbelievable," recalls Diane, fifty-one. At the time her father was diagnosed with Alzheimer's disease there was relatively little public awareness of this devastating brain affliction. "We'd never heard of it," says Diane, who later founded New Orleans's first chapter of the Alzheimer's Association.

We thought my father-in-law had suffered from this one condition, called hardening of the arteries, and that Daddy had a different disease, called Alzheimer's. But as his disease progressed, we realized they were the same

thing. I asked the doctor, "What's going to happen? Is it going to get worse?" "Yes," he said, "it's going to get worse." "Well, what can we expect?" He answered, "I don't know. I can't tell you." The only information he was able to give us was, "It's the same disease Rita Hayworth has."

Just like my father-in-law, my father lived five more years, spent his last six months in a nursing home, and also died at the age of sixty-six.

Clarence Lindstrom of Columbus, Ohio, was just fifty when he was diagnosed with Parkinson's disease, a disabling neurological disorder normally associated with old age. "He'd probably had it a good five years before that," says his seventy-eight-year-old widow, Betty, a retired social worker.

460

My husband was a strong, healthy, independent person. So it was especially dreadful for him, being an engineer, when he couldn't write anymore and, being an outdoorsman, when he couldn't walk anymore. Parkinson's disease isn't easy for anybody, but it always seemed particularly unfair for him to have it.

We had some very good years. But after he retired, he went downhill fairly rapidly. The last five years were very bad: He was quite dependent, then he became housebound, then he was bedfast for the last two and a half years. He could do nothing for himself.

Few illnesses inspire more terror than amyotrophic lateral sclerosis (ALS), a degenerative condition that eventually imprisons its victims in their own bodies, unable to move, speak, eat, or breathe unassisted. For Jack LaCava, an energetic seventy-year-old businessman and avid golfer from Marblehead, Massachusetts, the first signs that something was wrong surfaced in 1990.

"My father began to notice that he was losing his balance a little bit when playing golf," says his daughter, Debra Bulkeley, a reporter and editor. "On one tee he swung his club and fell flat on his keister, as he put it." Without telling his family, Jack saw a neurologist at Boston's New England Medical Center. A battery of tests revealed he had ALS, giving him two to five years to live. "Yours seems to be slow," he was told, "so maybe you'll live ten years." Jack kept the news a secret.

I really noticed how much my father was dragging his left foot. I would ask him about it but could never get more than two words out of him.

I finally called his doctor. "I want to know what's wrong with my father," I said. "He's not getting any better."

And he said, "Well . . . in his condition, he's not going to be getting any better."

"What condition?"

That's when he realized I had no

idea. He said, "I can't say anything else about it. You'll have to talk to your father." This was at four o'clock on a Monday afternoon. I put my daughter in the car and drove out to Marblehead in rush-hour traffic and confronted him.

"Look," I said, "I spoke to your doctor, and he told me there's something wrong. What is it?"

My father was very upset. "Have you ever heard of Lou Gehrig's disease?" he asked.

Diseases of the nervous system afflict 5.5 million Americans*—more than any ailment except heart disease. Four million of those suffer from Alzheimer's; 500,000 from Parkinson's. Although neither is terminal in and of itself, both disorders eventually confine patients to bed, thus opening the door to potentially deadly complications such as infections and respiratory distress. ALS, another degenerative neurological disease, seizes far fewer victims (40,000) but invariably pursues a fatal course. Medical science has yet to discover successful strategies for halting the progression of these conditions. Their causes, too, remain obscure.

Certainly neurological diseases rank among the most nightmarish of illnesses in terms of how they disrupt families' lives, drain finances, and subject those involved with the patient's care to enormous stress. Because the person's physical and/or mental faculties deteriorate over time, he may require round-the-clock care for years on end. This chapter concentrates on the crises commonly seen in the latter

---

* We've chosen to look at Alzheimer's and Parkinson's because of their prevalence, and ALS because of its deadliness. Other adult neurological diseases, such as epilepsy, multiple sclerosis, muscular dystrophy, and myasthenia gravis, tend to be more chronic; Huntington's chorea, an inherited, incurable degenerative brain disease that affects both movement and intellectual faculties, frequently ends in death but is relatively rare.

stages of these diseases, which leave loved ones dependent on their caregivers for even the most basic of tasks: eating, going to the bathroom, keeping their air passages free of mucus.

"It's continual care," reflects Betty Lindstrom, who nursed her husband at home for five years. He died of complications from Parkinson's on New Year's Eve, 1984. "There isn't much day and there isn't much night. And when you get to that point, it's a downward spiral. You become tired. Then you start to feel guilty about the fact that you get angry sometimes and feel as if you're trapped."

The Central Nervous System

The central nervous system consists of the *brain*, a spongy three-pound mass of tissue, blood vessels, and nerve cells surrounded by a protective membrane, and the *spinal cord*, a network of nerve fibers encased in the bony spinal column. The brain orchestrates everything we do, from conscious actions like walking and talking to the automatic functions of breathing and digesting food; the spinal cord distributes its messages throughout the body via branches of *peripheral nerves*, which serve muscles as well as organs.

Nerves belong to one of three categories. *Sensory nerves* convey sensations of heat, cold, and pain as well as other information from the outside world to the brain and spinal cord, while *motor nerves* carry instructions from the central nervous system to the muscles. And *mixed nerves*, composed of both types, transmit messages in both directions simultaneously.

All thoughts, memories, sensations, and emotions travel the body as electrical impulses, passing along chains of billions and billions of nerve cells, or *neurons*. A neuron resembles a tree with a tall, slender trunk; the signal enters at the top and proceeds downward. So that impulses can traverse the gap *(synapse)* between one neuron and a neighboring cell, neurons discharge *neurotransmitters*. These chemicals not only act as bridges—adhering to adjoining cells and allowing signals to cross—but they stimulate the receiving neuron to release *its* neurotransmitters. In the space of an instant, one nerve cell after another "fires," speeding messages on their way at two hundred miles an hour.

Alzheimer's disease, Parkinson's disease, and amyotrophic lateral sclerosis all stem from the progressive, irreversible degeneration of a specific type of nerve cell in the brain or spinal cord. In Alzheimer's and Parkinson's, the neuron destruction subsequently brings about a shortage of crucial neurotransmitters.

Alzheimer's Disease

Few things are more heartbreaking than witnessing the mental deterioration from Alzheimer's disease. I watched it rob my uncle Billy, a successful mortgage banker with a wicked sense of humor, of his memory, his intellect, his personality, his *essence*. He and my aunt Kitty were married forty-two years. She first noticed signs of the disease several years before Billy died. For the last six months, she says, "he was like a baby," incapable of feeding or dressing himself.

One in ten men and women over sixty-five and nearly *half* of those eighty-five or older, will develop Alzheimer's disease, the most prevalent cause of dementia in the elderly. *Dementia*, a term that has come to replace *senility*, is defined as a marked, permanent decline in the ability to think, reason, and remember.

Compounding the tragedy of this disease is the financial burden it imposes. People can live with Alzheimer's anywhere from three to twenty years. Neither Medicare nor most private insurance policies pays for the long-term-care services that Alzheimer's patients need at home or in residential

---

**Nursing Home Care for Alzheimer's Patients on
Medicaid or Veterans' Medical Benefits**

Alzheimer's patients eligible for Medicaid may be entitled to nursing home benefits and, in some states, limited community long-term-care services. For more information contact the state Medicaid agency, which is usually under the aegis of the Department of Social Services or the Department of Welfare. ◄ *See "Medicaid," page 279.*

☎ If you can't find its telephone number in the white pages' State Government listings, call the federal Health Care Financing Administration in Baltimore at 410-786-3000.

About one-third of the 172 medical centers nationwide of the Department of Veterans Affairs provide inpatient and/or outpatient health care for former military men and women suffering from Alzheimer's or other forms of dementia. Services offered may include adult day care, home nursing care, acute hospital care, and long-term care, either in a VA center nursing home unit or in a nursing home under contract to the Department of Veterans Affairs. ◄ *See "Veterans and Military Dependents," page 280.*

☎ Eligibility requirements are complex. To learn if someone you love qualifies, call the Division of Veterans' Benefits and Services at 800-827-1000 or contact the nearest VA medical center.

---

facilities. Nursing home care averages a staggering $36,000 per year and can exceed $70,000—a major reason why seven in ten Alzheimer's patients are nursed at home by family and friends. According to the Alzheimer's Association, patients and families shoulder 90 percent of the expenses related to Alzheimer's.

You've probably heard someone attribute an elderly person's forgetfulness or confusion to "hardening of the arteries." *Atherosclerosis*, the hardening and thickening of blood vessels, has nothing to do with Alzheimer's disease, though it can bring about dementia by triggering a stroke. In this case, either a blood clot obstructs a diseased cranial artery, depriving part of the brain of blood—and, subsequently, oxygen—or one of the vessels ruptures, inundating the brain. Both sudden events decimate brain tissue.

By contrast, Alzheimer's insidiously weaves its way through the brain, leaving behind bundles of useless nerve cells (called *neurofibrillary tangles*) and abnormal chemical deposits *(neu-*

ritic plaques). This is what Dr. Alois Alzheimer, a German psychiatrist, discovered in 1906 when he autopsied the brain of a deceased woman who had suffered from a prolonged, unidentified mental illness. Her symptoms were the ever-worsening impairments of intellect, emotions, and behavior that are recognized today as the signature of Alzheimer's.

Neurologists can accurately diagnose nine in ten cases of Alzheimer's based on the patient's clinical symptoms plus several tests to rule out any of seventy other conditions that impair memory and intellect. These include stroke, brain cancer, traumatic brain injury, viral and bacterial brain infections, AIDS dementia, hepatic encephalopathy, multiple sclerosis, side effects of medications, nutritional deficiencies, anemia, and even severe depression. But a brain autopsy remains the only measure for definitively confirming the disease. Patients don't die of Alzheimer's directly but from related complications; Diane Young's bed-bound father-in-law ultimately succumbed to pneumonia.

Early Signs of Alzheimer's Disease

Neurologist Steven DeKosky, director of the Alzheimer Disease Research Center at the University of Pittsburgh, compares the slow onset of symptoms from Alzheimer's to the all but imperceptible movement of a clock's hour hand. "You don't really notice the changes from Alzheimer's day to day," he says, "but rather over the course of three-, six-, or nine-month intervals. People will remark something to the effect of 'Last summer I began to notice that Dad wasn't remembering things as well as he used to.' "

Alzheimer's disease originates in the brain's memory bank, a nub of tissue called the *hippocampus*. Classically, a deficit in short-term memory is the first sign to emerge. Mild memory loss, Dr. DeKosky emphasizes, is a natural consequence of aging. "But in normal aging, it's usually a case of people being unable to recall a name, which they subsequently remember later. The problem doesn't worsen or interfere with the activities of daily living."

Diane Young recalls how her father-in-law would mow the lawn three times in one afternoon, forgetting he'd already cut it. "Or he'd take out food to eat, put it on the stove to defrost, then forget to eat it. At the time, his wife was dying of leukemia. Not knowing anything about the disease, I just figured he was distracted and wasn't paying attention."

Next, the disease typically consumes neurons in the brain's outer layer, the tough, rindlike *cerebral cortex*, where the majority of information processing takes place. Alzheimer's seems especially to raid areas that oversee cognitive functions such as language, reasoning, and abstract thinking.

"My father and father-in-law did such bizarre things," reflects Diane. "You'd wonder sometimes if they weren't doing them on purpose. Of course, now I know they weren't." She recalls having to climb into the bathtub to bathe her elderly father because he no longer knew how. "I'd hand him the soap and washcloth, and he'd just stand there looking at them, not knowing what to do with them. You can't believe that a person's mind can deteriorate so."

Ten Warning Signs of Alzheimer's Disease

Because Alzheimer's disease is so prevalent in older people, many of us are liable to find ourselves caring for a sick person who in addition to his serious illness begins to exhibit signs of mental decline. Have you observed any of the symptoms, compiled by the Alzheimer's Association, listed below?

1. Recent, frequent memory loss: forgetting telephone numbers, people's names, assignments at work.
2. Misplacing things: not merely losing the car keys but stashing items in inappropriate places—a toaster in the freezer or a watch in the sugar bowl.
3. Difficulty performing familiar tasks: preparing a meal but forgetting to serve it.
4. Language problems: forgetting simple words, using incorrect words, or an inability to form a coherent sentence.
5. Disorientation of time and place: not knowing the day of the week, forgetting a destination, or becoming lost in familiar places.
6. Impaired judgment: wearing several shirts or blouses at once.
7. Problems with abstract thinking: being unable to balance a checkbook.
8. Abrupt mood swings: careening from calm to anger to tears for no apparent reason.
9. Changes in personality: uncharacteristic confusion, fear, paranoia.
10. A passive demeanor and loss of initiative: retreating into a shell.

If more than two apply, arrange for your loved one to see a neurologist. As

Dr. DeKosky points out, "Even without a cure, there are things that can be done to aid in feeding and caring for people with Alzheimer's and for the emotional well-being of both the patient and family.

"We have a tremendous prejudice in this country about what passes for normal age-related loss of mental function, whereby old people are often allowed to become absolutely daft without anyone's thinking there is anything wrong." Physicians, he adds, aren't necessarily immune from the same antiquated attitudes. "If a doctor says to you, 'Oh, he's just senile. Take him home, there's nothing we can do,' that's extremely unfair to the patient *and* to the family. Seek another physician."

The most important reason not to ignore evidence of dementia is that one in five suspected cases of Alzheimer's turns out to be another medical condition, which in some instances may be treatable.

Parkinson's Disease

It wasn't until the 1960s—150 years after the British physician Dr. James Parkinson first described the disease that later was to bear his name—that neurologists discovered how the disorder disables its victims.

Parkinson's disease obliterates nerve cells in a broad area of the inner brain: the *basal ganglia*. It particularly targets the dark-pigmented neurons in a tiny but essential segment known as the *substantia nigra*. The nerve cells of the basal ganglia and substantia nigra produce the chemical messenger *dopamine*, which enables the substantia nigra to interact with the *striatum*, the part of the brain responsible for controlling movement, balance, and walking.

Dopamine is an *inhibitory* neurotransmitter—that is, it works to suppress other cells and counteract the stimulating effect of *excitatory* neurotransmitters such as *acetylcholine*. Parkinson's disease results from an imbalance between these two powerful brain chemicals: Neurons in the basal ganglia degenerate, depleting the dopamine content and leading to a relative upsurge in acetylcholine activity. The nerve cells fire chaotically, causing shaking, rigidity, and other abnormal movements.

Early Signs of Parkinson's Disease

"Many Parkinson's patients go undiagnosed for a while because the typical complaints and findings are so subtle that physicians don't always recognize the signs," notes Dr. Lucien Côté, a neurologist at New York's Columbia Presbyterian Medical Center. It usually isn't until the striatum's dopamine reserve has dwindled to about 20 percent that symptoms become evident. Parkinson's classic trio of features includes tremors, muscular rigidity, and bradykinesia.

Tremors. Dr. Parkinson titled his historic 1817 treatise "Essay on the Shaking Palsy." Indeed, the first sign patients or their loved ones often notice is a mild trembling of the hands that becomes more pronounced when resting them, say, on a table. Interestingly, handwriting can provide a tipoff that someone has the stirrings of Parkin-

---

INSIDE INFORMATION

We don't want men or women with tremors to cut themselves while shaving. Be sure to replace straight-edge razors with electric shavers. Also, help loved ones avoid spilling hot food or beverages on themselves by serving these in large half-filled mugs instead of cups or bowls.

Tricks for Easing Tremors

Have the person lie face down on the floor and relax her entire body while taking slow, deep breaths through her mouth. The shaking should subside within five to fifteen minutes.

When hand tremors come on, give the person a rubber ball to squeeze.

Encourage the person to use both hands for tasks that normally require one.

Show the person how to grip a spoon firmly with the thumb, then curl the other fingers around it.

Tremor in one arm? Suggest the person sleep on her side, with the affected hand under the pillow. The weight should halt the tremor.

---

son's disease: After the first few words, the letters typically appear cramped and gnarled. In time, the tremors may involve the feet, head, neck, face, and jaw.

Rigidity. It is the dynamic tension between pairs of muscles that generates movement. When we flex an elbow, for example, the biceps contract while their counterparts, the triceps, relax. In Parkinson's, the opposing muscles turn rigid; hence the stiff, ratchetlike motions of the arms and legs.

Bradykinesia. The disease's most disabling trait, bradykinesia, refers to the sluggish movement identified with Parkinson's. Drug treatment to replace dopamine often grants several more years of mobility, but eventually the bradykinesia will overtake the body, leaving the person "frozen," unable to walk or stand. This is called *akinesia.*

Many times Parkinson's patients experience bradykinesia of the nerves that control the facial muscles, giving their faces a stolid, masklike appearance. Your loved one may feel distraught or overjoyed, yet her face will register no emotion. Likewise, should the condition later affect the nerves and muscles necessary for speech, the voice assumes a flat, expressionless tone.

Each of these manifestations usually affects one side of the body, then infiltrates the other side within a year or two. According to the United Parkinson Foundation, if the disease remains confined to the original side for about five years even when medication is withheld, the patient is unlikely to develop symptoms on both sides. Although stress in no way causes Parkinson's disease, extreme emotional upset (or anything that sets off a rush of adrenaline —a slamming door, a car horn) can intensify the stiffness, sluggish movement, and other symptoms.

Amyotrophic Lateral Sclerosis

Lou Gehrig's disease, named for the New York Yankees' Hall of Fame first baseman who died of ALS in 1941 at the age of thirty-seven, can be viewed as the mirror image of Alzheimer's: The motor neurons in the spinal cord and brain stem that innervate the skeletal muscles shut down, eventually rendering them useless; yet, as evidenced by Stephen Hawking, the mind survives intact. Remarkably, the British astrophysicist and author has lived with ALS for three decades. Of the five thousand men and women diagnosed annually, four in five are destined to die within two to five years. Like marionettes whose strings have been snipped, they lose one function after another as the muscles waste away. "Typically," says Dr.

Richard Gan, director of the ALS Clinic at Boston University Medical Center, "patients become so debilitated in terms of mobility, swallowing, and breathing, they die."

Early Signs of ALS

As with Alzheimer's and Parkinson's diseases, the initial symptoms of ALS are often so subtle, they go undetected. Patients' common complaints concern weakness and cramping of the extremities, limping, difficulty swallowing, impaired speech, and a rippling of muscles beneath the skin called *fasciculations*.

The appearance of symptoms—and patients' longevity—depends largely on where the disease takes root. Within amyotrophic lateral sclerosis are four classes of motor-neuron degeneration:

1. *Progressive muscular atrophy* affects the lower motor neurons of the spinal cord that sustain the skeletal muscles.
2. *Primary lateral sclerosis* affects the upper motor neurons in the brain's cerebral cortex.
3. *Progressive bulbar palsy* arises in the brain stem.
4. In *amyotrophic lateral sclerosis*, neurons begin to wither and die in all three locations.

Of the four, progressive muscular atrophy is the least aggressive, with patients able to survive as long as ten years. Progressive bulbar palsy carries the bleakest prognosis because it affects the muscles that control swallowing early on. People stricken by this form tend to deteriorate radically within one year. Whichever course the disease takes, the outcome is the same: near-total paralysis and death. Although Lou Gehrig's disease is progressive overall, a loved one will plateau in between stages of dramatic decline.

Jack LaCava first felt the effects of ALS in his left foot, says Debra Bulkeley. "From there it progressed up the left side of his body, then down the right side. It really didn't affect him too much the first couple of years. For a while we had high hopes that he had the slow-moving form. But in the last two years it really began to have an impact on my parents' lives. He had to give up driving. Then my mother had to do chores around the house, like taking out the garbage, because he couldn't do that anymore." The debilitating nature of the disease "truly hit me," she reflects, the day she noticed her father had so little strength in his left arm, "he could no longer clip the fingernails on his right hand.

"I can't tell you how many times I went to bed at night and said, 'God, just make it stop *now*. If it stops now, it's okay.' But the disease doesn't stop."

How Neurological Diseases Are Diagnosed

Most of the tests customarily ordered to help diagnose Alzheimer's, Parkinson's, and ALS do so indirectly, by ruling out other conditions with identical characteristics. A tumor of the central nervous system, for instance, can produce symptoms that resemble all three diseases. In view of this, you should expect your loved one's neurologist to take a detailed history and conduct a thorough physical exam. "In spite of all the fancy tests we have," says Dr. Côté, "the most valuable way to diagnose a disease is to listen to the patient and examine him."

How Neurological Diseases Are Treated

The best that medicine can offer people with Alzheimer's or Parkinson's disease is therapy to control symptoms, while the sole treatment for ALS is a drug that extends patients' lives by a few months. At present, nothing can halt the progression of any of these three diseases.

Common Tests for Diagnosing Alzheimer's Disease, Parkinson's Disease, and Amyotrophic Lateral Sclerosis

Procedure	Purpose
Lumbar puncture (spinal tap)	• To analyze the *cerebrospinal fluid* for evidence of cancer or an inflammation of the brain. A sample of this fluid, which cushions the brain and flows through the central canal of the spinal cord, is withdrawn from the lower spine via a syringe.
Electroencephalography (EEG)	• To study brain function by recording brain waves in various areas of the brain. Electrodes, attached to the skull, relay the impulses to a machine that represents their pattern on paper.
One or more imaging studies: head X ray brain scan CT scan PET scan MRI scan	• To visualize central nervous system tumors or evidence of a cerebrovascular stroke. • To reveal brain atrophy or shrinkage. • To detect spinal stenosis, a condition in which the cavity in the spinal column narrows, compressing the spinal cord.
Electromyography/nerve conduction velocity test (EMG/NCV)	• To record muscles' electrical activity and measure the speed at which nerves conduct impulses; it is a two-part test.
Blood tests	• To exclude diseases that mimic AD and ALS: pernicious anemia, chronic low blood glucose, thyroid disease, liver disease, kidney disease, lymphoma, autoimmune diseases, and hexosaminidase-enzyme deficiency.
Mental status tests	• To assess memory, attention span, language, reasoning, comprehension, perception, and problem-solving abilities.
Eyedrops test	• To determine if a patient's pupils change slightly in size, indicating that Alzheimer's disease is present. This simple yet sensitive and specific test, still under investigation, employs eyedrops similar to the type routinely used to dilate the pupils during eye exams.

Alzheimer's Disease

Drug Therapy

Two *cholinesterase inhibitor* drugs, tacrine (brand name: Cognex) and donepezil (Aricept), have been approved by the FDA for mild to moderate Alzheimer's. Both improve some patients' thinking, memory, and language abilities by increasing the amount of acetylcholine in the brain. Neither medication benefits folks with late-stage disease, Dr. DeKosky explains, "because by then the neurotransmitter system it's trying to help is pretty much burned out. There are people who are clearly helped, but they make up a relatively small percentage." More effective medications are available for managing the noncognitive effects of Alzheimer's, such as depression, anxiety, sleeplessness, agitation, wandering, and aggression.

Parkinson's Disease

Drug Therapy

After it was discovered that dopamine deficiency caused Parkinson's symptoms, physicians tried replacing the compound, which is found in bananas and several other fruits. The strategy failed, says Dr. Côté, "because dopamine cannot get into the brain. But we can trick Mother Nature by giving patients its precursor, *dopa*." (Physicians may also refer to it as *L-dopa* or *levodopa*.) The synthetic amino acid penetrates the brain, where it gets transformed into dopamine.

Today's mainstay of therapy, a drug called Sinemet, combines levodopa and *carbidopa*. This substance, Dr. Côté explains, "runs interference for the dopa," preventing the liver, spleen, and kidneys from breaking it down before it reaches the brain. When levodopa travels the body unaccompanied by carbidopa, 90 percent of it converts to dopamine prematurely in the bloodstream and is denied entry to the brain.

The more potent Sinemet contains one-fifth the dose of levodopa, thus sparing patients adverse side effects such as nausea, heart irregularities, and low blood pressure.

Sinemet is not without its own side effects. A small percentage of patients do not tolerate the drug. They'll suffer from hallucinations, vivid dreams, or nightmares "even with just a small dose," says Dr. Côté. "What they see is extremely real to them. They may insist they see an army of soldiers marching to the house." ◀ *See "Delusional or Hallucinatory Behavior," page 204.*

Whether alone or combined with carbidopa, "levodopa helps patients immensely in terms of agility and being able to move better," says Dr. Côté. "But it does not alter the course of the disease." After about three to five years, the brain responds less and less to the levodopa. Whereas it once acted for perhaps four hours, it may now do so for one or two hours, or not work as quickly as before. It's at this point that people with Parkinson's disease begin to experience complications that hamper their mobility:

Dyskinesia, a sudden, uncontrollable twitching and jerking of the arms and legs as the medication either kicks in or wears off.

On-Off Syndrome, a temporary loss of motor function that ambushes patients in mere minutes. "A person with Parkinson's may be able to get himself a glass of water, tie his shoes, and so on," explains Dr. Côté. "Then, as if a curtain has descended, he's unable to do any of it.

"Very few caregivers understand Parkinson's," he continues. "They'll say to the patient, 'Don't fool me! You did this just two minutes ago. This is all psychological!' Even nurses don't always understand this." Betty Lindstrom recalls the time a home health aide scolded her husband while giving him a bath because he suddenly couldn't lift his arm. "She knew little about Parkinson's dis-

---

INSIDE INFORMATION

A sluggish digestive tract can detain oral levodopa from getting down to business. Parkinson's disease itself tends to slow the transit of food from the stomach to the intestines, where absorption into the circulation takes place and so does a class of drugs, *anticholinergics*, which are often prescribed to Parkinson's patients.

If your loved one's levodopa still works continuously, this isn't a source of concern. But if he has become dependent on each dose and the neurologist finds delayed gastric emptying to be a problem, you may have to time dosages with meals. The National Parkinson Foundation suggests that patients take oral levodopa on an empty stomach *and* at least 30 minutes before eating.

Some other tips for hastening digestion:

- Encourage the person to move about or exercise after taking the dose.
- Crush the tablet, mix it with water or soda, and have her drink it.
- Ask the doctor about possibly prescribing a *prokinetic* drug such as cisapride (Propulsid), which accelerates the motility of the stomach muscles.

---

ease and figured he was just being stubborn. She kept pushing Clarence's arm. I said, *'He can't raise his arm.'* She'd been quite rude to him, and he was upset. He had tears running down his cheeks."

Freezing, when the akinesia comes on in a flash, often when the person approaches doorways and other narrow spaces. Later on in this chapter we will show you ways to help avoid freezing and how to assist patients when it occurs.

Since levodopa's effectiveness eventually wanes, neurologists often prescribe it in combination with other anti-Parkinson drugs. Or they'll reserve the levodopa for when symptoms progress. In those instances where the disease's symptoms seem impervious to the medications *and* the patient is suffering profound side effects as well, the neurologist may recommend what's called a "drug holiday": Patients are hospitalized for at least five days during which all medications are withdrawn, to clear the brain and bloodstream. Then the drugs are carefully reintroduced. Ideally, by the time the person leaves the hospital, his dosage has been reduced by nearly half, with significant

side effects a thing of the past. In addition, his walking ability should have improved noticeably.

Surgery

Following the introduction of levodopa in 1967, physicians largely abandoned neurosurgery as treatment for Parkinson's disease. But now that the limitations of drug therapy have become apparent, the practice is experiencing a modest revival. Still, fewer than one in ten people with Parkinson's undergo any of the following surgical options:

Pallidotomy/Thalamotomy. Peculiar as it may seem, both these forms of *stereotactic* surgery involve destroying brain tissue with a cold-tipped probe. "There are at least two basic pathways in the brain," explains Dr. Côté. "Some of the symptoms of Parkinson's arise because one pathway overshadows the other. By making a lesion in a minute, specific area, we essentially reestablish the balance between the two."

In a pallidotomy, the neurosurgeon freezes tissue in the part of the brain known as the *globus pallidus*. The procedure dramatically reduces some patients' rigidity, twitching, and motor fluctuation. However, the gains tend to be temporary and may be accompanied by serious side effects such as impaired vision and cerebral bleeding. A brain hemorrhage can leave a person paralyzed, blind, demented, or comatose. Thalamotomy—applying extreme cold to a portion of the thalamus—appears to alleviate Parkinsonian tremor, but it, too, can result in neurological damage and is rarely offered.

Deep Brain Stimulation. This nondestructive, reversible technique uses electrical stimulation to ease severe tremor in people who no longer respond to conventional therapy. After the patient receives anesthesia, a stimulator wire is placed beneath the scalp and is then connected to a second wire that runs through the neck to the chest, where an activator unit is implanted, much like a cardiac pacemaker. Patients activate or deactivate the device by passing a magnet across it.

Fetal Tissue Implant Surgery. The theory behind this experimental procedure is that healthy brain cells, implanted in the brain of a person with Parkinson's, will grow and produce the dopamine he lacks. Both fetal tissue implant surgery and deep brain stimulation are rare.

Exercise

Exercising daily can help reduce the severity of the disease's disabling effects and enhance the response to anti-Parkinson's medications. Although patients certainly benefit from formal rehabilitation therapy, not all require it or are healthy enough to participate. The aim of *physical therapy* is to teach men and women with Parkinson's how to move about safely and efficiently; *occupational therapy* concentrates on fine coordination and techniques for better carrying out the skills of daily living: eating, dressing, personal hygiene, and so on.

Chances are, the neurologist will recommend only periodic visits to a rehabilitation facility, where trained therapists instruct and supervise patients in a moderate exercise regimen to be carried out at home. Before your loved one engages in any strenuous physical activity, be sure to discuss it with the physician or physical therapist.

Since Parkinson's disease limits range of motion, the goal of a conditioning program is to extend, rotate, and flex the muscles and joints. For instance, patients can improve their posture simply by reaching up and gripping the top of a door frame. Or how about this twisting exercise, which helps reduce stiffness during walking and makes rolling over in bed easier:

1. Have the person sit in a chair with her feet flat on the floor and her arms folded across her chest.
2. Ask her to turn her upper body to the left and bend forward until her right elbow touches her left knee.
3. Return to the upright position.
4. Now have her twist to the right, touching the left elbow to the opposite knee.
5. Repeat five times.

To locate a rehab program, ask your loved one's neurologist or call these Parkinson's disease patient-service organizations for referrals:

☎ The American Parkinson's Disease Association at 800-223-2732
☎ National Parkinson Foundation at 800-327-4545; in Florida, 800-433-7022
☎ Parkinson's Disease Foundation at 800-457-6676
☎ United Parkinson Foundation at 312-733-1893

Dr. Côté's booklet "Exercises for the Parkinson Patient," available free from the Parkinson's Disease Foundation, contains exercises for promoting chest expansion, knee flexibility, and manual dexterity, to name a few. The United Parkinson Foundation (UPF) publishes "The Exercise Program," a three-ring notebook of thirty-eight exercises designed by physical therapists under its medical advisory board.

All too often Parkinson's sufferers allow themselves to become inactive and reclusive, even well before symptoms reach the disabling stage. As long as loved ones are well enough to get out of the house, let's encourage them to attend one of the group exercise programs conducted by a number of patient support groups and adult day care centers. Both the American Parkinson's Disease Association and the National Parkinson Foundation sponsor groups around the country; the Parkinson's Disease Foundation and the United Parkinson Foundation do not but may be able to direct you to local patient organizations. Still another valuable resource for locating exercise and recreational activities geared toward seniors are community service organizations such as Catholic Charities USA, United Way of America, and the Area Agency on Aging. You'll find their telephone numbers in Appendix B under "Community Services."

Diet

Dietary protein can interfere with the bloodstream's absorption of levodopa, making for erratic motor responses. Some Parkinson's patients find that if they eat a protein-heavy meal (chicken, beef, or fish) shortly after taking their Sinemet, the medication doesn't work nearly as well and sometimes not at all. "The motor fluctuations are not only disabling but unpredictable," says Dr. William J. Weiner, director of the Movement Disorders Center at the University of Miami School of Medicine. "Someone may get frozen in a grocery store for two hours."

Sound familiar? If so, ask your loved one's neurologist about possibly trying a *restricted-protein diet*. The normal recommended daily allowance for protein is 55 grams per day, although most Americans far exceed that amount. This diet calls for 45 grams per day. More important than the quantity of protein, though, is how we allocate those 45 grams. Dr. Weiner suggests serving all but 10 at dinner, with breakfast and lunch containing 5 grams of protein apiece.

"The idea is to shift the protein to evening so that when people are out during the day, they might have a smoother, more consistent performance" from the levodopa. There's a tradeoff, of course: poorer motor function at night. But as Dr. Weiner points out, "It's easier for patients to deal with an episode of freezing at home."

The restricted protein diet applies only to patients taking Sinemet or levodopa who are experiencing motor fluctuations; dietary protein has no known effect on the action of the other types of drugs that may be prescribed for Parkinson's disease. "If after two weeks you don't notice a significant improvement in their response to the medications," Dr. Weiner stresses, "there's no point in continuing the diet."

Amyotrophic Lateral Sclerosis

Drug Therapy

In 1995 the FDA approved the world's first drug for Lou Gehrig's disease. Riluzole (brand name: Rilutek), an *antiglutamate* agent, has been found to prolong patients' lives by about three months, though it neither slows ALS's progression nor relieves symptoms.

Effects of Advanced Progressive Neurological Disease

The plot lines of Alzheimer's, Parkinson's, and amyotrophic lateral sclerosis vary somewhat from one another, but their final acts are tragically alike, with patients requiring twenty-four-hour-a-day care. The following pages describe the difficulties caregivers are likely to encounter and ways to manage them. First we highlight the symptoms unique to each illness, then those complications they share.

Effects of End-Stage Alzheimer's Disease

Alzheimer's is perhaps as agonizing for family and friends as it is for the victims themselves. Imagine watching someone you love all but reduced to a shell, devoid of personality and spirit, unable to communicate or recognize even those closest to him.

"It would be so awful to see Daddy," reflects Diane Young. "I'd drop my daughter off at school in the morning, then drive over to the nursing home. Usually I'd sit in the car and cry because I didn't want to go in, though I knew I had to. I don't think he knew who I was. I'd tell myself, *That's not Daddy.* My father almost didn't even look like himself anymore—so thin and expressionless, mumbling incoherently. Then I'd look at his hands; at least his hands never changed."

Hyperactivity

Ask any caregiver which aspect of Alzheimer's disease most turns their lives upside down, and chances are they'll say the incessant, aimless pacing and wandering that affects seven in ten Alzheimer's patients.

Why the hyperactivity? "We think it is due to a loss of inhibition of the motor system so that patients get restless and want to move," explains Dr. DeKosky. "Sometimes it happens because the person doesn't recognize his surroundings and wants to go home, even though he *is* home." It's not unusual for an Alzheimer's patient to suddenly get up and, without a word, stride purposefully out the door. My uncle Billy used to circle the block repeatedly for hours on end. This puts caregivers in the stressful position of having to constantly monitor the person's whereabouts.

Compounding the problem is the fact that the disease frequently disrupts the sleep-wake cycle so that patients may wander at night and sleep sporadically during the day—rarely for more than an hour at a time. "And if the patient doesn't sleep," says Dr. DeKosky, "obviously the caregiver doesn't, either." Fortunately for my aunt, the neighbors all kept an eye on Billy, so his daily spins around the block afforded her a desperately needed break.

How It Is Managed

We don't want to routinely give an Alzheimer's patient sleep aids, since they can further dull mental function and heighten confusion. Reserve them for those nights where you're verging on a meltdown from sleep deprivation. (When caring for someone with Alzheimer's, that could describe almost any night.) The antihistamine Benadryl, while effective, can induce headaches and grogginess; you might ask the physician to prescribe chloral hydrate, a milder, short-acting oral sedative. Over-the-counter brands can be useful, too, but get the doctor's approval first, since these products may interact with certain anti-Parkinson drugs. ◄ *See "Insomnia and Other Sleep Disorders," page 172.*

Sorry to say, the interlinked problems of hyperactivity and sleep-cycle disruption have no ideal long-term solution.

Dr. DeKosky suggests taking loved ones out for a walk during the day, "which essentially tires them out and lets them relax." Uncle Billy's marathon walks used to exhaust him, which curbed his restlessness for a while.

Distraction, too, can prove effective. As Dr. DeKosky points out, "The person's poor short-term memory is an ally here." Give them repetitive tasks to do. Alzheimer's patients can occupy themselves folding and unfolding clothes or balling and unballing socks. If these seem like tactics for dealing with childlike behavior, essentially they are. That's the sad reality of end-stage Alzheimer's.

What's a Memory Book? The Pittsburgh Alzheimer Disease Research Center has had some success with something called a memory book, a collection of personal photos and magazine pictures from the patient's past. "With Alzheimer's, remote memories remain far more intact than recent memories," Dr. DeKosky explains. "Memory books can distract patients. And because people with Alzheimer's have a short-term memory problem, they can look at them again and again without remembering that they did so ten minutes ago."

To Discourage Wandering. To discourage wandering, outfit all doorknobs leading outside with plastic safety covers, just as if you had an adventurous toddler. These covers require a fair amount of hand strength and manual dexterity to open. Other precautions include installing intricate locks and latches or simply placing a chair in front of the door—anything to complicate the task of opening it.

Still, as long as an Alzheimer's patient is mobile, it's wise to enroll him in the Alzheimer's Association Safe Return program. For $25 your loved one is registered in a nationwide database. Should he ever wander away from home, you call a special toll-free number to report him missing. Safe Return then alerts a network of 17,000 local law enforcement agencies across the country. You'll receive a wallet ID, clothing labels, and a bracelet or necklace for the person to wear. ◄ *See "Wandering," page 207.*

☎ For more information, call Safe Return at 800-272-3900.

Hiding Objects

Not only do people with Alzheimer's frequently lose objects, they deliberately hide them, then forget *where*. One explanation for this behavior is that stashing away items brings a feeling of security to a patient who is painfully aware of all the disease has taken from him. You can imagine, though, the frustration for the caregiver: reaching into the kitchen drawer for the car keys, only to find them missing. While nothing can be done to change our loved one's behavior, there are steps we can take to make this less of a problem:

- Store papers, jewelry, and other valuables in a box or safe that is locked away someplace where the person won't easily find it.
- Keep spare sets of keys, glasses, and other essential items in the house.
- Get into the habit of checking wastebaskets before you empty them.
- First check your loved one's favorite hiding spots when objects vanish.
- Always put important articles such as glasses and dentures in the same place to help the person locate them.

Combative Behavior

Everyone who knew Billy Smith adored him. He and my aunt had no children of their own, so they doted on their nieces and nephews. Whenever Billy visited them at college, he'd always slip the young person a $100 bill with a wink. Alzheimer's disease turned this gentle, charming man into a suspicious and, at times, violent stranger.

After our father's funeral, my brother David stayed on in Mobile to help Aunt Kitty care for her husband, who by then was thoroughly demented and only weeks away from death himself. "Billy had never been jealous in his life," she says, "but he grew insanely jealous. I could never be out of his sight." To give you an idea of how completely the mind can unravel, he no longer recognized David and became convinced that the young man sleeping in the guest bedroom was his wife's *lover.*

Aggressive behavior toward family members flares up "only occasionally," says Dr. DeKosky, "but when it does, naturally it's very upsetting, because the patient is agitated and can't listen to reason." One morning at five o'clock Billy kicked open David's door and barked, "I told you to get out!"

My brother knew to try to calm him by speaking softly and clearly. "Okay, Uncle Bill," he replied. "Just give me time to pack."

"Well, hurry up!" Billy spluttered before stalking off down the hall.

David says, "I closed the door and went back to sleep, figuring he'd forget about it. Which he did, for a while. Half an hour later he kicked at the door again! This time Billy hauled me out of bed with a sudden burst of strength and pushed me all the way to the back door. And whereas he hadn't been able to turn the doorknob in months, he managed to open it and shove me outside, then Kitty! I had to laugh, but my aunt was so scared that from then on she had me sleep on a cot in her room."

How It Is Managed

The demented person's blip of an attention span is our ally. Minutes after throwing David and Kitty out of the house, Billy's anger evaporated, as if his brain had changed channels. What made the incident remarkable, in fact, was that he'd kept this train of thought on track for as long as he did.

Effects of End-Stage Parkinson's Disease

In advanced Parkinson's disease the progressive loss of voluntary movement begins to cast its shadow across the mechanisms controlling speech and swallowing, as well as the gastrointestinal tract, the respiratory tract, and other body systems. Nowhere is the functional decline more dramatic than in mobility.

Impaired Mobility

While the tremors from Parkinson's may remain about the same, the muscle rigidity and sluggish movement worsen, reducing a patient's stride to a slow shuffle. You've probably noticed that people with Parkinson's take short, mincing steps and pitch forward, as if leaning into a fierce wind. This is to compensate for the failing sense of balance. Further impairing stability, many patients no longer swing their arms in rhythm with the opposite leg while walking. Instead, the arms hang at their sides, partially flexed.

All these problems combine to make Parkinson's sufferers extremely vulnerable to dangerous falls. Remember, most of these folks are elderly, with porous, fragile bones, or osteoporosis. "They tend to get hurt when they fall," notes Dr. Côté, "breaking hips and damaging shoulders." A prolonged convalescence in bed can lead to pneumonia and other life-threatening complications. Thus, taking steps to minimize the chances of a fall becomes a chief concern.

Tips for Preventing Falls When a Loved One Has Parkinson's Disease

Walking. As a result of perpetually tilting forward, Parkinson's patients tend to walk on the balls of their feet instead of their heels. When a loved one lapses into this shuffling gait, coach her in the following steps, recommended by the American Parkinson's Disease Association:

1. Stand still.
2. Spread your feet about eight inches apart.
3. Envision yourself taking a broad step.
4. Bring one foot up high as if you were marching.
5. Lift up your toes and set your heel down first.
6. Roll onto the ball of your foot and toes.
7. Now do the same with the other foot.
8. As you stride, swing your arms in cadence: left arm with right foot, right arm with left foot.

Parkinson's sufferers have fewer mishaps if they concentrate solely on the act of walking. Trying to do two things at once often makes them lose their balance or freeze in place. Remind loved ones to stop walking if they want to converse or look at something.

Never pull the person. Stand to one side and offer an arm for support.

Many PD patients are so anxious about tripping, they affix their eyes to the floor while walking. Doing so actually contributes to falls. Encourage the person to focus straight ahead and assure her that even with the head held erect, she'll be able to see what's on the ground.

Similarly, patients often veer away from furniture for fear of having an accident. In fact, touching or holding on to chairs and tables provides stability and alleviates tension.

When turning, people with Parkinson's should keep their feet spread, take baby steps, and rock gently from side to side, facing *into* the turn and taking care not to cross one leg in front of the other.

A cane or walker may prove to be more detrimental than beneficial, always getting in the way. Also, walkers can contribute to stooped posture.

Getting In or Out of a Chair. When sitting down, the person should back up slowly until her legs touch the chair. She can then bend her knees and slowly lower herself into the seat.

Standing up too quickly can lead to a fall, not only on account of the waning sense of balance but because PD sufferers are prone to dizziness from *orthostatic hypotension*, a decline in blood pressure upon standing. The following steps are recommended:

1. Slide forward to the edge of the seat.
2. Place both feet on the floor, one in front of the other, ten inches or so apart.
3. Put weight on the ball of the closest foot.
4. Sway back and forth for momentum.
5. With a count of "one, two, three, go!" push down on the arm rests and stand up.
6. Once upright, stand still to regain balance.

Make sure all chairs are heavy enough so that they won't slide back when the person gets up.

Have the person hold a telephone directory or heavy book in front of her while getting up from a sitting position; this helps maintain equilibrium.

You can assist by gently pushing a loved one's back as she rises from the chair. As with walking, never pull someone by the arms.

A satin pillow on any seat prevents pants and skirts from sticking. For practical—and aesthetic—reasons, *discard all plastic slipcovers immediately!* People stick to them, and this can cause them to fall while getting up.

Getting Out of Bed. Most Parkinson's sufferers feel particularly stiff and rigid in the morning. When your loved one is ready to get out of bed, she should do the following:

1. Lie on her side at the edge of the bed.
2. Dangle her legs over the side.

3. Using an elbow and the opposite hand, push down on the mattress.
4. Lift her head as she rises to her feet.

A sturdy night table gives the person something to lean on for support. Some folks grasp a knotted rope tied to the foot of the bed and pull themselves upright.

Elevate the head of the bed by placing four-inch blocks under the front legs or headboard. The angle makes it easier for patients to get up. ◀ *See "Tips for Preventing Falls," page 134.*

When a Parkinson's Patient Falls

Chapter 3 describes the correct way to assist a person who has fallen, but with Parkinson's there's an added complication. "When Parkinson's patients fall," explains Dr. Côté, "many become so paralyzed, they cannot even begin to help themselves get up. The best thing to do is calm the patient, give him a pillow, cover him up, and let him rest. After a few minutes he will regain his strength and be able to help you in getting him to his feet."
◀ *See "What to Do if a Patient Falls," page 135.*

When Freezing Occurs

Akinesia typically leaves men and women with Parkinson's stooped over, their knees bowed and heels off the ground. Trying to move only throws off their balance further. To help themselves "thaw out," patients should do as follows:

1. Relax back on their heels and raise their toes.
2. Straighten their posture.
3. Tap the side of the leg they intend to move first.
4. Rock gently from side to side or take a few steps backward.
5. March in place, counting, "One, two, three, four."

6. Start moving forward, heel first.
7. Keep the feet about eight inches apart.

Seeing an obstacle in one's path frequently triggers akinesia. Yet strangely enough, you can often help jump-start a patient who is frozen by placing an object (your foot or the handle of a cane if he uses one) in front of him.

Trying to open a door while walking is also a common cause of freezing. Instruct your loved one to walk up as close to the door as she can, stop, open the door, then walk through—four separate actions.

Sometimes the touch of another person is all it takes to release the tension of akinesia and allow patients to resume movement.

Chronic Constipation

Several factors predispose virtually all Parkinson's patients to constipation. The intestines' muscular contractions slow down, and the anticholinergic drugs often prescribed for PD sufferers tend to aggravate this problem. In addition, once Parkinson's encroaches on swallowing ability, patients aren't able to take in adequate amounts of roughage and fluid.

Constipation poses problems for people with Lou Gehrig's disease and bedbound patients in general, but in a Parkinsonian it can mushroom into a potentially fatal *fecal impaction*, where the hardened stool builds up dangerously in the bowel. Betty Lindstrom counsels PD patients as a full-time volunteer in two support groups. "In just the last two years," she says, "we've had four people die from severe constipation."

Preventive Management

Think prevention! "Once constipation develops," Dr. Côté warns, "patients become very uncomfortable, their Parkinson's symptoms grow much worse, and it's a nightmare to treat." The most natural method for keeping things moving, so to speak, is dietarily, by seeing to it that loved ones drink water throughout the day and, if they are able to swallow, eat fiber-rich foods and natural laxatives such as figs, prunes, and prune juice. Daily fiber supplements and stool softeners can also help prevent stool from backing up in the bowel.

How It Is Managed

Doctor-prescribed laxatives are used. Should an impaction form, don't delay in contacting a physician or nurse, who will use a finger to carefully extricate the mass. This is not something to attempt yourself without direct medical supervision. ◄ See "Constipation and Gas," page 167.

Dependent Edema

Swelling of the feet and legs from an accumulation of fluid is a familiar problem for all immobilized patients but especially so for Parkinson's sufferers, who may sit statuelike for hours without moving, their feet seemingly cemented to the floor. What's more, their increasingly rigid leg muscles don't adequately push blood from the feet back up to the heart.

Preventive Management

◄ See "Circulatory Complications," page 178.

Eye Irritation

Although we hardly notice it, we blink our eyes eight to twelve times every minute. Parkinson's patients, however, blink only two to four times per minute, thus giving them the appearance of constantly staring. While this can be disconcerting to others, more important, the sporadic blinking leads to conjunctivitis: dryness and infectious inflammation of the delicate membrane lining the eyelids and protecting the eyeball.

At the same time, men and women with Parkinson's may experience the opposite problem, where the eyelids shut involuntarily. This is called blepharospasm. For reasons that defy explanation, patients can sometimes get their eyes to reopen simply by touching their nose or face.

How It Is Managed

Like a windshield wiper, each blink of the eye swabs tears across the conjunctiva. Part of a PD patient's daily care includes regularly soothing and lubricating the eyes with artificial tears, available in any pharmacy, or an ointment recommended by an ophthalmologist.

Conjunctivitis is treated with antibiotic eye drops or ointments. Blepharospasm is often relieved with levodopa alone. In severe cases an ophthalmologist injects a tiny amount of botulinum toxin around the eye to paralyze the spasming optic muscles.

Seborrhea/Seborrheic Dermatitis

While by no means one of Parkinson's more severe effects, seborrhea is a nuisance, leaving an oily coating on the face and scalp. When accompanied by redness and scaling, as often happens, the condition is called seborrheic dermatitis. It is unclear why Parkinson's disease predisposes patients to both skin disorders.

How It Is Managed

Encourage loved ones to bathe and shampoo at least every other day, and to avoid oil-based soaps and lotions. Topical cortisone creams and prescription shampoos should bring relief. Over-the-counter shampoos, too, can achieve good results. The American Academy of Dermatology recommends looking for products containing tar, zinc pyrithione, selenium sulfide, sulfur, or salicylic acid. Unfortunately, seborrheic dermatitis is incurable and will most likely recur periodically.

Dementia

Dr. James Parkinson's original description of the disease made no mention of cognitive impairment, but between 25 and 50 percent of Parkinson's patients eventually exhibit Alzheimer's-like symptoms. According to Dr. Côté, "It's unclear whether this is Alzheimer's disease waiting in the wings or a type of dementia specific to Parkinson's disease." Given that one in ten people over sixty-five has Alzheimer's, the two diseases inevitably overlap in some senior citizens. The incidence of dementia is greater in people who develop Parkinson's after age sixty. ◀ *See "When a Loved One Suffers from Brain Function Impairment," page 202.*

Depression

While depression is an understandable response to any debilitating illness, a disproportionately high number of PD patients—as many as one in two—sink into despair. Not all are reacting solely to their progressive disabilities. In the same way that Parkinson's upsets the crucial balance between the neurotransmitters that facilitate motor function, it also depletes two brain chemicals that influence mood: *norepinephrine* and *serotonin*. So a PD patient's depression is as likely to be chemical as well as "reactive."

Interestingly, a sense of melancholy often descends on patients "a year or two before they develop physical signs that we neurologists can diagnose," says Dr. Côté, though it usually goes unrecognized as a precursor of Parkinson's. Besides acting depressed, people with early-stage disease may grow uncharacteristically quiet and withdrawn.

How It Is Managed

Not only does depression intensify a patient's distress, in Parkinson's it can

---

Antidepressants Commonly Prescribed for Parkinson's Patients

Tricyclics
Amitriptyline (brand names: Elavil, Endep)
Desipramine (Norpramin)
Imipramine (Tofranil)
Nortriptyline (Pamelor)
Protriptyline (Vivactil)

Nontricyclics
Bupropion (Wellbutrin)
Fluoxetine (Prozac)
Trazodone (Desyrel)

---

exacerbate the physical symptoms of the disease. (For that matter, so can extreme emotions of any kind, even elation.) If you observe depressive behavior, alert the doctor.

One dividend of Sinemet and another anti-Parkinson's drug, Parlodel, is that they alleviate depression. Should the physician feel your loved one could benefit from antidepressant medication, she will probably choose one of the drugs listed in the sidebar.

Effects of End-Stage Amyotrophic Lateral Sclerosis

"In general, I'm not a big fan of assisted suicide," says a prominent East Coast neurologist. "But advanced ALS is one of the few diseases where I feel comfortable with that, if the patient is ready for it. Many neurologists routinely put ALS patients in contact with societies that can help them with euthanasia.

"ALS is not a comfortable way to die," he adds. "It's a terrible disease and a terrible thing to have to watch." Patients typically spend the twilight of their lives immobilized, fighting for breath, and choking on their own mucus. Worst of all, they are acutely aware of everything that is happening, and capable of sensing pain and discomfort.

Impaired Mobility

For the last months of Jack LaCava's life, his mobility was limited to shifting from bed to a wheelchair and back again. "He needed help just to sit up in bed," says his daughter, Debra Bulkeley. "From there he could sort of pull himself upright with the aid of a walker and go right into the wheelchair. That was the extent of his movement."

How It Is Managed

Nothing can be done to forestall the near total paralysis that will set in unless a patient dies beforehand of infection, respiratory failure, or some unrelated cause—a blessing, many would say. But as long as a loved one with ALS is ambulatory, consider renting or purchasing special equipment that can enhance his comfort and ability to maneuver. These range from wheelchairs and walkers to sophisticated mechanical lifts and portable wheelchair ramps. ◄ *See "Modifying the Home," page 78.* ► *See Appendix B: "Adaptive Technology," page 504.*

Symptoms Common to Advanced AD, PD, and ALS

Once bed-bound, patients become tempting targets for pneumonia and other complications: urinary-tract infections, bedsores, pneumonia, indigestion, thrombophlebitis, dependent edema, chronic constipation, foot drop, fever, venous thrombosis (blood clots in the legs), and bone, muscle, and joint pain.

Incontinence

Both Alzheimer's and Parkinson's directly inhibit urinary control. Parkinson's disease has a double-barreled effect on the bladder: The bulblike organ's muscular walls become increasingly rigid and bradykinetic, weakening the contractions that expel urine through the urethra and out of the body. (Lou Gehrig's disease rarely touches the smooth muscles of the bladder and other internal organs.) Second, the brain occasionally instructs the bladder to contract involuntarily. Most PD patients are elderly, of course; not all have the sphincter muscle control to prevent an accident.

Alzheimer's-related incontinence is also *neurogenic* in nature—that is, prompted by damage to the central nervous system—although this symptom generally doesn't emerge until extremely late in the course of the disease. By then, cognitive function is often so thoroughly erased, patients may no longer perceive the once-familiar urge to use the bathroom. For that matter, they may not remember *where* the bathroom is or what it is for. "At night," Diane Young recalls, "my father would just get up and urinate at the side of the bed."

How It Is Managed

Chapter 3 contains strategies for controlling incontinence. One of the most effective ways to avoid accidents is to simply remind loved ones to use the toilet (or, if they're confined to bed, a portable urinal) every two to three hours. If the person is still mobile but has trouble finding the bathroom, tape a picture of a toilet or a sign reading TOILET in large bold letters to the bathroom door. Also, because people suffering from dementia are easily distracted, keep the bathroom free of magazines and other objects that might grab their attention.

As these disabling illnesses progress,

trips to the bathroom or using bedpans and urinals may eventually become too demanding for caregivers and patients alike. At this point we start relying on adult diapers. Men have the option of wearing condom catheters, disposable thin rubber sheaths that slip over the penis and collect the urine. ◀ *See "Incontinence," page 170.*

Contracture

Anyone immobilized for a prolonged period of time falls prey to *contracture,* where muscles and tendons literally shrink from disuse and lose their elasticity. The joints, too, may grow stiff or freeze altogether. In advanced Alzheimer's, the sight of a bedridden patient curled up in the fetal position, hands clenched and toes splayed like a baby's, is tragically common. At this late stage in the brain's deterioration, only the primitive reflexes we're born with remain.

PD and ALS sufferers can develop contracture while still considerably mobile. As muscles grow rigid from Parkinson's, for example, many patients tend to neglect certain joints. Not only do the underused joints themselves turn rigid, but muscles in the area contract, further restricting mobility. That's why keeping physically active is so important in helping to retain as much dexterity, functional strength, and lean muscle mass as possible. Similarly, a right-handed person with early-stage ALS may walk perfectly well yet experience contracture of the left wrist because she doesn't exercise it adequately. The expression "Use it or lose it" definitely applies.

Preventive Management

Chapter 3 explains how to minimize contracture by flexing, rotating, and extending a bed-bound patient's joints. The doctor, nurse, or physical therapist can demonstrate these *passive range-of-motion exercises* for you. No matter how sick someone is, we do this several times a day for five to ten minutes. While loved ones are bound to lose a degree of muscle tone, "keeping the joints more mobile will make it easier to take care of the person," says nurse-practitioner Audrey MacMillan, clinical coordinator at the Pittsburgh Alzheimer Disease Research Center. "Once they're severely contracted, turning, bathing, and changing all become even more difficult." ◀ *See "Preventing Muscle Contracture and Foot Drop," page 135.*

Muscle Cramping

Parkinson's disease and ALS may subject patients to muscle aches and cramping in the legs, feet, toes, and thighs. Many people with PD will tell you their discomfort is most acute in the morning or as their levodopa or levodopa-carbidopa is wearing off.

How It Is Managed

Time to work with your hands: Gently massaging loved ones' legs, calves, and thighs (both front and back) at night helps relieve leg cramps, while a warm tub bath, sponge bath, or hot-water bottle can soothe muscle spasms. ◀ *See "Nonpharmaceutical Pain Management," page 156.*

Parkinson's Disease. The aches and cramps often subside with the next dose of levodopa or Sinemet. But then there are patients—particularly those on heavy doses—who suffer a persistent deep muscle pain that Dr. Côté describes as agonizing. "They may also develop a pain related to the spasmlike movements of the extremities," he says, "especially the toes and ankles."

The only effective remedy is for the physician to lower the dosage. Doing so essentially substitutes one set of symptoms for another, as the effects of the Parkinson's itself will intensify. "Painkillers don't work very well," Dr. Côté explains, "because they tend to constipate." For severe discomfort the physician may try baclofen (brand name: Lioresal), a muscle relaxant and antispastic drug, or anticholinergics such as trihexyphenidyl (Artane) or benztropine (Cogentin).

ALS. Here, too, painkillers present a problem because they depress breathing. So do barbiturates, opiates, and sleeping pills. Always check with the doctor before administering any of these medications. The cramping associated with Lou Gehrig's disease frequently responds to baclofen.

When Paralysis Sets In

Once a loved one loses use of his legs, they may "flop" outward when he's lying down. This can produce a painful sensation in the groin and leg joints. Use pillows to bolster both legs. If you need something sturdier, try the inexpensive vinyl cushions and wedges that hospitals often use to position patients. You should be able to find these products at most surgical supply dealers.

Insomnia

The reversed sleep patterns seen with Alzheimer's disease also plague a number of Parkinson's patients. They nap intermittently during the day and toss and turn at night, then meet the dawn bleary-eyed and exhausted. "That's a real problem," notes Dr. Côté, "because if they don't get a good night's sleep, their Parkinson's symptoms are much worse the next day." ALS isn't known to disrupt the sleep cycle per se, but its common end-stage complications—choking, respiratory distress, and difficulty shifting position in bed—hamper the chances of sleeping through the night.

How It Is Managed

The doctor may prescribe a short-acting sedative like zolpidem (brand name: Ambien) or chloral hydrate, or amitrip-tyline (Elavil), an antidepressant with sedative properties. If you're experimenting with nonprescription sleep aids, consult the doctor first, since Unisom, Sominex, Nytol, and others may interact with anti-Parkinson's drugs.

The Parkinson's Patient at Night

The fitful movements of Parkinson's present another obstacle to sleep. It's not unusual for patients to wake up entangled in the bedsheets and blankets or marooned in an awkward position, unable to roll over.

Silky rayon pajamas and sheets make it easier for patients to turn in bed.

Dressing loved ones in heavy bedclothes such as wool socks, sweatshirts, and sweatpants keeps them warm with fewer covers.

Some PD patients bite their tongue in their sleep. Wearing a rubber mouth guard (the type used by boxers and football players) can prevent a painful accident. ◄ See *"Insomnia and Other Sleep Disorders," page 172.*

Speech/Language Loss (Aphasia)

Aphasia is a broad term encompassing an array of physical and cognitive problems that impede the ability to communicate. A person with Parkinson's or Lou Gehrig's disease knows what she wants to say, but damage to nerves and muscles necessary for speech may impair articulation and projection. In Alzheimer's, the opposite occurs: While the voice mechanism survives intact, the disease scrambles the brain's speech, language, thinking, and memory centers. Eventually patients can no longer process information, express themselves coherently, or remember from one moment to the next, although glimmers of lucidity still appear much of the time. At my father's funeral, Uncle Billy kept whispering, "Where's Bob? What are all these people doing here?" Yet when my cousin Ginny drove him to

Dad's house while the rest of us were attending the burial, he directed her like an air-traffic controller bringing in a crippled airliner. "We didn't miss a turn," she marveled later.

How It Is Managed

Speech-Language Therapy. Nothing can be done to undo the intellectual deterioration from Alzheimer's or the motor dysfunction loss from ALS that ultimately renders patients mute. Parkinson's sufferers, half of whom experience speech problems, can often benefit from sessions with a *speech-language pathologist*, who will teach exercises for limbering up the tongue, lips, cheeks, and jaw, and techniques for improving speech, such as speaking in shorter sentences so they don't run out of breath, proper breathing techniques to prevent words from running together, and accentuating important words and raising the pitch at the end of questions to offset the monotonal delivery characteristic of PD patients.

☎ Your loved one's neurologist should be able to recommend a speech-language facility or private speech pathologist in your area. You can also call the American Speech-Language-Hearing Association Information Resource Center (800-638-8255) for free referrals to ASHA-certified members.

Telephone Amplification Devices. For less than $1 a month, AT&T leases a special receiver with a built-in amplifier, ideal for folks who can't muster sufficient volume to talk on the phone. The handset plugs into any standard desk model. (You can also purchase it for about $20.)

☎ To rent, call AT&T at 800-555-8111; to buy, call 800-222-3111.

Computer Technology for ALS Patients. Lou Gehrig's disease spares only the eye muscles, which connect to the central nervous system differently from other muscles. A remarkable computer system, the Asyst 3000 Communi-Mate, enables patients to communicate by moving their eyebrows or an ear muscle or whatever muscle still functions, thereby activating a sensor attached to a headband. The machine displays letters, words, and phrases on a video monitor or synthesizes the person's own voice, sampled from old tape recordings. It can even be programmed to regulate the thermostat and other household appliances.

Depending on how it's customized, the Communi-Mate lists for between $4,500 and $8,000. While this puts it well beyond the reach of most families, local chapters of the Amyotrophic Lateral Sclerosis Association and other foundations purchase a number of the computers and rent them to patients for a nominal fee. "The first thing we do when we receive a call is see if the person can get the equipment through a foundation," says Steve Wells, codesigner of the Asyst 3000.

A less expensive, albeit less sophisticated alternative is Crestwood Company's Talking Laser Beam, a cap fitted with—you guessed it—a battery-operated laser beam. Patients must retain some degree of head movement in order to be able to aim the red light at an alphabet board (for spelling out words) or at objects up to one hundred feet away. The cost is $214.95.

If the person can still point or in some way indicate yes or no, cutting-edge technology is not required. Simple *talking pictures* that illustrate basic needs such as "hungry," "thirsty," "bathroom," and so on, remain an excellent tool for helping speech-impaired patients express themselves. Chapter 4's section on impaired communications skills tells you where to buy the cards or how to make them yourself.

For more information contact the following:

☎ The Amyotrophic Lateral Sclerosis Association, 21021 Ventura Boulevard, Suite 321, Woodland Hills, CA 91364-2206; 800-782-4747.

☎ Asyst Communications Company, 39 Crestland Road, Indian Creek, IL 60061; 888-779-9998/847-816-8580.

☎ Crestwood Company, 6625 N. Sidney Place, Milwaukee, WI 53209-3259; 414-352-5678.

▶ *See Appendix B: "Adaptive Technology," page 504.*

Difficulty Swallowing (Dysphagia)

A major concern for caregivers. When someone cannot swallow properly, he may inadvertently inhale food or liquid into the larynx, down the windpipe, and into the lungs. This can give rise to *aspiration pneumonia*, a leading cause of death for people with a chronic progressive neurological disease.

"The last year of Clarence's life," says Betty Lindstrom, "he was hospitalized with aspiration pneumonia three times." As with speech impairment, the dysphagia that occurs in late-stage Parkinson's or ALS stems from one or more physical malfunctions: The tongue loses its strength to adequately push food into the throat, and the undulating muscle contractions that normally nudge food down the throat and esophagus en route to the stomach weaken. Patients frequently complain that food lodges in their throat. On top of this, the valve that permits food to enter the stomach may not always close properly. Acidic digestive juices then back up into the esophagus, causing inflammation. The burning sensation and fullness from *esophagitis* is treatable with antacids.

Diane Young's father, too, developed aspiration pneumonia. Strange as it may sound, people with advanced Alzheimer's find it difficult to swallow not because of muscle failure but because they simply don't know *how* to anymore.

"We used to feed my dad liquids through a straw," Diane recalls. "But he would blow into the straw instead of inhaling! How do you explain to

someone whose memory is impaired how to suck? So I'd dip the straw in the cup, place my finger over the opening of the straw, and use it like an eyedropper to give him tiny amounts of liquid."

How It Is Managed

Chapter 3 contains techniques for feeding loved ones unable to swallow normally, such as pureeing solid food. "That helped a lot," says Betty Lindstrom. "My husband couldn't get down anything thicker than pudding." Conversely, some liquids can be too thin, trickling easily down the wrong pipe, so to them we add special thickening products. (Tip: Mixing in dry baby cereals or instant mashed potato flakes works equally as well.)

Even with these precautions, during meals we need to watch loved ones and encourage them to chew their food thoroughly. A person with Parkinson's or ALS has to expend so much energy chewing, he may get lazy on occasion and try to gulp down a piece of partially chewed food. The larger it is, the greater the chance of its catching in the throat or windpipe. In late-stage Alzheimer's, patients tend to hold bites of food in their mouth, so get used to repeatedly reminding them to swallow.

Suctioning. It's wise to have a mechanical suctioning device, or *aspirator*, on hand for those emergencies when someone is choking on runny food or liquid. Ask the doctor to write out a prescription. "Without that little machine," says Betty, "my husband would have been in the hospital even more than three times that last year."

✱ *Never use the aspirator to suction out a piece of solid food. Either dislodge it with your fingers or perform the Heimlich maneuver.*

Tube Feeding. In the event that dysphagia becomes so severe it interferes with adequate nutrition, a feeding tube (discussed below) may be the only solution. ◄ *See "Difficulty Swallowing (Dysphagia), page 165; "Using a Suction Device to Clear the Airway," page 177; and "The Heimlich Maneuver," page 182.*

Appetite Loss/Wasting

Between dysphagia and difficulty handling utensils, patients often lose interest in eating. (With Parkinson's, this may also be due to the disease's effect on the hypothalamus, the portion of the brain that regulates appetite, among other functions.) It is common for weight to plummet up to thirty pounds. The resulting lack of fatty tissue for cushioning leaves loved ones dangerously susceptible to bedsores.

How It Is Managed

Any of these diseases can dampen a patient's appetite well before death beckons. Until that time arrives, we're concerned with getting them sufficient nourishment. The basic game plan:

- Instead of breakfast, lunch, and dinner, serve five or six smaller meals, which are less tiring for patients.
- Puree food or cut it into small pieces to reduce the risk of choking and also to spare patients some of the effort of chewing.
- Make the most of what they *can* eat by serving foods rich in protein and high in calories.
- Buy utensils and dishes specially designed for people unable to grip properly—for example, forks with built-up handles and plates with suction cups on the bottom to prevent slipping.
- Saintly patience! Be prepared to set aside more time than usual for meals. "It took Clarence so long to chew and swallow," reflects Betty Lindstrom, "he might start eating lunch at eleven o'clock and not finish until after one. And this was when he was still able to get to the table."

Also expect that one day you will have to spoon-feed, as my aunt Kitty did the last three months of Uncle Billy's life. "He could not feed himself anymore," she recalls. "He would take his fork and just poke and poke, but could never get the food on the fork. I would let him play with his food a bit while *I* ate, then I'd reach over and put a spoonful in his mouth."

✳ *At mealtime try not to become so obsessed with feeding a debilitated loved one that you neglect your own diet. Eat!*

Tube Feeding. Most people with Parkinson's or Alzheimer's manage to continue eating without the aid of a tube. But as Lou Gehrig's disease progresses, a *gastrostomy* will inevitably be necessary. In a surprisingly simple surgical procedure conducted using local anesthesia, a flexible tube is placed in the stomach through a small incision. You should realize, however, that no amount of calories and nutrients will alter the muscle atrophy and wasting from this disease. ◄ *See "Tricks for Stimulating Appetite," page 159; "Tube Feeding and Total Parenteral Nutrition (TPN)," page 166.* ► *See Appendix B: "Adaptive Technology," page 504.*

Difficulty Expelling Secretions

The fading muscle tone from ALS and Parkinson's that hampers swallowing also makes it difficult to cough up mucus and saliva. Especially with ALS, patients suffer chronic discomfort and gagging from secretions that pool in the back of the throat. The problem is compounded by the fact that Lou Gehrig's disease—and to a lesser extent Parkinson's—cause excessive drooling.

How It Is Managed

As you can imagine, many loved ones find the recurrent choking sensation unbearable. Positioning them on their side helps keep secretions from collecting in the throat. When phlegm does congest the airway, cup your hand and lightly tap on their back. "Often that will loosen it up and bring it to the surface," explains Marianne Kelly, a nurse at Boston University Medical Center, "so that you can suction that much more of it and make the person more comfortable."

In addition, ask the doctor about prescribing medications to dry up secretions. "I'll usually give patients Elavil [amitriptyline] to be taken at bedtime," says Dr. Richard A. Gan, "or something with strong anticholinergic properties." Drugs from that category often prescribed for this purpose include atropine (available under several brand names), trihexiphenidyl (Artane), and propantheline (Pro-Banth-Ane). ◄ *See "Using a Suction Device to Clear the Airway," page 177.*

Difficulty Breathing (Dyspnea)/Respiratory Failure

Parkinson's and ALS have the same effect on muscles crucial to breathing as they do on other muscles of the body. Of the two, Parkinson's produces less serious respiratory symptoms. The chest wall muscles that normally stretch, allowing the lungs to expand, become rigid and move slowly. According to Dr. Côté, "patients tend to breathe shallowly. Plus, it takes them longer than normal to draw air into their lungs. Many of them complain they feel short of breath whenever they exert themselves."

ALS paralyzes these muscles. Most seriously of all, it weakens the *diaphragm*, the large convex muscle that lies beneath both lungs. The diaphragm's contractions enable the two airbags to inflate during inhalation. Then the abdominal muscles force it back into position, which expels air from the lungs and up the respiratory tract. Eventually ALS compromises the respiratory system so severely that patients can barely breathe unassisted.

How It Is Managed

The following are possibilities:

Pulmonary Rehabilitation. PD patients can enhance their breathing ability by practicing exercises designed to help them rely more on their diaphragm, improve chest expansion, and exhale more forcefully. Ask a respiratory therapist or nurse to demonstrate.

The benefits of a pulmonary rehabilitation program are less concrete for people with advanced ALS. "At that stage," says Nurse Kelly, "you're looking at the quality of life and what's going to make them feel most comfortable. If it's something they are physically able to do and are willing to do, it's certainly worth a shot."

For free referrals to a pulmonary rehab progam, call

☎ The American Association of Cardiovascular and Pulmonary Rehabilitation in Middleton, Wisconsin, at 608-831-6989.

Oxygen Therapy. To assist the patient's breathing, the physician may recommend using a portable oxygen tank or a *bilevel positive airway pressure* machine. Not unlike a mechanical ventilator (see below), the BIPAP automatically drives air down the throat and into the lungs.

Mechanical Ventilation. By early 1995, says Debra Bulkeley, "the disease began to affect my father's breathing muscles. He no longer had the strength to push air in and out of his lungs." From the start Jack LaCava had made it clear to family members that he did not want mechanical respiration or a feeding tube used; shortly after he was diagnosed with ALS, he executed both a living will and a power of attorney stating his wishes in writing.

Many people with Lou Gehrig's disease, aware of what is to come, reach the same decision. Going on long-term artificial respiration entails an invasive procedure called a *tracheostomy*, in which a surgeon makes an artificial opening through the neck and into the windpipe, then implants a permanent tube that attaches to the ventilator and delivers oxygen to the lungs. However, "in my experience," says Dr. Gan, "most patients opt not to have a tracheostomy and ventilatory support." ◄ *See "Difficulty Breathing (Dyspnea)," page 174; "Administering Supplemental Oxygen," page 175; and "Mechanical Ventilation," page 175.*

Debra Bulkeley: *Starting around the end of February, my father had some episodes where he passed out from not being able to breathe. He landed in the hospital a couple of times. My mother ended up getting very ill herself, so we put him in a rehab facility for a week to give her some respite and to hire some home nursing care and so forth.*

That last week my father was in the hospital, he was getting respiratory therapy to try to loosen up all the pleghm in his lungs. He tried like hell to get that stuff up—he was a real trouper to the very last minute—but he was just too weak from the ALS. He died of respiratory failure on April 24, 1995.

Recommended Reading

The following is available free from the ALS Association (800-782-4747):
 • "Basic Home Care for ALS Patients"

The following is available free from the Alzheimer's Disease Education and Referral Center (800-438-4380):
 • "Alzheimer's Disease"

The following is available free from the American Parkinson's Disease Association (800-223-2732):
 • "Parkinson's Disease Handbook"

The following are available free from the National Parkinson Foundation (800-327-4545):
 • "Patient Perspectives on Parkinson's"
 • "The Parkinson Handbook"

The following is available free from the Parkinson's Disease Foundation (800-457-6676):
 • "Exercises for the Parkinson Patient, with Hints for Daily Living"

The following is available free from the United Parkinson Foundation (312-733-1893):
 • "Parkinson's Disease: A Guide for Patients"

APPENDIX A

Recommended Resources

The organizations and agencies listed here can be of great help to patients and caregivers. Besides raising funds for medical research, most offer informative pamphlets and other educational materials free of charge and maintain toll-free information hot lines. People there can often direct you to medical specialists, community services for eligible patients, buyers clubs, and patient assistance programs for medications, clinical trials, and support groups. Some provide limited financial assistance. Funding typically varies from chapter to chapter, as do the types of services available.

We suggest you consider becoming a member of those organizations pertinent to your loved one's illness. Most publish newsletters, available at a nominal fee, that contain invaluable tips on patient care. Perhaps most important of all, they bring patients and caregivers together with others facing a similar crisis.

Most resources are designed to serve the needs of patients with a particular condition and their caregivers. We've arranged these alphabetically by disease, followed by general resources for patients and care partners.

AIDS/HIV

AIDS Clinical Trials Information Service (ACTIS)
800-874-2572
HIV/AIDS Treatment Information Service (ATIS)
800-448-0440
Monday through Friday, 9:00 A.M. to 7:00 P.M. ET

Both ACTIS and ATIS are cooperative projects of several government agencies, including the Centers for Disease Control and Prevention (CDC).

Trained ATIS staffers can answer your questions about federally approved treatments and send you print information. A patient at any stage of HIV infection may be eligible for experimental drugs and other therapies. ACTIS can tell you which studies are

---

Information on the Internet

Many of the associations listed here have also set up shop along the information superhighway—a great help when you need information after hours. You can either call an organization directly for its Internet address or type in the name and conduct a search via your on-line service or Internet access provider.

---

open, their location and eligibility requirements, and the names and telephone numbers of the contact persons. Subscribers to the on-line databases AIDSTRIALS and AIDSDRUGS, available through the National Library of Medicine, may access this information directly via the Internet or by purchasing a user-friendly software package known as Grateful Med. Call 800-638-8480 for more details.

AIDS Treatment Data Network

611 Broadway, Suite 613, New York, NY 10012-2809; 800-734-7104

Monday through Friday, 10:00 A.M. to 6:00 P.M. ET; messages can be left after hours

The Network can apprise you of approved, experimental, and alternative treatments for AIDS and HIV, including those available through your state's Medicaid program, AIDS drug assistance programs, and access programs sponsored by pharmaceutical companies. In addition to distributing print information, Network counselors are available to explain treatment options or simply to talk. Request the nonprofit organization's newsletter, "Treatment Review," published eight times a year, and "The Experimental Treatment Guide," which comes with a handbook entitled "Should I Enter an AIDS Drug Trial?"

American Foundation for AIDS Research

733 Third Avenue, 12th Floor, New York, NY 10017; 800-392-6327 or 212-682-7440

Monday through Friday, 8:30 A.M. to 6:00 P.M. ET

AmFar, the country's leading private organization dedicated to AIDS research and education, publishes the *AIDS/HIV Treatment Directory*. Issued every ninety days, this comprehensive, up-to-date resource describes treatments in development for AIDS and HIV infection, and related opportunistic infections and tumors. Anyone who cannot afford a subscription ($55 a year) may obtain a free copy through the CDC National AIDS Clearinghouse (800-458-5231), which operates from 9:00 A.M. to 7:00 P.M. ET, Monday through Friday.

Catholic Charities USA

1731 King Street, Suite 200, Alexandria, VA 22314; 703-549-1390

Monday through Friday, 9:00 A.M. to 5:00 P.M. ET

Many of the more than fourteen hundred Catholic Charities aid homeless men and women with AIDS/HIV and their families. The Brooklyn, New York, agency's Supportive Living Apartment Program is one of the most comprehensive. A permanent caseworker assigned to each patient arranges for free furnished housing, then continues to assist the patient or family, whether it be registering children in school or obtaining public entitlements. The Brooklyn Catholic Charities also offers free legal services, short-term individual and family counseling, crisis intervention, and support groups. Other Catholic Charities may provide housing and referrals but not the same level of follow-up care. For the name and number of the Catholic Charities agency nearest you, call the organization's headquarters.

CDC National HIV/AIDS Hotline

800-342-2437

Operates twenty-four hours a day, seven days a week

This toll-free hot line can answer general questions about AIDS and send you free educational materials about the disease. For certain free publications, the information specialist may have you call the toll-free CDC National AIDS Clearinghouse (800-458-5231, 9:00 A.M. to 7:00 P.M. ET, Monday through Friday).

One of its most valuable services is assisting callers in finding a physician knowledgeable about AIDS. The hot line can also refer you to a local case manager, who in turn can inform you of entitlement programs and community services that may be helpful.

Gay Men's Health Crisis

119 West 24th Street, New York, NY 10011; 212-367-1000

Monday through Friday, 10:00 A.M. to 6:00 P.M. ET

Legal services: 212-367-1040

Monday through Friday, 10:00 A.M. to 6:00 P.M. ET

Hot line: 212-807-6655

Monday through Friday, 10:00 A.M. to 8:00 P.M. ET

Gay Men's Health Crisis, founded in 1981, offers an array of services for New Yorkers with AIDS, including case management, legal assistance, referrals to HIV/AIDS entitlements, nutritional counseling, and group and individual therapy. On the national level, its hot line can send you free educational materials and answer questions about AIDS and treatment. A monthly newsletter, "The Gay Men's Health Crisis Newsletter of Experimental AIDS Therapies," is available at no cost to people with AIDS, although donations are appreciated (recommended: $30 for individuals, $60 for international subscriptions).

People With AIDS Coalition of New York

50 West 17th Street, 8th floor, New York, NY 10011; 800-828-3280 or 212-647-1420

Monday through Friday, 10:00 A.M. to 6:00 P.M. ET

Twelve People With AIDS coalitions exist throughout the United States, each independent of the others. While these coalitions primarily serve locally, they do administer some national programs.

For example, the New York Coalition operates a toll-free AIDS Hotline and Treatment Information Bureau staffed exclusively by men and women with AIDS/HIV. PWAC handles thousands of calls annually from patients seeking treatment-related information or an understanding ear. In addition to answering questions over the phone, the staff can mail you relevant scientific studies and other medical information.

The coalition publishes a monthly magazine, *Newsline*, and *SIDAahora*, a Spanish/English bimonthly. Subscriptions ($35 a year) also bring you PWAC's quarterly guide to free or low-cost AIDS/HIV services in the New York Metropolitan area. Patients unable to afford either magazine are placed on the mailing list free of charge.

Other People With AIDS coalitions are in Dallas, Texas; Detroit, Michigan; Hammond, Indiana; Macon, Georgia; Philadelphia, Pennsylvania; Washington, D.C.; and in Fort Lauderdale, Jacksonville, Oakland Park, Orlando, and Tampa, Florida.

Project Inform Treatment Hotline

1965 Market Street, Suite 220, San Francisco, CA 94103; 415-558-8669

National hot line: 800-822-7422

Local and international hot line: 415-558-9051 (administrative offices)

Monday through Friday, 9:00 A.M. to 5:00 P.M. PT; Saturday, 10:00 A.M. to 4:00 P.M.

The Project Inform Treatment Hotline fields thousands of calls a month. Established to update people with AIDS and their caregivers on the latest in treatment news, it distributes free fact sheets and discussion papers that explain specific treatments and offer perspectives on such issues as how to manage HIV disease and misinformation on AIDS in the media. The "PI Briefing Paper," published three times a year, reports on drugs in development, standards of care, and other late-breaking news. Many national hot line services, including the CDC National HIV/AIDS Hotline, regularly refer callers to Project Inform, which was founded in 1985.

Alzheimer's Disease

Alzheimer's Disease Education and Referral Center

P.O. Box 8250, Silver Spring, MD 20907-8250; 800-438-4380

Monday through Friday, 8:30 A.M. to 5:00 P.M. ET

This service of the National Institute on Aging is affiliated with a network of research centers and can refer you to those conducting clinical trials. An information specialist can also steer you to organizations and state agencies that provide services to patients and caregivers.

Alzheimer's Disease and Related Disorders Association

919 North Michigan Avenue, Suite 1000, Chicago, IL 60611-1676; 800-272-3900 or 312-335-8700

Monday through Friday, 8:00 A.M. to 5:00 P.M. CT

The Alzheimer's Association, founded in 1980, has more than 220 chapters nationwide; to locate the one nearest you, call its toll-free twenty-four-hour information and referral line. Your local chapter can direct you to area day care centers, respite care, elder-law attorneys, clinical trials, and the nearest Alzheimer's Association support group. Membership costs $15 annually and brings you the association's quarterly newsletter and monthly chapter newsletters.

The Alzheimer's Association sponsors a program called Safe Return, conceived to help return memory-impaired men and women who have wandered away from home. For $25 the patient is registered in a national database. Loved ones can report a missing patient to a toll-free number that connects them with a nationwide network of seventeen thousand local law enforcement agencies. In addition to keeping a detailed description of the patient on file, Safe Return sends you wallet cards, clothing labels, and a bracelet or necklace (available in three styles) for the patient to wear.

National Institute of Neurological Disorders and Stroke

P.O. Box 5801, Bethesda, MD 20824; 800-352-9424 or 301-496-5751

Monday through Friday, 8:00 A.M. to 5:00 P.M. ET

Ask to be sent the institute's free information packet on Alzheimer's disease.

Amyotrophic Lateral Sclerosis

The Amyotrophic Lateral Sclerosis Association

21021 Ventura Boulevard, Suite 321, Woodland Hills, CA 91364-2206; 800-782-4747 or 818-340-7500

Monday through Friday, 7:30 A.M. to 4:00 P.M. PT

ALSA publishes a free newsletter, "Link," three times a year, and its toll-free patient hot line can answer questions and make referrals.

The association's 135 chapters and support groups offer various levels of service. For example, its largest chapter, in Philadelphia, lends medical equipment, provides transportation to and from medical appointments, and evaluates patients' homes for safety and accessibility. Each chapter has at least one support group for patients, family members, and friends.

Les Turner Amyotrophic Lateral Sclerosis Foundation

8142 Lawndale Avenue, Skokie, IL 60076; 847-679-3311

Monday through Friday, 8:30 A.M. to 4:30 P.M. CT; messages can be left after hours

The Les Turner Amyotrophic Lateral Sclerosis Foundation, founded in memory of a young man who died of the disease in 1978, provides a range of services to patients at its Lois Insolia ALS Center at Northwestern University Medical School in Evanston, Illinois. These include home visits by nurses and occupational therapists, loans of medical and communication equipment, and support groups. On the national level, it distributes complimentary literature, answers questions, and can route you to clinical trials and support groups near you. Anyone can receive the foundation's free newsletter for patients and family members, "Dialogue," which appears three times a year. When calling the above number, ask to speak to the patient service coordinator.

National Institute of Neurological Disorders and Stroke

P.O. Box 5801, Bethesda, MD 20824; 800-352-9424 or 301-496-5751

Monday through Friday, 8:00 A.M. to 5:00 P.M. ET

Ask to be sent the institute's free information packet on ALS.

Cancer

American Cancer Society

1599 Clifton Road, N.E., Atlanta, GA 30329; 800-227-2345 or 404-320-3333

Monday through Friday, 9:00 A.M. to 5:00 P.M. (all time zones)

Calling the toll-free number above connects you directly to your local division of the American Cancer Society, a volunteer health organization. Either a nurse or the medical affairs director has access to an up-to-date database on all forms of cancer and can answer questions and make referrals regarding diagnosis, treatment, second opinions, and available clinical trials. ACS can also make you aware of community resources for cancer patients, although as you can see below, it offers a number of free services and aid directly.

Contact your division to learn which of the following services it offers:

• Free transportation to and from treatment sessions for ambulatory patients. If volunteer drivers are not available, ACS will reimburse public-transportation expenses.

• Short-term crisis counseling (four to six sessions) for patients and/or family members who do not have insurance for professional therapy and cannot otherwise afford it.

• Look Good, Feel Better, a free program developed by the Cosmetic, Toiletry and Fragrance Association (CTFA), teaches cancer patients undergoing chemotherapy or radiation how to use makeup, wigs, and other accessories to enhance their self-image and self-confidence. The single-session program is usually held at a hospital.

• Intervention in health insurance disputes. For instance, if a patient considered cured of cancer is denied future coverage, the ACS might bring the case before the state insurance commissioner.

• The ACS lends free wigs to anyone experiencing hair loss from treatment and partially reimburses patients who purchase their own. Women who have undergone a mastectomy and are considering buying a breast prosthesis can be shown the models available, by appointment, at their division office. Free prostheses are available for patients unable to afford them.

• Extremely limited financial assistance is available for home health care, medical equipment, child care, and pain medication for patients without health insurance or with limited coverage.

• ACS sponsors several support groups designed to serve specific cancer populations and/or their caregivers.

Reach to Recovery is a short-term visitation program that links a newly diagnosed breast cancer patient with a breast cancer survivor. The trained volunteer visits the patient in the hospital, home, American Cancer Society office, or other mutually agreed upon site. The purpose is to provide emotional support and practical tips based on experience, but never medical advice.

The *CanSurmount* program, available upon request, also provides one-to-one support, both patient to patient and family member to family member.

I Can Cope is an education program for helping cancer patients and their families make informed medical decisions. During the eight-week course, consisting of weekly two-hour sessions, doctors, nurses, social workers, and other health care professionals explain the nature of the disease and its treatment, offer practical suggestions, and answer questions.

ACS also sponsors support groups for men and women whose voice boxes had to be surgically removed (laryngectomy) due to cancer of the larynx; colon cancer patients and bladder cancer patients who have undergone colostomies and ileostomies, respectively; and mastectomy patients suffering from lymphedema. This rare but sometimes permanent surgical side effect causes a buildup of lymph fluid, which brings about swelling in the arm and hand.

Cancer Information Service

800-422-6237 (800-4-CANCER)

Monday through Friday, 9:00 A.M. to 7:00 P.M. (all time zones). In Oahu, Hawaii: 524-1234; call collect from other Hawaiian islands.

The Cancer Information Service, a program of the National Cancer Institute, is a nationwide telephone service for both the public and health professionals. Dialing the toll-free number connects you to one of nineteen regional offices. The trained cancer information specialists there have access to the NCI's comprehensive up-to-date database known as Physician's Desk Query, or PDQ.

You can receive free informative booklets and pamphlets about each cancer. Particularly useful for an overview of the disease and its treatment are the PDQ state-of-the-art treatment information statements for more than seventy-five forms of cancer. Statements are geared specifically to patients or physicians. The patient statements average six pages and contain current data on staging, treatment, and prognosis.

In addition to sending you printed materials, your regional office can refer you to

• medical centers, physicians, and organizations that provide cancer care;

• pain management specialists at hospitals and pain management clinics;

• community organizations that offer patient services;

• support groups;

• clinical trials;

• smoking cessation programs.

If you have access to a fax machine, you can have PDQ statements faxed immediately by calling CancerFax at 301-402-5874. This free service (you pay only for the cost of the call to the CancerFax computer in Bethesda, Maryland) operates twenty-four hours a day, seven days a week.

Brain Cancer

American Brain Tumor Association

2720 River Road, Des Plaines, IL 60018; 800-886-2282 (patient line) or 847-827-9910

Monday through Friday, 8:30 A.M. to 5:00 P.M. CT; messages can be left after hours

The ABTA, founded in 1973, publishes nearly two dozen excellent booklets on brain tumors, treatment, help, and resources, as well as information about support groups and clinical trials. All are free, as is its newsletter, "Message Line," which is published three times a year. The toll-free information line can refer you to community services and aid for patients and caregivers. Although the association does not run support groups per se, it sponsors

Connections, a pen pal program for men and women with brain tumors.

The Brain Tumor Society

84 Seattle Street, Boston, MA 02134-1245, 800-770-8287 or 617-783-0340

Monday through Friday, 8:00 to 5:00 P.M. ET

In addition to funding research, the Brain Tumor Society will send you its quarterly newsletter, "Heads Up," and helpful resource booklet, "Color Me Hope," free of charge. Call the organization for referrals to brain tumor support groups throughout the country or to take advantage of its Patient/Family Telephone Network program, in which patients, former patients, and family members volunteer to share their experiences and offer support by phone.

National Brain Tumor Foundation

785 Market Street, Suite 1600, San Francisco, CA 94103; 800-934-2873 or 415-284-0208

Monday through Friday, 9:00 A.M. to 5:00 P.M. PT; messages can be left after hours

A group of brain tumor patients and their families started the National Brain Tumor Foundation in 1981. Call for referrals to medical institutions specializing in brain tumors and to one of the more than 120 brain tumor support groups in the United States. In addition, the support line can put you in touch with people who have had the disease. A free newsletter, "Search," comes out three times a year.

Leukemia, Lymphomas, and Multiple Myeloma

International Myeloma Foundation

2120 Stanley Hills Drive, Los Angeles, CA 90046; 800-452-2873 (800-452-CURE) or 213-654-3023

Monday through Friday, 8:00 A.M. to 5:00 P.M. PT

The IMP can send you information about multiple myeloma and treatment options, as well as its quarterly newsletter, "Myeloma Today."

Leukemia Society of America

600 Third Avenue, New York, NY 10016; 800-955-4572 (800-955-4LSA) or 212-573-8484

Operates twenty-four hours a day, seven days a week

The Leukemia Society of America distributes literature about leukemia and related diseases at no cost; its free newsletter is published three times a year. The toll-free information line can also refer you to your local chapter.

Patients undergoing treatment for leukemia, lymphomas, or multiple myeloma are eligible for $750 a year in financial assistance from the LSA's Patient Aid Program. This money may be used for services not covered by other sources, including:

- outpatient chemotherapy using any of approximately four dozen approved drugs;
- processing, typing, screening, and cross-matching of blood components for transfusions;
- transportation (mileage reimbursement, parking fees, tolls, cab fare) to and from a doctor's office, hospital, or treatment center;
- initial induction radiation therapy for men and women with Hodgkin's disease, in amounts up to $300;
- up to $300 of cranial radiation therapy for people with acute leukemia;
- testicular therapy treatment for relapsed acute lymphocytic leukemia, up to $300 annually

Lung Cancer

American Lung Association

1740 Broadway, New York, NY 10019-4374; 800-586-4872 or 212-315-8700

Monday through Friday, 8:30 A.M. to 4:30 P.M. ET

The ALA, founded in 1904 to fight tuberculosis, has affiliates in every state. Calling its toll-free number connects you to a health educator who can answer questions about lung diseases and treatment options, refer you to pulmonary specialists in your area, and send you helpful literature free of charge. Although some affiliates may be able to assist patients in financial need (for instance, obtaining oxygen for them), the ALA is primarily a research and educational voluntary health organization.

Skin Cancer

American Academy of Dermatology
930 North Meacham Road, Schaumburg, IL 60173-4965; 847-330-0230
Monday through Friday, 8:30 A.M. to 5:00 P.M. CT
Call the AAD for local referrals to dermatologists, physicians specializing in diagnosing and treating skin diseases, including cancers of the skin.

Skin Cancer Foundation
245 Fifth Avenue, Suite 1403, New York, NY 10016; 212-725-5176
Monday through Friday, 9:00 A.M. to 5:00 P.M. ET
The Skin Cancer Foundation focuses primarily on prevention and early detection. It can, however, send you free information on treatment options, including methods currently under investigation.

Cardiovascular Disease

American Heart Association
7272 Greenville Avenue, Dallas, TX 75231-4596; 800-242-8721 or 214-373-6300
Monday through Friday, 8:30 A.M. to 5:00 P.M. (all time zones); messages can be left after hours
Mended Hearts support group: 214-706-1442
Monday through Friday, 8:30 A.M. to 5:00 P.M. CT
The American Heart Association, founded in 1924 by six cardiologists, is primarily dedicated to prevention through research and education. Dialing its toll-free number routes you to your nearest AHA office. (Each state has its own affiliate, as do several major cities, and there are also hundreds of divisions and branches.) AHA can answer basic questions about heart condi-

tions and mail you relevant literature. It can also refer you to its affiliated support network, Mended Hearts, which has over 250 groups nationwide.

National Heart, Lung and Blood Institute Information Center
P.O. Box 30105, Bethesda, MD 20824-0105; 301-251-1222
Monday through Friday, 8:30 A.M. to 5:00 P.M. ET
The National Heart, Lung and Blood Institute's information center publishes free booklets and fact sheets on cardiovascular disease, most of which concern prevention. If you're seeking information on a rare disorder, request what is called a specialized inquiry: An information specialist will search the NHLBI's library for medical journal articles and other materials at no cost.

American Association of Cardiovascular and Pulmonary Rehabilitation
7611 Elmwood Avenue, Suite 201, Middleton, WI 53562; 608-831-6989
Monday through Friday, 9:00 A.M. to 5:00 P.M. CT
Call this association for referrals to cardiovascular rehabilitation programs for post–heart attack patients.

Cerebrovascular Stroke

National Stroke Association
96 Inverness Drive, Suite I, Englewood, CO 80112; 800-787-6537 or 303-649-9299
Monday through Thursday, 8:00 A.M. to 4:30 P.M. MT; Friday, 8:00 A.M. to 4:00 P.M. MT
The National Stroke Association's Stroke Information and Resource Center Hotline is staffed by a nurse who can refer you to stroke specialists, rehabilitation centers, community and government services, and support groups. "Be Stroke Smart," the NSA's quarterly newsletter, regularly publishes information about clinical trials that may benefit stroke patients. Membership costs

$20 annually, although no one is denied enrollment.

Stroke Connection of the American Heart Association
7272 Greenville Avenue, Dallas, TX 75231-4596; 800-553-6321 or 214-706-1777
Monday through Friday, 8:30 A.M. to 5:00 P.M. CT
The American Heart Association raises funds for research and education pertaining to stroke as well as heart disease. Its Stroke Connection can answer basic questions about stroke and send you literature. There are also more than nine hundred Stroke Connection support groups throughout the country for patients and their families. *Stroke Connection Magazine*, published bimonthly, is available for $8 a year; any patient unable to afford a subscription will receive the magazine as a courtesy.

Chronic Obstructive Pulmonary Disease (Emphysema)

American Lung Association
1740 Broadway, New York, NY 10019-4374; 800-586-4872 or 212-315-8700
Monday through Friday, 8:30 A.M. to 4:30 P.M. ET
◀ *See "Lung Cancer," page 495.*

National Heart, Lung and Blood Institute Information Center
P.O. Box 30105, Bethesda, MD 20824-0105; 301-251-1222
Monday through Friday, 8:30 A.M. to 5:00 P.M. ET
The National Heart, Lung and Blood Institute's information center publishes a small number of free booklets on COPD and other pulmonary diseases. If you're seeking information on a rare disorder, request what's called a specialized inquiry: An information specialist will search the NHLBI's library for medical journal articles and other materials at no cost.

American Association of Cardiovascular and Pulmonary Rehabilitation
7611 Elmwood Avenue, Suite 201, Middleton, WI 53562; 608-831-6989
Monday through Friday, 9:00 A.M. to 5:00 P.M. CT
Call this association for referrals to pulmonary rehabilitation programs.

Diabetes

American Diabetes Association
1660 Duke Street, Alexandria, VA 22314; 800-342-2383 (800-DIABETES)
Monday through Friday, 9:00 A.M. to 4:30 P.M. ET
By calling the American Diabetes Association's information hot line, you can receive free literature about diabetes, nutrition, potential complications, management techniques, and testing. A trained staffer or volunteer can also direct you to ADA support groups in your area. ADA has over eight hundred affiliates and chapters in the United States and Puerto Rico.
Diabetes Forecast, a monthly lifestyle magazine, contains inspirational stories, information on diabetes-related products, recipes, research findings, and other news of interest to diabetics and their families. It comes with a $24 annual membership. Members also receive discounts on ADA publications, such as its popular meal-planning series and cookbooks.

National Diabetes Information Clearinghouse
1 Information Way, Bethesda, MD 20892-3560; 301-654-3327
Monday through Friday, 9:00 A.M. to 5:00 P.M. ET
A service of the National Institute of Diabetes and Digestive and Kidney Diseases, the National Diabetes Information Clearinghouse distributes many free publications about the disease, such as "The Diabetes Dictionary," an illustrated glossary of more than 350 diabetes-related terms. Also ask to re-

ceive the NDIC's quarterly newsletter, "Diabetes Dateline."

Head Injury

Brain Injury Association

1776 Massachusetts Avenue, N.W., Suite 100, Washington, DC 20036; 800-444-6443 or 202-296-6443

Monday through Friday, 9:00 A.M. to 5:00 P.M. ET

The Brain Injury Association, begun as a small grassroots organization in 1980, now has forty-five state associations and a network of over 450 support groups. Call its family help line for the number of your state association and/or affiliate, which in turn can refer you to head injury specialists, rehabilitation facilities, sources of financial assistance and patient services, free hospital care, clinical trials, and support groups. Members receive the quarterly magazine *TBI Challenge!* (Membership costs $35; for brain-injured patients of limited means, $5.)

Kidney Disease

American Association of Kidney Patients

100 South Ashley Drive, Suite 280, Tampa, FL 33602; 800-749-2257

Monday through Friday, 8:30 A.M. to 5:00 P.M. ET

For an annual membership fee of $15, patients receive "Bulletin," the AAKP's quarterly newsletter, and *Renalife* magazine, which is published three times a year. Each of the organization's twenty-five chapters runs a support group for kidney patients and their families. The association is active in legislative issues of concern to people with renal disease and also assists patients individually, insofar as helping them obtain health insurance and access to medications at reduced cost.

American Kidney Fund

6110 Executive Boulevard, Suite 1010, Rockville, MD 20852; 800-638-8299 or 301-881-3052

Monday through Friday, 8:30 A.M. to 5:00 P.M. ET

The American Kidney Fund's help line can answer general questions about kidney disease as well as provide referrals to support groups. Its free newsletter appears monthly. More so than any other kidney disease–related organization, the AKF runs a number of financial aid programs for needy patients with end-stage renal disease:

- Individual Grants Program. Eligible patients may receive financial aid for medications, transportation, kidney donor assistance, special dietary needs, and other treatment-related services and expenses. Patients must be referred by their physician and their social worker.
- Emergency Fund Program. Cash grants for emergency transportation, medications, or other treatment-related emergencies may be available through dialysis and transplant facilities. The AKF funds eligible facilities, enabling staff members to assist patients financially when the need arises.
- Disaster Relief Program. End-stage renal disease patients who have suffered major losses due to a natural disaster can receive grants for replacing clothing and household items, paying for food or utility deposits, and other essential relief services.
- Sherer Travel-Related Dialysis Program. Should a renal patient have to travel due to an emergency and require dialysis while away, this program pays the 20 percent of costs not covered by Medicare or another source of insurance.

End Stage Renal Disease Network
Health Care Financing Administration

The Health Care Financing Administration oversees the End Stage Renal Disease Network, made up of seventeen regional offices throughout the United States. The ESRD acts as a clearinghouse for information and referrals about end-stage renal disease. One of its main functions is to monitor and work with kidney dialysis facilities on improving the quality of care and to investigate patient complaints about treatment. Newly diagnosed end-stage renal disease patients can be put in touch with a social worker, who can help them obtain benefits. ESRD offices also arrange for second opinions by local nephrologists.

ESRD regional offices (from East to West):

- Connecticut, Maine, Massachusetts, New Hampshire, Rhode Island, Vermont
  203-387-9332
- New York
  212-289-4524
- New Jersey, Puerto Rico, U.S. Virgin Islands
  609-395-5544
- Delaware, Pennsylvania
  412-647-3428
- District of Columbia, Maryland, Virginia, West Virginia
  804-794-3757
- Georgia, North Carolina, South Carolina
  919-876-7545
- Florida
  813-251-8686
- Alabama, Mississippi, Tennessee
  601-936-9260
- Illinois, Indiana, Kentucky, Ohio
  317-257-8265
- Michigan, Minnesota, North Dakota, South Dakota, Wisconsin
  612-644-9877
- Iowa, Kansas, Missouri, Nebraska
  816-880-9990
- Arkansas, Louisiana, Oklahoma
  405-843-8688
- Texas
  972-503-3215
- Arizona, Colorado, Nevada, New Mexico, Utah, Wyoming
  303-831-8818
- Alaska, Idaho, Montana, Oregon, Washington
  206-448-1803
- American Samoa, Guam, Hawaii, Northern California, Mariana Islands
  415-472-8590
- Southern California
  213-962-2020

**National Kidney
and Urologic Diseases
Information Clearinghouse**
3 Information Way, Bethesda, MD 20892-3580; 301-654-4415
Monday through Friday, 9:00 A.M. to 5:00 P.M. ET
Request the clearinghouse's free information packet about kidney diseases.

The National Kidney Foundation
30 East 33rd Street, 11th Floor, New York, NY 10016; 800-622-9010 or 212-889-2210
Monday through Friday, 8:30 A.M. to 5:30 P.M. ET; messages can be left after hours

Call the National Kidney Foundation's headquarters for a referral to one of its fifty-two affiliates or more than two hundred chapters. Your local affiliate can direct you to area kidney specialists and NKF support groups for patients and family members, and steer you to available public and private services. The National Kidney Foundation publishes two quarterly newspapers: *Family Focus*, tailored to dialysis patients; and *Transplant Chronicles*, for transplant patients.

Programs vary, but those below are offered at most affiliates.

• Predialysis Education Program. Taught by a certified instructor, this multisession program for newly diagnosed kidney patients explains treatment options in depth.

• Patient-to-Patient Counseling. Patients can be put in touch with other kidney patients.

• Patient aid includes Medic Alert jewelry and cards issued free to patients and financial aid for transportation to and from dialysis units. Affiliates also refer patients to drug assistance programs or help pay for prescriptions directly.

• Nutritional Support Program. Affiliates donate nutritional supplements to dialysis units for distribution to patients; affiliates may also arrange for free food vouchers at area supermarkets.

Liver Disease

American Liver Foundation
1425 Pompton Avenue, Cedar Grove, NJ 07009; 800-223-0179 or 201-256-2550
Monday through Friday, 8:30 A.M. to 5:00 P.M. ET

The American Liver Foundation's toll-free hot line answers questions about hepatitis and its treatment, as well as mails free brochures and information sheets about this and other forms of liver disease. The hot line can also refer callers to liver specialists nationwide. "Progress," a newsletter published two or three times annually, keeps members informed of new research, clinical trials, and other pertinent information. (Membership costs $25 a year.) There are over two dozen chapters around the country, some of which run support groups.

National Digestive Diseases Information Clearinghouse
2 Information Way, Bethesda, MD 20892-3570; 301-654-3810
Monday through Friday, 9:00 A.M. to 5:00 P.M. ET

Ask to be sent the NDDIC's list of free fact sheets and information packets, such as "Cirrhosis of the Liver" and "Liver Diseases—General Information."

Parkinson's Disease

The American Parkinson's Disease Association
1250 Hylan Boulevard, Suite 4B, Staten Island, NY 10305; 800-223-2732 or 718-981-8001
Monday through Friday, 9:00 A.M. to 5:00 P.M. ET

There are over eighty chapters of the American Parkinson's Disease Association, which was established in 1961. In addition, every state has an APDA information and referral center, housed in a hospital. These centers dispense educational manuals, can inform you of clinical trials, and will give you names and telephone numbers of three Parkinson's specialists in your area, as well as reha-bilitation facilities. All chapters sponsor free symposia and conferences on coping with the disease and new medical treatments. Membership in a chapter costs $10 a year, but all services are free, including the association's quarterly newsletter and its 350 support groups.

National Parkinson Foundation
1501 N.W. 9th Avenue, Bob Hope Road, Miami, FL 33136-1494; 800-327-4545 or 305-547-6666
In Florida: (800) 433-7022
Monday through Friday, 8:00 A.M. to 5:00 P.M. ET; messages can be left after hours

Staff members at the National Parkinson Foundation's toll-free information line can refer you to Parkinson's disease specialists, clinical trials, physical rehabilitation, prescription drug patient-assistance programs, and any of some six hundred support groups. Ask to receive the NPF's free quarterly newsletter, "The Parkinson Report."

The foundation lends equipment on a limited basis.

Patients receive physical, occupational, and speech therapies at the foundation's Miami headquarters regardless of their ability to pay; most of the twenty medical facilities the NPF has designated Centers of Excellence (thirteen in the U.S., seven aboard) also treat indigent Parkinson's patients free of charge.

Parkinson's Disease Foundation
William Black Medical Research Building, Columbia-Presbyterian Medical Center, 710 West 168th Street, New York, NY 10032; 800-457-6676 or 212-923-4700
Monday through Friday, 9:00 A.M. to 8:00 P.M. ET

Founded in 1957 primarily to raise funds for medical research, the Parkinson's Disease Foundation sends free educational literature and can answer general questions about Parkinson's; a clinical specialist is on staff to answer more technical inquiries. Call PDF for referrals to Parkinson's disease specialists, physical rehabilitation, community services and government aid, clinical trials, discount pharmacies and indigent-patient prescription programs, and support groups. The foundation runs several support groups of its own in New York City. Request a free subscription to the quarterly newsletter.

United Parkinson Foundation
833 West Washington Boulevard, Chicago, IL 60607; 312-733-1893
Monday through Friday, 9:45 A.M. to 6:00 P.M. CT
The United Parkinson Foundation can refer you to movement-disorder specialists, community services, physical rehabilitation, occupational therapists, major medical centers, clinical trials, discount drug programs, and support groups. Its "Quarterly UPF Newsletter" comes with the $25 membership; patients are asked to contribute whatever they can.

Rare Disorders

National Organization for Rare Disorders
P.O. Box 8923, New Fairfield, CT 06812-8923; 800-999-6673 or 203-746-6518
Monday through Friday, 9:00 A.M. to 5:00 P.M. ET; messages can be left after hours

The National Organization for Rare Disorders answers more than 75,000 inquiries each year from around the world, drawing on its Rare Disease Data Base (RDB) on more than 5,000 "orphan" disorders. (You can access the RDB directly through the CompuServe electronic information system.) A call to NORD's 800 line brings you two free reports on a particular disorder; additional reports cost $4 per copy. These reports outline symptoms, causes (if known), standard and investigational treatments, and resources to contact for further in-depth information. The organization can refer you to patient assistance drug prescription programs. Although NORD does not run support groups per se, patients who wish to contact others afflicted with the same rare disorder may enlist in its networking program. For the $25 membership fee you receive the newsletter "Orphan Disease Update," which is published three times a year.

APPENDIX B

Miscellaneous Resources

These resources, from *Acupuncture* to *Viatical Settlements*, are arranged alphabetically except for *Community Services*. We've listed this category first because Area Agencies on Aging and Catholic Charities can be lifelines for patients and caregivers, providing an array of essential services.

Community Services

Area Agencies on Aging
Eldercare Locator
   800-677-1116
   Monday through Friday, 9:00 A.M. to 11:00 P.M. ET
   Eldercare Locator, administered by the National Association of Area Agencies on Aging, refers callers to their Area Agency on Aging, of which there are more than 650 in the United States. You should also be able to find your AAA's phone number in the Community Service Numbers section of the white pages. (Your AAA may be re-ferred to as the Administration on Aging, Senior Citizen's Division or another title.)
   As mandated by the Older Americans Act, Area Agencies on Aging arrange services for senior citizens, either directly or through contractors. Many are free; others are based on the person's ability to pay. Programs vary, but all AAAs provide
   • home-delivered meals;
   • transportation to and from medical visits;
   • homemaker and chore-mainte-nance services;
   • adult day care;
   • respite care;
   • home health care;
   • telephone reassurance: regularly scheduled phone calls from volunteer seniors to frail, homebound elderly persons who live alone;
   • legal assistance;
   • caregiver support groups;
   • home modification.

Your Area Agency on Aging may also offer:

- nursing home placement;
- mental health services;
- case management;
- assistance with medical billing, filing claims and appeals, and resolving problems with Medicare, Medicaid, and Social Security supplemental insurance programs.

Catholic Charities USA

1731 King Street, Suite 200, Alexandria, VA 22314; 703-549-1390

Monday through Friday, 9:00 A.M. to 5:00 P.M. ET

Catholic Charities USA, the country's largest private social service network, serves over 10 million people of all religious and ethnic backgrounds through its more than fourteen hundred local agencies and institutions. (These may go under such names as Catholic Social Services or Associated Catholic Charities.) The organization's headquarters can refer you to the Catholic Charities nearest you. Some programs are free; others have sliding scale fees, based on the person's ability to pay. Among the services that may be offered are

- hospice care;
- respite care;
- adult day care;
- residential care;
- transportation services;
- child day care and after-school care;
- individual, marital, family, and group counseling;
- family mediation;
- legal assistance for people with AIDS/HIV.

United Way of America

701 North Fairfax Street, Alexandria, VA 22314-2045; 703-836-7100

Monday through Friday, 8:30 A.M. to 5:30 P.M. ET

There are more than twelve hundred United Way offices throughout the United States. Primarily a fund-raising foundation, United Way is a great source of information and referrals to community care programs, from chore services to Meals on Wheels to respite care. Check the white pages for the United Way in your area or call the organization's headquarters.

Other potential sources of information or referrals:

- Support group members
- Local chapters of disease-related organizations
- Social workers at hospitals, dialysis centers, nursing homes, and hospices
- Community Chest organizations
- Religious organizations: check with local churches and synagogues
- Civic clubs such as the Elks, Kiwanis, and Rotary
- Other caregivers and patients

Acupuncture

For Relieving Pain, Nausea, and Anxiety

American Academy of Medical Acupuncture

5820 Wilshire Boulevard, Suite 500, Los Angeles, CA 90036; 800-521-2262

The academy will mail you, free of charge, a list of members in your state who have completed at least two hundred hours of training in medical acupuncture.

National Certification Commission for Acupuncture and Oriental Medicine

1424 16th Street, N.W., Suite 501, Washington, DC 20036; 202-232-1404

For a list of certified acupuncturists in your state, send a $3 check or money order and a self-addressed stamped envelope.

Other potential sources of information or referrals:

- The department of social work, psychiatry, or psychology at a local hospital
- Support group members
- Local chapters of disease-related organizations
- Other caregivers and patients
- Your state's licensing board for acupuncture, to find out if a practitioner is state licensed

Adaptive Technology

Adaptive technology refers to products and services designed to aid patients and those caring for them: everything from portable commodes to grab bars installed around the home, to mechanical lifts and ramps.

Abledata
8455 Colesville Road, Suite 935, Silver Spring, MD 20910-3319; 800-227-0216 or 301-608-8998
Monday through Friday, 8:00 A.M. to 6:00 P.M. ET
A free service of the National Rehabilitation Information Center, Abledata is an extensive data base that describes some 21,000 patient products. Abledata fact sheets outline the many devices available and their manufacturers, while its consumer guides contain references to product reviews and studies on each product class. You may access this information twenty-four hours a day via the Internet; ask an Abledata information specialist for instructions.

Assistive Technology Funding and Systems Change Project
800-827-0093
Monday through Friday, 9:00 A.M. to 5:00 P.M. ET
The Assistive Technology Funding and Systems Change Project, a free referral service sponsored by the United Cerebral Palsy Association, assists families with trying to locate funding for home modifications for patients.

Other potential sources of information or referrals:

- Support group members
- Local chapters of disease-related organizations
- The patient's physician
- Other caregivers and patients

Assisted Suicide

The Hemlock Society
P.O. Box 101810, Denver CO 80250-1810; 800-247-7421
Monday through Friday, 8:00 A.M. to 5:00 P.M. MT
Derek Humphry founded the Hemlock Society, a right-to-die advocacy group, in 1980, five years after he had helped his cancer-stricken wife, Jean, end her life. His books *Let Me Die Before I Wake* and *Final Exit*, both available through the society, explicitly describe methods of self-deliverance and the legal ramifications of assisting in a terminal patient's suicide.
Callers to the toll-free number seeking recipes for a painless death are instead encouraged to discuss thoughts of suicide with loved ones and a physician. Very often the mortally ill contemplate suicide out of fear of dying in pain or in a hospital, unaware that there exist alternatives to both. A crisis-intervention counselor will send them a packet of material describing effective methods of pain control and other settings for dying, such as hospice care.

Bereavement

Counseling

▶ *See "Mental Health Services," page 510.*

Support Groups

The THEOS Foundation
1301 Clark Building, 717 Liberty Avenue, Pittsburgh, PA 15222; 412-471-7779
Monday through Thursday, 9:00 A.M. to 4:00 P.M. ET; messages can be left after hours
This network of support groups for widowed men and women has more

than 144 chapters in the United States and Canada. *THEOS* is the Greek word for God and an acronym for They Help Each Other Spiritually. However, the foundation is ecumenical and does not promote a particular church or religion. For $15 you will receive "The Communicator," a quarterly newsletter. To be directed to your nearest chapter, call THEOS international headquarters.

Widowed Persons Service
American Association of
Retired Persons
601 E Street, N.W., Washington, DC 20049; 202-434-2277
Monday through Friday, 9:00 A.M. to 5:00 P.M. ET
Widowed Persons Service programs can be found in more than 230 communities. Conceived by the American Association of Retired Persons, the nation's leading organization for people over fifty, WPS works with local religious organizations, social service and mental health agencies, and other groups to establish programs for widowed men and women. These include support groups, one-to-one support from a trained volunteer who also lost a spouse or partner, and a directory to community services that can help survivors cope better with grief and suddenly finding themselves alone. For information about the Widowed Persons Service, call your regional office or the association's headquarters. Membership in AARP costs $8 a year. WPS is open to anyone.
AARP regional offices (from East to West):
Northeast Region
Connecticut, Delaware, Maine, Massachusetts, New Hampshire, New Jersey, New York, Pennsylvania, Rhode Island, Vermont
617-723-7600
Southeast Region
Alabama, District of Columbia, Florida, Georgia, Kentucky, Maryland, Mississippi, North Carolina, Puerto Rico, South Carolina, Tennessee, U.S. Virgin Islands, Virginia, West Virginia
404-888-0077

Midwest Region
Illinois, Indiana, Iowa, Michigan, Minnesota, Nebraska, North Dakota, Ohio, South Dakota, Wisconsin
773-714-9800
Southwest Region
Arizona, Arkansas, Colorado, Kansas, Louisiana, Missouri, New Mexico, Oklahoma, Texas, Utah
214-265-4060
West Region
Alaska, California, Guam, Hawaii, Idaho, Montana, Nevada, Oregon, Washington, Wyoming
206-517-9349

Biofeedback

For Relieving Pain, Nausea, and Anxiety

Association for Applied
Psychophysiology and Biofeedback
10200 West 44th Avenue, #304, Wheat Ridge, CO 80033-2840
For referrals to certified biofeedback therapists in your area, send an SASE to the association.

Other potential sources of information or referrals:
• The department of social work, psychiatry, or psychology at a local hospital
• Support group members
• Local chapters of disease-related organizations
• Other caregivers and patients

Bone Marrow Transplantation

National Marrow Donor Program
500 Broadway Street, N.E., Minneapolis, MN 55413; 800-526-7809
Monday through Friday, 8:00 A.M. to 4:00 P.M. CT
Hot line: 800-627-7692
Monday through Friday, 8:00 A.M. to 6:00 P.M. CT
The federally funded National Marrow Donor Program maintains an inter-

national registry of nearly 3 million volunteer unrelated bone marrow donors. Founded in 1987, the organization matches donors and recipients, coordinates the blood tests necessary for determining genetic compatibility, and assists with facilitating transplantation arrangements. Potential donors and recipients should call the toll-free hot line for information.

Other potential sources of information or referrals are staff members at a hospital transplant unit or the hospital social worker.

CPR (Cardiopulmonary Resuscitation)

American Red Cross
431 18th Street, N.W., Washington, DC 20006; 703-206-7090
Monday through Friday, 9:00 A.M. to 5:00 P.M. ET
All the nearly two thousand Red Cross chapters nationwide offer courses in CPR taught by trained, certified instructors. The four-hour course in adult CPR costs $30; the five-hour course in infant-child CPR, $34. (Prices may vary slightly.) To locate your local chapter, consult the Community Service Numbers sections of the white pages or call the office of public inquiries at the society's headquarters.

Other potential sources of information or referrals:
• Local hospitals, which may offer CPR instruction
• Other caregivers and patients

Credit and Debt Problems

National Foundation for Consumer Credit Referral Line
800-388-2227
Operates twenty-four hours a day, seven days a week
To locate a consumer-credit counseling service in your area, call the National Foundation for Consumer Credit's automated referral line.

Dietitians

American Dietetic Association's Consumer Nutrition Hotline
216 West Jackson Boulevard, Chicago, IL 60606-6995; 800-366-1655
Monday through Friday, 9:00 A.M. to 4:00 P.M. CT
Diet figures prominently in the management of many life-threatening illnesses, such as diabetes, kidney disease, and cardiovascular disease. The ADA's consumer nutrition hot line, staffed exclusively by registered dietitians, can refer you to registered dietitians in your area.

Funeral, Burial, and Cremation

Funeral Service Consumer Assistance Program
P.O. Box 27641, Milwaukee, WI 53227; 800-662-7666
Monday through Friday, 9:00 A.M. to 4:00 P.M. CT
Should a disagreement arise over a funeral service contract, contact the Funeral Service Consumers Assistance Program. This free service of the National Research and Information Center acts as an impartial third party to help mediate complaints as well as answer general questions.

Cremation Association of North America
401 North Michigan Avenue, Chicago, IL 60611; 312-644-6610
Monday through Friday, 9:00 A.M. to 5:00 P.M. CT
More than half of the 1,100 crematories in the United States and Canada belong to CANA, which requires that they sign a code of ethics. Call for a list of members in your area. The association will also send you informative free pamphlets about cremation; an SASE is requested.

Funeral and Memorial Societies of America

P.O. Box 10, Hinesburg, VT 05461; 800-765-0107 or 802-482-3437

Messages can be left twenty-four hours a day, seven days a week

Over 500,000 people in the United States belong to memorial societies, the main goal of which is to help members plan ahead for simple, dignified, and affordable funerals. Funeral and Memorial Societies of America has 147 societies in 40 states. Some survey area funeral homes and distribute price lists to members; others contract one or more funeral homes, enabling members to purchase services at a substantial discount.

FAMSA is also a consumer advocate group, helping to bring about the 1984 Federal Trade Commission Funeral Rule. Expect to pay a onetime enrollment fee of $10 to $30. In addition, some societies charge annual dues, usually no higher than $10. To locate the memorial society nearest you, call the toll-free number above.

Hypnotherapy

For Relieving Pain, Nausea, and Anxiety

American Society of Clinical Hypnosis

2200 East Devon Avenue, Suite 291, Des Plaines, IL 60018; 847-297-3317

Send an SASE for a list of licensed hypnotherapists in your area (not broken down by specialty).

Other potential sources of information or referrals:
- The department of social work, psychiatry, or psychology at a local hospital
- Support group members
- The patient's physician
- Local chapters of disease-related organizations
- Other caregivers and patients
- Your state's licensing board for medicine/psychiatry, psychology, or social work, to find out if a practitioner is state licensed

Incontinence

National Association for Continence

P.O. Box 8310, Spartanburg, SC 29305-8310; 800-252-3337 or 864-579-7900

Monday through Friday, 8:00 A.M. to 5:00 P.M. ET

The National Association for Continence, founded in 1982 as Help for Incontinent People (HIP), is a national information and resource center. Its quarterly newsletter regularly addresses issues of interest to anyone caring for an incontinent patient, such as tips on using self-adhesive condom catheters. You'll find discount coupons on incontinence-related products and addresses of manufacturers who provide free samples. As part of the $15 annual membership, you also receive The Resource Guide—Products and Services for Incontinence.

The Simon Foundation for Continence

P.O. Box 835, Wilmette, IL 60091; 800-237-4666 or 847-864-3913

Monday through Friday, 8:30 A.M. to 5:00 P.M. CT

Cheryle B. Gartley, an incontinence sufferer, started The Simon Foundation in 1983. It now has several hundred support groups across the country for incontinent men and women. You can call the foundation with questions about managing incontinence. Staff members can often refer callers to physicians and nurses specializing in incontinence treatment and control. For $15 annually, members receive a quarterly newsletter, "The Informer."

Other potential sources of information or referrals:
- Hospital and home-care nurses
- Other caregivers and patients

Job Discrimination

Equal Employment Opportunity Commission

800-669-4000

Monday through Friday, 8:30 A.M. to 5:00 P.M. (all time zones)

The federal Equal Employment Opportunity Commission answers questions about patients' and caregivers' rights under the Americans With Disabilities Act. Although the EEOC does not offer legal advice or opinions about the merits of a specific case over the phone, it can help you figure out avenues of redress and show you how to initiate a complaint.

Other potential sources of information or referrals:
• Your local human rights commission, the number of which appears in the white pages' Government Listings.

Legal Services

AARP Legal Hotline

601 E Street, N.W., Washington, DC 20049; 800-424-3410

Monday through Friday, 9:00 A.M. to 5:00 P.M. ET

A service of the American Association of Retired Persons, this hot line offers people age sixty and older telephone consultations with an attorney about virtually any legal matter, including estate planning and other end-of-life issues. Of the ten states plus the District of Columbia participating in the program as of 1998, only Pennsylvania charges a sliding-scale fee; the others are free.

Area Agencies on Aging

Eldercare Locator

800-677-1116

Monday through Friday, 9:00 A.M. to 11:00 P.M. ET

All Area Agencies on Aging offer legal assistance to senior citizens. Eldercare Locator can refer you to your AAA, the number of which is listed in the white pages.

National Academy of Elder Law Attorneys

1604 North Country Club Road, Tucson, AZ 85716; 520-881-4005

Monday through Friday, 8:00 A.M. to 5:00 P.M. MT

The National Academy of Elder Law Attorneys publishes a registry of some five hundred elder law attorneys, listing them by state and areas of expertise, such as disability planning, Medicaid, Medicare, guardianships/conservatorships, estate planning, and long-term-care issues. *The Experience Registry* can be purchased by check, money order, or credit card for $25.

Other potential sources for information or referrals:
• Local chapters of disease-related organizations
• State bar associations, some of which now have elder law sections and offer referrals
• Social workers at hospitals, dialysis centers, nursing homes, and hospices
• Other caregivers and patients

Living Wills and Durable Power of Attorney

Choice in Dying

200 Varick Street, 10th Floor, New York, NY 10014-4810; 800-989-9455 or 212-366-5540

Monday through Friday, 9:00 A.M. to 5:00 P.M. ET

Each year Choice in Dying, a national, nonprofit organization, distributes more than a quarter of a million preprinted forms for establishing a living will and for appointing a durable power of attorney for health care. The documents are updated regularly to reflect changes in each state's laws regarding advance directives (a general term for living wills and durable power of attorney for health care). Call the toll-free number above for a free copy of each.

Meals on Wheels

**National Meals on
Wheels Foundation**
2675 44th Street, S.W., Suite 305, Grand Rapids, MI 49509; 616-531-9909
Monday through Friday, 8:30 A.M. to 4:30 P.M. CT
Roughly twenty thousand federally funded and privately sponsored Meals on Wheels programs deliver nutritious meals to homebound senior citizens. Exact services vary from one community to another, but generally you can count on a hot lunch (and possibly a cold dinner as well) five days a week. In some states the programs are free; at most, expect to donate $5 or less per meal. Meals on Wheels provides more than food. For patients and caregivers hungry for contact with others, the regular visits by MoW volunteers help brighten up the day.

Eligibility depends on need and the demands on the program. If an elderly person has someone in the household to do the cooking, he probably won't qualify, especially if there's a waiting list. The national foundation can put you in touch with the program serving your loved one's community, as can the Area Agencies on Aging/Eldercare Locator and United Way of America.
◄ *See "Community Services," page 502.*

Medicaid

**Health Care
Financing Administration**
7500 Security Boulevard, Baltimore, MD 21244-1850; 410-786-3000
Monday through Friday, 6:00 A.M. to 6:00 P.M. ET
Call HCFA with general questions about Medicaid; ask for the Medicaid manual, which explains the program.

The office can give you the number of your state Medicaid agency.

Other potential sources of information or referrals:
• Dial your state Medicaid agency directly. This federal program is administered at the state level by either the Department of Social Services or the Department of Welfare. Check the Government Listings section of the white pages for their numbers.
• Social workers at hospitals, dialysis centers, nursing homes, and hospices
• Care managers
• Your Area Agency on Aging
• Other caregivers and patients

Medicare

**Health Care Financing
Administration Medicare Hotline**
800-638-6833
Monday through Friday, 8:00 A.M. to 8:00 P.M. ET
HCFA's Medicare Hotline can answer questions about enrollment, claims, coverage, and eligibility, and send you the "Medicare Handbook."

Social Security Administration
Baltimore, MD 21235; 800-772-1213
Monday through Friday, 7:00 A.M. to 7:00 P.M. ET
Although Medicare is administered by the Health Care Financing Administration, the Social Security Administration's toll-free information line also addresses Medicare-related questions and complaints. For more information on the Medicare program, ask for the free "Medicare Handbook."

Other potential sources of information or referrals:
• Your Area Agency on Aging
• Social workers at hospitals, dialysis centers, nursing homes, and hospices
• Care managers
• Other caregivers and patients

Mental Health Services

American Cancer Society
1599 Clifton Road, N.E., Atlanta, GA 30329; 800-227-2345 or 404-320-3333

Monday through Friday, 9:00 A.M. to 5:00 P.M. (all time zones)

Many American Cancer Society chapters offer short-term crisis counseling (four to six sessions) for patients and/or family members who do not have insurance for professional therapy and cannot otherwise afford it.

American Medical Association
515 North State Street, Chicago, IL 60610; 312-464-5000

Monday through Friday, 9:00 A.M. to 5:00 P.M. CT

Call the AMA for referrals to psychiatrists or psychologists.

American Psychiatric Association
1400 K Street, N.W., Washington, DC 20005; 202-682-6000

Monday through Friday, 9:00 A.M. to 5:00 P.M. ET

The American Psychiatric Association's referral line will route you to your local APA chapter, which can assess your needs and refer you to appropriate psychiatrists in your area.

American Psychological Association
750 First Street, N.E., Washington, DC 20002-4242; 202-336-5500

Monday through Friday, 8:30 A.M. to 5:00 P.M. ET

The national office will refer you to your state's American Psychological Association affiliate, which can help you find a suitable psychologist.

Catholic Charities USA
1731 King Street, Suite 200, Alexandria, VA 22314; 703-549-1390

Monday through Friday, 9:00 A.M. to 5:00 P.M. ET

Catholic Charities USA arranges for individual, marital, family, and group counseling and family mediation at sliding-scale fees. Its headquarters can refer you to one of more than fourteen hundred Catholic Charities agencies and institutions around the country.

National Association of Social Workers
750 First Street, N.E., Suite 700, Washington, DC 20002-4241; 800-638-8799 or 202-408-8600

Monday through Friday, 8:30 A.M. to 6:00 P.M. ET

The NASW will give callers three referrals to social workers in their area. Its registry denotes members' areas of specialization, such as bereavement counseling.

Other potential sources of information or referrals:
- The department of social work, psychiatry, or psychology at a local hospital
- Your state or county department of mental health
- Your Area Agency on Aging
- Local chapters of disease-related organizations
- United Way of America
- Other caregivers and patients
- Your state's licensing board for medicine/psychiatry, psychology, or social work, to find out if a practitioner is state licensed

Ostomies

American Cancer Society
1599 Clifton Road, N.E., Atlanta, GA 30329; 800-227-2345 or 404-320-3333

Monday through Friday, 9:00 A.M. to 5:00 P.M. (all time zones)

The American Cancer Society sponsors support groups for colon cancer patients and bladder cancer patients who have undergone colostomies and ileostomies.

United Ostomy Association
19772 MacArthur Boulevard, Suite 200, Irvine, CA 92612; 800-826-0826 or 714-660-8624

Monday through Friday, 7:00 A.M. to 4:30 P.M. PT

People with ostomies can find support and information through the United Ostomy Association's nearly six hundred chapters. Call its California headquarters for referrals to enterostomal nurses. Membership in a chapter costs $15.50 annually. For a $25 associate membership, you receive the UOA's informative magazine, *Ostomy Quarterly*, which contains tips on ostomy care, nutrition, and other essential topics, as well as advertisements for ostomy-related products.

Other potential sources of information or referrals:
- Support group members
- Hospital and home-care nurses
- Other caregivers and patients

Pain Management

When pain management is inadequate and the patient is told nothing more can be done for his or her pain, request a consultation with a pain management team. The ideal team is multidisciplinary, consisting of an anesthesiologist, an internist, a neurologist, a psychiatrist and/or psychologist, and a social worker, but few teams will have all these components. Your best bet is to contact your nearest major medical center in addition to the numbers below.

American Pain Society
4700 West Lake Avenue, Glenview, IL 60025-1485; 847-375-4731
Monday through Friday, 9:00 A.M. to 5:00 P.M. CT
The American Pain Society, made up of pain management professionals from different disciplines, publishes a directory of more than five hundred pain centers and clinics nationwide. These include specialists in acute pain, chronic pain, and cancer pain. The society will photocopy and send patients the directory listings for their state free of charge.

Cancer Information Service
800-422-6237 (800-4-CANCER)
Monday through Friday, 9:00 A.M. to 7:00 P.M. (all time zones). In Oahu, Hawaii: 524-1234; call collect from other Hawaiian islands.
Among its many referrals, the Cancer Information Service of the National Cancer Institute directs callers to pain management clinics and pain specialists at hospitals.

Prescription Drug Patient-Assistance Programs

American Cancer Society
1599 Clifton Road, N.E., Atlanta, GA 30329; 800-227-2345 or 404-320-3333
Monday through Friday, 9:00 A.M. to 5:00 P.M. (all time zones)
Some ACS chapters offer limited financial assistance for pain medication for patients without health care or with limited coverage.

American Kidney Fund
6110 Executive Boulevard, Suite 1010, Rockville, MD 20852; 800-638-8299 or 301-881-3052
Monday through Friday, 8:30 A.M. to 5:00 P.M. ET
Patients may receive financial aid for medications through the AKF's Individual Grants and Emergency Fund programs.

Leukemia Society of America
600 Third Avenue, New York, NY 10016; 800-955-4572 (800-955-4LSA) or 212-573-8484
Operates twenty-four hours a day, seven days a week
Patients qualifying for the LSA's Patient Aid Program receive $750 annually, which may be used toward outpatient chemotherapy.

The National Kidney Foundation

30 East 33rd Street, 11th Floor, New York, NY 10016; 800-622-9010 or 212-889-2210

Monday through Friday, 8:30 A.M. to 5:30 P.M. ET; messages can be left after hours

Many NKF affiliates help pay for prescriptions.

Pharmaceutical Research and Manufacturers of America

1100 Fifteenth Street, N.W., Washington, DC 20005; 202-835-3400

Monday through Friday, 8:30 A.M. to 5:30 P.M. ET

PhRMA, which represents more than one hundred pharmaceutical companies, publishes an annual directory of programs that provide prescription drugs for patients who cannot afford them. The free booklet lists the name, address, and phone number of each manufacturer, as well as the products covered by each program and its eligibility requirements. *All requests must be made by the patient's physician.*

Other potential sources of information or referrals:
• Support group members
• Local chapters of disease-related organizations
• The patient's physician
• Other caregivers and patients

Social Security

Retirement Benefits, Disability Benefits, Supplemental Security Income, and Survivors Benefits

Social Security Administration

Baltimore, MD 21235; 800-772-1213

Monday through Friday, 7:00 A.M. to 7:00 P.M. ET

Social Security Administration service representatives are available to assist Social Security recipients and to answer questions about SSA programs, eligibility, and how to file for benefits.

Also call this number to be routed to one of the SSA's thirteen hundred local offices. Request any or all of these free guidebooks about Social Security programs: "Retirement," "Disability," "SSI," "A Guide to Social Security and SSI Disability Benefits for People with HIV Infection," and "Survivors."

Other potential sources of information or referrals:
• Social workers at hospitals, dialysis centers, nursing homes, and hospices
• Your Area Agency on Aging
• Other caregivers and patients
• Care managers

Speech-Language Therapy

American Speech-Language-Hearing Association Information Resource Center

10801 Rockville Pike, Rockville, MD 20852-3279; 800-638-8255

Monday through Friday, 8:00 A.M. to 5:00 P.M. ET

ASHA certifies over 65,000 speech-language pathologists nationwide. Call its toll-free information line for referrals to members in your area.

Other potential sources of information or referrals are the departments of speech therapy and social work at the hospital or rehabilitation center.

Support Groups (Not Specific to a Disease)

Children of Aging Parents

1609 Woodbourne Road, Suite 302-A, Levittown, PA 19057-1511; 800-227-7294 or 215-945-6900

Monday through Friday, 9:00 A.M. to 3:00 P.M. ET; messages can be left after hours

Despite its name, this nonprofit support group serves anyone caring for an elderly patient. All staff persons who answer the phone have experience caring for an ailing loved one. They can refer you to nursing care, hospice care, and other health care facilities in your area. There are only six Children of Aging Parents support groups outside the Philadelphia area; a staff person can give you names and numbers of similar groups in your section of the country.

With membership ($20 a year; $40 for you and up to two family members), you receive the organization's bimonthly newsletter, "CAPsule," and a 15 percent discount on all CAPS manuals and fact sheets.

Make Today Count

1235 East Cherokee, Springfield, MO 56804-2263; 417-885-2000 (ask for Make Today Count)

Monday through Friday, 9:00 A.M. to 5:30 P.M. CT

There are two hundred Make Today Count support groups around the country for patients with a life-threatening illness, their families, and their friends. The national office distributes free educational literature written for both patients and caregivers. A social worker is available to advise callers of services in their community, indigent patient prescription drug programs, and so on. Request the group's free monthly newsletter, "The Messenger."

National Family Caregivers Association

9621 East Bexhill Drive, Kensington, MD 20895-3104; 301-942-6430

Monday through Friday, 9:00 A.M. to 6:00 P.M. ET; messages can be left after hours

The National Family Caregivers Association was founded in 1992 to assist all family caregivers. It can direct you to caregiver support groups as well as send you free information on how to start your own caregivers group. The quarterly NFCA newsletter, "Take Care!," comes with a $15 annual membership.

National Self-Help Clearinghouse

25 West 43rd Street, Room 620, New York, NY 10036; 212-354-8525

Monday through Friday, 9:00 A.M. to 5:00 P.M. ET; messages can be left after hours

The National Self-Help Clearinghouse will refer you to one of approximately fifty regional clearinghouses, all of which maintain directories of area support groups. Should you reside in a state not served by a regional office, the national clearinghouse would put you in touch with the headquarters of a support network, such as the Alzheimer's Association or the American Cancer Society.

Transplant Recipients International Organization

1000 Sixteenth Street, N.W., Suite 602, Washington, DC 20036; 800-874-6386 or 202-293-0980

Monday through Friday, 8:00 A.M. to 6:00 P.M. ET

TRIO was begun in 1983 by Brian Reames, a heart transplant recipient from Pittsburgh. It has since evolved into a nationwide organization of more than seventy support groups for organ transplant recipients, candidates, donor family members, and health care professionals. TRIO keeps members abreast of developments in organ and tissue donation, transplantation, medications, social issues, and finances through its newsletter, "Lifelines," published six times a year. National membership costs $25 a year.

Well Spouse Foundation

601 Lexington Avenue, Suite 814, New York, NY 10022-6005; 800-838-0879 or 212-644-1241

Monday through Friday, 10:00 A.M. to 4:00 P.M. ET

Founded in 1988, Well Spouse Foundation is a self-help organization dedicated to providing emotional and practical support for partners of the chronically ill and/or disabled, as well as for men and women whose partners have died. With a yearly membership ($20), you receive a bimonthly newsletter written by and for care partners. WSF also sponsors more than fifty-five support groups nationwide. Anyone without a support group nearby may participate in round-robin letter-writing chains, exchanging letters with five or six members.

Other potential sources for information or referrals:
- Local hospitals, which run support groups for patients and caregivers
- Your Area Agency on Aging
- Social workers at hospitals, dialysis centers, nursing homes, and hospices
- Other caregivers and patients

◄ *See "Bereavement: Support Groups," page 504.*

Veterans' and Military Dependents' Health Benefits

Department of Veterans Affairs, Division of Veterans' Benefits and Services
800-827-1000
Monday through Friday, 8:00 A.M. to 4:30 P.M. (all time zones)
If an ailing loved one once served in the military, call the Department of Veterans Affairs with any questions you may have regarding his eligibility for medical care, pension, and other benefits. Dialing the toll-free number above automatically routes you to your regional VA office.

Civilian Health and Medical Program of the Department of Veterans Affairs
P.O. Box 65023, Denver, CO 80206-5023; 800-733-8387

Monday through Friday, 7:30 A.M. to 11:30 A.M. MT
CHAMPVA is a health-benefits program for dependents of veterans who sustained a permanently disabling injury or became ill while on active military duty.

Civilian Health and Medical Program of the Department of the Uniformed Services
Aurora, CO 80045-6900; 303-361-1126
Monday through Friday, 7:30 A.M. to 4:00 P.M. MT
CHAMPUS, administered by the Department of Defense, covers military retirees and their dependents as well as families of deceased servicemen or those on active military duty.

Other potential sources for information or referrals are the military health-benefits advisors at the 172 VA medical centers.

Viatical Settlements

National Viatical Association
1200 G Street, N.W., Washington DC 20005, 202-347-7361
Monday through Friday, 9:00 A.M. to 5:30 P.M. ET
The National Viatical Association can send you a free list of viatical-settlement companies: groups of investors that purchase life-insurance policies of terminally ill people. Depending on how long the person is expected to live, viators pay between 50 and 80 percent of the policy's face value.

APPENDIX C

For Referrals to Home Health Care, Hospice Care, Long-Term Care, Adult Day Care, Respite Care, and Rehabilitation Facilities

American Health Care Association

1201 L Street, N.W., Washington, DC 20005-4014; 202-842-4444

Monday through Friday, 9:00 A.M. to 6:00 P.M. ET

More than eleven thousand long-term-care facilities belong to AHCA, the largest federation of nursing homes and long-term health care facilities in the United States. Its national office can route you to its affiliate in your state, which can then refer you to local AHCA member facilities. These include home-based care, adult day care, and assisted living care.

Catholic Charities USA

1731 King Street, Suite 200, Alexandria, VA 22314; 703-549-1390

Monday through Friday, 9:00 A.M. to 5:00 P.M. ET

Adult day care, respite care, hospice care, residential care, and child day care and after-school care are just some of the services offered by the more than fourteen hundred Catholic Charities agencies and institutions nationwide.

Hospicelink

190 Westbrook Road, Essex, CT 06426-1511; 800-331-1620; for those in CT and AK, 860-767-1620

Monday through Friday, 9:00 A.M. to 4:00 P.M. ET

Hospicelink, a free referral service of the Hospice Education Center, maintains a computerized directory of hospices and palliative care services nationwide.

National Association for Home Care

228 Seventh Street, S.E., Washington, DC 20003; 202-547-7424

Monday through Friday, 9:00 A.M. to 6:00 P.M. ET

For a list of state-licensed home-care agencies, contact the NAHC. The national office will refer you to the association serving your state.

National Citizens Coalition for Nursing Home Reform

1424 16th Street, N.W., Suite 202, Washington, DC 20036-2211; 202-332-2275

Monday through Friday, 8:30 A.M. to 5:00 P.M. ET

If you have a complaint regarding a patient's quality of care in a long-term facility, the National Citizens Coalition for Nursing Home Reform can refer you to your state's agency responsible for investigating and resolving such matters. The NCCNHR, a consumer-advocacy organization, distributes free pamphlets on how to choose a nursing home, while staff members with medical backgrounds and experience in long-term care can advise you on quality of care and quality of life conditions.

National Institute on Adult Day Care

409 Third Street, S.W., Washington, DC 20024; 202-479-1200

Monday through Friday, 9:00 A.M. to 5:00 P.M. ET

Write the National Institute on Adult Day Care for referrals to day care centers in your county. Should the institute not maintain a list for your county, expect to be referred to your Area Agency on Aging.

National Hospice Organization

1901 North Moore Street, Suite 901, Arlington, VA 22209; 800-658-8898 or 703-243-5900

Monday through Friday, 8:30 A.M. to 5:30 P.M. ET

The National Hospice Organization's help line refers callers to hospices in their area and informs them whether or not a facility or agency is state licensed and Medicare certified.

Nursing Home Information Service

8403 Colesville Road, Suite 1200, Silver Spring, MD 20910; 301-578-8938

Messages can be left twenty-four hours a day, seven days a week

This referral service of the National Council of Senior Citizens maintains national directories not only of nursing homes but of adult day care programs, and agencies and organizations that assist the disabled. Bear in mind that the NHIS does not rate facilities for quality.

Visiting Nurse Associations of America

11 Beacon Street, Suite 910, Boston, MA 02108; 888-866-7673

Monday through Friday, 7:00 A.M. to 6:00 P.M. ET

This organization represents over four hundred Visiting Nurse Associations that offer skilled nursing care, home health aides, hospice care, social work and counseling, and other in-home health services. Skilled nursing care, performed by registered nurses, encompasses intravenous therapy, injections, wound management, colostomy care, oxygen therapy, catheter care, and supervising medications. Call the toll-free national referral line above for a referral to the VNA nearest you.

Other potential sources for information or referrals:

• Your Area Agency on Aging
• Support group members
• Local chapters of disease-related organizations
• The patient's physician
• Social workers at hospitals, dialysis centers, nursing homes, and hospices
• United Way of America
• Other caregivers and patients

Accreditation Organizations

The following organizations evaluate and accredit health care facilities and services. When considering health care of any kind, make sure it is accredited by at least one of the organizations below; simply call and ask. While accreditation by no means ensures superior care for patients, it at least tells you that the institution or service meets certain standards. What's more, you then have a monitoring body with which to register complaints.

Commission on Accreditation of Rehabilitation Facilities

4891 East Grant Road, Tucson, AZ 85712; 520-325-1044

Monday through Friday, 8:00 A.M. to 4:30 P.M. MT

Send an SASE to CARF to receive a free list of accredited rehabilitation facilities in your area.

Community Health Accreditation Program

350 Hudson Street, New York, NY 10014; 800-669-1656 or 212-989-9393

Monday through Friday, 8:30 A.M. to 5:30 P.M. ET

CHAP, a subsidiary of the National League for Nursing, reviews and accredits several hundred home and community health care organizations. These organizations may provide one or more services, among them nursing, hospice care, home health aides, home medical equipment, infusion therapy, respiratory therapy, and physical therapy.

Foundation for Hospice and Homecare

228 Seventh Street, S.E., Washington, DC 20003; 202-547-7424

Monday through Friday, 8:00 A.M. to 6:00 P.M. ET

The Foundation for Hospice and Homecare not only accredits several hundred agencies but certifies tens of thousands of home-care aides and hospice aides. To qualify for certification, aides must accumulate at least seventy-five hours of training, demonstrate their skills in front of a registered nurse, and pass a written exam. The foundation can run a computer check for you at no charge to see if the aide you're considering hiring is indeed certified.

Joint Commission on Accreditation of Healthcare Organizations

One Renaissance Boulevard, Oakbrook Terrace, IL 60181; 630-792-5000

Department of Home Care Accreditation Services: 630-792-3004

Complaint Office: 630-792-5642

Monday through Friday, 7:00 A.M. to 5:00 P.M. CT

The largest accreditation organization of its kind, the JCAHO accredits more than 5,200 hospitals and 6,000 other health care organizations, including nursing homes, hospices, home-care agencies, home medical equipment companies, rehabilitation facilities, pharmaceutical services, and clinical respiratory services.

To find out if an individual health care practitioner is state licensed, call directory assistance for your state capital and request the number of the licensing board for that particular profession: the state licensing board for practical nursing, the state licensing board for physical therapy, and so forth. The only information you need supply is the person's last name, although a Social Security number or, better yet, state license number may speed up the search. (Ask the person you're considering hiring for his or her professional license number, which, incidentally, is public information; we'd be wary of anyone who resisted giving it to you.)

Professional Care Management

National Association of Professional Geriatric Care Managers

1604 N. Country Club Road, Tucson, AZ 85716-3195; 520-881-8008

Monday through Friday, 8:00 A.M. to 5:00 P.M. MT

The social workers, nurses, and psychologists who belong to this association, founded in 1986, act as private consultants. Depending on the patient's and caregiver's needs, they offer a wide range of services, among them screening, arranging, and monitoring in-home help; assisting with financial, legal, or medical issues; and providing counseling and support.

A list of GCM members costs $25 (payable by credit card over the phone);

private care managers charge an average of $75 per hour, with the typical case requiring an hour and a half for an initial assessment.

Free or Low-Cost Health Care

Hospitals, Nursing Homes, Outpatient Facilities, Rehabilitation Facilities, Public Health Centers, and Mental Hospitals

Hill-Burton Program
Department of Health
and Human Services
  Rockville, MD 20857; 800-638-0742
  In Maryland: 800-492-0359

Monday through Friday, 1:30 P.M. to 3:30 P.M. ET; messages can be left after hours

Under a 1946 congressional law, hospitals that have received what are called Hill-Burton funds must care for indigent patients. There are approximately eighteen hundred of these facilities in the United States. Each determines which services it will offer for free or at reduced cost. *Only the facility costs are covered, not private physician's bills.* For information on eligibility and a list of Hill-Burton programs in your area, call the toll-free hot line.

Bibliography

Books

Anderson, Patricia. *Affairs in Order.* New York: Macmillan Publishing Company, 1991.

Buckman, Dr. Robert. *"I Don't Know What to Say..."* New York: Vintage Books, 1989.

Burns, Stanley B., M.D. *Sleeping Beauty: Memorial Photography in America.* Altadena, Calif.: Twelvetrees Press, 1990.

Cahill, Matthew, executive editor. *Patient Teaching.* Springhouse, Pa.: Springhouse Corporation, 1987.

Cole, Harry A., with Martha M. Jablow. *One in a Million.* Boston: Little, Brown and Company, 1990.

Grief, Judith, and Beth Ann Golden. *AIDS Care at Home.* New York: John Wiley & Sons, 1994.

Miller, Dr. Benjamin F., and Claire Brackman Keane, R.N., B.S., M.Ed. *Encyclopedia and Dictionary of Medicine, Nursing, and Allied Health,* 4th ed. Philadelphia: W. B. Saunders Company, 1987.

Nuland, Sherwin B. *How We Die.* New York: Alfred A. Knopf, 1994.

Rando, Therese A., Ph.D. *How to Go On Living When Someone You Love Dies.* New York: Bantam Books, 1991.

Rob, Caroline, R.N., with Janet Reynolds, G.N.P. *The Caregiver's Guide.* Boston: Houghton Mifflin Company, 1991.

Senak, Mark S., J.D. *HIV, AIDS and the Law.* New York: Plenum Publishing Company, 1996.

Sommers, Tish, and Laurie Shields. *Women Take Care: The Consequences of Caregiving in Today's Society.* Gainesville, Fla.: Triad Publishing Company, 1987.

Tapley, Donald F., M.D., et al. *The Columbia University College of Physicians and Surgeons Complete Home Medical Guide,* rev. ed. New York: Crown Publishers, 1989.

Selected Newspapers, Periodicals, Medical Journals, Reports, and Other Sources

"About Metastatic Tumors to the Brain and Spine." American Brain Tumor Association, 1993.

"Acute Lymphocytic Leukemia." Leukemia Society of America, 1991.

"Acute Myelogenous Leukemia." Leukemia Society of America, 1987.

"Advanced Cancer: Living Each Day." National Cancer Institute, 1992.

"Alzheimer's Disease." National Institutes of Health, 1994.

"Alzheimer's Disease: A Guide to Federal Programs." National Institutes of Health, 1993.

"Around the Clock with COPD." American Lung Association, 1994.

"Atrial Fibrillation and Stroke." National Stroke Association, 1994.

"Basic Home Care for ALS Patients." The Amyotrophic Lateral Sclerosis Association, 1992.

Battista, Carolyn. "The Modern Way of Dying." *Yale Medicine*, summer 1994.

"Bone Marrow Transplantation Research Report." U.S. Department of Health and Human Services, 1991.

"Brain and Spinal Cord Tumors." National Institute of Neurological Disorders and Stroke, 1993.

"Brain Tumors: A Guide." National Brain Tumor Foundation, 1994.

"Cancer Facts and Figures—1997." American Cancer Society, 1997.

"Cancer of the Lung Research Report." U.S. Department of Health and Human Services, 1993.

"Cancer of the Stomach Research Report." U.S. Department of Health and Human Services, 1988.

"Cancer of the Uterus: Endometrial Cancer Research Report." U.S. Department of Health and Human Services, 1991.

"The Care Partner Seesaw: Understanding Your Limits." Sandoz Pharmaceuticals Corporation, 1993.

"Chemotherapy and You." U.S. Department of Health and Human Services, 1991.

"Chronic Lymphocytic Leukemia." Leukemia Society of America, 1992.

"Chronic Myelogenous Leukemia." Leukemia Society of America, 1991.

"Chronic Obstructive Pulmonary Disease." National Heart, Lung and Blood Institute, 1993.

"Cirrhosis of the Liver." National Institutes of Health, 1991.

"Coping Effectively." National Kidney Foundation, 1992.

"Coping with a Brain Tumor, Part I: From Diagnosis to Treatment." American Brain Tumor Association, 1994.

"Coping with a Brain Tumor, Part II: During and After Treatment." American Brain Tumor Association, 1994.

"Coping Needs of the Parkinson Care Partner." Sandoz Pharmaceuticals Corporation, 1994.

"Depression Is a Treatable Illness." U.S. Department of Health and Human Services, 1993.

"Diabetes in Adults." National Institutes of Health, 1990.

"The Diabetes Dictionary." National Institutes of Health, 1994.

"Diabetes Overview." National Institutes of Health, 1994.

"The Doable Renewable Home." American Association of Retired Persons, 1991.

Dorros, Sid, and Donna Dorros. "Patient Perspectives on Parkinson's." National Parkinson's Foundation, 1992.

"End-Stage Renal Disease: Choosing a Treatment That's Right for You." National Institutes of Health, 1994.

"Exchange Lists for Meal Planning." American Diabetes Association and the American Dietetic Association, 1995.

"Exercises for the Parkinson Patient, with Hints for Daily Living." Parkinson's Disease Foundation.

"Facts About Angina." National Heart, Lung and Blood Institute, 1992.

"Facts About Arrhythmias/Rhythm Disorders." National Heart, Lung and Blood Institute, 1992.

"Facts About Coronary Heart Disease."

National Heart, Lung and Blood Institute, 1993.

"Facts About Heart and Heart/Lung Transplants." National Heart, Lung and Blood Institute, 1990.

"Facts About Heart Failure." National Heart, Lung and Blood Institute, 1994.

"Flawed Treatment of Head Injuries Found." *The New York Times*, October 16, 1991.

"Gehrig's Disease Drug Approved." *The New York Times*, December 13, 1995.

Gorner, Peter. "Scientists Hail Discovery of Gene That Triggers ALS." *Chicago Tribune*, March 1, 1993.

"Head Injury: Hope Through Research." National Institute of Neurological and Communicative Disorders and Stroke, 1984.

"Heart and Stroke Facts." American Heart Association, 1993.

"Heart and Stroke Facts: 1994 Statistical Supplement." American Heart Association, 1993.

"High Blood Pressure and Stroke." National Stroke Association, 1994.

"Hodgkin's Disease and the Non-Hodgkin's Lymphomas." Leukemia Society of America, 1991.

"Home Exercises for Stroke Survivors." National Stroke Association, 1994.

"Insulin-Dependent Diabetes." National Institutes of Health, 1990.

"Know Your Brain." National Institutes of Health, 1992.

"Legal Answers About AIDS." Whitman-Walker Clinic, Inc.

Lieberman, Abraham N., M.D., et al. "Parkinson's Disease Handbook." American Parkinson Disease Association, Inc.

"Living at Home After a Stroke." National Stroke Association, 1994.

"Lung Disease Data 1994." American Lung Association, 1994.

"Mastectomy: A Treatment for Breast Cancer." U.S. Department of Health and Human Services, 1990.

McCaul, Mary E., Ph.D., and Janice Furst, Ph.D. "Alcoholism Treatment in the United States." *Alcohol Health & Research World*, vol. 18, no. 4, 1994.

"Melanoma Research Report." U.S. Department of Health and Human Services, 1992.

"Mental Health/Mental Illness: A Consumer's Guide." U.S. Department of Health and Human Services, 1992.

"Mesothelioma Research Report." U.S. Department of Health and Human Services, 1988.

"Monthly Vital Statistics Report." Centers for Disease Control and Prevention/National Center for Health Statistics, December 8, 1994.

"Multiple Myeloma (MM)." Leukemia Society of America, 1992.

"NCI Fact Book." U.S. Department of Health and Human Services, 1992.

"Neurological Disorders: Voluntary Health Agencies and Other Patient Resources." National Institutes of Health, 1994.

"Noninsulin-Dependent Diabetes." National Institutes of Health, 1992.

Nott, Phil. "Dying at Home: A Manual for People with AIDS Who Wish to Die at Home." Commonwealth Department of Human Services and Health, Australia, 1994.

"The Parkinson Handbook." National Parkinson Foundation, 1994.

"Parkinson's Disease: A Guide for Patients." United Parkinson Foundation, 1983.

"Parkinson's Disease and the Benefits of Personal Financial Planning." Sandoz Pharmaceuticals Corporation, 1994.

"Parkinson's Disease: Hope Through Research." National Institutes of Health, 1983.

"A Patient's Guide." Memorial Sloan-Kettering Cancer Center, 1991.

"PCP Prophylaxis." Project Inform Fact Sheet, October 12, 1993.

Perneger, Thomas V., M.D., Ph.D., Paul K. Whelton, M.D., M.Sc., and Michael J. Klag, M.D., M.P.H. "Risk of Kidney Failure Associated with the Use of Acetaminophen, Aspirin and Nonsteroidal Antiinflammatory Drugs." *New England Journal of Medicine*, vol. 331, no. 25, December 22, 1994.

"Personal Perspectives on Parkinson's Disease: Personal Relationships." Sandoz Pharmaceuticals Corporation, 1994.

"Post-Stroke Rehabilitation: Assessment, Referral, and Patient Management." Agency for Health Care Policy and Research, 1995.

"Preventing Pressure Ulcers: A Patient's Guide." Agency for Health Care Policy and Research, 1992.

"The Prevention and Treatment of Complications of Diabetes: A Guide for Primary Care Practitioners." National Institutes of Health, 1991.

"A Primer of Brain Tumors." American Brain Tumor Association, 1991.

"A Profile of Older Americans." American Association of Retired Persons and the Administration on Aging, 1993.

"Progress Report on Alzheimer's Disease 1995." National Institutes of Health, 1995.

"Quality Care for Life: A Proposal for Long Term Care Financing Reform." American Health Care Association, 1994.

"Questions and Answers About Breast Lumps." U.S. Department of Health and Human Services, 1992.

"Radiation Therapy and You." U.S. Department of Health and Human Services, 1993.

"Recovering After a Stroke." Agency for Health Care Policy and Research, 1995.

"Recurrent Stroke." National Stroke Association, 1994.

"Reducing Risk and Recognizing Symptoms." National Stroke Association, 1994.

Shay, Art. "Opening the Lines to Communication." Chicago Tribune, August 8, 1993.

"Skin Cancer Fact Sheet." American Academy of Dermatology, 1993.

"Skin Cancers: Basal Cell and Squamous Cell Carcinomas Research Report." U.S. Department of Health and Human Services, 1990.

"Social Security Handbook 1993," 11th ed. U.S. Department of Health and Human Services/Social Security Administration, 1993.

"Stroke: Hope Through Research." National Institute of Neurological and Communicative Disorders and Stroke, 1983.

"Stroke Is a Brain Attack!" National Stroke Association, 1994.

"Stroke Treatment and Recovery." National Stroke Association, 1994.

"Surgery Can Reduce the Risk of Stroke, Researchers Say." The New York Times, October 1, 1994.

"Taking Time: Support for People with Cancer and the People Who Care About Them." National Cancer Institute, 1993.

"Talking with Your Doctor: A Guide for Older People." National Institute on Aging, 1994.

"Transfusion Alert: Use of Autologous Blood." National Institutes of Health, 1994.

"Treating Pressure Sores." Agency for Health Care Policy and Research, 1994.

"Treatment Strategy: Project Inform Discussion Paper No. 1," May 17, 1993.

"Understanding HIV." Agency for Health Care Policy and Research, 1994.

"Understanding Speech and Language Problems After Stroke." National Stroke Association.

"Urologic Problems After Stroke (Part I)." Stroke: Clinical Updates, September 1993, vol. 4, issue 3.

"Urologic Problems After Stroke (Part II)." Stroke: Clinical Updates, November 1993, vol. 4, issue 4.

"What You Need to Know About Diabetes." American Diabetes Association, 1984.

Wright, Michael. "Project Inform Guide to the Management of Opportunistic Infections," March 15, 1995.

Index

Page numbers in *italics* refer to tables.

AAT (alpha-1-antitrypsin), 379, 382
abandonment, fear of, 311
acceleration/deceleration injury, 357
acetaminophen, 138, 178, 180, 248, 312, 365, 442
acidosis, 103, 104
Actifed, 117, 152
Actigall (ursodiol), 432
Activase (tissue plasminogen activator), 359
acupuncture, 156, 157, 235, 425
acyclovir (Zovirax), 109–10, 423
adult day care (ADC), 253
advance directives, 99, 184, 283, 284, 298–299, 300, 301–3
Advera, 160, 250
Advil, 155, 442
AF (atrial fibrillation), 345, 354
Agency for Health Care Policy and Research, 367, 369, 373, 375, 423
AIDS (acquired immunodeficiency syndrome), 27–28, 45, 106, 109, 115, 160, 165, 169, 187, 199, 229, 269, 413–28
  chronic diarrhea and, 424
  clinical trials and, 423–24
  cryptosporidiosis and, 418–19, 422
  drug assistance programs for, 276
  financial aid sources for, *274*
  getting clinical trials information on, *233*
  illnesses of, 416–20
  indicator diseases of, 415–16
  Kaposi's sarcoma and, 419–20, 422

  managing symptoms and side effects of, 424–27
  medications for, 418, 419, 421–23
  mortality rate of, 413
  mycobacterium avium complex and, 418, 423
  nature of, 415–16
  peripheral neuropathy and, 424–25
  pneumocystis carinii pneumonia and, 416–18
  pressure ulcers and, 424
  resources, 489–92
  stigma of, 425–26
  symptoms of illnesses of, *426–27*
  toxoplasmosis and, 419
  treatment and prevention of, 422–23
  tuberculosis and, 418, 423
AIDS clinical trials information service, *233*, 489
AIDS Treatment Data Network, *233*, 428, 490
Aid to Families with Dependent Children (AFDC), 272
akinesia, 466
Al-Anon, 437
Alcoholics Anonymous, 199, 436
alcoholism, 430
  encephalopathy and, 434
  rehabilitation and, 435–37
  see also liver disease
Aleve (naproxen), 138

allergic reactions, 117, 184
  anaphylactic shock and, 142
  management of, 151–52
  symptoms of, 151
alopecia, 333–34
alprazolam (Xanax), 260, 382
ALS, see amyotrophic lateral sclerosis
altered taste, 160–61, 447
alternative therapies, 235–38
  charlatans and, 235–36
  guidelines to research on, 236–37
Alupent (metaproterenol), 381
Alzheimer's disease, 32, 36, 115, 165, 173,
    196, 200, 201, 202, 208, 230, 460–87
  appetite loss in, 485
  brain abnormalities in, 463
  brain injury and incidence of, 374
  combative behavior in, 474–75
  contracture in, 481
  diagnosis of, 463
  diagnostic tests for, 468
  drug therapy for, 469
  end-stage, 469–75
  getting clinical trials information on,
    233
  health insurance and, 462–63
  hiding objects and, 474
  hyperactivity in, 473
  incontinence in, 480–81
  insomnia in, 482
  memory book for, 474
  nursing home care and, 463
  paralysis in, 482
  sleep disturbance in, 473–74
  speech/language loss in, 482–83
  swallowing problems in, 484–85
  symptoms of, 464–65
  wandering and, 474
  warning signs of, 464–65
  wasting in, 485
  see also dementia
Alzheimer's Disease and Related Disorders
    Association, 208, 233, 460, 463, 492
Alzheimer's Disease Education and Referral
    Center, 233, 487, 492
Ambien (zolpidem), 482
ambulance, calling for, 182–84
American Academy of Dermatology, 478,
    496
American Academy of Medical
    Acupuncture, 157, 503
American Association of Cardiovascular
    and Pulmonary Rehabilitation, 344, 381,
    486, 496, 497
American Association of Kidney Patients,
    448, 498
American Association of Retired Persons,
    78, 80, 81, 226, 279, 290, 449
  Legal Hotline of, 286, 508

  Pharmacy Service of, 275
  Widowed Persons Service of, 319, 505
American Brain Tumor Association, 233,
    337, 494–95
American Cancer Society, 32, 127, 200, 225,
    226, 233, 274, 332, 334, 510, 511
  services of, 493–94
American College of Physicians, 139
American Diabetes Association, 233, 397,
    399, 403, 412, 497
American Dietetic Association, 399, 412,
    457, 459, 506
American Foundation for AIDS Research,
    233, 428, 490
American Health Care Association, 245, 253,
    515
American Heart Association, 200, 233, 340,
    344, 351, 375, 496
American Kidney Fund, 274, 450, 498, 511
American Liver Foundation, 85, 233, 439,
    500
American Lung Association, 85, 274, 381,
    386, 390, 495–96, 497
American Medical Association, 193, 261,
    435, 510
American Pain Society, 158, 511
American Parkinson's Disease Association,
    233, 471, 472, 476, 487, 500
American Psychiatric Association, 193, 261,
    319, 510
American Psychological Association, 193,
    261, 319, 510
American Red Cross, 103, 181, 184, 506
American Society of Clinical Hypnosis, 157,
    507
American Speech-Language-Hearing
    Association Information Resource
    Center, 372, 483, 512
Americans with Disabilities Act (ADA) of
    1990, 293, 294
aminophylline, 350
amitriptyline, 362, 425, 482, 486
amnesia, 434
amyotrophic lateral sclerosis (ALS), 162,
    165, 174, 176, 208, 230, 274, 460–87
  appetite loss and, 485
  breathing problems in, 486–87
  computer technology for, 483–84
  contracture in, 481
  diagnostic tests for, 468
  drug therapy for, 472
  early signs of, 467
  end-stage, 479–80
  expelling secretions and, 485–86
  impaired mobility in, 480
  incontinence in, 480–81
  insomnia in, 482
  motor-neuron degeneration in, 467
  muscle cramping in, 481, 482

paralysis and, 482
respiratory failure in, 486–87
speech/language loss in, 482–83
swallowing problems in, 484–85
symptoms of, 467
wasting in, 485
Amyotrophic Lateral Sclerosis Association, 32, 75, 228, *223, 274,* 483, 487, 492
anaphylactic shock, 142
anaphylaxis, 151, 152
anemia, 331, 332, 350, 445
aneurysm, 356
surgery and, 358–59
anger, 188–89, 254–55
angina pectoris, 145, 175
administering nitroglycerine for, 341–342
myocardial ischemia and, 339
angioplasty, balloon, 343
Angiotensin Converting Enzyme (ACE), inhibitors, 350, 411
Antabuse (disulfiram), 436–37
antibiotics, 106, 110, 168, 297, 387, 409
anticipatory grief, 194
anxiety, 155, 156, 189
among dying, 311
management of, 258–61
aphasia (speech/language loss), 208, 365–366, 405, 482–83
appetite, 385, 485
radiation therapy and, 328–29
stimulation of, 159–60
see also diet; food
Approaching Death: Improving Care at the End of Life, 301
apraxia, 365
Aquaphor, 328
Area Agency on Aging, 33, 75, 193, 225, 253, 273, 279, 286, 472, 502–3, 508
Aricept (donepezil), 469
Aristocort, 134
arrhythmias, 104, 141, 339, 342, 344–47, 354, 390, 404, 444
causes of, 345
CPR and, 345
defibrillation and, 296
diagnosis of, 345–46
mechanics of, 344–45
medication for, 346, 390
monitor for, 346
pacemaker for, 346–47
symptoms of, 345
treatment of, 346–47
see also cardiovascular disease
Artane (trihexyphenidyl), 482, 486
arteriovenous fistula, 450, 451
arteriovenous malformation (AVM), 356
artificial life support, *see* extraordinary life support measures

artificial respiration, 295–96
ascites, 433, 437, 444–45
aspirational pneumonia, 60, 165, 361, 484
aspirin (salicylic acid), 138, 155, 178, 180, 248, 343, 355, 443
Assistive Technology Funding and Systems Change Project, 80, 504
Association for Applied Psychophysiology and Biofeedback, 156, 505
asthma, 142, 174, 377
Asyst 3000 Communi-Mate, 483
atherosclerosis, 339, 343, 345, 354, 373, 398, 442, 463
Ativan, 331
atrioventricular (AV) node, 344
atrophy, 364–65
attorney-in-fact, 291, 292, 299
autologous blood donation, 45–46
autologous BMT, 335
azathioprine (Imuran), 458–59

background retinopathy, 411
baclofen (Lioresal), 482
bacteria, 106
overuse of antibiotics and, 110
Bactrim (trimethoprim-sulfamethoxazole), 418
balloon angioplasty, 343
Barri-Care, 116
baths, bathing, 112–16
basin, 115
bed, 114–15
of dementia patients, 115–16
entering of, 113
equipment for, 113
exiting of, 114
radiation therapy and, 326
bedpads, 119
bedpans, 124
bedsores, *see* pressure ulcers
Benadryl, 117, 152, 172, 174, 331, 473
beta-blockers, 342, 374, 435
Better Breathers of Utah, 199
bilevel positive airway pressure machine (BIPAP), 486
biofeedback, 156, 235, 410
urinary incontinence and, 170
biological therapy, 334
biopsy, 325, 443
bite blades, 180–81
bladder training, 170, 362–63
bleeding, 179–80
variceal, 434–35
blepharospasm, 478
blood:
disorders of, 105, 129, 331–33
donation of, 45–48
types of, *47*
see also platelets

blood clots, 178
  chemotherapy and, 179, 332–33
  congestive heart failure and, 348
  heart attack and, 340, 342
  medication for, 354, 355, 361–62
  stroke and, 361–62
  symptoms of, 179–80
blood platelet deficiency
    (thrombocytopenia), 129
blood poisoning (septicemia), 105, 172, 296
blood pressure, measuring, 140–41
blood urea nitrogen (BUN), 394
bone marrow transplantation:
  for cancer, 335–36
  cost of, 336
  rejection and, 336
  types of, 335
Bowes and Church's Food Values of
    Portions Commonly Used
    (Pennington), 457
bradycardia, 140, 345, 346
brain, parts of, 363, 462
"brain attack," 353
brain function impairment, see dementia
brain injury, 352–75
  as acceleration/deceleration injury, 357
  Alzheimer's disease and, 374
  aneurysm surgery for, 358–59
  apathy and, 366
  atrophy and, 364–65
  carotid endarterectomy for, 358
  causes of, 356–57
  cerebral edema in, 359
  as closed head injury, 356–57
  coma and, 356
  complications and management of, 359–
    360
  contracture and, 364–65
  contusions, hematomas and, 357
  craniotomy and, 358
  defined, 356
  depression and, 362, 366–67
  diagnosis of, 357–59
  diffuse lesions and, 357
  drug therapy and, 359
  dysarthria and, 366
  emotional lability and, 366
  focal lesions and, 357
  frequency of, 353
  hemispheric neglect and, 365
  ICP monitoring and, 359–60
  impaired respiration and, 361–62
  incontinence and, 362–63
  infection and, 360
  life-threatening complications of, 373–75
  long-term effects of, 363–67
  as open head injury, 357
  paralysis/weakness and, 363–64
  personality, behavior changes and, 366
    potential impairments from, 364
    pulmonary embolism and, 361–62
    PVS and, 360
    rehabilitation and, 367–73
    speech/language loss and, 365–66
    swallowing problems and, 361
    treatment of, 357–59
    what happens in, 356–57
Brain Injury Association, 233, 356–57, 498
Brain Trauma Foundation, 360
Brain Tumor Society, 495
BRAT diet, 170
breath rate, monitoring, 141–42
Broadway Cares/Equity Fights AIDS, 24, 42,
    44, 306, 319–20
bronchitis, 178
    see also chronic obstructive pulmonary
      disease
bronchodilators, 174, 177, 381
Broviac, 150
bullectomy, 386
bypass surgery, 343

cachexia, see wasting
calcium acetate (PhosLo), 446
cancer, 160, 190, 229, 323–37
    benign tumors vs., 324
    biological therapy for, 334
    biopsy and, 325
    bone marrow transplantation for, 335–36
    chemotherapy for, 329–34
    complications of, 336
    diagnosis of, 325
    financial aid sources for, 274
    getting clinical trials information on, 233
    hormonal therapy for, 334
    immunotherapy for, 334
    incidence of, 324
    radiation therapy for, 326–29, 331
    remission and, 325–26
    resources, 493–96
    staging of, 325–26
    surgery and, 326
    survival time of, 323–24
    symptoms of, 324–25
    wasting in, 336
Cancer Information Service, 158, 494
candidiasis, 420, 421
Capoten (captopril), 350
carbohydrates, 397, 400
cardiomyopathy, 348
cardioplasty, 350
cardiopulmonary resuscitation (CPR), 181–
    182, 506
    arrhythmia and, 345
    as extraordinary measure, 294, 295
cardiovascular disease, 140–41, 338–51
    causes of, 339–40
    palpitations and, 344

potential complications of, 350–51
sudden cardiac death and, 351
see also arrhythmias; congestive heart
 failure; heart attack; *specific conditions*
cardioversion, 296, 345, 346, 354
cardioverter defibrillator implantation, 346
Cardizem (diltiazem), 342
caregivers, 247–65
 adult day care and, 253
 children and, 262–64
 dehydration and, 249
 eating habits and, 248–50
 emotional coping and, 254–58
 exercises for, 251–52
 faith, religion and, 260
 marital maintenance and, 261–62
 medical, dental appointments and, 252
 medications for, 260–61
 mental health referrals for, 261
 nutritional supplements and, 250
 physical stamina and, 247–48
 professional counselors for, 260
 respite care and, 253
 rest for, 248, 253–54, 258–59
 romantic partner and, 261–62
 skin care and, 250–51
 sleep habits and, 248
 stress, anxiety and, 258–61
 support groups and, 259–60
 weight loss and, 249
caregiving:
 accepting help with, 216–17, 223–24
 availability for, 213–14
 communicating with medical team and,
  88–90
 complaints and, 68–70
 criticism, friction and, 222–23
 dialysis and, 450–51
 discontinuing therapy and, 237–38
 distributing work of, 212–15
 emotions and, *see* emotions, coping with
 employer and, 44–45
 excessive, overstaying visitors and, 64
 family conference on, 214–15
 family disappointments and, 220–21
 foul-ups and, 67–68
 histrionic visitors and, 221–22
 home modification and, 78–80
 home safety measures and, 76–78
 hospital discharges and, 74–76
 hospital visitation policies and, 70–71
 infantilizing of patient by, 37, 111
 journal of, 89
 medical visits and, 73–74
 men and, 217–19
 need for, 42–43
 notetaking and, 89
 pain relief and, 66–67
 preparation for, 44–45, *45*

procedures and, 72–73
 rehabilitation and, *see* rehabilitation
 resentments and, 219, 221
 scheduling appointments and, 71–72
 teens, children and, 219–20
 venipuncture and, 64–66
 see also nursing skills
carotid endarterectomy, 355, 358
Catholic Charities USA, 75, 225, 240, 253,
 273, *274*, 472, 490, 503, 510, 515
CDC National AIDS Clearinghouse, 428, 491
CDC National HIV/AIDS Hotline, 85, 276
Center for Medical Consumers, 232
Center for Substance Abuse, 436
Centers for Disease Control and Prevention,
 392, 398, 406, 414, 424
Centerwatch Clinical Trials Listing Service,
 232
central venous catheter, 65–66
cerebral embolism, 354
cerebral thrombosis, 354
cerebral vascular accident (CVA), *see* stroke
channel blockers, 342, 374
chemotherapy, 329–34
 blood disorders and, 331–33
 clotting problems and, 332–33
 cycles of, 330
 hair loss and, 333–34
 immunosuppression and, 332
 for Kaposi's sarcoma, 419–20
chest pain, 183
chest percussion, 384
chest physiotherapy, 177
chicken pox, 108, 109, 110
children:
 caregivers and, 262–64
 caregiving and, 219–20
 custody of, 283, 287–88
Children of Aging Parents (CAPS), 83, 195,
 213, 259, 260, 512–13
Chloroseptic, 162
chlorpropamide (Diabinese), 401
Choice in Dying, 299, 508–9
choking, 165, 166
 on medication, 145–46
 see also Heimlich maneuver
cholangitis, 431
cholecystectomy, 433
cholesterol, 339, 340, 354, 398
chronic obstructive pulmonary disease
 (COPD), 376–90, 348, 376–90
 appetite loss in, 385
 causes of, 378–79
 chronic coughing in, 384
 cor pulmonale and, 389
 depression in, 385–86
 diagnosis of, 379
 drug therapy for, 381–82, 384
 dyspnea in, 379–80

chronic obstructive pulmonary disease
(COPD) (cont.)
expelling secretions in, 384
hydration in, 384
inhalation therapy for, 384
insomnia in, 385
life-threatening complications of, 386–90
lungs and, 377–78
lung transplantation for, 386
mechanical ventilation for, 383–84
oxygen therapy for, 382–83
pulmonary infections and, 387, 389
pulmonary rehabilitation and, 380–81
respiratory acidosis and, 387–88
respiratory failure and, 389
secondary polycythemia and, 388–89
smoking and, 378–79, 380
symptoms of, 379
ventilatory failure in, 389
Cipro IV (ciprofloxacin), 418
circulatory problems, 178–80
bleeding, bruising and, 179–80
circulatory shock, 68
circulatory system, 339
cirrhosis, 430
alcoholism and, 431, 435
causes of, 432
see also liver disease
cisapride (Propulsid), 410, 470
civic organizations, 80, 225, 226
Civilian Health and Medical Program of the
Department of Uniformed Services
(CHAMPUS), 280, 450
Civilian Health and Medical Program of the
Department of Veterans Affairs
(CHAMPVA), 450, 458, 514
clinical trials, 229–35
finding out about, 231–32
funding of, 230
health insurance and, 230
HIV/AIDS and, 423–24
information sources on, 233
informed consent and, 231
participating in, 232–34
phases of, 230–31
process of, 230–31, 231
questions to ask about, 234–35
clofazimine (Lamprene), 418
closed head injury, 356–57
codeine, 155
Cogentin (benztropine), 482
Cognex (tacrine), 469
cold compresses, 157
colony-stimulating factors, 47, 334
colostomy, 126
coma, 356, 361
diabetic, 405–6, 407
extraordinary measures and, 297–
298

Commission on Accreditation of
Rehabilitation Facilities, 371, 517
commodes, 125
Community Action Agency (CAA), 269–70,
273
Community Health Accreditation Program,
241, 245, 517
Community Prescription Service, 275
community support services, 224–27
cost of, 225
locating of, 225
resources, 502–3
transportation and, 224, 226
Compazine, 152, 163, 311
complete blood count (CBC), 331
computed tomography, 358
condom catheter, 171
Confident, 126
congestive heart failure, 159, 173, 174, 175,
178, 179, 296, 339, 347–50, 445
aging and, 348
blood clots and, 348
brain injury and incidence of, 374
congenital defect and, 348
cor pulmonale and, 389
diagnosis of, 349–50
edema in, 347, 348–49
hypertension and, 348
lung disease and, 348
other heart conditions and, 348
pleural effusion in, 348–49
shortness of breath in, 349
symptoms of, 348
transplant and, 350
treatment of, 350
conjunctivitis, 446, 478
Consolidated Omnibus Budget
Reconciliation Act (COBRA) of 1986,
277
constipation, 103
diabetic neuropathy and, 410
digestive disorders and, 166, 167–68
Parkinson's disease and, 477–78
Continuous Ambulatory Peritoneal Dialysis
(CAPD), 454
continuous blood-cell processor, 48
Continuous Cycling Peritoneal Dialysis
(CCPD), 454
contracture, 135–36, 364–65, 481
contusions, brain, 357
convulsions, 180, 183
coronary artery bypass graft, 343
coronary care unit (CCU), 52
coronary thrombosis, 340
coronary vasodilators, 342
cor pulmonale, 348, 361, 389
corticosteroids, 381, 382
coughing:
chronic, 178

controlled, 384
    medications and, 145–46
    weak, 176–77
Coumadin (warfarin), 169, 342–43, 354, 359
CPR, *see* cardiopulmonary resuscitation
craniotomy, 358
creatinine, 443
credit cards, 268
creditors, 268, 288
Cremation Association of North America,
    290, 506
Crestwood Company, 483, 484
critically ill, defined, 29
crixivan (Indinavir), 422
cryptococcosis, 419
cryptosporidiosis, 108, 169, 418–19
cyanosis, 383, 388
cyclosporine (Sandimmune), 336, 458–59
cytomegalovirus, 420
Cytovene (ganciclovir), 110, 423

daily hygiene, 110–33
    bathing in, 112–16
    dressing patient in, 129–31
    grooming in, 127–28
    hair care in, 128–29
    itching and, 116, 117
    mindset for, 110–12
    nail, cuticle care in, 129
    odors and, 112
    oral hygiene in, 123
    pressure sores and, 117–20
    privacy in, 111–12
    shaving in, 129
    skin care in, 116–17
    squeamishness in, 110–11
    toileting in, 123–27
    see also nursing skills
Dapsone, 423
Daraprim (pyrimethamine), 419
Darvon, 155
death, dying, 306–20
    acceptance of, 308–9
    closure and, 307
    death watches and, 311–12
    depression after, 318
    environment for, 310–11
    eulogy and, 317
    fear of abandonment and, 311
    funeral and, 316–17
    grieving after, 318–19
    at home, 309–10
    making peace and, 307–8
    moment of, 314–16
    notifications of, 316–18
    obituary and, 316
    privacy and, 310–11
    visitors and, 310
Decadron (dexamethasone), 381

deep brain stimulation, 471
defibrillation, 296
dehydration, 102–5, 106, 167
    of caregiver, 249
    dying patient and, 303
    signs of, 103
    skin care and, 116
    symptoms of, 103, 169
Deltasone (prednisone), 134, 458
dementia:
    agitated, paranoid behavior and, 205–6
    bathing patients with, 115–16
    causes of, 202
    combative behavior and, 206–7
    communication and, 208–9
    coping with, 202–4
    dangerous situations and, 203
    defined, 202, 462
    delusional hallucinatory behavior and,
        204–5
    dressing patients with, 130–31
    extraordinary measures and, 297–98
    HIV, 419
    memory loss and, 203–4, 208, 209
    "pseudo," 202
    signs of, 202
    toileting patients with, 125
    wandering and, 207–8
    see also Alzheimer's disease
denial, 185, 186–87
dependent edema, 178, 409
depression, 155, 189, 191–94
    in brain injured patients, 366–67
    of caregiver, 261
    COPD and, 385–86
    after a death, 318
    defined, 191
    dialysis and, 447–48
    health insurance and, 194
    heart attacks and, 344
    kidney disease and, 447–48
    loss of libido and, 262
    major, 191
    neuropathy and, 408
    Parkinson's disease and, 478
    reactive, 191
    roots of, 191–92
    signs of, 192–93
    in stroke patients, 366–67
    suicide and, 304
    survival and, 192
    traumatic brain injury and, 362, 366–67
    treatment of, 193–94
dermatitis, 478–79
detoxification, 436
diabetes, 109, 159, 161, 167, 169, 391–412
    adult-onset, 392–93
    blood glucose monitoring in, 394, 395–97,
        399

diabetes (*cont.*)
  coma and, 405–6, 407
  complications of, 404
  constipation in, 410
  diagnosis of, 393–94
  diarrhea in, 410
  diet in, 397–401
  foot ulcers in, 408–9
  forms of, 392–93
  gastroparesis in, 391–92, 409–10
  heart attack and, 411
  hypertension and, 411
  incontinence in, 410
  infection in, 404
  insulin regimen for, 401–3
  ketoacidosis in, 405–6
  life-threatening complications of, 411–12
  long-term complications of, 407–8
  nature of, 392–93
  neuropathy in, 408, 441–42
  obesity in, 393
  preventive management of, 411–12
  publications available on, 412
  renal diet in, 457
  renal disease in, 411, 441–42
  retinopathy in, 410–11
  sources of clinical trials information on, *233*
  stroke and, 411
  symptoms of, 393
  treatment of, 394–95
  vascular disorders and, 407–8
Diabinese (chlorpropamide), 401
diagnosis:
  checklist following, *32*
  inquiries to make at time of, 90
  see also specific diseases and conditions
diagnosis-related groups (DRGs), 101
dialysis, 294, 296, 411, 440, 441, 442, 444, 446, 447–56
  caregiver and, 450–51
  depression and, 447–48
  health insurance and, 449–50
  hemodialysis method of, 448–52
  HMOs and, 454
  life support and, 296
  measurements required in, 451
  peritoneal method of, 448–49, 454–55, 456
  questions on, 453–54
  shoddy practices and, 452–54
  side effects of, 451–52
diaper rash, 171
diaphoresis, 389
diarrhea:
  AIDS and, 424
  diabetes and, 410
  digestive disorders and, 166, 168, 169–70
  management of, 169–70
diastolic blood pressure, 140, 354

didanosine (ddI) (Videx), 421
diet:
  BRAT, 170
  diabetic, 397–401
  HIV wasting syndrome and, 420
  insulin and, 400–401
  kidney disease and, 455, 459
  liquid, *61*, 169
  liver disease and, 434, 437–38
  Parkinson's disease and, 472
  renal, 455–57
  restricted, *61*
  soft, *61*
  specialized, *61*
  see also food
dieticians, 239–40
diffuse axonal injury, 357
diffuse lesions, 357
Diflucan (fluconazole), 423
digestive disorders, 158–70
  altered taste and, 160–61
  anorexia and, 158–59
  appetite loss and, 158–60
  constipation and, 166, 167–68
  dementia patients and, 162
  diarrhea and, 166, 168, 169–70
  dry heaves and, 165
  dry mouth and, 161
  fecal impaction and, 167, 168
  gas and, 167, 168–69
  indigestion and, 162–63
  nausea and, 162–64, 166
  nutritional supplements for, 160
  peritonitis and, 167
  physically impaired patients and, 162
  sore mouth, throat and, 161–62
  swallowing problems in, 165–67
  TPN and, 166–67
  tube feeding and, 166–67
  vomiting and, 164–65
  wasting and, 159
digitalis glycosides, 350, 445
digoxin (Lanoxin), 350, 390
dilaudid, 155
diltiazem (Cardizem), 342
Directory of Physicians in the United States, 85
disability, defined, 271
disulfiram (Antabuse), 426–37
diuresis, 103
diuretics, 105, 174, 179, 296, 349, 350, 374, 390, 433, 445
"Doable Renewable Home, The: Making Your Home Fit Your Needs" (AARP), 81
doctors:
  advance directives and, 99
  adversarial stance with, 83
  and attitude toward illness and dying, 27–28

changing of, 98–100, 153, 302
choosing of, 83–86
communicating with, 88–90, 96
dissatisfaction with, 96–98, 100
DNR orders and, 298, 300, 301–3
elevated status of, 82–83
expectations of, 83
hospital routine and, 57–58
inadequate symptom control by, 99
medical language of, *91–95*
negligence, incompetence of, 98
questions on choosing of, 85–86
referrals to, 85
second opinions and, 86–88
toxic chemistry with, 99
tracking down, 96
types of, 52–55
donepezil (Aricept), 469
Donnatal (phenobarbital), 181
Do Not Resuscitate (DNR) order, 298, 301–3
dopamine, 465, 466, 469
drawsheet, 115, 124
making and using of, 132
dressings:
application of, 122–23
supplies for, 121
types of, 121
"drug fever," 138
dry heaves, 163, 165
dry mouth (xerostomia), 103, 123, 161, 175, 447
dry shampoos, 128
Duoderm dressing, 121
dysarthria, 366
dyskinesia, 469
dysnomia, 365
dyspepsia, 163
dysphagia, 103, 165–67, 361, 484–85
dysphasia, 159
dyspnea, 174, 176
congestive heart failure and, 349
COPD and, 379–80
management of, 349
treating, 175–76

echocardiogram, 349
Economic Opportunity Act of 1964, 269
edema, 104, 174, 176, 177, 350, 389
cerebral, 297, 359
congestive heart failure and, 347, 348–49
dependent, 178, 409
kidney disease and, 444–45
liver disease and, 433
oxygen therapy for, 349
Parkinson's disease and, 478
peripheral, 178
pulmonary, 142, 159, 296, 347
stroke and, 359
symptoms of, 348

elastase, 378–79
Elavil (amitriptyline), 362, 425, 482, 486
Eldercare Locator referral service, 33, 225, 253, 286
electrocardiogram (EKG), 342, 345, 346, 349, 411, 443
electrocautery, 347
electrolytes, 103, 104, 105, 169, 345, 394, 404, 434
electrophysiologic studies (EPS), 346
emergency room (ER), 52
emotional lability, 366
emotions, coping with, 185–94
acceptance and, 194
activities and, 197
altered body image and, 195
anger, resentment and, 188–89, 254–55
anticipatory grief and, 194
bargaining and, 190–91
common fears and, 198
communication aids for, 209–10
decision making and, 195
dementia patient and, *see* dementia
denial and, 185, 186–87
depression and, *see* depression
faith, religion and, 200–201
false cheerfulness and, 195
family life and, 196
goals and, 190–91, 197
grief and, 257–58
guilt and, 255–56
helplessness and, 257
isolation, loneliness and, 256
listening and, 188, 197–99
long-standing conflicts and, 201
normality and, 196–97
objectifying patients and, 195
passive-aggressive behavior and, 189
perceived loss of status and, 195
personal relationship and, 195
physical contact and, 199
sense of shock and, 254
stress, anxiety and, 255, 258–61
support systems and, 199–200
surrender of control and, 195
unconscious patient and, 201–2
worry and, 256–57
emphysema, 129, 142, 175, 176, 177, 178
bullous, 386
see also chronic obstructive pulmonary disease
EMS (emergency medical service), 53, 184
dying patient and, 304
encephalitis, 106
encephalopathy, 419, 434
endocarditis, 106
endorphins, 251
endoscopy, 325
endotracheal tube, 295–96, 349

end-stage renal disease (ESRD), 441–42, 444–48, 498–99
  see also kidney disease
Endura, 105
enemas, 167–68
Ensure, 160, 250, 385
enzyme-linked immunosorbent assay (ELISA), 421
epidural catheter, 156
epinephrine, 152, 296
Epivir (lamivudine) (3TC), 421
Epogen (epoetin alfa), 332, 445
Equal Employment Opportunity Commission (EEOC), 292, 294, 508
equipment and products:
  for ALS, 480, 483–84
  for arrhythmias, 346–47
  for bathing, 113
  for bedroom, 119
  for blood glucose monitoring, 396
  for communication problems, 209–10
  for dialysis, 452, 454
  for dressings, 121
  for grooming and dressing, 131
  health insurance and, 80
  for incontinence, 171
  for insulin injection, 402
  for lifting patients, 134
  loans sources for, *274*
  for measuring blood pressure, 141
  for ostomy care, 127
  pressure-release mattress, 119
  for respiratory failure, 486
  sources of, 119
  speech/language, 483
  for tracking medications, 144
"Essay on the Shaking Palsy" (Parkinson), 465
estrogen, 334
ethambutol (Myambutol), 418
Excedrin, 155, 180, 442
"Exchange Lists for Meal Planning," 399
exercise EKG (stress) test, 346
exercises for caregiver, 251–52
"Exercises for the Parkinson's Patient" (Côté), 472
experimental therapies, *see* clinical trials
extraordinary life support measures, 294–305
  cardioversion, 296
  coma, dementia and, 297–98
  CPR, 294, 295
  defibrillation, 296
  dialysis, 296
  emergency surgery, tests and, 296–97
  food, hydration and, 303–4
  intubation, 295–96
  IV feeding, 296
  living trusts and, 291

mechanical ventilation, 295–96
  pharmaceutical life support, 296, 297
  transfusions, 296

faith, 200–201, 260
falls, prevention of, 135, 475–77
famciclovir, 110
family:
  advance directives and, 300–301
  and coping with emotions, 196
  DNR orders and, 302
  home care and, 239
Family and Medical Leave Act of 1993, 43–44
  "Compliance Guide to the Family and Medical Leave Act," 43
Family Caregiver Alliance, 202
family conference, 214–15
  checklist for, *216–17*
fasciculation, 467
fasting blood glucose test, 394, 443
fats, 398, 404–5, 457
fecal impaction, 167, 168, 477
Federal Trade Commission, 289
feeding tubes, 166, 296
fee for service coverage, 277–78
fentanyl, 155
fetal tissue implant surgery, 471
fever, 103, 183
  chills and, 139
  convulsions and, 180
  "drug," 138
  food and, 139
  high-grade, 138
  infection and, 138
  keeping records of, 139
  low-grade, 138
  management of, 138–39
  medications for, 138–39
  pressure ulcers and, 139
  "quad," 138
  symptoms of, 138
filgrastim (Neupogen), 332
Final Exit (Humphry), 305, 504
finances, 265–81
  AFDC and, 272
  bankruptcy and, 270
  buyers' clubs and, 275
  cash flow maintenance and, 267–69
  COBRA and, 277
  counselor services and, 270
  credit cards and, 268
  creditors and, 268, 270
  family disability benefits and, 271–72
  financial-assistance programs and, 270–273
  food stamps and, 272
  fraternal organizations and, 273
  health insurance and, 277–81

IRAs and, 269
legal affairs file and, 267
life insurance loans and, 269
medical insurance file and, 267
mortgage loans and, 268–69
pensions and, 273
prescription drugs and, 273–76
privately funded programs and, 272–273
resources file and, 266–67
Social Security benefits and, 270–72
survivors benefits and, 272, 273
unpaid bills file and, 267
utility company programs and, 269–70
veterans and, 280
viatical sales and, 269
first aid, 180–84
    CPR and, 181–82
    Heimlich maneuver and, 182–83
    for seizures and convulsions, 180–81
fluconazole (Diflucan), 423
fluoroscopy, 343
focal lesions, 357
food, 60
    caregiver and, 249–50
    COPD and, 385
    in diabetic diet, 397–99
    dying patient and, 303–4
    fever and, 139
    and home meals programs, 226
    preparation and storage of, 107–8
    stimulating appetite with, 159–60
    see also diet
Food and Drug Administration (FDA), 229, 230–31, 350, 421, 469
food poisoning, 107
food stamps, 272
foot drop, 136
Fortovase (saquinavir), 422
Foundation for Hospice and Homecare, 241, 517
functional incontinence, 170
Funeral and Memorial Societies of America, 289, 507
funerals, 316–17
    prearrangement of, 289–91
Funeral Service Consumer Assistance Program, 291, 506
fungi, 106

gallstones, 432–33
ganciclovir (Cytovene), 110, 423
Garamycin, 122
gas, 167, 168–69
gastroparesis, 167, 391–32
    diabetes and, 391–92, 409–10
    symptoms of, 409
gastrostomy tubes (G tubes), 166, 361, 485
Gatorade, 105, 169

Gay Men's Health Crisis, 24, 415, 423, 425, 428, 491
    Hotline of, *233*
giardia, 108
glomerulonephritis, 441, 442
gloves, disposable, 107, 112, 121
glucagon, 407
glucocorticoid drugs, 134
glycogen, 392, 430, 438
glycohemoglobin test, 396–97
grab bars, 78
graft-versus-host disease (GVHD), 336
grand mal seizures, 180, 436
granulocytopenia, 422
grief, coping with, 257–58
grooming and dressing, 127–28
guided visualization/imagery, 156
guilt, coping with, 255–56

hair care, 128–29
hair loss (alopecia), 333–34
hairy leukoplakia, 423
Halcion, 174
handwashing, 106, 107
Health and Human Services Department, U.S., 230, 518
Health Care Financing Administration, 278, 279, 372, 453, 459, 498, 509
health care proxy, 50, 267, 283, 284, 299–300
    enforcement of, 301–2
health insurance, 265–66, 276–81
    Alzheimer's disease and, 462–63
    clinical trials and, 230
    COBRA and, 277
    dialysis coverage and, 449–50
    emergency room visits and, 51
    getting most from, 280–81
    government funded, 278
    home modification and, 80
    kidney transplants and, 458
    lifting devices and, 134
    medical equipment and, 80
    open enrollment and, 277
    psychiatric coverage by, 194
    rehabilitation programs and, 372–73
    types of, 277–78
    see also Medicaid; Medicare; Medigap insurance
Health Maintenance Organizations (HMOs), 274, 277, 278, 279, 454
"Healthy Food Guide, A," 457
heart, structure of, 339
heart attack (infarction), 339–44
    angina and, 342
    balloon angioplasty for, 343
    blood clots and, 340, 342
    bypass surgery for, 343
    depression and, 344
    diagnosis of, 342

heart attack (infarction) (*cont.*)
  rehabilitation and, 344
  responding to, 340–41
  risk factors for, 353–54
  stroke and, 361
  symptoms of, 340
  treatment of, 342–43
  see also cardiovascular disease
Heimlich maneuver, 146, 178
  performance of, 182–83
Help for Incontinent People, 170
helplessness, coping with feelings of, 257
hematomas, 357, 288
hemiparesis, 363
hemiplasia, 405
hemiplegia, 363, 419
Hemlock Society, 305, 504
hemochromatosis, 431
hemorrhagic stroke, 355–56
Heparin, 150, 343, 359
hepatic encephalopathy, 434
hepatitis:
  A, 45
  alcoholism and, 430
  B, 45, 46, 430
  C, 46, 429, 430–31, 438–39
  treatment of, 431
  see also liver disease
hepatorenal syndrome, 433
herpes zoster (shingles), 109, 110, 153, 421
Hickman catheter, 150
high blood pressure, *see* hypertension
HIV (human immunodeficiency virus), 45,
    229, 413–28
  antiviral medications for, 421–22
  clinical testing and, 423–24
  diagnosis of, 420–21
  encephalopathy and, 419
  nature of, 415–16
  resources, 489–92
  stigma of, 425–26
  treatment of, 422–23
  wasting syndrome of, 420
  see also AIDS
HIV/AIDS Treatment Information Service
    (ATIS), 489–90
Hivid (zalcitabine) (ddC), 421
Holter monitor, 346
home:
  dying at, 309–10
  modifying of, 78–80
  safety measures for, 76–78
home care, 28, 238–39
  civic organizations and, 225
  community support services for, 224–27
  contracting for, 241–42
  culture clashes and, 242–44
  family life and, 239
  licensing, certification and, 240–41

locating agencies and programs for, 240
  meals programs and, 226
  Medicare and, 239, 241
  personnel for, 239–40, 242
  phone networking tips for, 226–27
  private agencies for, 225
  professional case managers and, 227–28
home equity loans, 268–69
home health aides, 239
homemaking, 239
hormonal therapy, 334
hospice care, 240
Hospicelink, 240, 515
hospital, 41–81
  admitting office registration in, 48–51, *49*
  asking questions in, 97
  checklist for patient care in, *63*
  choice of, 84
  clothing suitable for, 131
  complaint procedures in, 68–70
  daily life in, 57–58
  discharge from, 74–76
  documents needed for, 48, *49*, 50
  first day in, 51–52
  flowers in, 58
  health history for, 51
  medical visits to, 73–74
  medication in, 66–67
  ordering meals in, 60
  outpatient appointments and tests in, 71–
      72
  pain relief situations in, 66–67
  personal care in, 62
  personalizing room in, 58–59
  preadmission tours of, 46
  preparing for stay at, 45–48, *49*
  PRN order in, 66–67
  procedures preparation and, 72–74
  relating to nursing staff in, 60–61, 66–67
  restricted diets in, *61*
  roommates in, 60, 62
  social workers in, 56–57
  staff of, 56–57
  technicians in, 56
  types of nurses in, 55–56
  types of physicians in, 52–54
  venipuncture situations in, 64–66
  visiting patients in, 59, 62, 64
  see also medical team
human leukocyte antigens, 335
humidifiers, 175, 177
hydration, 102–5, 106, 159
  COPD and, 384
  dying patient and, 303–4
  as extraordinary measure, 296
  and getting patients to drink, 104–5
  secretions and, 177
Hydrodiuril (hydrochlorothiazide),
    350

Hygiene 1, 126
hyperalimentation, 167
hyperfractionated radiation, 329
hyperglycemia, 394–95, 397, 403–5
    coma and, 404–5
hyperglycemic hyperosmolar nonketotic
    coma, (HHNK), 405
hyperkalemia, 444
hyperphosphatemia, 446
hypertension, 340, 345, 354, 374, 398
    congestive heart failure and, 348
    diabetes and, 411
    medication for, 374, *374*, 411, 442–43
    portal, 433, 434
    renal disease and, 441–42
hyperthermia, 137–38
hyperventilation technique, 360
hypervolemia, 347
hypnotherapy, 156, 236
hypoglycemia, 249, 394–95, 401, 404
    intensive insulin therapy for, 402
    management of, 406–7
hypotension, 452
hypoventilation, 378
hypovolemia, *see* edema
hypoxemia, 382
hypoxia, 382

ibuprofen, 138, 155, 178, 442
ice packs, 157, 180
ileostomy, 126
imaging, 325
imipramine (Tofranil), 362
immunosuppression, 332, 439
    chemotheraphy and, 332
    kidney disease and, 446
    medication for, 458–59
immunotherapy, 334
Imodium, 169
Imuran (azathioprine), 458
incompetence, declaration of, 292
incontinence:
    ALS and, 480–81
    Alzheimer's disease and, 480–81
    causes of, 170
    coughing and, 178
    diabetic bladder dysfunction and, 410
    functional, 170
    overflow, 170, 362
    Parkinson's disease and, 480–81
    skin care and, 116
    stress, 170, 178, 362, 384
    stroke-induced, 362–63
    traumatic brain injury and, 362–63
    types of, 170
    urge, 170
Inderal (propranolol), 342
Indinavir (crixivan), 422
individual retirement account (IRA), 269

infection, 105–10
    airborne transmission of, 108–9
    of blood, 105
    diabetes and, 404
    direct transmission of, 106–7
    fever and, 138
    food preparation, storage and, 107–8
    immunocompromised patients and, 110
    indirect transmission of, 107–8
    inflammation and, 106
    pets and, 110
    pulmonary, 387
    susceptibility to, 105–6, 109–10
    types of, 106
    urinary-tract, 172
    waste disposal and, 123
inflammation, 106
    from radiation therapy, 327–28
influenza, 106, 108
inhalation therapy, 384
injections:
    administering of, 146–47
    of insulin, 401–3
    intravenous, *see* intravenous injection
    minimizing pain and fear of, 148–49
    preventing bleeding from, 388
inoculations, 109, 110
insomnia, 172–74
Institute of Medicine, 301
insulin, 144, 392, 399
    diet and, 400–401
    infusion pump for, 402
    injection of, 401–3
    ketone production and, 405
    resistance to, 393
    types of, *402*
intensive care unit (ICU), 52
interferon, 334
    for liver disease, 431
interleukin-2, 334
Intermittent Peritoneal Dialysis (IPD), 454
International Myeloma Foundation, *233*, 495
interstitial nephritis, 442
intracerebral hemorrhage, 355, 357
intracoronary thrombolysis therapy, 296,
    342–43
intracranial pressure (ICP), 359–60
intrathecal catheter, 156
intravenous injection, 144–45
    backflow of blood and, 150
    central venous catheter for, 150–51
    common problems of, 149–50
    infusion rates and, 149
    permanent port for, 151
    shunt for, 150
intubation, 295–96
Invirase (saquinavir) 422
ischemic stroke, 353–55
isolation, sense of, 256

isoniazid (INH), 423
Isuprel (isoproterenol), 381
itching, 116, 117, 447

jaundice, 432
jejunostomy tubes (J tubes), 410
Joint Commission on Accreditation of
    Healthcare Organizations, 241, 245, 371,
    517
joint tenancy, 291–92

Kaiser Permanente, 454
Kaposi's sarcoma, 419–20, 422
Kayexalate (sodium polystyrene sulfonate),
    444
ketoacidosis, 405–6
ketone bodies, 404–5
Ketostix, 406
kidney disease, 440–59
    anemia and, 445
    causes of, 441–42
    complications of, 444–48
    depression in, 447–48
    diabetics and, 457
    diagnosis of, 443
    dialysis and, see dialysis
    diet and, 455, 459
    edema in, 444–45
    health insurance and, 458
    hyperkalemia and, 444
    immunosuppression and, 446
    itching in, 447
    kinds of, 440–42
    metabolic acidosis and, 445, 47
    neuropathy and, 446
    renal osteodystrophy and, 445–46
    role of kidneys and, 441
    sexual dysfunction in, 448
    stages of renal failure in, 440–41
    transplantation and, 441, 457–58
    treatment of, 448–49
    uremia and, 444
KT/V measurement, 451

Lactaid, 168
lamivudine (3TC) (Epivir), 421
Lamprene (clofazimine), 418
Lanoxin (digoxin), 350, 390
left side neglect, 365
left ventricular assist device (LVAD), 350
legal matters, 282–305
    advance directives and, 283, 284, 298–99,
        300, 301–3
    asset distribution and, 288
    child custody and, 283, 287–88
    creditors and, 288
    declaration of incompetence and, 292
    discrimination against sick and disabled
        and, 292–93

documents needed for, 284–86
    extraordinary measures and, 294–305
    finding an attorney for, 286
    funeral arrangements and, 289–91
    health care proxy and, 283, 284, 299–302
    inventory checklist for, 285
    joint tenancy and, 291–92
    living wills and, 293, 299–301, 302
    physician assisted suicide and, 304–5
    powers of attorney and, 283, 291
    safe-deposit box and, 284–86
    wills and, 283, 286–89
    withholding, withdrawing treatment and,
        305
lesions:
    brain, 357
    diffuse, 357
    focal, 357
Les Turner Amyotrophic Lateral Sclerosis
    Foundation, 233, 493
leukemia, 329
    bone marrow transplant for, 335
Leukemia Society of America, 274, 337, 495,
    511
leukocytes (white blood cells), 47, 331, 336,
    422
LeVeen shunt, 433
levodopa (L-dopa), 469, 472, 478, 481
licensed practical nurses (LPNs), 55
Lifeline Systems, 184
Lioresal (baclofen), 482
lipodystrophy, 403
liquid diet, 61, 169
listening, 188, 197–99
liver disease, 429–39
    alcoholism and, 430, 435–37
    amnesia in, 434
    ascites in, 433, 437
    cirrhosis and, 430–32
    diagnosis of, 431–32
    diet and, 434, 437–38
    edema in, 433
    gallstones and, 432–33
    hepatic encephalopathy and, 434
    hepatitis and, 429, 430–31
    interferon for, 431
    jaundice and, 432
    life-threatening complications of, 433–35
    liver function and, 430
    management of, 432–33
    medication for, 431, 432, 433, 434, 439
    symptoms of, 431–33
    transplantation and, 431, 438–39
    treatment of, 435–37
    variceal bleeding and, 434–35
living trust, 288, 291
living will, 50, 283, 299–301, 302
Lomotil, 169
Low Income Weatherization, 269

lungs:
   COPD and, 377–78
   transplantation of, 386
lung volume reduction surgery, 386
luteinizing hormone-releasing hormone
   (LHRH), 334

macrovascular disease, 408
magnetic resonance imaging (MRI), 325,
   342, 358
major depression, 191
Make Today Count, 513
malignancy, primary and secondary, 324
manometer, 140–41
Mantoux method (PPD) skin test, 418
Marax (theophylline), 381, 383
marijuana, 160, 420
   medical use of, 164
   prescription form of, 164
Marinol, 160, 164
masks, surgical, 108, 109
massage, 157, 236
Meals on Wheels, 509
mechanical ventilation, 175–76, 295–96,
   383–84, 389, 486
Medicaid, 75, 80, 240, 244, 245, 279
   advance directives and, 299
   dialysis coverage and, 449, 453
   kidney transplant and, 458
   prescription drugs and, 274
   qualifying for, 279
   rehabilitation and, 372
   Spousal Impoverishment Act and, 279
Medic Alert, 184, 208, 450, 499
medical records, transfer of, 87–88
medical specialists, 53
   directory of, *54–55*
medical team:
   advance directives and, 284, 300
   changing doctors and, 98
   communicating with, 88–90
   directory of specialists for, *54–55*
   DNR orders and, 301, 302
   doctors on, 52–55
   establishing rapport with, 52, 66–67
   initial contact with, 52
   nurses on, 55–56
   pharmacist in, 143
   see also hospital
Medicare, 75, 80, 266, 268, 274
   advance directives and, 299
   Alzheimer's disease and, 462–63
   diabetic foot disease and, 409
   dialysis coverage by, 449
   disability eligibility and, 271
   fixed fees of, 101
   home care and, 239, 241
   Hotline of, 278, 372
   kidney transplant and, 458

mental health coverage by, 194
pneumococcal vaccinations and, 108
prescription drugs and, 273
rehabilitation and, 344, 372
   see also Medigap insurance
"Medicare Handbook, The," 372
medication, 142–52, 248
   aerosol administration of, 145
   allergic reactions to, 151–52
   for angina, 341–42
   antinausea, 163, 164
   beta-blocking, 342, 374, 435
   blood disorders and, 332
   for bone marrow transplantation, 336
   of care givers, 260–61
   channel-blocking, 342, 374
   choking on, 145–46
   for circulatory problems, 179
   "compassionate use" of, 231
   constipation from, 155
   cost-dosage savings on, 145
   cough, 145–46, 178, 384
   dependency, addiction and, 153
   depression from, 192
   "drug" fever and, 138
   for fever, 138–39
   financial assistance for, 273–75
   in hospital, 66–67
   for immunocompromised patients, 109–
      110
   injections of, 146–49
   intramuscular administration of, 144,
      147–48
   intravenous injection of, 144–45, 149–51
   life support and, 296, 297
   metered-dose inhaler for, 382
   new prescriptions of, 142–43
   oral administration of, 144, 145–46
   patient-assistance programs for, 275–76
   PCA systems and, 155–56
   recordkeeping and tracking of, 143–44
   routes of administration of, 144–45
   for secretions, 177
   for seizure control, 181
   side effects of, 143, 145, 155
   subcutaneous administration of, 144,
      148
   suppository administration of, 144, 146
   terminal sedation and, 304
   tolerance level of, 154
   in transdermal patches, 146
   see also chemotherapy; clinical trials;
      specific conditions and diseases
Medigap insurance, 266, 274, 278–79
   dialysis coverage and, 449
Medi-Mail, Inc., 275
meditation, 156
Medrol, 134
Megace, 160

Memorial Sloan-Kettering Cancer Center, 230, 327–28
memory book, 474
Mended Hearts program, 200
metabolic acidosis, 434, 445, 447
metabolism, 392
Metamucil, 155, 167, 410
metaproterenol (Alupent), 381
metered-dose inhaler, 382
metoclopramide (Reglan), 163, 410
Mexitil (mexiletine), 425
microvascular disease, 407
monoclonal antibodies, 334
morphine, 155, 297, 315, 382, 350, 382
mortgages, 268–69
Mothers' Voices, 414
Motrin (ibuprofen), 138, 155, 178, 442
mouth, sore, 161–62
mucolytics, 174, 177
Myambutol (ethambutol), 418
mycobacterium avium intracellulare complex (MAC), 418, 423
Mycobutin (rifabutin), 418, 423
Mylanta, 163, 168
Mylicon, 168
myocardial infarction, see heart attack
myocardial ischemia, 339, 343, 353

naproxen, 138
narcosis, 297
narcotics, 174, 384
nasogastric (NG) tubes, 296, 361
National Academy of Elder Law Attorneys, 286, 508
National Association for Continence, 170, 171, 507
National Association for Home Care, 240, 515
National Association of Professional Geriatric Care Managers, 228, 517–18
National Association of Social Workers, 193, 261, 319, 510
National Brain Tumor Foundation, 233, 495
National Certification Commission for Acupuncture and Oriental Medicine, 157, 503
National Citizens Coalition for Nursing Home Reform, 246, 516
National Diabetes Information Clearinghouse, 233, 412, 497–98
National Digestive Diseases Information Clearinghouse, 439, 500
National Family Caregivers Association, 217, 222, 260, 513
National Foundation for Consumer Credit, 270, 506
National Heart, Lung and Blood Institute, 45, 348, 351, 379, 383, 385, 390, 496, 497
National Hospice Organization, 240, 516

National Institute on Adult Day Care, 253, 516
National Institute on Aging, 108
National Institute on Neurological Disorders and Stroke, 358, 373, 492, 493
National Institutes of Health (NIH), 230, 235, 379, 452
National Kidney Foundation, 32, 75, 184, 200, 274, 448, 449, 450, 459, 499–500, 512
National Marrow Donor Program, 335, 505–506
National Meals on Wheels Foundation, 226, 509
National Organization for Rare Disorders, 233, 501
National Parkinson Foundation, 233, 274, 470, 471, 472, 487, 500
National Rehabilitation Information Center, 79, 113, 210, 291
National Self-Help Clearinghouse, 33, 226, 513
National Stroke Association, 85, 233, 353, 365, 367, 375, 496–97
National Viatical Association, 269, 514
nausea, 156
   causes of, 163
   digestive disorders and, 162–64, 166
   dry heaves and, 163
   marijuana and, 160, 164
   nonpharmaceutical techniques and, 164
   pain and, 154–55
NebuPent (pentamidine), 423
necrosis, 340
nelfinavir (Viracept), 422
neoadjuvant therapy, 326
Neosporin, 122
nerve disease (diabetic neuropathy), 408
nerve growth factor (NGF), 425
nerves, types of, 462
Neupogen (filgrastim), 332
neuralgia, 152–53
neurological disease, 460–87
   central nervous system and, 462–63
   diagnostic tests for, 468
   incidence of, 461
   treatment of, 467–68
   see also Alzheimer's disease; amyotrophic lateral sclerosis; Parkinson's disease
neuropathy:
   AIDS and, 424–25
   depression and, 408
   diabetes and, 408, 441–42
   kidney disease and, 446
neurotransmitters, 462
nevirapine (Viramune), 422
New England Journal of Medicine, 46, 235, 359
New York Times, 414, 452, 454

nitroglycerin, 145
  administering of, 341–42
Norvir (ritonavir), 422
nosocomial infections, *63*
NPO order, 60
NSAIDS (nonsteroidal anti-inflammatory
    drugs), 155, 248, 442–43
Nu-Gard, 116
Nuprin, 155
nurses:
  caregivers taught by, 102
  establishing rapport with, 52, 66–67
  home care role of, 239
  private duty, 69
  types of, 55–56
nursing home care:
  checklist for inspection of, 246
  contracting for, 245–46
  cost of, 238–39, 244
  health insurance, Medicare and, 244
  locating of, 245
  rectifying problems with, 246
Nursing Home Information Service, 245, 253
nursing skills, 101–84
  allergic reactions and, 151–52
  ambulance calling and, 183–84
  basic first aid and, 180–84
  circulatory complications and, 178–80
  contracture and, 135–36
  CPR and, 181–82
  for daily hygiene, *see* daily hygiene
  digestive disorders and, *see* digestive
    disorders
  falls prevention and, 134–35
  foot drop prevention and, 136
  Heimlich maneuver and, 182–83
  home safety and, 134–35
  hydration, dehydration and, 102–5, 106
  infections and, *see* infection
  making occupied bed and, 132–33
  for maneuvering patient, 132–33
  medication and, *see* medication
  pain management and, *see* pain, pain
    management
  personal emergency response systems
    and, 184
  range-of-motion exercises and, 136
  respiratory complications and, 174–76
  secretions difficulties and, 176–78
  sleep disorders and, 172–74
  urinary tract complications and, 170–72
  vital signs measurement and, *see* vital
    signs
  walking safety and, 134–35
Nutren, 160
Nytol, 482

obesity, diabetes and, 393, 398
obituary, 316

occupational therapy, 239–40, 368, 471
odors:
  daily hygiene and, 112
  ostomy care and, 126–27
  of vomit, 165
*Official American Board of Medical
    Specialties Directory of Board
    Certified Specialists*, 85
Older Americans Act of 1973, 225
Older Women's League (OWL), 212, 218,
    242, 253
One in a Million (Cole), 373
One Touch II blood glucose meter, 396
on-off syndrome, 469
oophorectomy, 334
open head injury, 357
oral glucose tolerance test, 394, 443
Orchid Fresh, 126
orchiectomy, 334
Orinase (tolbutamide), 401
orthopnea, 349
orthostatic hypotension, 133–34, 178, 179,
    368, 476
osteoporosis, 134, 446, 475
ostomy care, 126–27
overflow incontinence, 170, 362
oxygen, administering of, 175
oxygen therapy, 349, 382–83, 389, 390, 486

pacemaker, 296, 297, 346–47
pain, pain management, 152–58, 189
  attitudes toward, 153–54
  chronic, 156
  cold compresses for, 157
  dependency, addiction and, 153
  describing of, 158
  dying person and, 297
  forms of, 152–53
  fundamentals of, 154–55
  gas, 168–69
  ice packs for, 157
  of injections, 148–49
  local, 152
  massage and, 157
  medication for, 154–55, 442–43
  moist heat for, 157
  narcotics and, 155
  nausea and, 154–55
  nonpharmaceutical methods for, 156–57
  nonprescription medications for, 155
  patterns of, 154
  PCA systems and, 155–56
  perception of, 157–58
  poorly controlled, 157–58
  splinting and, 157, 178
  suicide and, 304
  TENS and, 157
  threshold of, 153, 157–58
pallidotomy, 470–71

palpitations, heart, 344–45
pancreatitis, 422
paracentesis, 433
"parking lot syndrome," 74
Parkinson's disease, 32, 78, 129, 135,
    167, 173, 174, 202, 208, 230, *274*,
    460–87
  appetite loss in, 485
  bradykinesia and, 465, 466
  brain abnormalities and, 465
  breathing problems in, 486–87
  chronic constipation in, 477–78
  contracture in, 481
  dependent edema in, 478
  dermatitis and, 478–79
  diagnostic tests for, *468*
  drug therapy for, 469
  dyskinesia and, 469
  early signs of, 465–66
  end-stage, 475–79
  expelling secretions in, 485–86
  eye irritation in, 478
  falls and, 475–77
  freezing and, 470, 477
  impaired mobility and, 475
  incontinence in, 480–81
  muscle cramps in, 481–82
  neurosurgery for, 470–71
  on-off syndrome and, 469
  paralysis in, 482
  respiratory failure in, 486–87
  rigidity in, 465, 466
  sleep disturbance in, 482
  sources of clinical trials information on,
    233
  speech/language loss in, 482–83
  swallowing problems in, 484–85
  symptoms of, 465–66
  tremors in, 465–66
  wasting in, 485
Parkinson's Disease Foundation, *233*, 471,
    472, 487, 500–501
Parlodel, 479
patency, 451
patient advocate, 36–37, 57, 67, 70
patient-controlled analgesia (PCA) systems,
    155–56
"Patient's Bill of Rights, A," 50, 52
Patient Self-Determination Act of 1990, 298,
    299
PCP prophylaxis, 423
Penlet, 395
pensions, 273
Pentam (pentamidine), 418
pentamidine, 423
pentoxifylline (Trental), 409
People with AIDS Coalition of New York,
    233, 491
Percocet/Percodan, 155

percutaneous endoscopic gastrostomy
    (PEG), 166
percutaneous transluminal coronary
    angioplasty (PTCA), 343
Periactic, 160
Peri-Care, 116
peripheral edema, 178
peristalsis, 409
peritonitis, 106, 167, 168, 297, 454
permanent blood-access port, 65
persistent vegetative state (PVS), 297–98,
    356, 360
petit mal seizures, 180
Pharmaceutical Research and
    Manufacturers of America, 276, 512
Phenergan, 163
phenobarbital, 181
phlebitis, 147, 150, 178
phlebotomy, 46, 48
PhosLo (calcium acetate), 446
photocoagulation, 411
physical therapy, 239–40, 367–68, 471
physician-assisted suicide, 304–5
physicians, *see* doctors
Physicians' Desk Reference, 232, 276
Pittsburgh Alzheimer Disease Research
    Center, 115, 136
plaque, 339, 344, 354, 398
platelets (thrombocytes), 129, 179
  cancer therapies and, 331, 332
  donation of, 47–48
pleural effusion, 179, 348–49
pneumocystis carinii pneumonia (PCP),
    416–18
pneumonia, 105, 108, 142
  aspirational, 60, 165, 361, 484
  infections and, 387
  pneumocystis carinii, 416–18
  types of, 106
pneumothorax, 349
polycystic kidney disease, (PCK), 442
polycythemia, 388
Polysporin, 122
polyuria, 443
Port-O-Cath, 150
postural bronchial drainage, 384
PowerBar, 250
powers of attorney, 267, 291, 299, 302
prednisone, 192, 382, 458–59
Preferred Provider Organizations (PPOs),
    278
Preferred Rx, 275
"Prescription Drug Patient Assistance
    Programs, Directory of," 276
pressure-release mattress, 119
pressure ulcers (bedsores), *63*, 103, 171
  AIDS and, 424
  common sites of, 117
  fever and, 139

healing of, 122
prevention of, 118–20
symptoms of, 118
treatment of, 120
Primatene, 383
PRN (*pro re nata*) order, 66–67
Pro-Banth-Ane (propantheline), 486
Procrit (epoetin alfa), 332, 445
products, *see* equipment and products
progressive relaxation, 156
Project Inform, *233*, 423, 428, 491–92
propranolol (Inderal), 342
Propulsid (cisapride), 410, 470
protein, 397–98, 455–56
pseudo dementias, 202
psittacosis, 110
psychoeducational group model, 199
Public Health Service, U.S., 108
pulmonary edema, 142, 159, 296, 347
pulmonary effusion, 348–49
pulmonary embolism, 179, 348
pulmonary fibrosis, 348
pulmonary function tests, 379
pulmonary rehabilitation, 380–81, 486
pulse, taking of, 139–40
pyelonephritis, 442
pyrimethamine, 419

"Quad Fever," 138
Quadrinal (phenobarbital), 181, 383
"Questions and Answers about AIDS," 415

radiation therapy, 326–29, 331
bathing and, 326
hyperfractionated, 329
internal, 329
for Kaposi's sarcoma, 419
rale, 348–49
random blood glucose test, 394, 443
range-of-motion (ROM) exercises, 136, 179,
    365, 367, 481
Reach to Recovery program, 200
reactive depression, 191
red blood cells (erythrocytes), 47
chemotherapy and, 331, 332
overabundance of, 388
registered nurses (RNs), 55
home care role of, 239
Reglan (metoclopramide), 163, 410
rehabilitation:
alcoholism and, 435–37
choosing program for, 369–72, *370–71*
health insurance and, 372–73
from heart attack, 344
Parkinson's disease and, 471–72
pulmonary, 380–81, 486
setting for, 368–69
from stroke, 367–73
religion, 200–201, 260

remission, 325–26
renal failure, *see* kidney disease
renal osteodystrophy, 445–46
resentment, coping with feelings of, 254–55
respiration, monitoring, 141–42
respirator, 176, 294, 295, 315, 349, 383–84,
    388
respiratory acidosis, 387–88
respiratory complications:
administering oxygen and, 175
breathing problems in, 174–76
mechanical ventilation and, 175–76
trach care and, 176
respiratory system, 377
respiratory therapy technicians, 239–40
respite care (RC), 253
resting heart rate, 140
Restoril, 174
restraints, 207
restricted diet, *61*
retinopathy, diabetic, 410–11
Retrovir (zidovudine)(ZDV), 421
reverse mortgage, 269
rheumatic fever, 106
rheumatic heart disease, 348
rifabutin (Mycobutin), 418, 423
Right to Die movement, 27, 305
Rilutek, 472
ritonavir (Norvir), 422
Robert Wood Johnson Foundation, 298
Rolaids, 163
Rostrix (capsaicin), 408

safe-deposit box, 284–86
Safe Return program, 208, 474, 492
salicylic acid (aspirin), 138, 155, 178, 180,
    248, 342, 355, 443
saline solution, 120
Sandimmune (cyclosporine), 336, 458–59
saquinavir, 422
sclerotherapy, 435
scopolamine, 177
seborrhea, 478–79
secondary caregiver, 43
secondary polycythemia, 388–89
second mortgages, 268–69
second opinion, 86–88
medical records and, 87–88
secretions, 176–78, 384
seizures, 180–81, 436
self-help group model, 199
septicemia (blood poisoning), 105, 172, 296
septic shock, 68, 105
Septra (trimethoprim-sulfamethoxazole),
    418
"sharps" container, 148
shaving, 129
shingles (*herpes zoster*), 109, 110, 153, 421
shock, sense of, 254

shortness of breath, *see* dyspnea
shunts, 150, 358, 433, 435, 451
silences, 197–99
Simon Foundation for Continence, 171,
    507
Sinemet, 469, 472, 479, 487
sinoatrial (SA) node, 344, 345
Skin Cancer Foundation, 496
skin care, 116–17
    of caregiver, 250–51
    dehydration and, 116
    incontinence and, 171
    kidney disease and, 447
    liver disease and, 432
    radiation therapy and, 327–28
    "weeping" and, 327
    see also pressure ulcers
sleep disorders, 155, 172–74, 189
    causes of, 173
sleepwear, 117
smoking, 340, 378–79, 380
Social Security Administration, 270, 509,
    512
    disability as defined by, 271
    disability insurance of, 75, 271–72
    Information Line of, 278
    retirement benefits and, 270–71
social workers, 56–57, 74, 75, 273, 448
    home care role of, 240
sodium polystyrene sulfonate (Kayexalate),
    444
soft diet, *61*
Sominex, 482
sore throat, 106, 161–62, 175
specialized diets, *61*
speech/language loss (aphasia), 208, 365–
    366, 405, 482–83
speech-language therapy, 368
spider naevi, 435
splinting, 157, 178
Spousal Impoverishment Act, 279
Stadtlanders Pharmacy, 275
stavudine (d4T) (Zerit), 421
stereotactic surgery, 470–71
sterile technique, 107, 120–23
stomas, 120, 126
    cleaning of, 127
stool softener, 167
strep throat, 106, 108
streptokinase, 342
stress, management of, 258–61
stress incontinence, 170, 178, 362, 384
stroke, 115, 176, 352–75
    aneurysm surgery for, 358–59
    apathy and, 366
    atrophy and, 364–65
    blood clots and, 361–62
    carotid endarterectomy for, 358
    cerebral edema and, 359

communication and, 208–9
complications and management of, 359–
    360
contracture and, 364–65
craniotomy and, 358
depression and, 362, 366–67
diagnosis of, 357–59
drug therapy for, 359
emotional lability and, 366
first injury and, 359
frequency of, 353
heart attack and, 361
hemispheric neglect and, 365
hemorrhagic, 355–56
high blood pressure and, 354
ICP monitoring and, 359–60
impaired respiration and, 361–62
incontinence and, 362–63
infection and, 360
ischemic, 353–55
life-threatening complications of, 373–75
long-term effects of, 363–67
paralysis/weakness and, 363–64
personality, behavior changes and, 366
potential impairments from, *364*
pulmonary embolism and, 361–62
PVS and, 360
rehabilitation and, 367–73
risk factors for, 353–54
second, 374
secondary injury and, 355
sources of clinical trials information on,
    233
speech/language loss and, 365–66
stress and, 374
swallowing problems and, 361
symptoms of, 354–55
transient ischemic, 355
treatment of, 357–59
    see also brain injury
Stroke Connection of the American Heart
    Association, *233*, 497
subarachnoid hemorrhage, 355
subdural hematoma, 357
suction catheter, 177–78
sudden cardiac death (SCD), 351
suicide, physician assisted, 304–5
submaximal EKG exercise test, 344
Supplemental Security Disability Income
    (SSDI), 270, 271
Supplemental Security Income (SSI), 270,
    272
support groups, 32, 33–36, 199–200
    for caregivers, 259
    resources, 504–5, 512–13
    table of, *34–35*
support services, *see* community support
    services
survivors benefits, 272

Sustacal, 160, 250
swallowing problems (dysphagia), 103, 165–167, 361, 484–85
symptoms:
of AIDS illnesses, *426–27*
of allergic reaction, 151
of ALS, 467
of Alzheimer's disease, 464–65
of anemia, 445
of arrhythmia, 345
of ascites, 433
of blood clots, 179–80
of bradycardia, 345
of brain hemorrhage, 356
of cancer, 324–25
of clotting disorders, 179–80
of compromised platelets, 331
of congestive heart failure, 348
of COPD, 379
of cor pulmonale, 389
of dehydration, 103, 169
of dementia, 202
of depression, 192–93
describing of, 89–90
of diabetes, 393
of electrolyte imbalance, 169
of fever, 138
of gastroparesis, 409
of head injury, 135
of heart attack, 340
of heart failure, 348
of HHNK, 405
of hyperkalemia, 444
for immediate medical assistance, 183
of immunocompromised white cells, 331
of internal hemorrhaging, 183
of ischemic stroke, 354–55
of liver disease, 431–33
of low blood sugar, 406
of metabolic acidosis, 445
of Parkinson's disease, 465–66
of polycythemia, 388
of pressure ulcers, 118
of pulmonary edema, 348
of respiratory failure, 389
of respiratory infection, 387
of secondary polycythemia, 388
of septic shock, 106
slow onset of, 184
of tachycardia, 345
of transient ischemic stroke, 355
of ventilatory failure, 389
of wasting, 420
syngeneic BMT, 335
systolic blood pressure, 140, 354

tachycardia, 345, 346, 351
tacrine (Cognex), 469
Tagamet, 155, 163, 249

Talking Laser Beam, 483
tamoxifen, 334
taste, altered, 160–61, 447
telephone amplification device, 210, 483
temperature, 137–38
terminally ill, defined, 29
terminal sedation, 153, 304
testosterone, 334
tetracycline, 110
tetrahydrocannabinol (THC), 164
thalamotomy, 470–71
theophylline (Marax), 381, 383
THEOS Foundation, 319, 504–5
thermometers, *137*
3TC (lamivudine) (Epivir), 421
thrombocytes, *see* platelets
thrombolysis therapy, 342–43
thrombophlebitis, 178–79
thrush (*Candida*), 106
thyroxicosis, 350
Ticlid (ticlopidine), 355
tissue plasminogen activator (TPA) (Activase), 342, 359
T lymphocytes, 336
Tofranil (imipramine), 362
toileting, 124–27
bedding and, 124
cleaning and, 125–26
commode and, 125
of dementia patients, 125
ostomy care and, 126–27
routine for, 170–71
and using bedpan, 124
and using urinal, 124
tolbutamide (Orinase), 401
total lung capacity, 378
total parenteral nutrition (TPN), 166–67
toxemia, 296
toxoplasma gondii protozoan, 110
toxoplasmosis, 419
tracheostomy, 175–76, 296, 383, 487
tranquilizers, 382
transcatheter therapy, 347
transcutaneous electrical nerve stimulation (TENS), 157
transdermal patches, 146
transfusions, 296
transient ischemic attack (TIA), 355
transient ischemic stroke, 355
Transplant Recipients International Clearinghouse, 513
traumatic brain injury (TBI), *see* brain injury
Trental (pentoxifylline), 409
trihexyphenidyl (Artane), 486
Triple Care, 116
tube feeding, 166–67, 484–85
tuberculosis, 108, 418
AIDS and, 418, 423